Health, United States, 2003

With Chartbook on Trends in the Health of Americans

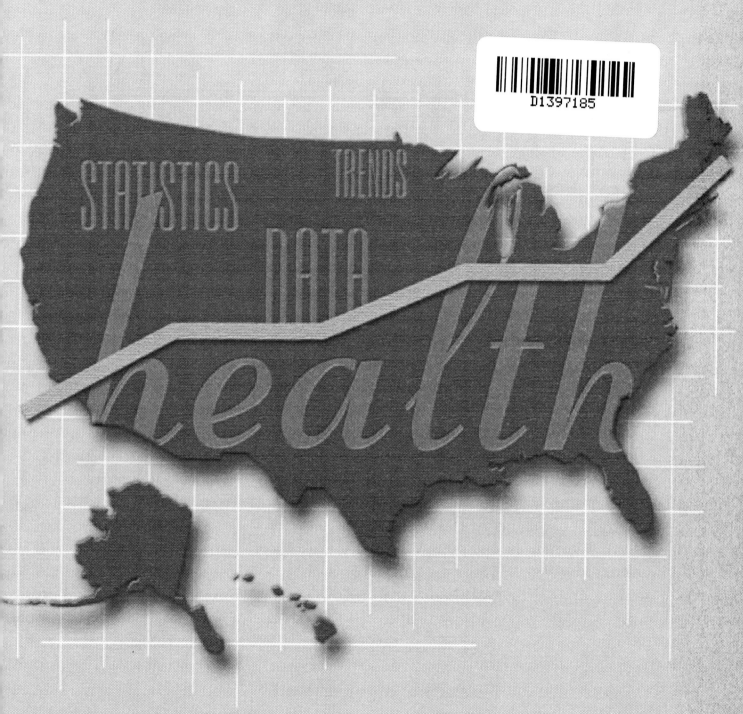

U.S. DEPARTMENT OF HEALTH AND HUMAN SERVICES
Centers for Disease Control and Prevention
National Center for Health Statistics

Copyright Information

Suggested Citations

National Center for Health Statistics.
Health, United States, 2003.
Hyattsville, Maryland: 2003.

Freid VM, Prager K, MacKay AP, Xia H.
Chartbook on Trends in the Health of Americans.
Health, United States, 2003. Hyattsville, Maryland:
National Center for Health Statistics. 2003.

Library of Congress Catalog Number 76–641496
For sale by Superintendent of Documents
U.S. Government Printing Office
Washington, DC 20402

Health, United States, 2003

With Chartbook on Trends in the Health of Americans

U.S. DEPARTMENT OF HEALTH AND HUMAN SERVICES
Centers for Disease Control and Prevention
National Center for Health Statistics

September 2003
DHHS Publication No.2003-1232

U.S. Department of Health and Human Services

Tommy G. Thompson
Secretary

Centers for Disease Control and Prevention

Julie Louise Gerberding, M.D., M.P.H.
Director

National Center for Health Statistics

Edward J. Sondik, Ph.D.
Director

Preface

Health, United States, 2003 is the 27th report on the health status of the Nation, and is submitted by the Secretary of the Department of Health and Human Services to the President and Congress of the United States in compliance with Section 308 of the Public Health Service Act. This report was compiled by the National Center for Health Statistics (NCHS), Centers for Disease Control and Prevention (CDC). The National Committee on Vital and Health Statistics served in a review capacity.

The *Health, United States* series presents national trends in health statistics. Major findings are presented in the highlights section. The report also includes a chartbook, trend tables, extensive appendixes, and an index.

Chartbook

The second *Chartbook on Trends in the Health of Americans* updates and expands information in last year's chartbook. In addition to assessing the Nation's health by presenting trends and current information on selected determinants and measures of health status, the 2003 chartbook includes a feature on diabetes with charts on prevalence, utilization of ambulatory and inpatient health services by persons with a diagnosis of diabetes, and mortality due to diabetes. Information was expanded to include more data by race and ethnicity in charts where sample size is sufficiently large, a more inclusive measure of physical activity for adults that takes into account both leisure-time and usual daily activity, limitation in activities of daily living by Medicare beneficiaries, and trends in poverty by age. Determinants of health considered in the chartbook include demographic factors, health insurance coverage, health behaviors and risk factors, and preventive health care. Measures of health status include mortality and limitations of activity due to chronic health conditions. Many measures are shown separately for persons of different ages because of the strong effect of age on health, as well as differences in causes of morbidity and mortality across the age span. Selected figures also highlight differences in determinants and measures of health status by such characteristics as sex, race, and Hispanic origin.

Trend Tables

The chartbook section is followed by 151 trend tables organized around four major subject areas: health status and determinants, health care utilization, health care resources, and health care expenditures. A major criterion used in selecting the trend tables is availability of comparable national data over a period of several years. The tables report data for selected years to highlight major trends in health statistics. Earlier editions of *Health, United States* may present data for additional years that are not included in the current printed report. Where possible, these additional years of data are available in Excel spreadsheet files on the *Health, United States* Web site. Tables with additional data years are listed in Appendix III.

Racial and Ethnic Data

Many tables in *Health, United States* present data according to race and Hispanic origin consistent with Department-wide emphasis on expanding racial and ethnic detail when presenting health data. Trend data on race and ethnicity are in the greatest detail possible, after taking into account the quality of data, the amount of missing data, and the number of observations. The large differences in health status by race and Hispanic origin documented in this report may be explained by several factors including socioeconomic status, health practices, psychosocial stress and resources, environmental exposures, discrimination, and access to health care. New standards for Federal data on race and ethnicity are described in Appendix II under *Race*.

Changes in This Edition

Each volume of *Health, United States* is prepared to maximize its usefulness as a standard reference source while maintaining its continuing relevance. Comparability is fostered by including similar trend tables in each volume. Timeliness is maintained by adding new tables each year to reflect emerging topics in public health and improving the content of ongoing tables. New to *Health, United States, 2003* is a table on screening for cervical cancer (table 81) based on National Health Interview Survey (NHIS) data and a table that compares the distribution of medical expenditures by age between 1987 and 1998–99 (table 119) based on data from the National Medical Expenditure Survey (1987) and Medical

Expenditure Panel Survey (1998–99). Medicare coverage in table 130 is now differentiated between those with Medicare managed care through an HMO and those with only Medicare fee-for-service, based on NHIS data.

Other changes were prompted by the availability of population estimates that were revised to reflect the 2000 census. Population estimates in table 1 include bridged-race intercensal population estimates for 1991–99, and bridged-race population estimates for 2000 and 2001 that were produced under a collaborative arrangement with the U.S. Census Bureau. Mortality rates in tables 29, 35–42, and 44–47, and birth rates in table 3 were recalculated based on these revised population estimates. Hospital discharge rates for 2000 and 2001 in tables 90–92 and 94 are also based on the 2000 census.

Appendixes

Appendix I describes each data source used in the report and provides references for further information about the sources. Appendix I is reorganized with data sources listed alphabetically within two broad categories: Government Sources, and Private and Global Sources.

Appendix II is an alphabetical listing of terms used in the report. It also presents standard populations used for age adjustment (tables I, II, and III); ICD codes for causes of death shown in *Health, United States* from the Sixth through Tenth Revisions and the years when the Revisions were in effect (tables IV and V); comparability ratios between ICD-9 and ICD-10 for selected causes (table VI); ICD-9-CM codes for external cause-of-injury, diagnostic, and procedure categories (tables VII, IX, and X); industry codes from the Standard Industrial Classification Manual (table VIII); and sample tabulations of NHIS data comparing the 1977 and 1997 Standards for Federal data on race and Hispanic origin (tables XI and XII).

Appendix III lists tables for which additional years of trend data are available electronically in Excel spreadsheet files on the *Health, United States* home page and CD-ROM, described below under Electronic Access.

Index

The Index to Trend Tables is a useful tool for locating data by topic. Tables are cross-referenced by such topics as Child and adolescent health; Women's health; Nutrition-related data; State data; American Indian, Asian, Black, and Hispanic origin populations; Education; Poverty status; Disability; and Metropolitan/nonmetropolitan data.

Electronic Access

Health, United States may be accessed on the World Wide Web at www.cdc.gov/nchs/hus.htm. From the *Health, United States* Web site, one may also register for the *Health, United States* electronic mailing list to receive announcements about release dates and notices of updates to tables.

Health, United States, 2003, the chartbook, and each of the 151 individual trend tables are available as separate Acrobat .pdf files on the Web. Individual tables are downloadable as Excel spreadsheet files. Pdf and spreadsheet files for selected tables will be updated on the Web if more current data become available near the time when the printed report is released. Readers who register for the electronic mailing list will be notified of these table updates. Previous editions of *Health, United States* and chartbooks, starting with the 1993 edition, also may be accessed from the *Health, United States* Web site.

Health, United States is also available on CD-ROM, where it can be viewed, searched, printed, and saved using Adobe Acrobat software on the CD-ROM.

Copies of the Report

Copies of *Health, United States, 2003* and the CD-ROM may be purchased from the Government Printing Office through links to GPO on the *Health, United States* Web site.

Questions?

For answers to questions about this report, contact:

Data Dissemination Branch
National Center for Health Statistics
Centers for Disease Control and Prevention
3311 Toledo Road, Fifth Floor
Hyattsville, Maryland 20782
Phone: 301-458-INFO
E-mail: nchsquery@cdc.gov
Internet: www.cdc.gov/nchs

Acknowledgments

Overall responsibility for planning and coordinating the content of this volume rested with the Office of Analysis, Epidemiology, and Health Promotion, National Center for Health Statistics (NCHS), under the general direction of Amy B. Bernstein and Diane M. Makuc.

Health, United States, 2003 highlights, trend tables, and appendixes were prepared under the leadership of Kate Prager. Trend tables were prepared by Amy B. Bernstein, Alan J. Cohen, Margaret A. Cooke, La-Tonya D. Curl, Catherine R. Duran, Virginia M. Freid, Ji-Eun Lee, Andrea P. MacKay, Mitchell B. Pierre, Jr., Rebecca A. Placek, Anita L. Powell, Kate Prager, Laura A. Pratt, and Henry Xia, with assistance from Stephanie Furr and Ryan Sheely. Appendix tables and index to trend tables were assembled by Anita L. Powell. Production planning and coordination of trend tables were managed by Rebecca A. Placek. Administrative and word processing assistance were provided by Carole J. Hunt, Lillie C. Featherstone, and Anne E. Mann.

The *Chartbook on Trends in the Health of Americans* was prepared by Virginia M. Freid, Kate Prager, Andrea P. MacKay, and Henry Xia. This year's chartbook updates and expands on information presented in last year's edition prepared by Patricia N. Pastor, Diane M. Makuc, Cynthia Reuben, and Henry Xia. Data and analysis for specific charts were provided by Patricia M. Barnes, Margaret A. Cooke, Deborah D. Ingram, Ellen A. Kramarow, Patricia N. Pastor, and Charlotte A. Schoenborn. Graphs were drafted by La-Tonya D. Curl. Technical assistance was provided by Liming Cai, Alan J. Cohen, Catherine R. Duran, Mark S. Eberhardt, Lois A. Fingerhut, Ji-Eun Lee, Hanyu Ni, Elsie R. Pamuk, Mitchell B. Pierre, Jr., Rebecca A. Placek, Felicity Skidmore, and Gregory Spencer of the U.S. Census Bureau.

Publications management and editorial review were provided by Thelma W. Sanders and Linda L. Bean. The designer was Sarah M. Hinkle. Graphics were supervised by Stephen L. Sloan. Production was done by Jacqueline M. Davis and Zung T. Le. Printing was managed by Joan D. Burton and Patricia L. Wilson.

Electronic access through the NCHS Internet site and CD-ROM were provided by Christine J. Brown, Michelle L. Bysheim, Jacqueline M. Davis, Zung T. Le, Sharon L. Ramirez, and Thelma W. Sanders.

Data and technical assistance were provided by staff of the following NCHS organizations: *Division of Health Care Statistics:* Catharine W. Burt, Donald K. Cherry, Barbara J. Haupt, Lola Jean Kozak, Karen L. Lipkind, Linda F. McCaig, Robert Pokras, Susan M. Schappert, Alvin J. Sirrocco, Genevieve W. Strahan, and David A. Woodwell; *Division of Health Examination Statistics:* Margaret D. Carroll, Rosemarie Hirsch, and Clifford L. Johnson; *Division of Health Interview Statistics:* Patricia F. Adams, Barbara Bloom, Viona I. Brown, Pei-Lu Chiu, Robin A. Cohen, Richard H. Coles, Nancy G. Gagne, Cathy C. Hao, Kristina Kotulak-Hays, Susan S. Jack, Jane B. Page, John R. Pleis, Eve Powell-Griner, Charlotte A. Schoenborn, Mira L. Shanks, Anne K. Stratton, and Luong Tonthat; *Division of Vital Statistics:* Robert N. Anderson, Thomas D. Dunn, Brady E. Hamilton, Donna L. Hoyert, Kenneth D. Kochanek, Marian F. MacDorman, Joyce A. Martin, T.J. Mathews, Arialdi M. Minino, William D. Mosher, Sherry L. Murphy, Gail A. Parr, Manju Sharma, Stephanie J. Ventura, and Jim Weed; *Office of Analysis, Epidemiology and Health Promotion:* Lois A. Fingerhut, Deborah D. Ingram, Elizabeth W. Jackson, Richard J. Klein, Suzanne Proctor, and Thomas C. Socey; *Office of International Statistics:* Juan Rafael Albertorio-Diaz and Francis C. Notzon; and *Office of Data Standards, Program Development and Extramural Programs:* Donna Pickett.

Additional data and technical assistance were also provided by the *National Center for HIV, STD, and TB Prevention, CDC:* Tim Bush, Hazel D. Dean, Melinda Flock, and Luetta Schneider; *Epidemiology Program Office, CDC:* Samuel L. Groseclose and Patsy A. Hall; *National Center for Chronic Disease Prevention and Health Promotion, CDC:* Laurie Elam-Evans, Jo Anne Grunbaum, Sherry Everett Jones, and Lilo T. Strauss; *National Immunization Program, CDC:* Lawrence Barker, Emmanuel Maurice, and Dave Sanders; *National Institute of Occupational Safety and Health, CDC:* Rochelle Althouse and Robert M. Castellan; *Agency for Health Care Research and Quality:* David Kashihara and Steven Machlin; *Health Resources and Services Administration:* Stuart Bernstein; *Substance Abuse and Mental Health Services Administration:* Joanne Atay, Judy K. Ball, Joseph C. Gfroerer, Ronald Manderscheid, and Deborah Trunzo; *National Institutes of Health:* James D. Colliver and Lynn A. G. Ries; *Centers for Medicare & Medicaid Services:* Cathy A. Cowan, Frank Eppig, David A. Gibson, Deborah W. Kidd, Helen C. Lazenby, Katharine R. Levit, Anna Long, Anne B. Martin, Anthony C. Parker, and Carter S. Warfield;

Office of the Secretary, DHHS: Mitchell Goldstein; *Census Bureau:* Joseph Dalaker and Bernadette D. Proctor; *Bureau of Labor Statistics:* Alan Blostin, Kay Ford, Daniel Ginsburg, John Stinson, and Peggy Suarez; *Department of Veterans Affairs:* Michael F. Grindstaff; *Alan Guttmacher Institute:* Rebecca Wind; *Association of Schools of Public Health:* Mah-Sere K. Sow; *InterStudy:* Richard Hamer; *University of Michigan:* Patrick O'Malley; *Cowles Research Group:* C. McKeen Cowles; and *CSR Incorporated:* Gerald D. Williams.

Contents

List of Chartbook Figures

Special Feature: Diabetes

Highlights

Major Findings From *Health, United States, 2003*

Health, United States, 2003 is the 27th report on the health status of the Nation. It assesses the Nation's health by presenting trends and current information on selected determinants and measures of health status in a chartbook followed by 151 trend tables organized around four major subject areas: health status and determinants, health care utilization, health care resources, and health care expenditures. The 2003 Chartbook on Trends in the Health of Americans features a section on diabetes, a serious and increasingly common chronic health condition and a significant cause of illness, disability, and death in the United States. Highlights on the featured topic, diabetes, follow other major findings from the report.

Health Status and Determinants

Population characteristics

Important changes in the U.S. population will shape future efforts to improve health and health care. Two major changes in the demographic characteristics of the U.S. population are the growth of the older population and the increasing racial and ethnic diversity of the Nation.

From 1950 to 2000 the proportion of the **population age 65 years and over** rose from 8 to 12 percent. By 2050 it is projected that one in five Americans will be 65 years of age or over (figure 2).

The **racial and ethnic composition** of the Nation has changed over time. The Hispanic population and the Asian and Pacific Islander population have grown more rapidly than other racial and ethnic groups in recent decades. In 2000 more than 12 percent of the U.S. population identified themselves as Hispanic and 4 percent as Asian or Pacific Islander (figure 3).

In 2001 the overall percent of Americans living in **poverty** was 11.7 percent, up from 11.3 percent in 2000, the first increase in the poverty rate since 1993. In 2001 more than one-half of black and Hispanic children under 18 years and

more than one-half of the black and Hispanic population age 65 years and over were either poor or near poor (figures 4 and 5 and table 2).

Fertility

Birth rates for teens continued their steady decline while birth rates for women 30–44 years of age increased in 2001.

The **birth rate for teenagers** declined for the 10th consecutive year in 2001, to 45.3 births per 1,000 women aged 15–19 years, the lowest rate in more than six decades. The birth rate for 15–17 year olds in 2001 was 34 percent lower than in 1990, and the birth rate for older teens 18–19 years of age was 14 percent lower than the rate in 1990 (table 3).

In 2001 the **fertility rate** for Hispanic women (96.0 births per 1,000 Hispanic women 15–44 years) was 66 percent higher than for non-Hispanic white women (57.7 per 1,000) (table 3).

Between 1995 and 2001 the **birth rate for unmarried women** was relatively stable, about 44–45 births per 1,000 unmarried women ages 15–44 years. The birth rate for unmarried black women declined steadily over the past decade to 70.1 per 1,000 in 2001, and the birth rate for unmarried Hispanic women increased for the third year in a row to 98.0 per 1,000 (table 9).

Health Behaviors and Risk Factors

Health behaviors and risk factors have a significant effect on health outcomes. Cigarette smoking increases the risk of lung cancer, heart disease, emphysema, and other respiratory diseases. Overweight and obesity increase the risk of death and disease as well as the severity of disease. Regular physical activity lessens the risk of disease and enhances physical functioning. Heavy and chronic use of alcohol and use of illicit drugs increase the risk of disease and injuries. Environmental exposures also affect health. For example, air pollution contributes to respiratory illness, cardiovascular disease, and some cancers.

Since 1990 the percent of **adults who smoke cigarettes** has declined only slightly. In 2001, 25 percent of men and 21 percent of women were smokers. Cigarette smoking by adults is strongly associated with educational attainment. Adults with less than a high school education were nearly three times as likely to smoke as were those with a bachelor's degree or more education in 2001 (figure 12 and tables 59 and 60).

Between 1997 and 2001 the percent of **high school students who reported smoking cigarettes** in the past month declined from 36 percent to 29 percent, reversing an upward trend that began in the early 1990s (figure 12).

Cigarette smoking during pregnancy is a risk factor for poor birth outcomes such as low birthweight and infant death. In 2001 the proportion of mothers who smoked cigarettes during pregnancy declined to 12 percent, down from 20 percent in 1989. In 2001 the smoking rate during pregnancy for mothers ages 18–19 years (19 percent) remained higher than that for mothers of other ages (figure 12 and table 11).

In 2001, 38 percent of female **high school students** and 24 percent of male high school students did not engage in the recommended amounts of moderate or vigorous **physical activity**, about the same as in 1999 (figure 13).

In 2000 the percent of adults 18 years of age and over who were **inactive during their usual daily activity and leisure time** was higher for women than men (12 percent and 7 percent, age adjusted) and increased sharply with age. Nearly one-fifth of men age 65 years and over and more than one-quarter of women age 65 years and over were inactive (figure 14).

The prevalence of **overweight and obesity among adults** 20–74 years of age increased from 47 percent in 1976–80 to 65 percent in 1999–2000. During this period the prevalence of obesity among adults 20–74 years of age increased from 15 to 28 percent (percents are age adjusted) (figures 15 and 16 and table 68).

The prevalence of **obesity** among adults varies by **race and ethnicity**. In 1999–2000, 50 percent of non-Hispanic black women 20–74 years of age were obese, compared with 40 percent of women of Mexican origin and 30 percent of non-Hispanic white women (percents are age adjusted). Obesity among black women increased more than 60 percent since 1976–80, from 31 percent to 50 percent (figure 16 and table 68).

Between 1976–80 and 1999–2000 the prevalence of **overweight among children** 6–11 years of age more than doubled from 7 to 15 percent and the prevalence of overweight among **adolescents** 12–19 years of age more than tripled from 5 to 16 percent (figure 15 and table 69).

In 2001 among current drinkers age 18 years and over, 41 percent of men and 20 percent of women reported drinking **five or more alcoholic drinks** on at least 1 day in the past year (age-adjusted). This level of alcohol consumption was most common among young adults 18–24 years of age (table 65).

Between 2000 and 2001 the prevalence of **illicit drug use** within the past 30 days among youths 12–17 years of age increased 1 percentage point to 11 percent. The percent of youths reporting illicit drug use increased with age, from 4 percent among 12–13 year olds to 11 percent among those age 14–15 years and 18 percent among those 16–17 years in 2001 (table 62).

Between 1991 and 2001 the number of **cocaine-related emergency department episodes** per 100,000 population nearly tripled for persons 35 years and over, to 76 episodes per 100,000. The age group 26–34 years has the highest episode rate, 176 per 100,000 in 2001. The same patient may be involved in multiple drug-related episodes (table 64).

Air pollution causes premature death, cancer, and long-term damage to respiratory and cardiovascular systems. The presence of unacceptable levels of ground-level **ozone** is the largest source of air pollution. In 2001 approximately 41 percent of the U.S. population lived in areas designated as nonattainment areas for established health-based standards for ozone (table 51).

Morbidity

Limitation of activity due to chronic health conditions, limitations in activities of daily living, and self-assessed (or family member-assessed) health status are summary measures of morbidity presented in this report. Additional measures of morbidity that are presented include the incidence of specific diseases, injury-related emergency department use, and suicide attempts.

Limitation of activity due to chronic health conditions among children was more common among boys than among girls and was more than twice as high among school-age children (5–11 and 12–17 years of age) as among preschoolers (under 5 years of age) during the period 1999–2001. More than 9 percent of school-age and adolescent boys had an activity limitation compared with about 5 percent of girls, with the majority classified as having a limitation based on participation in special education. Between 1997 and 2001 levels of activity limitation among children remained about the same (figure 17 and table 56).

Limitations in handling personal care needs such as bathing (**activities of daily living or ADLs**) and routine needs such as shopping (**instrumental activities of daily living or IADLs**) increase sharply with age among the noninstitutionalized population. In 2001, about 14 percent of all Medicare beneficiaries 65 years of age and over were limited in at least one of six ADLs. Among noninstitutionalized persons age 65 years and over, about 10 percent had difficulty and received help or supervision with at least one ADL (figure 20).

Mental illness is a significant **cause of activity limitation** among working-age adults living in the community. In 1999–2001 mental illness was the second most frequently mentioned causal condition for activity limitation among adults 18–44 years of age and third among adults 45–54 years (figure 19).

In 2001 the percent of persons reporting **fair or poor health** was more than three times as high for persons living below the poverty level as for those with family income more than twice the poverty level (21 percent and 6 percent, age adjusted) (table 57).

New **pediatric AIDS cases** have been declining steadily since 1994 when U.S. Public Health Service guidelines recommended testing and treatment of pregnant women and neonates to reduce perinatal HIV transmission. The vast majority of pediatric AIDS cases occur through perinatal exposure. In 2001 fewer than 200 new AIDS cases were reported among children under the age of 13 years, compared with 745 in 1995 (table 53).

In 2001 **tuberculosis** incidence declined for the 9th consecutive year to 5.7 cases per 100,000 population, but the rate of decline slowed in 2001 compared with the previous 5 years (table 52).

Untreated **chlamydial infections** can lead to pelvic inflammatory disease (PID) with potentially serious complications including infertility, chronic pelvic pain, and life-threatening tubal pregnancy. In 2001 the reported rate for chlamydial infection was 278 cases per 100,000 persons. Rates of reported chlamydial infection have been increasing annually since the late 1980s when public programs for screening and treatment of women were first established to avert pelvic inflammatory disease and related complications (table 52).

Incidence rates for **all cancers combined** declined in the 1990s for males. Between 1990 and 1999 age-adjusted cancer incidence rates declined on average nearly 2 percent per year for Hispanic males, non-Hispanic white males, and black males. Although there was no significant change in cancer incidence for females overall, among Hispanic females rates decreased on average 1 percent per year, and among Asian or Pacific Islander females rates increased 1 percent per year (table 54).

The most frequently diagnosed **cancer sites in males** are prostate, followed by lung and bronchus, and colon and rectum. Cancer incidence at these sites is higher for black males than for males of other racial and ethnic groups. In 1999 age-adjusted cancer incidence rates for black males exceeded those for white males by 58 percent for prostate, 48 percent for lung and bronchus, and 10 percent for colon and rectum (table 54).

Breast cancer is the most frequently diagnosed cancer among females. Breast cancer incidence is higher for non-Hispanic white females than for females in other racial and ethnic groups. In 1999 age-adjusted breast cancer incidence rates for non-Hispanic white females exceeded those for black females by 24 percent, for Asian or Pacific Islander females by 48 percent, and for Hispanic females by 80 percent (table 54).

Injuries accounted for 37 percent of all visits to emergency departments (ED) in 1999–2000. The proportion of ED visits that were injury-related declined with age from 41 percent for children and adults under 45 years of age to 33 percent for persons 45–64 years and 26 percent for those 65 years and over. In 1999–2000 falls was the most often cited reason for injury-related ED visits among persons 45 years of age and older (tables 82 and 83).

Between 1993 and 2001, the percent of high school students who reported attempting suicide (8–9 percent) and whose **suicide attempts** required medical attention (about 3 percent) remained fairly constant. Girls were more likely than boys to consider or attempt suicide and were also more likely to make an attempt that required medical attention. However in 2000 adolescent boys (15–19 years of age) were nearly five times as likely to die from suicide as were adolescent girls, in part reflecting their choice of more lethal methods, such as firearms (tables 46 and 58).

Mortality Trends

Life expectancy and infant mortality are measures often used to gauge the overall health of a population. Life expectancy shows a long term upward trend and infant mortality attained a record low in 2000 and remained unchanged in 2001.

In 2001 **life expectancy** at birth for the total population reached a record high of 77.2 years, based on preliminary data, up from 75.4 years in 1990 (table 27).

In 2001 the **infant mortality** rate did not change from its 2000 record low of 6.9 infant deaths per 1,000 live births, based on preliminary data (figure 22 and table 22).

Since 1950 **mortality among teens and young adults age 15–24 years** has declined by 38 percent to 80 deaths per 100,000 population in 2000. Overall mortality at ages 15–24 years has declined, in part, due to decreases in death rates for unintentional injuries, cancer, heart disease, and infectious diseases. Homicide and suicide rates generally increased over this period, but have declined since the mid-1990s (figures 24 and 25).

Between 1950 and 2000 **mortality among adults age 25–44 years** declined by 44 percent overall, to 155 deaths per 100,000 population. Death rates for unintentional injuries, cancer, heart disease, and tuberculosis decreased substantially during this period. Suicide rates rose through 1980 and have since declined slightly. HIV disease was the leading cause of death in this age group in the mid-1990s; with decreasing HIV disease death rates, it dropped to the fifth leading cause of death between 1997 and 2000 (figures 26 and 27).

Since 1950 **mortality among adults age 45–64 years** has decreased by 49 percent overall, to 648 deaths per 100,000 population in 2000. During this period death rates for heart disease, stroke, and unintentional injury decreased while cancer mortality rose slowly through the 1980s and then declined. Cancer was the leading cause of death for 45–64 year olds in 2000, accounting for more than one-third of deaths in this age group (figures 28 and 29).

During the past 50 years **mortality among persons 65 years of age and over** has dropped by 35 percent to 5,169 deaths per 100,000 population in 2000. During this period death rates for heart disease and stroke have declined sharply while the death rate for cancer rose until 1995 and has since decreased slightly (figures 30 and 31).

Disparities in Mortality

Despite overall declines in mortality, racial and ethnic disparities in mortality, as well as gender disparities, persist. The gap in life expectancy between the sexes and between the black and white populations has been narrowing. As a result of revised death rates that incorporate information from the 2000 Census, some of the racial disparities in mortality are not as large as previously reported, while others are wider.

Infant mortality rates have declined for all **racial and ethnic groups**, but large disparities remain. In 2000 the infant mortality rate was highest for infants of non-Hispanic black mothers (13.6 deaths per 1,000 live births) and lowest for infants of mothers of Chinese origin (3.5 per 1,000 live births) (table 19).

Infant mortality increases as **mother's level of education** decreases. In 2000 the mortality rate for infants of mothers with less than 12 years of education was 58 percent higher than for infants of mothers with 13 or more years of education. This disparity was more marked among non-Hispanic white infants, for whom mortality among infants of mothers with less than a high school education was more than twice that for infants of mothers with more than a high school education (table 20).

Between 1990 and 2001 **life expectancy at birth** increased by more than 2 years for **males** and by 1 year for **females**. The difference in life expectancy between males and females narrowed from 7 years in 1990 to 5.4 years in 2001 (based on preliminary data) (figure 21 and table 27).

Between 1990 and 2001 **mortality from lung cancer** declined for **men** and increased for **women.** Although these trends reduced the sex differential for this cause of death, the age-adjusted death rate for lung cancer was still 86 percent higher for men than for women in 2000 and 83 percent higher in 2001 (preliminary data) (table 39).

Since 1990 mortality from **chronic lower respiratory diseases** remained relatively stable for **men** while it increased for **women.** These trends reduced the gap between the sexes for this cause of death. In 1990 the age-adjusted death rate for males was more than 100 percent higher than for females. In 2000 the difference between the rates had been reduced to 49 percent, and in 2001, to 44 percent (preliminary data) (table 41).

Between 1990 and 2001 **life expectancy at birth** increased more for the **black** than for the **white population**, thereby narrowing the gap in life expectancy between these two racial groups. In 1990 life expectancy at birth was 7 years longer for the white than for the black population. By 2000 the difference had narrowed to 5.7 years, and by 2001, to 5.5 years (preliminary data) (table 27).

Overall mortality was 31 percent higher for **black Americans** than for white Americans in 2001 compared with 37 percent higher in 1990. In 2001 age-adjusted death rates for the black population exceeded those for the white population by 40 percent for **stroke**, 29 percent for **heart disease**, 25 percent for **cancer**, and nearly 800 percent for **HIV disease** (based on preliminary data) (table 29).

The **5-year survival rate** for black females diagnosed in 1992–98 with breast cancer was 15 percentage points lower than the 5-year survival rate for white females (table 55).

In 2000 **breast cancer mortality** for black females was 31 percent higher than for white females, and in 2001, 34 percent higher, based on preliminary data, compared with 15 percent higher in 1990 (tables 40).

Homicide rates among young black males 15–24 years of age and among **young Hispanic males** were about 50 percent lower in 2000 than in the early 1990s when homicide rates peaked for these groups. In spite of these downward trends, homicide was still the leading cause of death for young black males and the second leading cause for young Hispanic males in 2000, and homicide rates for young black and Hispanic males remained substantially higher than for young non-Hispanic white males (table 45).

Since 1995 death rates for **HIV disease** declined sharply for **Hispanic males and black males** 25–44 years of age. In spite of these declines, HIV disease was still the second leading cause of death for Hispanic males 25–44 years of age and the third leading cause for black males 25–44 years of age in 2000, and HIV death rates remained much higher for Hispanic and black males than for non-Hispanic white males in this age group (table 42).

In 2000 death rates for **motor vehicle-related injury and suicide for young American Indian males** 15–24 years of age were about 45 percent higher than the rates for those causes for young white males. Death rates for the American Indian population are known to be underestimated (tables 44 and 46).

Overall mortality was almost 40 percent lower for **Asian males** than for white males throughout most of the 1990s. In 2000 age-adjusted death rates for **cancer and heart disease** for Asian males were 38–41 percent lower than corresponding rates for white males, whereas the death rate for **stroke** was only 3 percent lower. Death rates for the Asian population are known to be underestimated (tables 35–38).

Death rates vary by **educational attainment**. In 2000 the age-adjusted death rate for persons 25–64 years of age with fewer than 12 years of education was nearly three times the rate for persons with 13 or more years of education (table 34).

Occupational Health

Improvements in workplace safety constitute a major public health achievement in the twentieth century. Despite important accomplishments, preventable injuries and deaths continue to occur.

In 2001 the **occupational injuries with lost workdays** rate, 2.6 per 100 full-time equivalents (FTEs) in the private sector, was at its lowest level in three decades. The industries reporting the highest injury rates in 2001 were transportation, communication, and public utilities (4.2) and construction (3.9) (table 50).

Of the total 8,786 fatal work injuries in 2001, one-third resulted from the September 11th terrorist attacks. Excluding the September 11 fatalities, the **occupational injury death rate** in 2001 was the same as in 2000, 4.3 deaths per 100,000 employed workers. Mining (including oil and gas extraction), the industry with the highest death rate in 2001 (30.0 per 100,000), accounted for 3 percent of occupational injury deaths, excluding deaths from the September 11th attacks. The industry accounting for the largest percentage of occupational injury deaths, construction (21 percent), had a death rate of 13.3 per 100,000 (table 49).

A total of 2,859 **pneumoconiosis deaths**, for which pneumoconiosis was either the underlying or nonunderlying cause of death, occurred in 2000, compared with 4,151 deaths in 1980. Pneumoconiosis deaths are primarily associated with occupational exposures and can be prevented through effective control of worker exposure to occupational dusts (table 48).

Health Care Utilization and Health Care Resources

Major changes continue to occur in the delivery of health care in the United States, driven in part by changes in payment policies intended to rein in rising costs and by advances in technology that have allowed more complex treatments to be performed on an ambulatory basis. Use of hospital inpatient services has decreased while use of services such as outpatient surgery, home health care, and hospice care, has increased.

Between 1980 and 2000 the percent of all **office visits** to primary care physicians declined, while the percent of visits to specialty physicians increased. In 2000, 49 percent of all visits to physicians' offices were made to specialists, up from 43 percent in 1980 (table 84).

In 2001, 63 percent of all **surgical operations** in community hospitals were performed on outpatients, up from 51 percent in 1990 and 16 percent in 1980 (table 95).

Between 1985 and 2001 the **hospital discharge rate** declined 24 percent, from 151 to 115 discharges per 1,000 population, while **average length of stay** declined 1.7 days, from 6.6 to 4.9 days (data are age adjusted) (table 90).

Between 1995 and 2001, total **registered nurse graduates** per year declined from 97,000 to 69,000, **allopathic medicine graduates** remained stable at 16,000 per year, and **osteopathic medicine graduates** increased from 1,800 to 2,600 per year (table 103).

Between 1990 and 2001 the number of **community hospital beds** declined from about 927,000 to about 826,000. Community hospital occupancy, estimated at 64.5 percent in 2001, increased slightly from 62.5 percent in 1998, after declining from about 67 percent in 1990 (table 106).

Between 1996 and 2000 use of **home health care** by persons 65 years of age and over declined from 547 to 277 per 10,000 population, after increasing steadily between 1992 and 1996. The recent decline resulted in part from the Balanced Budget Act of 1997, which imposed stricter limits on the use of home health services funded by Medicare and interim limits on Medicare payments to home health agencies from October 1997 until a prospective payment system was implemented for Medicare home health agencies in October 2000 (data are age adjusted) (table 87).

Between 1994 and 2000 use of **hospice care** by persons 65 years of age and over increased by 83 percent to 25 patients per 10,000 population. Among persons age 65 and over, use of hospice services is slightly higher for males than for females (27 compared with 23 patients per 10,000 in 2000). Cancer is the most common diagnosis among hospice patients (data are age adjusted) (table 88).

In 1999 there were 1.5 million **nursing home residents** 65 years of age and over. More than one-half of the residents 65 years and over were at least 85 years of age and three-fourths were female. Between the mid-1970s and 1999, nursing home utilization rates increased for the black population and decreased for the white population (table 96).

In 2001 there were 1.8 million **nursing home beds** in facilities certified for use by Medicare and Medicaid beneficiaries. Between 1995 and 2001 nursing home bed occupancy in those facilities was relatively stable, estimated at 83 percent in 2001 (table 110).

Preventive Health Care

Use of preventive health services helps reduce morbidity and mortality from disease. Use of several different types of preventive services has been increasing. However disparities in use of preventive health care by race and ethnicity, and family income, remain.

The percent of mothers receiving **prenatal care** in the first trimester of pregnancy has continued to edge upward from 76 percent in 1990 to 83 percent in 2001. Although increases occurred for all racial and ethnic groups, in 2001 the percent of mothers with early prenatal care still varied substantially, from 69 percent for American Indian mothers to 90–92 percent for mothers of Japanese and Cuban origin (figures 8 and 9 and table 6).

In 2001, 77 percent of children 19–35 months of age received the combined **vaccination** series of four doses of DTaP (diphtheria-tetanus-acellular pertussis) vaccine, three doses of polio vaccine, one dose of MMR (measles-mumps-rubella vaccine), and three doses of Hib (Haemophilus influenzae type b) vaccine. Children living below the poverty threshold were less likely to have received the combined vaccination series than were children living at or above poverty (72 percent compared with 79 percent) (table 71).

Annual **influenza vaccination** can prevent influenza and its severe complications and one dose of **pneumococcal** vaccine can reduce the risk of invasive pneumococcal disease. Between 1989 and 1999 the percent of noninstitutionalized adults 65 years of age and over who reported an influenza vaccination within the past year more than doubled, to 66 percent and then decreased slightly to 63 percent in 2001. Between 1989 and 2001 the percent of older adults ever having received a pneumococcal vaccine increased sharply from 14 percent to 54 percent (figure 10).

Between 1987 and 2000 the age-adjusted percent of women 18 years and over who reported a **Pap smear** in the past 3 years increased from 74 percent to 81 percent. In 2000 Pap smear use was lower among women living below the poverty level compared with women with family incomes at or above the poverty level (72 percent and 84 percent). Pap smear use was lower among women 65 years and over than among younger women (table 81).

Access to Care

Access to care is important for preventive care and for prompt treatment of illness and injuries. Indicators of access to health services include having a usual source of health care and having a recent health care contact. Health insurance coverage, and the generosity of coverage, are major determinants of access to care.

The percent of the **population under 65 years of age with no health insurance coverage** (either public or private) fluctuated around 16–17 percent between 1994 and 2001. Among the under 65 population, poor and near poor persons whose family incomes were less than 200 percent of poverty were much more likely than others to be uninsured (figures 6 and 7 and table 129).

The likelihood of being uninsured varies substantially among the **States**. In 2001 the percent of the population under 65 years of age with **no health insurance coverage** varied from less than 10 percent in Massachusetts, Rhode Island, Wisconsin, Iowa, and Minnesota to 20 percent or more in Florida, Louisiana, Oklahoma, Texas, Arizona, New Mexico, and California (table 151).

In 2001, 11 percent of **children** under 18 years of age had **no health insurance coverage**. Between 2000 and 2001 among children with family income just above the poverty level (1–1.5 times poverty), the percent uninsured dropped from 26 to 19 percent. However children with low family

income remain substantially more likely than higher-income children to lack coverage (table 129).

Persons of Hispanic origin and American Indians who are under 65 years of age are more likely to have **no health insurance coverage** than are those in other racial and ethnic groups. In 2001 among the Hispanic-origin population, persons of Mexican origin were the most likely to lack health insurance coverage (39 percent). Non-Hispanic white persons were the least likely to lack coverage (12 percent) (figure 7 and table 129).

Six percent of **children** under 18 years of age had **no usual source of health care** in 2000–01. Hispanic and non-Hispanic black children were more likely to be without a usual source of care than non-Hispanic white children (14 percent and 7 percent compared with 4 percent) (table 74).

Thirteen percent of **children** under 18 years of age had **no health care visit** to a doctor or clinic within the past 12 months in 2000–01. Hispanic and non-Hispanic black children were more likely to be without a recent visit than non-Hispanic white children (20 percent and 15 percent compared with 10 percent) (table 73).

One in 5 **children** under 18 years of age had an **emergency department (ED) visit** within the past 12 months in 2001. Children with Medicaid coverage were more likely than those with private coverage or the uninsured to have had an ED visit within the past 12 months (29 percent compared with 19 percent and 17 percent) (table 75).

In 2001 nearly three-quarters of **children** 2–17 years of age had a **dental visit** in the past year. Use of dental care was lower among Hispanic children and non-Hispanic black children than among non-Hispanic white children (61 percent and 68 percent compared with 78 percent) (table 78).

Young adults 18–24 years of age are more likely than adults of other ages to have **no usual source of health care**. Twenty-six percent of young adults were without a usual source of health care in 2000–01 (table 76).

Working age-adults 18–64 years of age living below the poverty level were more than twice as likely as those with family income above twice the poverty level to have **no usual source of health care** in 2000–01 (27 percent and 12 percent). Among working-age adults living in poverty Hispanic persons were twice as likely as non-Hispanic white and black persons to be without a usual source of health care (44 percent compared with 22 percent and 21 percent) (percents are age adjusted) (table 76).

Use of hospital inpatient care is greater among the **poor** than among the nonpoor whose family income is at least twice the poverty level. In 2001 among persons under 65 years of age, the hospital discharge rate for the poor was almost twice the rate for nonpoor (168 and 87 per 1,000 population). Among those under 65 years of age, average length of stay was 1.4 days longer for poor than for nonpoor persons (5.1 and 3.7 days) (data are age adjusted) (table 89).

In 2001 among noninstitutionalized persons 65 years of age and over, those with Medicare fee-for-service coverage only were more likely to have had **no health care visits** within the past 12 months than were those with Medicare HMO, Medicaid, or private coverage (14 percent compared with 5–6 percent, data are age adjusted) (table 70).

In 2001 among noninstitutionalized persons 65 years of age and over, those with Medicaid coverage were twice as likely to be high volume users of the health care system with **10 or more visits within the past 12 months** than were those with Medicare HMO, private, or Medicare fee-for-service coverage only (44 percent compared to 21–25 percent, data are age adjusted) (table 70).

Health Care Expenditures

After 25 years of double-digit annual growth in national health expenditures, the rate of growth slowed during the 1990s. At the end of the decade the rate of growth started edging up again. Since the millennium, the rate has accelerated. This high rate of growth combined with a sluggish economy has resulted in health care expenditures claiming a larger share of the gross domestic product (GDP). The United States continues to spend more on health than any other industrialized country.

In 2001 **national health care expenditures** in the United States totaled $1.4 trillion, increasing 8.7 percent from the previous year compared with a 7.4 percent increase in 2000. In the mid-1990s annual growth had slowed somewhat, following an average annual growth rate of 11 percent during the 1980s (table 112).

The United States spends a larger **share of the GDP on health** than does any other major industrialized country. In 2000 the United States devoted 13.3 percent of the GDP to

health compared with 10.6–10.7 percent each in Germany and Switzerland and 9.1–9.5 percent in Canada and France, countries with the next highest shares (table 111).

In 2001 **health expenditures as a percent of the gross domestic product (GDP)** increased to 14.1 percent, up from 13.3 percent the previous year (table 112).

The rate of increase in the medical care component of the **Consumer Price Index** (CPI) was 4.7 percent in 2002 and 4.6 percent in 2001, compared with 3.4 percent per year during 1995–2000. During the last 3 years, the CPI for hospital services showed the greatest price increases (6–7 percent in 2000 and 2001 and 9 percent in 2002), compared with other components of medical care (table 113).

Expenditures by Type of Care and Source of Funds

During the last few years expenditures for prescription drugs have grown at a faster rate than any other type of health expenditure. The sources of funds for medical care differ substantially according to the type of medical care being provided.

Expenditures for hospital care accounted for 32 percent of all national health expenditures in 2001. Physician services accounted for 22 percent of the total in 2001, prescription drugs for 10 percent, and nursing home care for 7 percent (table 115).

Since 1995 the **average annual rate of increase for prescription drug expenditures** (on average 15 percent per year between 1995 and 2001) was higher than for any other type of health expenditure. During the first half of the decade expenditures for home health care increased more rapidly (19 percent per year between 1990 and 1995) than other types of expenditures (table 115).

In 2001 **prescription drug expenditures** increased 16 percent, and prescription drugs posted a 5-percent rate of price increase in the Consumer Price Index in both 2001 and 2002 (tables 113 and 115).

In 2001, 47 percent of **prescription drug expenditures** were paid by private health **insurance** (up from one-quarter at the beginning of the decade), 31 percent by out-of-pocket payments (down from 59 percent in 1990), and 17 percent by Medicaid. Although Medicare is the federal program that funds health care for persons age 65 years and over, and older persons are the highest per capita consumers of prescription drugs, Medicare paid only 2 percent of prescription drug expenses in 2001 (table 116).

In 1999, 88 percent of persons age 65 years and over in the civilian noninstitutionalized population had a **prescribed medicine expense**. The average annual out-of-pocket prescribed medicine expense per older person with expense was $614, an increase of 16 percent over the previous year (table 117).

In 1999, 95 percent of **persons age 65 years and over** in the civilian noninstitutionalized population reported **medical expenses** averaging about $6,300 per person with expense. Sixteen percent of expenses were paid out-of-pocket, 14 percent by private insurance, and two-thirds by public programs (mainly Medicare and Medicaid) (tables 117 and 118).

The burden of **out-of-pocket expenses** for health care varies considerably by age. In 1999 one-third of persons 75 years of age and over with expenses paid $1,000 or more in out-of-pocket expenses compared with 18 percent of those 45–64 years of age. Eight percent of those 18–44 years of age incurred out-of-pocket expenses of $1,000 or more in 1999, compared with only 1 percent of children under 6 years of age (table 119).

In 2001, 33 percent of **personal health care expenditures** were paid by the Federal Government and 11 percent by State and local government; private health insurance paid 35 percent and consumers paid 17 percent out-of-pocket (table 116).

In 2001 the major **sources of funds for hospital care** were Medicare (30 percent) and private health insurance (34 percent). **Physician services** were also primarily funded by private health insurance (48 percent) and Medicare (20 percent). In contrast, **nursing home care** was financed primarily by Medicaid (48 percent) and out-of-pocket payments (27 percent) (table 116).

In 1999 the average monthly charge per **nursing home** resident was $3,891. Residents for whom the primary source of payment was private insurance, family support, or their own income paid close to the average charge, compared with an average monthly charge of $5,800 when Medicare was the primary payor and $3,500 when Medicaid was the primary source of payment (table 124).

In 1998 less than one-fifth of **mental health expenditures** incurred by mental health organizations was for State and county psychiatric hospitals. In 1975 this share was nearly one-half of expenditures. The decline in the proportion of mental health expenditures for State and county psychiatric hospitals reflects the shift from inpatient to outpatient mental health care (table 125).

Publicly Funded Health Programs

The two major publicly funded health programs are Medicare and Medicaid. Medicare is funded through the Federal Government and covers persons 65 years of age and over and disabled persons for their health care. Medicaid is jointly funded by the Federal and State Governments to provide health care for certain groups of low-income persons. Medicaid benefits and eligibility vary by State.

In 2001 the **Medicare** program had 40 million enrollees and expenditures of $245 billion (table 134).

In 2001 **hospital insurance** (HI) accounted for 59 percent of **Medicare** expenditures. Expenditures for home health agency care decreased to 3 percent of HI expenditures in 2001, down from 13 percent in 1997 (table 134).

In 2001 **supplementary medical insurance** (SMI) accounted for 41 percent of **Medicare** expenditures. Seventeen percent of SMI expenditures in 2001 were payments to managed care organizations, compared with 20–22 percent in the previous 3 years. One-half of the $84 billion SMI paid for fee-for-service utilization in 2001 went to physicians under the physician fee schedule (table 134).

Of the 33 million **Medicare enrollees in the fee-for-service program** in 2000, 11 percent were 85 years of age and over and 15 percent were under 65 years of age. Among fee-for-service Medicare enrollees age 65 years and over, payments in 2000 increased with age from an average of $4,000 per year per enrollee for those age 65–74 years to $7,700 for those 85 years and over. Average payments per fee-for-service enrollee increased in 2000 after declining the previous 2 years (table 135).

In 1999, 81 percent of **Medicare beneficiaries** were non-Hispanic white, 9 percent were non-Hispanic black, and 7 percent were Hispanic. Some 20–24 percent of Hispanic and non-Hispanic black beneficiaries were persons under 65 entitled to **Medicare through disability**, compared with 11 percent of non-Hispanic white beneficiaries (table 136).

In 2000 **Medicare payments per fee-for-service enrollee** varied by State, ranging from less than $4,000 in Hawaii and New Mexico to more than $6,300 in New York, New Jersey, Maryland, the District of Columbia, and Louisiana (table 148).

In 2000 **Medicaid** vendor payments totaled $168 billion for 43 million recipients (table 137).

In 2000 children under the age of 21 years accounted for 46 percent of **Medicaid recipients** but only 16 percent of expenditures. Aged, blind, and disabled persons accounted for one-quarter of recipients and 70 percent of expenditures (table 137).

In 2000, 21 percent of **Medicaid payments** went to nursing facilities, 14 percent to inpatient general hospitals, 15 percent to capitated payment services, and 12 percent to prescribed drugs (table 138).

In 2000, **Medicaid payments per recipient varied by State** from less than $2,300 in California and Tennessee to $7,600 in New York. On average payments per recipient were lower in the Southeast, Southwest, and Far West States than in the New England and Mideast States (table 149).

In 2002 spending on health care by the **Department of Veterans Affairs** was $23 billion. Forty-one percent of inpatients and 34 percent of outpatients were low-income veterans without a service-connected disability (table 139).

Private Health Insurance

More than 70 percent of the population under 65 years of age has private health insurance, most of which is obtained through the workplace. In private industry, the share of employees' total compensation devoted to health insurance decreased in 2002.

Between 1995 and 2001 the age-adjusted proportion of the population under 65 years of age with **private health insurance** fluctuated between 71 and 73 percent after declining from 77 percent in 1984. More than 90 percent of private coverage was obtained through the workplace (a current or former employer or union) in 2001 (figure 6 and table 127).

In 2002 **private employers' health insurance costs** per employee-hour worked were $1.29, largely unchanged from $1.28 in 2001, and an increase from $1.09 in 2000. Among private employers the share of total compensation devoted to health insurance was 5.9 percent in 2002, down from

6.2 percent in 2001 but higher than the 2000 share, 5.5 percent (table 121).

Health Maintenance Organizations (HMOs)

An HMO is a prepaid health plan delivering comprehensive care to members through designated providers. More than one-quarter of all persons in the United States were enrolled in HMO in 2002. HMO enrollment peaked in 1999 and has declined slowly since then.

Enrollment in HMOs totaled 76 million persons or 26 percent of the U.S. population in 2002. HMO enrollment varied from 20–21 percent in the Midwest and South to 33 percent in the Northeast and 38 percent in the West. HMO enrollment increased steadily through 1999 but declined by more than 5 million between 1999 and 2002. The number of HMO plans decreased by 22 percent to 500 plans during these 3 years (table 132).

In 2002 the percent of the population enrolled in **HMOs** varied among the **States**, from 0 in Alaska to 51 percent in California. States with the next highest HMO enrollment were Massachusetts with 42 percent and Connecticut, Rhode Island, and Maryland, each with at least 35 percent (table 150).

In 2001, 27–29 percent of **children** under 18 years of age and **adults** age 18–44 and 45–64 years had health insurance coverage through a **private HMO**. Nine percent of children had coverage through a **Medicaid HMO** while less than 3 percent of adults under 65 years of age had this coverage (table 131).

State Health Expenditures

Total personal health care per capita expenditures and its components vary substantially among the States. State expenditures are affected by factors such as population age structure and health, payment rates, and supply of services.

Personal health care per capita expenditures averaged $3,800 in 1998, but varied among the States from $2,700 in Utah to $4,800 in Massachusetts. Higher expenditures were clustered in the New England and Mideast States, with lower per capita expenditures in the Rocky Mountain, Southwest, and Far West States (table 140).

The components of personal health care expenditures vary significantly by State. **Hospital care** per capita expenditures in 1998 ranged from $1,016 in Utah to $1,807 in Massachusetts. **Physician** and other professional services per capita expenditures varied from $763 in Utah to $1,347 in Minnesota. Per capita expenditures for **nursing home care** ranged from $90 in Alaska to $860 in Connecticut (tables 141–143).

Twenty-one percent of all personal health care expenditures were paid by **Medicare** in 1998, up from 17 percent in 1991. The Medicare share of State health expenditures in 1998 varied from 9 percent in Alaska to 25–26 percent in Mississippi, Louisiana, and Pennsylvania and 28 percent in Florida (table 145).

The share of personal health care expenditures paid by **Medicaid** increased from 13 percent in 1991 to 16 percent in 1995 through 1998. The Medicaid share of personal health care expenditures in 1998 ranged from less than 10 percent in Nevada and Virginia, to 21 percent in the District of Columbia, Rhode Island, and Maine, and 32 percent in New York (table 146).

Special Feature: Diabetes

Diabetes is characterized by high levels of blood glucose resulting from defects in insulin secretion, insulin action, or both. Diabetes can be associated with serious complications and premature death, especially if it is not well controlled. Complications can include disorders of the kidneys, nerves, blood vessels, and eye. Diabetes is a major contributing factor to blindness, end-stage renal disease, and lower extremity amputations. Complications, morbidity, and mortality associated with diabetes can be reduced through medical management of the disease. In addition, a healthy lifestyle—weight control, exercise, and healthy diet—can reduce or delay both incidence and complications.

The **age-adjusted prevalence of diagnosed diabetes** increased from 5.3 percent of the adult population in 1997 to 6.5 percent in 2002. Prevalence rises rapidly with age. Adults 65 years and over are more than twice as likely to have diabetes as are persons 45–54 years of age (figure 32).

Diabetes is a group of diseases characterized by high levels of blood glucose (sugar). Type 1 diabetes usually strikes children and young adults and accounts for 5–10 percent of all diagnosed cases. Type 2 diabetes accounts for about 90–95 percent of diagnosed cases. **Risk factors** for developing **type 2 diabetes** include obesity, being physically inactive, older age, and a family history of diabetes. The rise in diabetes prevalence is likely related, in part, to the rise in obesity among adults and overweight among children and adolescents (figures 15 and 32).

Most people with diabetes visit medical practitioners to become better educated about their condition, to discuss behavioral changes, to receive prescriptions for medications to control their blood sugar levels, or to be monitored and treated for complications of the disease. The rate of **visits to physician's offices or hospital outpatient departments** with any diagnosis of **diabetes** has increased for persons age 45 years and over. Between 1995–96 and 1999–2000, the number of physician visits with any diagnosis of diabetes per 1,000 population increased 35 percent among persons 45–54 and increased 43 percent among persons 55–64 years of age (figure 33).

Persons with diabetes are at increased risk of health complications and hospitalization. Among persons 45 years of age and over **hospital discharges** with any mention of **diabetes** accounted for 22 percent of discharges in 2000–01. Between 1990–91 and 2000–01 the rate of hospital discharges with any mention of diabetes increased for all age groups (figure 34).

Diabetes is a major cause of mortality. In 2000 **diabetes** was the fifth **leading cause of death** among women and the sixth leading cause among men. Diabetes was the underlying cause of death for nearly 70,000 deaths in 2000 and mentioned on the death certificates of at least twice as many additional deaths, contributing to deaths due to such underlying causes as heart disease, stroke, and kidney disease (figures 28 and 30 and table 31).

Chartbook on Trends in the Health of Americans

Monitoring the health of the Nation is essential for identifying and prioritizing health policy, program, and research initiatives. Current measures of the health status of the population, as well as its determinants, provide critical information about how the Nation's resources should be directed to improve the health of its population. Examination of emerging trends also identifies diseases, conditions, and risk factors that warrant study and intervention.

Many factors, including public health programs, advances in technology and medical science, and improved nutrition and economic status have contributed to increased life expectancy, reduced mortality and morbidity, and better overall health (1). However, the United States also spends more per capita than any other country on health and health care and the rate of increase in spending is increasing. Much of this spending is on health care—notable examples are prescribed medicines and cardiac operations—that control or reduce the impact of chronic diseases and conditions affecting an increasingly elderly population. Increasing prevalence of risk factors such as obesity also contribute to increased morbidity and its associated costs.

The *2003 Chartbook on Trends in the Health of Americans* assesses the current state of the Nation's health and how it is changing over time, both positively and negatively. This year's chartbook is an updated and revised version of the 2002 chartbook. Selection of the measures used in the chartbook was difficult because no single, limited set of measures can fully summarize the health of a large and diverse population. Any set of health measures involves some arbitrary choices and a good case could be made for including a number of other measures of health. In selecting overall measures, several factors were considered, including whether the measure was commonly used by health researchers and policy makers, whether the measure was easily understandable by a wide range of users, and whether information was available over time. As a group, the measures featured in the chartbook were selected to cover major topics of public health concern. In addition to sociodemographic information that provides the context within which to interpret health measures, the topics covered include: health insurance coverage, health-related risk factors, use of preventive care, disability, and mortality.

Because of the importance and availability of the measures selected for the 2002 chartbook, most have been included in this 2003 chartbook and will continue to be updated in future years. Each year, however, some charts will be replaced or revised to allow the inclusion of charts displaying new or emerging trends, and newly available or timely data. In addition, each year the *Chartbook on Trends in the Health of Americans* will include a special focus. This year's focus is on diabetes, a leading cause of morbidity and mortality that is affecting an increasing proportion of the population.

Organization of the Chartbook

Figures in the chartbook have been grouped into seven sections covering selected health determinants and outcomes. The first section (figures 1–5) presents major demographic, economic, and social factors influencing health: growth and aging of the national population, changing patterns of racial and ethnic diversity, and low income. The second section (figures 6–7) describes trends over time in health insurance coverage and characteristics of the uninsured. The third section (figures 8–11) presents trends in use of two types of preventive health care: prenatal care beginning during the first trimester of pregnancy and vaccination for influenza and pneumococcal disease among the elderly. The fourth section (figures 12–16) focuses on specific risk factors associated with increased risk of disease and death: cigarette smoking, overweight and obesity, and lack of physical activity. The fifth section (figures 17–20) shows the percent of children and working-age adults who have limitation of activity caused by chronic health conditions, and the prevalence of specific chronic health conditions causing activity limitation. It also contains a new chart on limitations in activities of daily living (ADLs) among elderly persons. The sixth section (figures 21–31) describes trends over time in mortality by showing changes in life expectancy at birth and at 65 years of age since 1901, changes in infant mortality since 1950, and age- and cause-specific death rates for persons ages 15 and over since 1950.

The seventh section, new this year, focuses on diabetes (figures 32–34). Diabetes is a serious chronic health condition and a significant cause of illness, disability, and death in the United States. Because of trends in obesity and aging of the population, diabetes is expected to reach almost epidemic proportions in coming years. This year's chartbook presents trends in prevalence of self-reported diabetes, as well as utilization of ambulatory and hospital care for persons diagnosed with this disease.

Many measures are shown separately for persons of different ages because of the strong effect age has on most health outcomes. Selected figures in the chartbook also highlight current differences in health and health determinants by variables such as sex, race, and Hispanic origin. Some estimates are age adjusted using the age distribution of the 2000 standard population. Line charts for which only selected years of data are displayed have dot markers on the data years. Line charts for which data are displayed for every year in the trend are shown without the use of dot markers. Time trends for some measures are shown on a logarithmic scale to emphasize the rate of change and to enable measures with large differences in magnitude to be shown on the same chart (figures 24, 26, 28, and 30). Other trends are shown on a linear scale to emphasize absolute differences over time (figures 1, 4, 6, 8, 10, 12, 15, 20, 21, 22, 32, 33, and 34). Time trends for some measures are not presented because of the relatively short amount of time that comparable national estimates are available (figures 13, 14, 17, 18, and 19). For some charts, data years are combined to increase sample size and reliability of the estimates. Changes in survey methodology, such as question wording, measures, sample size, and coding have also occurred, making comparability across years difficult in some instances. For example, the National Health Interview Survey was redesigned in 1997 to improve its efficiency and flexibility. These changes, however, make comparisons before and after 1997 problematic for many measures (see Appendix I, *National Health Interview Survey*).

Following the figures in the chartbook is a section containing data tables for each figure that show the data points graphed. For some measures, standard errors for the data points are provided and data not shown in the figures may be included. Additional information about the health measures is included in the notes to each data table as well as in Appendix II. Finally, the 151 trend tables in the body of *Health, United States, 2003* supplement the broad picture of the Nation's health presented in the chartbook by providing detailed data for many population groups within the United States. Additional measures of health status and determinants as well as information on health care use, health care resources, and health care expenditures are presented in these trend tables.

Chartbook Data Sources

Health-related and demographic data presented in this chartbook are from several national data systems. These are listed below and described in Appendix I.

Population counts and projections are from the U.S. Census Bureau. Poverty rates are based on data from the Current Population Survey. The National Health Interview Survey supplied data on health insurance coverage, adult cigarette smoking, adult physical inactivity, elderly vaccination, activity limitation due to chronic health conditions, and diagnosed diabetes prevalence. The National Ambulatory Medical Care Survey and the National Hospital Ambulatory Medical Care Survey data were used to estimate utilization of physician and hospital outpatient services by persons with diabetes. The National Hospital Discharge Survey provided data on hospitalizations by persons diagnosed with diabetes. The Youth Risk Behavior Survey provided data on smoking and physical activity among high school students. The Medicare Current Beneficiary Survey provided data on limitations in activities of daily living (ADLs) for the elderly population. The National Health and Nutrition Examination Survey was the source of data on overweight and obesity. Data from the National Vital Statistics System were used to estimate life expectancy, death rates, smoking during pregnancy, and use of early prenatal care. The National Linked File of Live Births and Infant Deaths provided data for estimates of infant mortality according to the race and Hispanic origin of the mother.

Conclusions

The health of our Nation has improved overall, in part due to the resources that have been devoted to health education, public health programs, health research, and health care. Over the past 50 years many infectious diseases have been controlled or their morbidity and mortality substantially reduced. However, other infectious diseases have re-emerged due to antibiotic resistant strains, while still other entirely new diseases have appeared as important threats to the Nation's health. Improved health care technologies, procedures, and medicines have also reduced mortality and morbidity associated with many chronic diseases and conditions. The cost of these advances, however, has been considerable (2).

Throughout the 21st century, efforts to improve health will be shaped by important changes in the U.S. population. As Americans meet this challenge, it will be in the context of a Nation that is growing older, and becoming more racially and ethnically diverse. The fraction of the population 65 years of age and over is increasing. With this increase, there will be more elderly Americans living longer, many with chronic health conditions or functional limitations. The Nation is becoming more diverse, with an increasing percent of Hispanic and other racial and ethnic groups who have historically been socioeconomically disadvantaged. Persons living in poverty and near poverty remain a segment of the national population at high risk for poor health outcomes and in need of greater access to health care. Socioeconomic and cultural differences among racial and ethnic groups in the United States will likely continue to influence patterns of disease, disability, and health care use in the future.

Recent improvements in health and increase in life expectancy reflect the influence of life style changes, greater use of some types of preventive care, public health efforts, new research findings, and advances in medicine. Decreased cigarette smoking among adults is a prime example of a risk factor for disease and death that has contributed to recent declines in mortality. Improvements in medical care and increased use of preventive health care have contributed to mortality reductions at all ages. A decline in the death rate from heart disease is an example of a major public health achievement, in part due to public education campaigns and increased use of cholesterol-lowering medications (3). The increasing percent of mothers who report beginning prenatal care during the first trimester of pregnancy and the increasing percent of elderly persons who have been vaccinated against influenza and pneumococcal disease illustrate the role for preventive health care throughout the life span. Public health and private efforts to improve motor vehicle transportation safety, as well as to increase safety in homes and workplaces, have contributed to lower death rates due to unintentional injuries for children and adults. Finally, the decline in the death rate for HIV disease in the 1990s demonstrates how new medical treatments can dramatically decrease the number of deaths caused by a particular disease.

For some important determinants of health, recent trends have not been favorable. Further lifestyle changes are needed to reduce risk factors for several chronic diseases. Even with decreases in cigarette smoking, in 2001 about 25 percent of men and 21 percent of women were smokers. Overweight and obesity, and physical inactivity among adults and children are significant risk factors for several chronic diseases, including diabetes and hypertension, and these indicators have not shown improvement—in fact, obesity is rising at an alarming rate. The rising prevalence of overweight in children and adolescents, and the high percent of both adults and adolescents not engaging in recommended amounts of physical activity raise additional concerns for future health outcomes (4–6).

Over the last half of the 20th century the prevalence of diabetes has steadily increased, and by 2002, more than 6 percent of the adult noninstitutionalized population reported they had diabetes (7,8). This is a conservative estimate of the true percentage of people who have the disease, as results from the National Health and Nutrition Examination Surveys in 1988–94 and 1999–2000 show that sizeable number of adults have undiagnosed diabetes (9,10).

Diabetes is a group of chronic diseases characterized by high levels of blood glucose (sugar). Type I diabetes accounts for 5–10 percent of diagnosed cases and the onset is generally in childhood or young adulthood. Type 2 diabetes accounts for 90–95 percent of diagnosed cases and is associated with older age, obesity, physical inactivity, and race/ethnicity. Prevalence rates of Type 2 diabetes are especially high among persons who are African American, Hispanic, or American Indian (11). Type 2 diabetes is also being diagnosed in an increasing number of adolescents and children (12).

Persons with diabetes are consuming an increasing amount of health care resources, including physicians' services and medications (13). Hospitalizations for persons with diabetes have also increased since 1990, while discharge rates for persons without diabetes remained stable or declined slightly during this time period. The importance of diabetes will substantially increase over time as the population ages, particularly if recent trends in obesity and physical inactivity continue.

This chartbook illustrates important trends in health and its associated risk factors, care, and resources. Many of the chartbook figures, as well as many of the 151 trend tables that follow the chartbook section provide more detailed information on these topics by racial, ethnic, and socioeconomic subpopulation. While many aspects of the health of the Nation have improved as a whole, the health of some subpopulations has lagged behind. Continued collection and dissemination of reliable and accurate information about health, its determinants, and resources expended will be critical for charting future trends, identifying how resources can be most effectively targeted, and prioritizing and evaluating programs and policies that will improve the health of all Americans.

References

1. Fielding JE. Public health in the twentieth century: Advances and challenges. Annu Rev Public Health (20):xiii–xxx. 1999.

2. Cutler DM, McClellan M. Is technological change in medicine worth it? Health Aff (Millwood) 20(5):11–29. 2001.

3. Achievements in Public Health, 1900–1999: Decline in deaths from heart disease and stroke—United States, 1900–99. MMWR 48(30):649–56. 1999.

4. Ogden CL, Flegal KM, Carroll MD et al. Prevalence and trends in overweight among US children and adolescents, 1999–2000. JAMA 288:1728–32. 2002.

5. Flegal KM, Carroll MD, Ogden CL et al. Prevalence and trends in obesity among US adults, 1999–2000. JAMA 288:1723–7. 2002.

6. Barnes PM, Schoenborn CA. Physical activity among adults: United States, 2000. Advance data from vital and health statistics; no 333. Hyattsville, Maryland: National Center for Health Statistics. 2003.

7. National Diabetes Data Group. Diabetes in America, 2nd Edition. Bethesda, Maryland: National Institutes of Health, (NIH publication no. 95–1468) 1995.

8. Ni H, Schiller J, Hao C, Cohen RA, Barnes P. Early release of selected estimates based on data from the 2002 National Health Interview Survey. Hyattsville, Maryland: National Center for Health Statistics. June 2003. Available from www.cdc.gov/nchs/nhis.htm.

9. Harris M, et al. Prevalence of diabetes, impaired fasting glucose, and impaired glucose tolerance in U.S. adults. Diabetes Care 21(4):518–24. 1998.

10. Centers for Disease Control and Prevention. Prevalence of diabetes and impaired fasting glucose in U.S. adults, 1999–2000. MMWR 52(35):833–7. 2003.

11. Centers for Disease Control and Prevention. 2002 National Diabetes Fact Sheet. Available from www.cdc.gov/diabetes/index.htm accessed on June 17, 2003.

12. Fagot-Campagna A, et al. Type 2 diabetes among North American children and adolescents: An epidemiologic review and a public health prospective. J Pediatr 136(5):664–72. 2000.

13. Centers for Disease Control and Prevention. National Center for Health Statistics, National Ambulatory Medical Care Survey, and National Hospital Ambulatory Medical Care Survey, unpublished analysis.

Figure 1. Total and elderly population: United States, 1950-2050

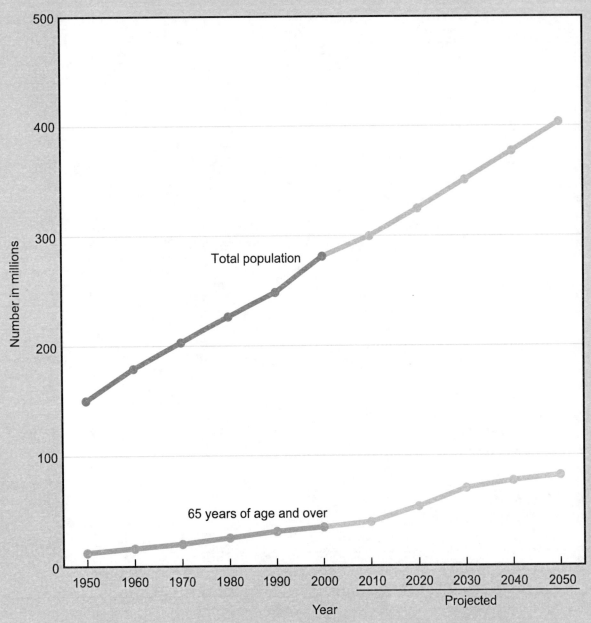

NOTE: See Data Table for data points graphed and additional notes.

SOURCES: U.S. Census Bureau, 1950-2000 decennial censuses and 2010-50 middle series population projections.

Age

From 1950 to 2000 the total resident population of the United States increased from 150 million to 281 million, representing an average annual growth rate of 1 percent (figure 1). During the same time period, the elderly population (65 years of age and over) grew twice as rapidly and increased from 12 to 35 million persons. Projections indicate that while both the total and elderly population will grow at a slower rate over the next 50 years the elderly population will continue to increase more rapidly than the total population.

During the past 50 years, the U.S. population has grown older (figure 2). From 1950 to 2000 the percent under 18 years of age fell from 31 percent to 26 percent while the percent elderly rose from 8 percent to 12 percent. From 2000 to 2050 a small decline in the percent of the population under 18 years of age is anticipated while a sizeable increase in the percent elderly is expected. Growth in the elderly population is projected to be particularly rapid as the "baby boom" generation turns 65 years of age beginning in 2011, with the rate of growth in the elderly population diminishing somewhat after 2030. By 2050 it is projected that one in five Americans will be elderly.

The aging of the population has important consequences for the health care system (1,2). As the elderly fraction of the population increases, more services will be required for the treatment and management of chronic and acute health conditions. Providing health care services needed by Americans of all ages will be a major challenge in the 21st century.

References

1. Wolf DA. Population change: Friend or foe of the chronic care system? Health Aff 20(6):28–42. 2001.

2. Goulding MR, Rogers ME, Smith SM. Health and aging: Trends in Aging—United States and worldwide. MMWR 52(06):101–6. 2003.

Figure 2. Percent of population in 3 age groups: United States, 1950, 2000, and 2050

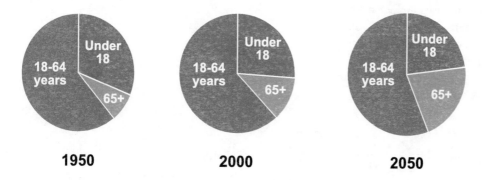

1950 **2000** **2050**

NOTE: See Data Table for data points graphed and additional notes.

SOURCES: U.S. Census Bureau, 1950 and 2000 decennial censuses and 2050 middle series population projections.

Race and Ethnicity

Changes in the racial and ethnic composition of the population have important consequences for the Nation's health because many measures of disease and disability differ significantly by race and ethnicity (*Health, United States, 2003*, trend tables). One of the overarching goals of U.S. public health policy is elimination of racial and ethnic disparities in health.

Diversity has long been a characteristic of the U.S. population, but the racial and ethnic composition of the Nation has changed over time. In recent decades the percent of the population of Hispanic origin and Asian or Pacific Islander race has risen (figure 3). In 2000 over one-quarter of adults and more than one-third of children identified themselves as Hispanic, black, Asian or Pacific Islander, or American Indian or Alaska Native.

In the 1980 and 1990 decennial censuses, Americans could choose only one racial category to describe their race (1). In the 2000 census the question on race was modified to allow the choice of more than one racial category. Although overall a small percent of persons of non-Hispanic origin selected two or more races in 2000, a higher percent of children than adults were described as being of more than one race. The number of American adults identifying themselves or their children as multiracial is expected to increase in the future (2).

In 2000 the percent of persons reporting two or more races also varied considerably among racial groups. For example, the percent of all persons reporting a specified race who mentioned that race in combination with one or more additional racial groups was 1.4 percent for white persons and 37 percent for American Indians or Alaska Natives (3).

References

1. Grieco EM, Cassidy RC. Overview of race and Hispanic origin. Census 2000 Brief. United States Census 2000. March 2001.

2. Waters MC. Immigration, intermarriage, and the challenges of measuring racial/ethnic identities. Am J Public Health 90(11):1735–7. 2000.

3. U.S. Census Bureau: Census 2000 Modified Race Data Summary File: 2000 Census of Population and Housing, September 2002.

Figure 3. Percent of population in selected race and Hispanic origin groups by age: United States, 1980-2000

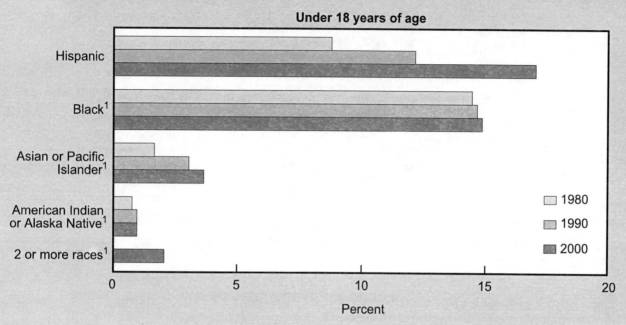

Under 18 years of age

Percent

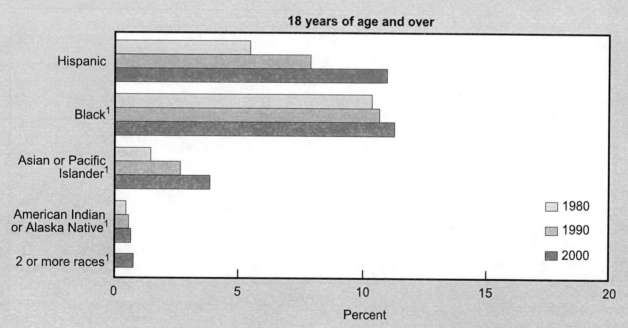

18 years of age and over

Percent

[1] Not Hispanic

NOTES: Persons of Hispanic origin may be of any race. Race data for 2000 are not directly comparable with data from 1980 and 1990. Individuals could report only one race in 1980 and 1990, and more than one race in 2000. Persons who selected only one race in 2000 are shown in single-race categories; persons who selected more than one race in 2000 are shown as having 2 or more races and are not included in single-race categories. In 2000 the category "Asian or Pacific Islander" includes Asian and Native Hawaiian or Other Pacific Islander. See Data Table for data points graphed.

SOURCE: U.S. Census Bureau, 1980-2000 decennial censuses.

Poverty

Children and adults in families with incomes below or near the Federal poverty level have worse health than those with higher incomes (see Appendix II, Poverty level for a definition of the Federal poverty level). Although, in some cases, illness can lead to poverty, more often poverty causes poor health by its connection with inadequate nutrition, substandard housing, exposure to environmental hazards, unhealthy lifestyles, and decreased access to and use of health care services (1).

In 2001 the overall percent of Americans living in poverty increased to 11.7 percent, up from 11.3 percent in 2000, reflecting the recession that started in the spring of 2000. This was the first increase in the poverty rate since 1993. Most of the increase in the poverty rate from 2000 to 2001 was accounted for by working-age adults who are less likely to receive income from government programs than are children and the elderly (2).

Starting in 1974 children have been more likely than either working-age adults or elderly persons to live in poverty (figure 4). Since 1974 poverty among children increased and remained at 20 percent or above from 1981 to 1997. Since then, the children's poverty rate has gradually declined to 16 percent.

Before 1974 the elderly were more likely to live in poverty than people of other ages. With the increasing dependence of the elderly on inflation adjusted government social insurance programs such as Social Security and Supplemental Security Income the poverty rate among the elderly declined rapidly until 1974 and has continued to decline gradually (3).

In 2001 the percent of persons living in poverty continued to differ significantly by age, race, and ethnicity (figure 5). At all ages, a higher percent of Hispanic and black persons than non-Hispanic white persons were poor or near poor

(100–199 percent of the poverty level). In 2001 more than one-quarter of Hispanic and black children were poor and more than one-half were either poor or near poor. In addition, more than one-half of elderly Hispanic and black persons were either poor or near poor. Persons of Asian and Pacific Islander descent had poverty rates slightly higher than those of non-Hispanic white persons but much lower than those of black and Hispanic persons. In 1999–2001 one in four American Indians and Alaska Natives lived in poverty. Poverty estimates for American Indians and Alaska Natives combine data for all age groups and several years in order to produce an estimate (2).

References

1. Pamuk E, Makuc D, Heck K, Reuben C, Lochner K. Socioeconomic Status and Health Chartbook. Health, United States, 1998. Hyattsville, Maryland: National Center for Health Statistics. 1998.

2. Proctor B, Dalaker J. Poverty in the United States: 2001. Current population reports, series P-60 no 219. Washington, DC: U.S. Government Printing Office. 2002.

3. Danziger S, Weinberg D. The historical record: trends in family income, inequality, and poverty. In Danziger S, Sandefur G, Weinberg D. (editors). Confronting Poverty: Prescriptions for Change. Cambridge, Massachusetts: Harvard University Press, 1994.

Figure 4. Poverty rates by age: United States, 1966-2001

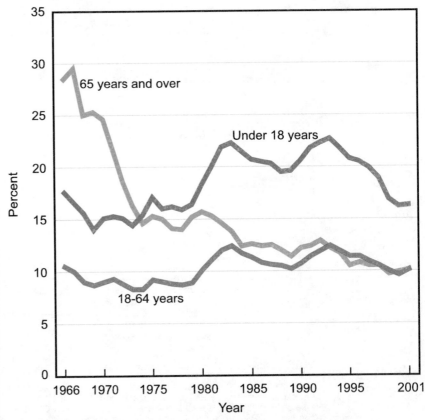

NOTES: Data shown are the percent of persons with family income below the poverty level. See Data Table for data points graphed and additional notes.

SOURCE: U.S. Census Bureau, Current Population Survey.

Figure 5. Low income population by age, race, and Hispanic origin: United States, 2001

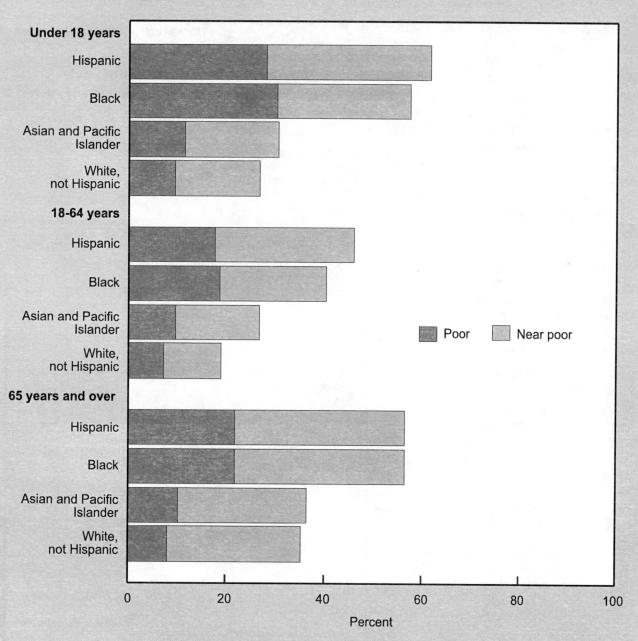

NOTES: Poor is defined as family income less than 100 percent of the poverty level and near poor as 100-199 percent of the poverty level. Persons of Hispanic origin may be of any race. Black, and Asian and Pacific Islander races include persons of Hispanic and non-Hispanic origin. See Data Table for data points graphed and additional notes.

SOURCE: U.S. Census Bureau, Current Population Survey.

Health Insurance

Health insurance coverage is an important determinant of access to health care (1). Uninsured children and nonelderly adults are substantially less likely to have a usual source of health care or a recent health care visit than their insured counterparts (*Health, United States, 2003*, tables 70, 73, 74, and 76). Uninsured persons are more likely to forgo needed health care due to cost concerns (2). The major source of coverage for persons under 65 years of age is private employer-sponsored group health insurance. Private health insurance may also be purchased on an individual basis, but it costs more and generally provides less coverage than group insurance. Public programs such as Medicaid and the State Children's Health Insurance Program provide coverage for many low-income children and adults.

Between 1984 and 1994 private coverage declined among the nonelderly population while Medicaid coverage and the percent of uninsured increased. Since 1994 the age-adjusted percent of the nonelderly population with no health insurance coverage has been between 16–17 percent, Medicaid between 9–11 percent, and private coverage between 70–73 percent (figure 6).

In 2001 more than 16 percent of Americans under 65 years of age reported having no health insurance coverage. The percent of nonelderly adults without health insurance coverage decreases with age. In 2001 adults 18–24 years of age were most likely to lack coverage and those 55–64 years of age were least likely (figure 7). Persons with incomes below or near the poverty level were at least three to four times as likely to have no health insurance coverage as those with incomes twice the poverty level or higher. Hispanic persons

and non-Hispanic black persons were more likely to lack health insurance than non-Hispanic white persons. Persons of Mexican origin were more likely to be uninsured than non-Hispanic black persons or other Hispanics. Access to health insurance coverage through employment is lowest for Hispanic persons (3).

References

1. Institute of Medicine. Committee on the Consequences of Uninsurance. Series of reports: Coverage matters: Insurance and health care; Care without coverage; Health insurance is a family matter. Washington, DC: National Academy Press. 2001–2002.

2. Ayanian JZ, Weissman JS, Schneider EC, et al. Unmet health needs of uninsured adults in the United States. JAMA 285(4):2061–9. 2000.

3. Monheit AC, Vistnes JP. Race/ethnicity and health insurance status: 1987 and 1996. Med Care Res Rev 57, Suppl 1:11–35. 2000.

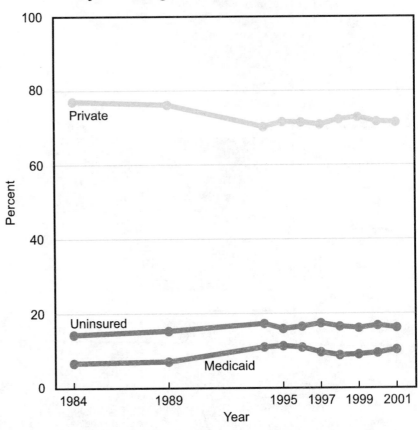

Figure 6. Health insurance coverage among persons under 65 years of age: United States, 1984-2001

NOTES: Percents are age adjusted. See Data Table for data points graphed, standard errors, and additional notes.

SOURCE: Centers for Disease Control and Prevention, National Center for Health Statistics, National Health Interview Survey.

Figure 7. No health insurance coverage among persons under 65 years of age by selected characteristics: United States, 2001

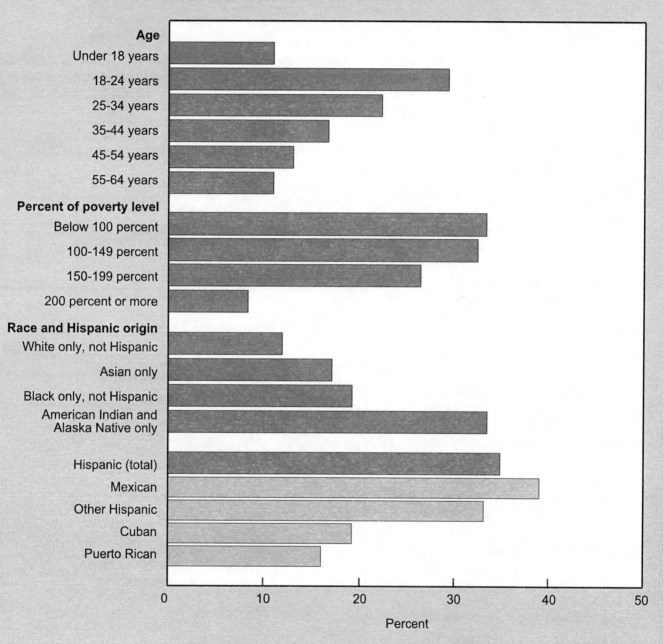

NOTES: Percents by poverty level, Hispanic origin, and race are age adjusted. Persons of Hispanic origin may be of any race. Asian, and American Indian and Alaska Native races include persons of Hispanic and non-Hispanic origin. See Data Table for data points graphed, standard errors, and additional notes.

SOURCE: Centers for Disease Control and Prevention, National Center for Health Statistics, National Health Interview Survey.

Prenatal Care

Prenatal care that begins in the first trimester and continues throughout pregnancy reduces the risk of maternal morbidity and poor birth outcomes. Appropriate prenatal care can enhance pregnancy outcome and long-term maternal health by managing preexisting and pregnancy-related medical conditions, providing health behavior advice, and assessing the risk of poor pregnancy outcome (1). Attitudes toward pregnancy, lifestyle factors, and cultural beliefs have been suggested as reasons women delay recommended prenatal care. Financial and health insurance problems are among the most important barriers to such care (2). Expansion of Medicaid coverage for pregnancy-related services has increased availability and use of prenatal care by low income women (3).

During the last three decades, the percent of mothers reporting prenatal care beginning in the first trimester has risen (figure 8). This upward trend reflects increases during the 1970s and the 1990s. By 2001, 83 percent of mothers reported receiving early prenatal care.

Increases in use of prenatal care beginning in the first trimester have been observed among mothers in all major racial and ethnic groups. Increases in use of prenatal care in the 1990s were greatest for those with the lowest rates of care: Hispanic, non-Hispanic black, and American Indian or Alaska Native women (*Health, United States, 2003*, table 6).

Important racial and ethnic differences in the percent of mothers reporting early prenatal care persist (figure 9). In 2001 the percent receiving early care was higher for non-Hispanic white women than for non-Hispanic black women, American Indian or Alaska Native women, and most groups of Hispanic women.

In 2001 about 4 percent of women began care in the third trimester of pregnancy or received no care at all, compared with 6 percent in 1990. The proportion of women receiving late or no prenatal care was highest among American Indian or Alaska Native women, non-Hispanic black women, and women of Mexican origin (6–8 percent) (*Health, United States, 2003*, table 6).

References

1. Martin JA, Hamilton BE, Ventura SJ, Menacker F, Park MM, Sutton PD. Births: Final data for 2001. National Vital Statistics Reports; Vol 51 no 2. Hyattsville, Maryland: National Center for Health Statistics. 2002.

2. Lewis CT, Mathews TJ, Heuser RL. Prenatal care in the United States, 1980–94. Vital Health Stat 21(54). Hyattsville, Maryland: National Center for Health Statistics. 1996.

3. Rowland D, Salganicoff A, Keenan PS. The key to the door: Medicaid's role in improving health care for women and children. Annu Rev Public Health 20:403–26. 1999.

Figure 8. Early prenatal care among mothers: United States, 1970-2001

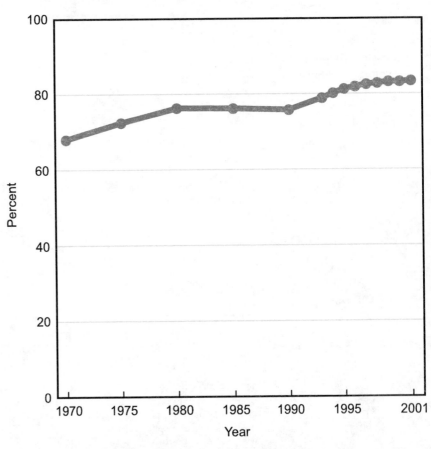

NOTES: Early prenatal care begins during the first trimester of pregnancy. See Data Table for data points graphed.

SOURCE: Centers for Disease Control and Prevention, National Center for Health Statistics, National Vital Statistics System.

Figure 9. Early prenatal care by detailed race and Hispanic origin of mother: United States, 2001

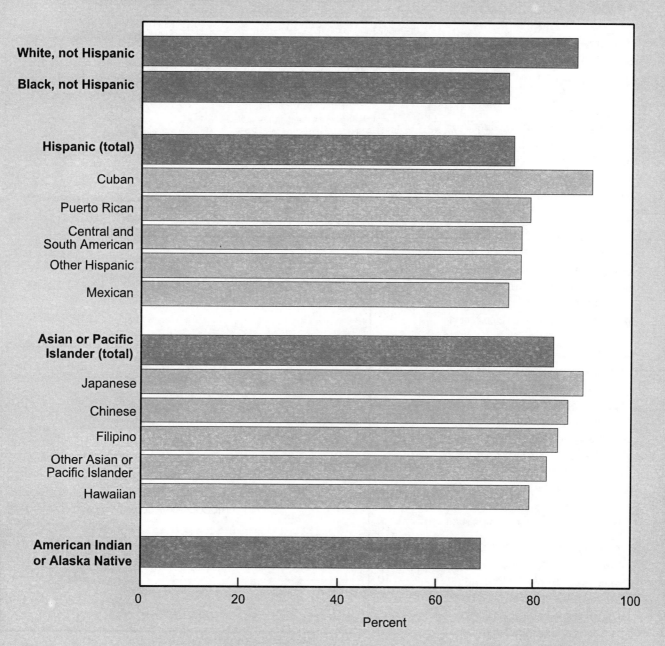

NOTES: Early prenatal care begins during the first trimester of pregnancy. Persons of Hispanic origin may be of any race. The race groups, Asian or Pacific Islander and American Indian or Alaska Native, include persons of Hispanic and non-Hispanic origin. See Data Table for data points graphed.

SOURCE: Centers for Disease Control and Prevention, National Center for Health Statistics, National Vital Statistics System.

Vaccination: Adults 65 Years of Age and Over

In the United States influenza resulted in the death of about 36,000 persons 65 years of age and over each year during the 1990s (1). Pneumococcal disease accounts for more deaths than any other vaccine-preventable bacterial disease. Annual influenza vaccination and one dose of pneumococcal polysaccharide vaccine can lessen the risk of illness and subsequent complications among elderly persons.

Between 1989 and 1999 the percent of noninstitutionalized elderly adults 65 years of age and over who reported an influenza vaccination within the past year more than doubled to 66 percent and then decreased slightly to 63 percent in 2001 (figure 10). During the same period the percent of elderly adults ever having received a pneumococcal vaccine increased sharply from 14 percent to 54 percent. Several factors have been suggested as contributing to these increases: greater acceptance of preventive health care by consumers and practitioners, improved Medicare coverage for these vaccines since 1993, and wider delivery of this care by health care providers other than physicians (2).

Vaccination levels varied by race and Hispanic origin in 1999–2001 (figure 11) but not by gender. Vaccinations against influenza were received by approximately two-thirds of non-Hispanic white and Asian, and approximately one-half of Hispanic and non-Hispanic black elderly adults. Vaccinations against pneumococcal disease were received by approximately one-half of non-Hispanic white, and approximately one-third of Asian, non-Hispanic black, and Hispanic elderly adults. Continued monitoring of vaccination rates for all racial and ethnic groups is needed to apprise efforts to improve rates overall and to reduce disparities in vaccination levels (3).

References

1. Thompson WW, et al. Mortality associated with influenza and respiratory syncytial virus in the United States. JAMA 289(2):179–86. 2003.

2. Singleton JA, et al. Influenza, pneumococcal, and tetanus toxoid vaccination of adults—United States, 1993–97. In: CDC Surveillance Summaries. MMWR 49(SS-9):39–62. 2000.

3. Fedson, DS. Adult immunization: Summary of the National Vaccine Advisory Committee report. JAMA 272(14):1133–7. 1994.

Figure 10. Influenza and pneumococcal vaccination among adults 65 years of age and over: United States, 1989-2001

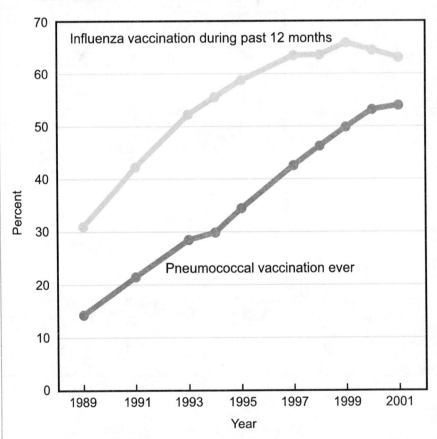

NOTES: Data are for the civilian noninstitutionalized population and are age adjusted. See Data Table for data points graphed, standard errors, and additional notes.

SOURCE: Centers for Disease Control and Prevention, National Center for Health Statistics, National Health Interview Survey.

Figure 11. Influenza and pneumococcal vaccination among adults 65 years of age and over by race and Hispanic origin: United States, 1999-2001

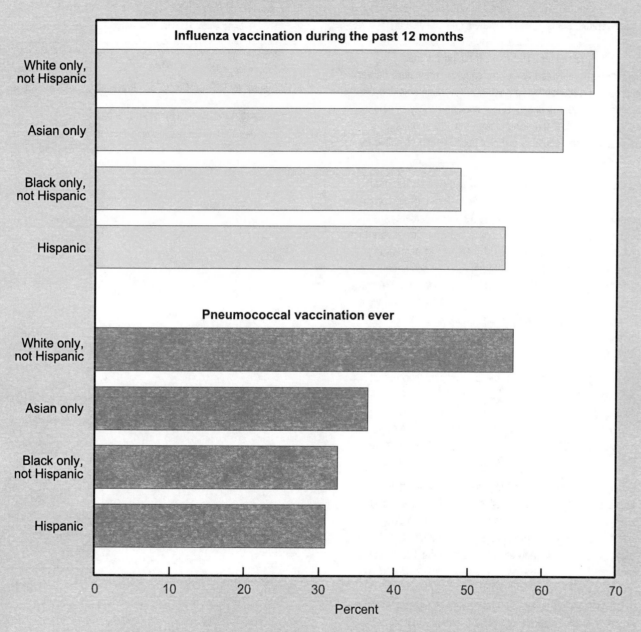

Smoking

As the leading cause of preventable death and disease in the United States, smoking is associated with significantly increased risk of heart disease, stroke, lung cancer, and chronic lung diseases (1). Smoking during pregnancy contributes to elevated risk of miscarriage, premature delivery, and having a low birthweight infant. Preventing smoking among teenagers is critical since smoking usually begins in adolescence (2). Decreasing cigarette smoking among adolescents and adults is a major public health objective for the Nation.

Cigarette smoking among adult men and women declined substantially following the first Surgeon General's Report on smoking in 1964 (figure 12). Since 1990 the percent of adults who smoke has continued to decline but at a slower rate than previously. In 2001, 25 percent of men and 21 percent of women were smokers. Cigarette smoking by adults continues to be strongly associated with educational attainment. Among adults, persons with less than a high school education were almost three times as likely to smoke as those with a bachelor's degree or more education (Health, United States, 2003, table 60).

Among high school students, the percent reporting recent cigarette smoking decreased between 1997 and 2001 after increasing in the early 1990s. During the last decade, a similar percent of male and female students reported smoking. In 2001 white and Hispanic students were more likely than black students to report current smoking (3).

Among mothers with a live birth, the percent reporting smoking during pregnancy declined between 1989 and 2001 (4). Twelve percent of mothers with a live birth in 2001 reported smoking during pregnancy. Maternal smoking declined for all racial and ethnic groups in the 1990s, but differences among these groups persist (Health, United States, 2003, table 11). In 2001 the percent of mothers reporting smoking during pregnancy was highest for American Indian or Alaska Native mothers (20 percent) and non-Hispanic white mothers (16 percent).

References

1. Centers for Disease Control and Prevention. Tobacco use—United States, 1900–1999. MMWR 48(43):986–93. 1999.

2. U.S. Department of Health and Human Services. Preventing tobacco use among young people: A report of the Surgeon General. Atlanta, Georgia: Centers for Disease Control and Prevention. 1994.

3. Centers for Disease Control and Prevention. Trends in cigarette smoking among high school students—United States, 1991–2001. MMWR 51(19):409–12. 2002.

4. Mathews TJ. Smoking during pregnancy in the 1990s. National vital statistics reports; vol 49 no 7. Hyattsville, Maryland: National Center for Health Statistics. 2001.

Figure 12. Cigarette smoking among men, women, high school students, and mothers during pregnancy: United States, 1965-2001

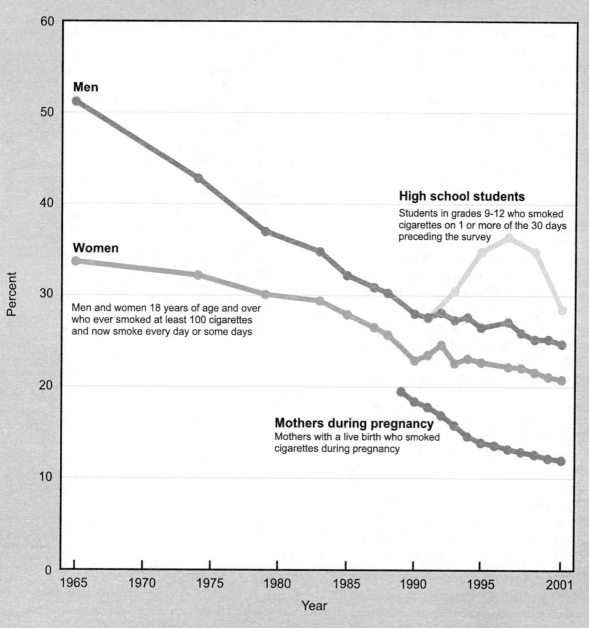

Men

Women

Men and women 18 years of age and over who ever smoked at least 100 cigarettes and now smoke every day or some days

High school students
Students in grades 9-12 who smoked cigarettes on 1 or more of the 30 days preceding the survey

Mothers during pregnancy
Mothers with a live birth who smoked cigarettes during pregnancy

Percent

Year

NOTES: Percents for men and women are age adjusted. See Data Table for data points graphed, standard errors, and additional notes.

SOURCES: Centers for Disease Control and Prevention, National Center for Health Statistics, National Health Interview Survey (data for men and women); National Vital Statistics System (data for mothers during pregnancy); National Center for Chronic Disease Prevention and Health Promotion, Youth Risk Behavior Survey (data for high school students).

Physical Activity

Many epidemiologic and clinical studies have shown the benefits of regular physical activity for reducing mortality, preventing cardiovascular disease, enhancing physical functioning, and controlling weight (1). Regular physical activity lessens the risk of heart disease, diabetes, colon cancer, high blood pressure, osteoporosis, arthritis, and obesity. It also improves symptoms associated with mental health conditions such as depression and anxiety. Although vigorous physical activity produces the greatest cardiovascular benefits, moderate amounts of physical activity are associated with lower levels of mortality. Among the elderly, even small amounts of physical activity may improve cardiovascular functioning (2).

In 2001, 38 percent of female high school students and 24 percent of male high school students reported a level of physical activity that did not meet the criteria for the recommended amount of either moderate or vigorous physical activity (figure 13, see data table for definition of physical activity levels). The percent reporting a lack of moderate and vigorous physical activity was higher among older students in 10th–12th grades than among younger students in 9th grade. Between 1999 and 2001 the percent of students reporting a lack of moderate and vigorous physical activity remained stable.

Overall physical activity level in adults was measured using questions about both leisure-time and usual daily activity. Respondents were categorized as being inactive, or having low, medium, medium/high, or high physical activity (see data table for figure 14, and reference 3). In 2000, 22 percent of men and 28 percent of women 18 years of age and over were either inactive or had low physical activity. A substantial proportion of adults in all age groups were either inactive or had low physical activity, taking into account both leisure-time and usual daily activity (figure 14).

The percent of adults who were inactive or with low activity increased with age, and was higher for women than men, due to gender and age differences in the percents who were inactive. In 2000, 12 percent of women compared with 7 percent of men were inactive. Inactivity increased with advancing age with nearly one-fifth of elderly men and more than one-quarter of elderly women being inactive.

Increasing physical activity during leisure-time is one way to counterbalance an otherwise sedentary lifestyle. However,

trends in leisure-time activity show the need for improvement. In 2000–01 about 38 percent of adults 18 years of age and over reported that they did not engage in physical activity during leisure time, about the same as in 1997–98 (4,5).

References

1. U.S. Department of Health and Human Services. Physical activity and health: A report of the Surgeon General. Atlanta, Georgia: Centers for Disease Control and Prevention. 1996.

2. Mensink GB, Ziese T, Kok FJ. Benefits of leisure-time physical activity on the cardiovascular risk profile at older age. Int J Epidemiol 28(4):659–66. 1999.

3. Barnes PM, Schoenborn CA. Physical activity among adults: United States, 2000. Advance data from vital and health statistics; no 333. Hyattsville, Maryland: National Center for Health Statistics. 2003.

4. Schoenborn CA, Barnes PM. Leisure-time physical activity among adults: United States, 1997–98. Advance data from vital and health statistics; no 325. Hyattsville, Maryland: National Center for Health Statistics. 2002.

5. Centers for Disease Control and Prevention. National Center for Health Statistics, National Health Interview Survey, unpublished analysis.

Figure 13. High school students not engaging in recommended amounts of physical activity (neither moderate nor vigorous) by grade and sex: United States, 2001

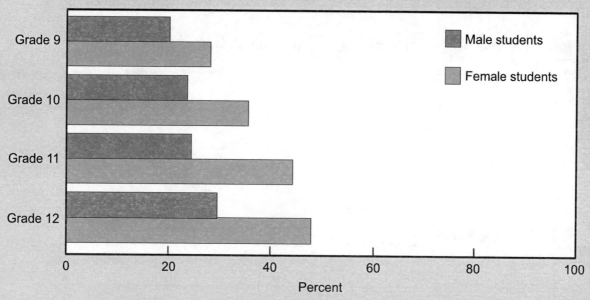

Percent

Figure 14. Adults who are inactive or have a low level of overall physical activity by age and sex: United States, 2000

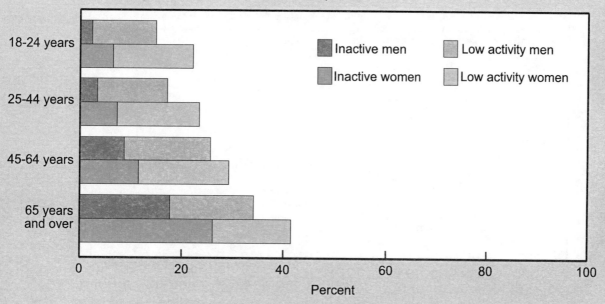

Percent

NOTE: See Data Table for data points graphed, standard errors, and additional notes defining moderate, vigorous, and overall activity level.

SOURCE for figure 13: Centers for Disease Control and Prevention, National Center for Chronic Disease Prevention and Health Promotion, Youth Risk Behavior Survey.

SOURCE for figure 14: Centers for Disease Control and Prevention, National Center for Health Statistics, National Health Interview Survey.

Figure 15. Overweight and obesity by age: United States, 1960-2000

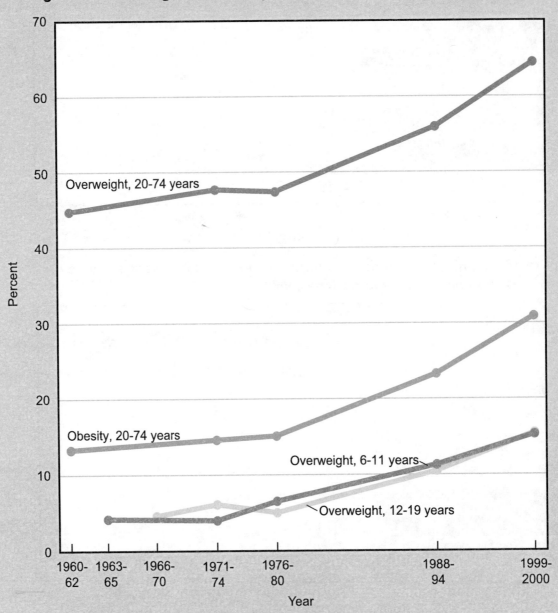

NOTES: Percents for adults are age adjusted. Overweight for children is defined as a body mass index (BMI) at or above the sex- and age-specific 95th percentile BMI cut points from the 2000 CDC Growth Charts: United States. Overweight for adults is defined as a BMI greater than or equal to 25 and obesity as a BMI greater than or equal to 30. Obesity is a subset of the percent with overweight. See Data Table for data points graphed, standard errors, and additional notes.

SOURCES: Centers for Disease Control and Prevention, National Center for Health Statistics, National Health Examination Survey and National Health and Nutrition Examination Survey.

Overweight and Obesity

Many epidemiologic and actuarial studies have shown that increased body weight is associated with excess morbidity and mortality (1). Among adults, overweight and obesity substantially elevate the risk of illness from heart disease, diabetes, and some types of cancer. Overweight and obesity are also factors that increase the severity of disease associated with hypertension, arthritis, and other musculoskeletal problems (2). Among children and adolescents, obesity increases the risk of high cholesterol, hypertension, and diabetes (3). Diet, physical activity, genetic factors, and health conditions all contribute to overweight in children and adults. The potential health benefits from reduction in overweight and obesity are of significant public health importance (4).

Results from a series of National Health and Nutrition Examination Surveys indicate that the prevalence of overweight and obesity changed little between the early 1960s and 1980 (figure 15). Findings from the 1988–94 survey, however, showed substantial increases in overweight and obesity among adults. The upward trend in overweight since 1980 reflects primarily an increase in the percent of adults who are obese. Estimates from the 1999–2000 survey indicate that overweight and obesity have continued to increase. In 1999–2000, 65 percent of adults were overweight with 31 percent obese.

Among children (6–11 years of age) and adolescents (12–19 years of age) the percent overweight increased after the mid-1970s. Estimates from the 1999–2000 survey indicate that about 15 percent of children and adolescents were overweight. The increase in overweight prevalence is highest among non-Hispanic black and Mexican-origin adolescents. More than 23 percent of non-Hispanic black and Mexican-origin adolescents were overweight in 1999–2000 (5).

The prevalence of obesity varies among adults by sex, race, and ethnicity (figure 16). In 1999–2000, 28 percent of men and 34 percent of women were obese. The prevalence of obesity among men differed little by racial and ethnic group; among women, non-Hispanic black women had a higher prevalence of obesity than did non-Hispanic white women. In 1999–2000 one-half of non-Hispanic black women were obese.

References

1. Allison DB, et al. Annual deaths attributable to obesity in the United States. JAMA 282(16):1530–8. 1999.

2. U.S. Department of Health and Human Services. The Surgeon General's call to action to prevent and decrease overweight and obesity. Rockville, Maryland. 2001.

3. Dietz WH. Health consequences of obesity in youth: Childhood predictors of adult disease. Pediatrics 101(3 Pt 2):518–25. 1998.

4. Flegal KM, et al. Prevalence and trends in obesity among US adults, 1999–2000. JAMA 288(14):1723–7. 2002.

5. Ogden CL, et al. Prevalence and trends in overweight among US children and adolescents, 1999–2000. JAMA 288(14):1728–32. 2002.

Figure 16. Obesity among adults 20-74 years of age by sex, race, and Hispanic origin: United States, 1999-2000

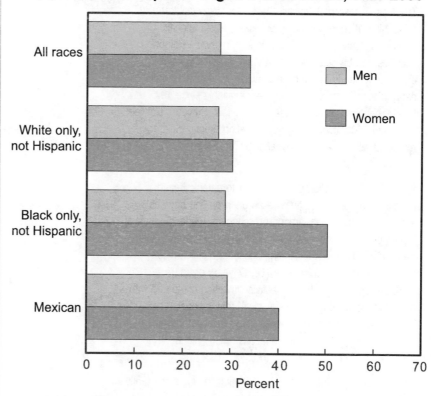

NOTES: Percents are age adjusted. Obesity is defined as a body mass index (BMI) greater than or equal to 30. Persons of Mexican origin may be of any race. See Data Table for data points graphed, standard errors, and additional notes.

SOURCE: Centers for Disease Control and Prevention, National Center for Health Statistics, National Health and Nutrition Examination Survey.

Limitation of Activity: Children

Limitation of activity due to chronic physical, mental, or emotional disorders or deficits is a broad measure of health and functioning. Among children chronic health conditions that limit activity include, but are not restricted to, hearing, visual, and speech problems; learning disabilities; mental retardation and other developmental problems (such as cerebral palsy); mental and emotional problems; and a variety of chronic health conditions (such as asthma). The long-term impact of activity limitation in children can often be ameliorated by use of health care and educational services.

The identification of activity limitation in children is sometimes uncertain because children are learning and mastering new activities as they develop. As a result some variation in children's activities may be due to differences in the pace of development. Estimates of the number of children with an activity limitation vary depending on the type of disabilities included and the methods used to identify them (1).

The National Health Interview Survey identifies children with activity limitation in two ways: by asking about specific limitations in play, self-care, walking, memory, and other activities and by determining if a child receives special education or early intervention services. Comparable national data on activity limitation have been available since 1997 (see Appendix | National Health Interview Survey). Between 1997 and 2001 levels of activity limitation among children remained about the same (*Health, United States, 2003*, table 56).

In 1999–2001 limitation of activity due to chronic health conditions occurred nearly twice as often among boys as among girls (figure 17). Among preschoolers (under 5 years of age) 4 percent of boys as compared with 2 percent of girls had an activity limitation. Among school-age children (5–11 years of age) and adolescents (12–17 years of age), 9–10 percent of boys had an activity limitation compared with about 5 percent of girls. Physiological, maturational, behavioral, and social differences between boys and girls have been suggested as explanations for the higher prevalence of activity limitation in boys (2).

The percent of children with activity limitation was significantly higher among school-age children and adolescents than among preschoolers. For boys and girls, the higher percent of school-age children and adolescents with activity limitation was largely explained by the number of children identified solely by participation in special education. About 7–8 percent of school-age and adolescent boys and approximately 4 percent of girls were classified as having activity limitation solely by their participation in special education.

References

1. Newacheck PW, Strickland B, Shonkoff JP, et al. An epidemiologic profile of children with special health care needs. Pediatrics 102(1):117–21. 1998.

2. Jans L, Stoddard S. Chartbook on women and disability in the United States: An InfoUse report. Washington, DC: U.S. National Institute on Disability and Rehabilitation Research. 1999.

Figure 17. Limitation of activity caused by 1 or more chronic health conditions among children by sex and age: United States, 1999-2001

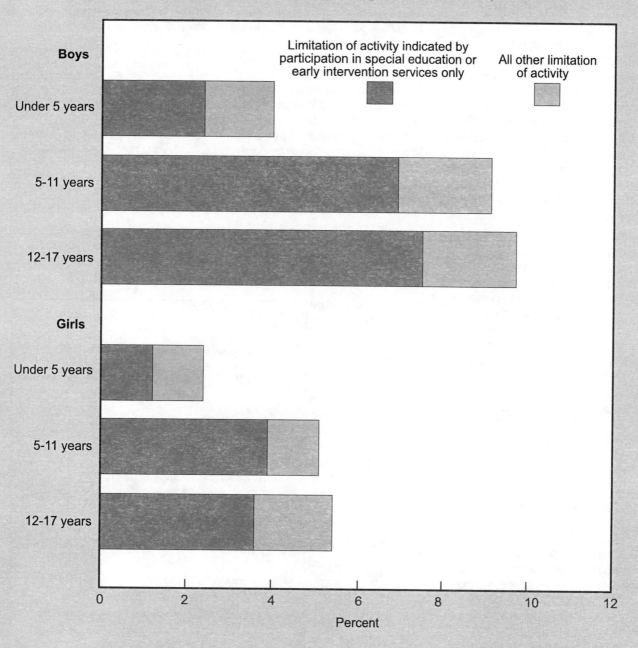

NOTES: Data are for noninstitutionalized children. Children with limitation of activity caused by chronic health conditions may be identified by enrollment in special programs (special education or early intervention services) or by some other activity limitation. The category "all other limitation of activity" may include children receiving special education or early intervention services. See Data Table for data points graphed and standard errors.

SOURCE: Centers for Disease Control and Prevention, National Center for Health Statistics, National Health Interview Survey.

Limitation of Activity: Working-Age Adults

Measuring limitations in everyday activities due to chronic physical, mental, or emotional problems is one way to assess the impact of health conditions on self-care and social participation (1). Chronic health conditions can alter the ability of adults to lead independent lives by affecting a person's capacity to carry out a variety of activities. The effect that chronic health conditions have on activity limitation may vary with the availability of supportive and health care services.

In the National Health Interview Survey, limitation of activity in adults includes limitations in handling personal care needs (activities of daily living), routine needs (instrumental activities of daily living), having a job outside the home, walking, remembering, and other activities. Comparable national data on activity limitation have been available since 1997 (see Appendix I National Health Interview Survey). Between 1997 and 2001 the percent of adults 18–64 years of age reporting any activity limitation caused by a chronic health condition remained relatively stable (*Health, United States, 2003*, table 56).

Among working-age adults, 6 percent of younger adults reported limitation in activity, in contrast to 21 percent of adults 55–64 years of age (figure 18). The percent of poor working-age adults reporting a limitation was three times that of adults with family income at 200 percent or more of the poverty level. After adjusting for differences in age, limitation of activity was about the same for men and women. Limitation of activity varies modestly by race and Hispanic origin from 8 percent of Hispanic persons to 12 percent of non-Hispanic black persons.

Health surveys that measure limitation of activity have typically asked about chronic conditions causing these restrictions. Health conditions usually refer to broad categories of disease and impairment rather than medical diagnoses and reflect the understanding the general public has of factors causing disability or limitation of activity (2). Persons who reported more than one chronic health condition as the cause of their activity limitation were counted in each category. Among younger and older working-age adults, arthritis and other musculoskeletal conditions were the most frequently mentioned chronic conditions causing limitation of activity (figure 19). Among persons 18–44 years of age, mental illness was the second most prevalent cause of activity limitation. Among older working-age adults (45–64 years), heart disease was the second most frequently mentioned condition.

References

1. Guralnik JM, Fried LP, Salive ME. Disability as a public health outcome in the aging population. Annu Rev Public Health 17:25–46. 1996.

2. Fujiura GT, Rutkowski-Kmitta V. Counting disability. In: Albrecht GL, Seelman KD, Bury M, eds. Handbook of disability studies. Thousand Oaks, California: Sage Publications, 69–96. 2001.

Figure 18. Limitation of activity caused by 1 or more chronic health conditions among working-age adults by selected characteristics: United States, 1999-2001

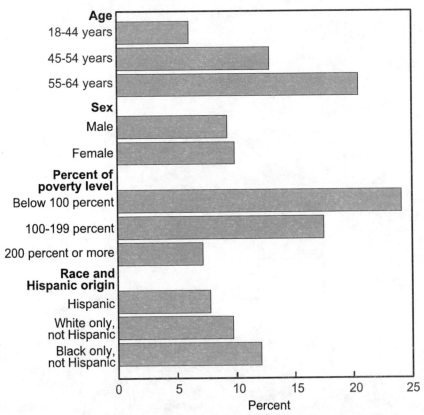

NOTES: Data are for the civilian noninstitutionalized population and are age adjusted. Persons of Hispanic origin may be of any race. See Data Table for data points graphed, standard errors, and additional notes.

SOURCE: Centers for Disease Control and Prevention, National Center for Health Statistics, National Health Interview Survey.

Figure 19. Selected chronic health conditions causing limitation of activity among working-age adults by age: United States, 1999-2001

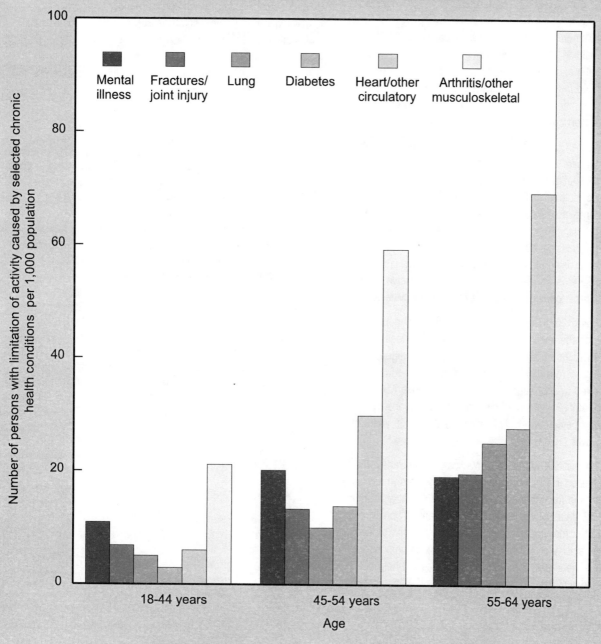

NOTES: Persons who reported more than one chronic health condition as the cause of their activity limitation were counted in each category. Selected chronic health conditions include the four leading causes of activity limitation among adults in each age group. See Data Table for data points graphed, standard errors, and additional notes.

SOURCE: Centers for Disease Control and Prevention, National Center for Health Statistics, National Health Interview Survey.

Limitation of Activity: Adults 65 Years of Age and Over

The ability to perform basic activities of daily living (ADL), such as bathing, dressing, and using the toilet is an indicator of the health and functional well-being of the older population. Being limited in ADLs compromises the quality of life of older persons and often results in the need for informal or formal caregiving services, including institutionalization.

The Medicare Current Beneficiary Survey reports the health and health care utilization of a representative sample of Medicare beneficiaries of all ages and in all types of residences, both institutional and noninstitutional. Respondents are asked about their level of difficulty and the kind of assistance received in performing six ADLs: bathing or showering, dressing, eating, getting in or out of bed or chairs, walking, and using the toilet. The definition of limitation here includes persons who have difficulty and who receive help or supervision performing at least one of the six activities.

From 1992 to 2001 the percent of all Medicare beneficiaries 65 years of age and over who were limited in at least one of six ADLs declined from 16 percent to 14 percent (figure 20). In 2001, 10 percent of noninstitutionalized persons had difficulty and received help or supervision with at least one ADL compared with 91 percent of institutionalized persons, who constitute 5 percent of all Medicare beneficiaries 65 years of age and over (1).

Among noninstitutionalized older Medicare beneficiaries, the percent limited in ADLs was higher for women than men and rises with age for women and men. For the oldest age group, persons 85 years of age and over, 27 percent of women and 21 percent of men received help or supervision with at least one basic activity of daily living in 2001. Among persons in institutions, nearly all, regardless of age, received help or supervision with ADLs (91 percent of men and 90 percent of women).

Some studies show that limitations in certain aspects of disability have declined among the older population, including the ability to perform physical tasks such as walking up steps and reaching arms overhead and the ability to perform instrumental activities of daily living (IADLs) such as shopping and managing money (2–5). Evidence on the trends in ADL limitation is mixed. The percent of noninstitutionalized Medicare beneficiaries 65 years of age and over who were limited in ADLs declined from 12 percent in 1992 to

10 percent in 2001. Among persons in institutions, however, the percent needing assistance increased from 86 percent to 91 percent during the same time period. Over time, the distinction between institutionalized and noninstitutionalized settings has blurred as "assisted living" facilities have become more prominent. More studies over a longer time period are needed to determine whether a sustained overall decline in ADL limitation is occurring.

References

1. Centers for Medicare and Medicaid Services, Medicare Current Beneficiary Survey, Access to Care files, unpublished analysis.

2. Freedman V, Martin L. Changing patterns of functional limitation among the older American population. AJPH 88:1457–62. 1998.

3. Lentzner HR, Weeks JD, Feldman JJ. Changes in disability in the elderly population: Preliminary results from the Second Supplement on Aging. Paper presented at the annual meetings of the Population Association of America. Chicago, Illinois: April 1998.

4. Crimmins E, Saito Y, Reynolds S. Further evidence on recent trends in the prevalence and incidence of disability among older Americans from two sources: The LSOA and the NHIS. J. Gerontol 52B(2): S59–71. 1997.

5. Manton KG, Gu, X. Changes in the prevalence of chronic disability in the United States black and nonblack population above 65 from 1982 to 1999. PNAS 98(11):6354–9. 2001.

Figure 20. Limitation in activities of daily living among Medicare beneficiaries 65 years of age and over: United States, 1992-2001

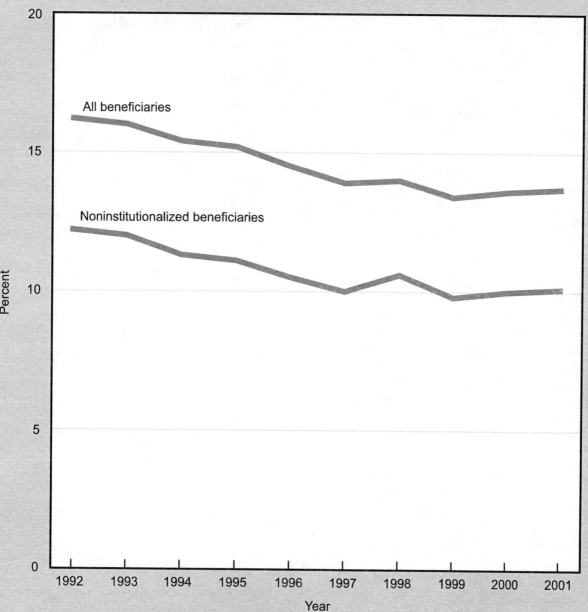

NOTES: Percents are age adjusted. Limitation in activities of daily living is defined as having difficulty and receiving help or supervision with at least one of the following six activities: bathing or showering, dressing, eating, getting in or out of bed or chairs, walking, and using the toilet. See Data Table for data points graphed, standard errors, and additional notes.

SOURCE: Centers for Medicare and Medicaid Services, Medicare Current Beneficiary Survey, Access to Care files.

Life Expectancy

Life expectancy is a measure often used to gauge the overall health of a population. As a summary measure of mortality, life expectancy represents the average number of years of life that could be expected if current death rates were to remain constant. Shifts in life expectancy are often used to describe trends in mortality. Life expectancy at birth is strongly influenced by infant and child mortality. Life expectancy later in life reflects death rates at or above a given age and is independent of the effect of mortality at younger ages (1).

During the 20th century, life expectancy at birth increased from 48 to 74 years for men and from 51 to almost 80 years for women (figure 21). Improvements in nutrition, housing, hygiene, and medical care contributed to decreases in death rates throughout the lifespan. Prevention and control of infectious diseases had a profound impact on life expectancy in the first half of the 20th century (2).

Life expectancy at age 65 also increased during the last century. Among men, life expectancy at age 65 rose from 12 to 16 years and among women from 12 to 19 years. In contrast to life expectancy at birth, which increased sharply early in the century, life expectancy at age 65 improved primarily after 1950. Improved access to health care, advances in medicine, healthier lifestyles, and better health before age 65 are factors underlying decreased death rates among the elderly (3).

While the overall trend in life expectancy for the United States has been upward throughout the 20th century, the gain in years of life expectancy for women generally exceeded that for men until the 1970s, widening the gap in life expectancy between men and women. The increasing gap during these years is attributed to increases in male mortality due to ischemic heart disease and lung cancer, both of which increased largely as the result of men's early and widespread adoption of cigarette smoking (4). After the 1970s the gain in life expectancy for men exceeded that for women and the gender gap in life expectancy began to narrow. During the 1990s the total gain in life expectancy for women was less than 1 year compared with more than 2 years for men, reflecting proportionately greater decreases in heart disease and cancer mortality for men than for women and proportionately larger increases in chronic lower respiratory disease mortality among women (4).

Longer life expectancies at birth in many other developed countries suggest the possibility of improving longevity in the United States (*Health, United States, 2003*, table 26). Decreasing death rates of less advantaged groups could raise life expectancy in the United States (*Health, United States, 2003*, table 27).

References

1. Arriaga EE. Measuring and explaining the change in life expectancies. Demography 21(1):83–96. 1984.

2. Centers for Disease Control and Prevention. Achievements in public health, 1900–99: Control of infectious diseases. MMWR 48(29):621–9. 1999.

3. Fried LP. Epidemiology of aging. Epidemiol Rev 22(1):95–106. 2000.

4. Arias E. United States life tables, 2000. National vital statistics reports; vol 51 no 3. Hyattsville, Maryland: National Center for Health Statistics. 2002.

Figure 21. Life expectancy at birth and at 65 years of age by sex: United States, 1901-2000

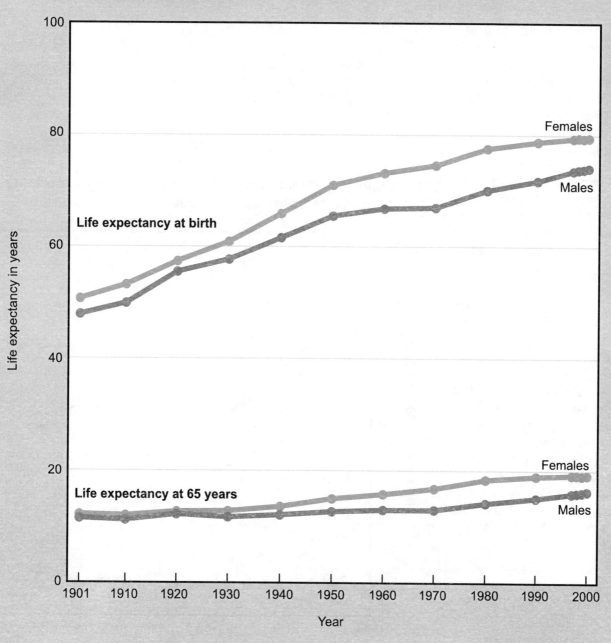

NOTE: See Data Table for data points graphed and additional notes.

SOURCE: Centers for Disease Control and Prevention, National Center for Health Statistics, National Vital Statistics System.

Infant Mortality

Infant mortality, the risk of death during the first year of life, is related to the underlying health of the mother, public health practices, socioeconomic conditions, and availability and use of appropriate health care for infants and pregnant women. Disorders related to short gestation and low birthweight, and congenital malformations are the leading causes of death during the first month of life (neonatal mortality). Sudden Infant Death Syndrome (SIDS) and congenital malformations rank as the leading causes of infant deaths after the first month of life (postneonatal mortality) (1).

Between 1950 and 2000 the infant mortality rate declined by more than 75 percent (figure 22).The overall 2000 infant mortality rate of 6.9 deaths per 1,000 live births represented a decline of 25 percent from 1990. Substantial declines occurred for both neonatal and postneonatal mortality. Two-thirds of all infant deaths occurred during the neonatal period (*Health, United States, 2003*, table 22). Declines in infant mortality have been linked to improved access to health care, advances in neonatal medicine, and educational campaigns such as the "Back to Sleep" campaign to curb fatalities caused by SIDS (2).

Infant mortality rates have declined for all racial and ethnic groups, but large disparities remain (*Health, United States, 2003*, table 19). During 1998–2000 the infant mortality rate was highest for infants of non-Hispanic black mothers (figure 23). Infant mortality rates were also high among infants of American Indian or Alaska Native mothers, Hawaiian mothers, and Puerto Rican mothers. Infants of mothers of Chinese

origin had the lowest infant mortality rates.

References

1. Anderson RN. Deaths: Leading causes for 2000. National vital statistics reports; vol 50 no 16. Hyattsville, Maryland: National Center for Health Statistics. 2002.

2. American Academy of Pediatrics Task Force on Infant Positioning and SIDS. Positioning and SIDS. Pediatrics 89(6):1120–6. 1992.

Figure 22. Infant, neonatal, and postneonatal mortality rates: United States, 1950-2000

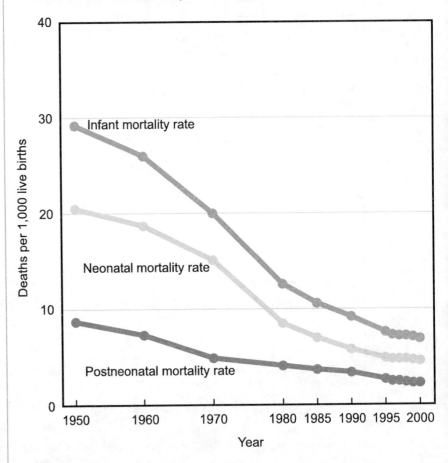

NOTES: Infant is defined as under 1 year of age, neonatal as under 28 days of age, and postneonatal as between 28 days and 1 year of age. See Data Table for data points graphed and additional notes.

SOURCE: Centers for Disease Control and Prevention, National Center for Health Statistics, National Vital Statistics System.

Figure 23. Infant mortality rates by detailed race and Hispanic origin of mother: United States, 1998-2000

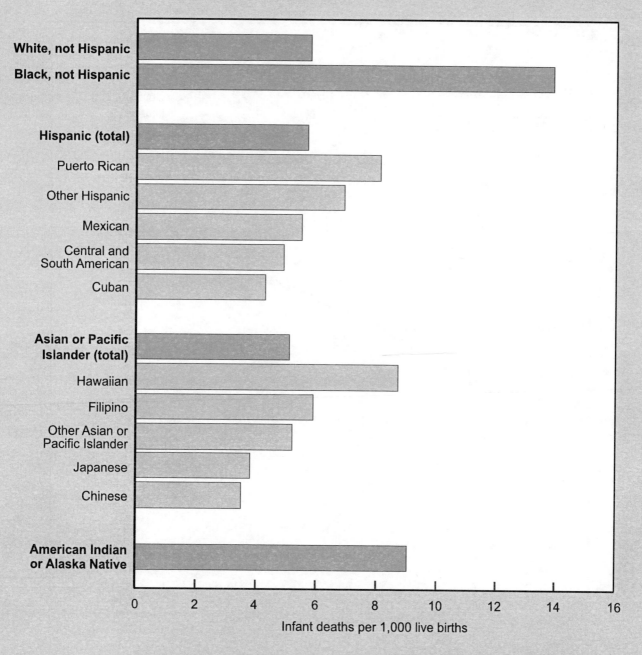

NOTES: Infant is defined as under 1 year of age. Persons of Hispanic origin may be of any race. Asian or Pacific Islander, and American Indian or Alaska Native races include persons of Hispanic and non-Hispanic origin. See Data Table for data points graphed and additional notes.

SOURCE: Centers for Disease Control and Prevention, National Center for Health Statistics, National Linked Birth/Infant Death Data Sets.

Figure 24. Death rates for leading causes of death among persons 15-24 years of age: United States, 1950-2000

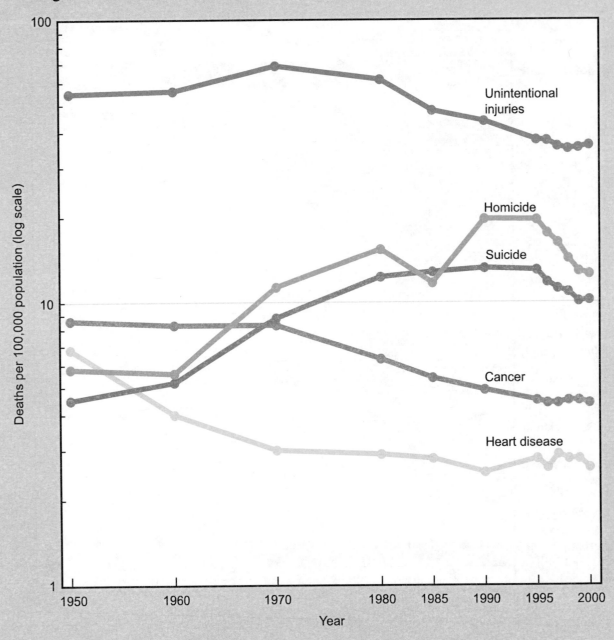

NOTES: Causes of death shown are the five leading causes of death among persons 15-24 years of age in 2000. See Data Table for data points graphed and additional notes.

SOURCE: Centers for Disease Control and Prevention, National Center for Health Statistics, National Vital Statistics System.

Teen and Young Adult Mortality: 15–24 Years of Age

During the past 50 years mortality among teens and young adults (15–24 years of age) has declined by almost 40 percent. In 2000 there were 31,000 deaths for this age group. The five leading causes of death in 2000 were related to either injury or chronic diseases. In 1950, in contrast, two of the five leading causes of death were infectious diseases (influenza/pneumonia and tuberculosis).

Unintentional injuries have been the leading cause of death for teens and young adults throughout the past 50 years. However, deaths rates for unintentional injuries have been declining since 1970 (figure 24). In 2000, 14,000 deaths among persons 15–24 years of age resulted from unintentional injuries accounting for 45 percent of all deaths to persons of this age group (figure 25). Nearly three-quarters of unintentional injury deaths for this age group resulted from motor-vehicle traffic related injuries (1).

Homicide and suicide were the second and third leading causes of death in this age group in 2000. Between 1960 and the mid-1990s, the homicide rate increased and then declined by more than one-third by 2000. Between 1950 and 1995 the suicide rate nearly tripled and then declined by 2000. Firearm-related injury deaths accounted for nearly three-fifths of suicides and four-fifths of homicides among teens and young adults in 2000 (2).

Homicide and suicide rates vary by sex and race among 15–24 year olds. Males 15–24 years of age are at substantially higher risk of homicide and suicide than

females. Homicide rates for young black males were more than eight times as great as for young white males in 2000 (*Health, United States, 2003*, tables 45 and 46).

Death rates for the other leading causes of death, cancer and heart disease, have also declined, with the greatest decline in cancer mortality occurring during 1970–95 and the greatest decline in heart disease mortality during 1950–70.

References

1. Centers for Disease Control and Prevention, National Center for Health Statistics, National Vital Statistics System, unpublished analysis.

2. Minino AM, Arias E, Kochanek KD, et al. Deaths: Final data for 2000. National vital statistics reports; vol 50 no 15. Hyattsville, Maryland: National Center for Health Statistics. 2002.

Figure 25. Percent of deaths due to leading causes of death among persons 15-24 years of age: United States, 2000

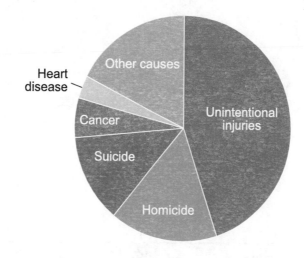

NOTE: See Data Table for data points graphed and additional notes.

SOURCE: Centers for Disease Control and Prevention, National Center for Health Statistics, National Vital Statistics System.

Figure 26. Death rates for leading causes of death among persons 25-44 years of age: United States, 1950-2000

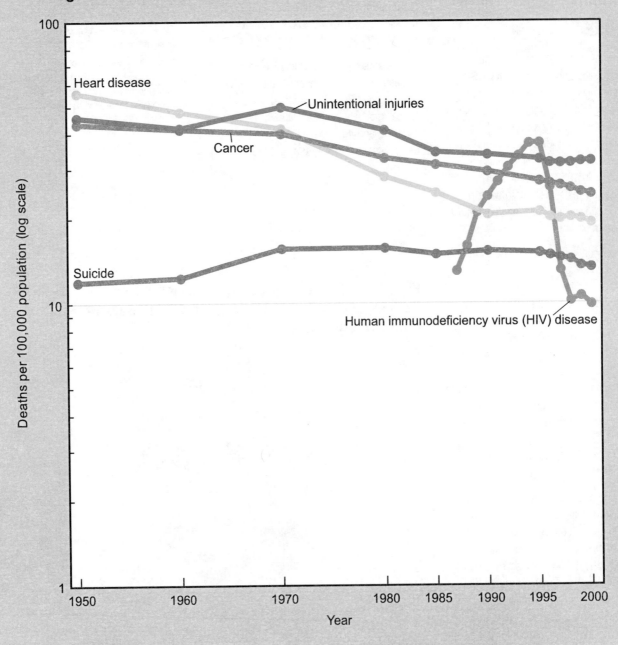

NOTES: Death rates are age adjusted. Causes of death shown are the five leading causes of death among persons 25-44 years of age in 2000. See Data Table for data points graphed and additional notes.

SOURCE: Centers for Disease Control and Prevention, National Center for Health Statistics, National Vital Statistics System.

Adult Mortality: 25–44 Years of Age

Since 1950 mortality among adults 25–44 years of age has declined by more than 40 percent. Underlying the overall decline in the death rate have been both favorable and unfavorable trends in the leading causes of death (figure 26). In 2000 there were approximately 130,000 deaths for this age group. Of the five leading causes of death in 2000, four were also leading causes of death in 1950. But tuberculosis, which was one of the top five causes of death in 1950, is no longer a significant cause of death for adults 25–44 years of age.

Mortality from heart disease has declined by about two-thirds since 1950, with most of the decrease occurring by 1990. Mortality from unintentional injury and cancer has also declined, with most of the decrease occurring after 1970. Altogether unintentional injury, cancer, and heart disease, the three leading causes of death among persons 25–44 years of age in 2000, accounted for about one-half of all deaths in this age group (figure 27).

In contrast to the declines for the top three causes of death, the suicide rate among persons 25–44 years rose between 1950 and 1980 but has declined slightly since 1980. Suicide, the fourth leading cause of death among young working-age adults in 2000, was responsible for 9 percent of deaths in this age group.

The fifth leading cause of death in 2000, human immunodeficiency virus (HIV) disease, has been an important cause of mortality among persons 25–44 years of age since the late 1980s (1). After rising rapidly in the late 1980s and the early

1990s, the HIV disease death rate began to fall sharply in the mid to late 1990s with the introduction of new antiretroviral therapies. Starting in 1998 the HIV death rate stabilized (2). In 2000 there were more than 8,000 deaths in this age group due to HIV disease.

HIV disease death rates among persons 25–44 years of age vary substantially by sex, race, and Hispanic origin. The risk of death is higher for males than females and is much higher for black and Hispanic persons than for those in other racial and ethnic groups. The HIV disease death rate for black males was

six times the rate for white males in 2000. For black females, the HIV disease death rate was more than 12 times the rate for white females (*Health, United States, 2003*, table 42).

References

1. Centers for Disease Control and Prevention. HIV and AIDS—United States, 1981–2000. MMWR 50(21): 430–4. 2001.

2. Centers for Disease Control and Prevention. HIV/AIDS Surveillance Report, 2000. 12(1):3–41. 2001.

Figure 27. Percent of deaths due to leading causes of death among persons 25-44 years of age: United States, 2000

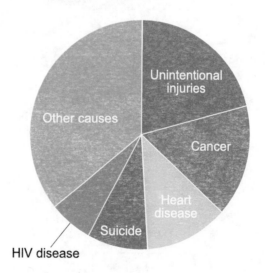

NOTE: See Data Table for data points graphed and additional notes.

SOURCE: Centers for Disease Control and Prevention, National Center for Health Statistics, National Vital Statistics System.

Figure 28. Death rates for leading causes of death among persons 45-64 years of age: United States, 1950-2000

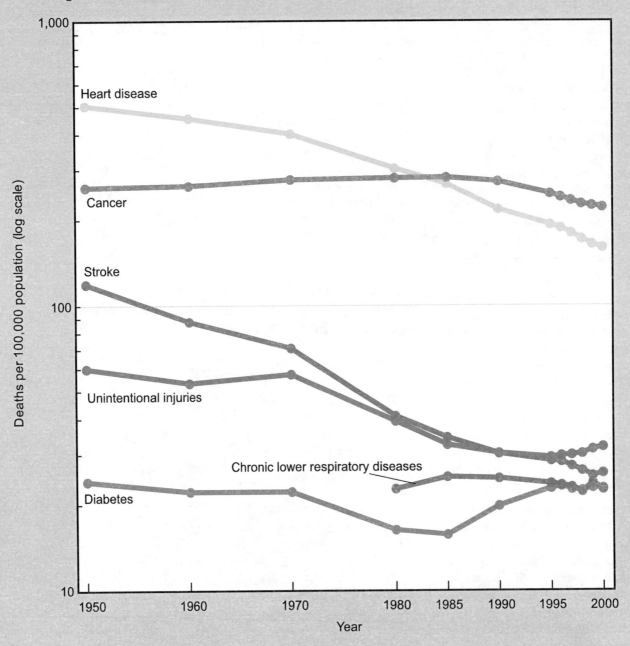

NOTES: Death rates are age adjusted. Causes of death shown are the six leading causes of death among persons 45-64 years of age in 2000. See Data Table for data points graphed and additional notes.

SOURCE: Centers for Disease Control and Prevention, National Center for Health Statistics, National Vital Statistics System.

Adult Mortality: 45–64 Years of Age

Death rates for persons 45–64 years of age have declined substantially over the past 50 years. Since 1950 mortality in this age group has decreased by almost 50 percent overall. In 2000 there were approximately 401,000 deaths for this age group. Of the five leading causes of death in 2000, four were also the leading causes of death in 1950. As with other age groups, tuberculosis, which ranked in the top five causes in 1950, was the cause of only a small number of deaths in 2000.

Among persons 45–64 years of age, the death rates for heart disease and stroke declined substantially between 1950 and 2000 (figure 28). During this period the death rate for heart disease declined by almost 70 percent and the death rate for stroke by nearly 80 percent. Advances in the prevention and treatment of heart disease and stroke rank among the major public health achievements of the 20th century (1).

In contrast to the large declines in heart disease and stroke mortality, the death rate for cancer among persons 45–64 years of age rose slowly through the 1980s and then declined. Cancer was the leading cause of death among persons 45–64 years of age, accounting for more than one-third of the deaths in this age group in 2000 (figure 29).

In 2000 the fifth leading cause of death for persons 45–64 years of age was diabetes. Diabetes was the underlying cause for more than 14,000 deaths in 2000. Diabetes was mentioned on the death certificates of almost twice as many additional deaths, contributing to deaths due to such underlying causes as heart disease, stroke, and kidney disease (2).

In 2000 cancer, heart disease, stroke, diabetes, and chronic lower respiratory diseases together accounted for 70 percent of all deaths in this age group. Biological and socioeconomic factors are strongly associated with death among older working-age adults. Men had a higher death rate than women, and adults with a high school education or less had a death rate more than twice as high as the rate for adults with more than a high school education in 2000 (3).

References

1. Centers for Disease Control and Prevention. Achievements in public health, 1900–99: Decline in deaths from heart disease and stroke—United States, 1900–99. MMWR 48(30):649–56. 1999.

2. Centers for Disease Control and Prevention, National Center for Health Statistics, National Vital Statistics System, unpublished analysis.

3. Minino AM, Arias E, Kochanek KD, Murphy SL, Smith BL. Deaths: Final data for 2000. National vital statistics reports; vol 50 no 15. Hyattsville, Maryland: National Center for Health Statistics. 2002.

Figure 29. Percent of deaths due to leading causes of death among persons 45-64 years of age: United States, 2000

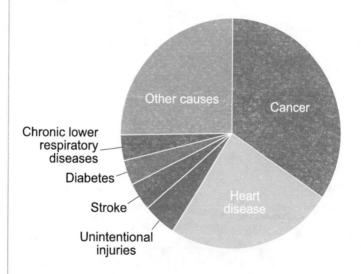

NOTE: See Data Table for data points graphed and additional notes.

SOURCE: Centers for Disease Control and Prevention, National Center for Health Statistics, National Vital Statistics System.

Figure 30. Death rates for leading causes of death among persons 65 years of age and over: United States, 1950-2000

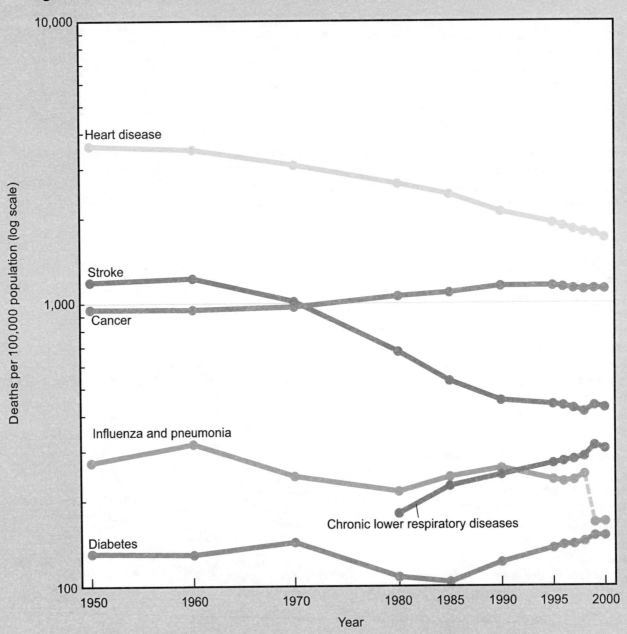

NOTES: Death rates are age adjusted. Causes of death shown are the six leading causes of death among persons 65 years of age and over in 2000. See Data Table for data points graphed and additional notes.

SOURCE: Centers for Disease Control and Prevention, National Center for Health Statistics, National Vital Statistics System.

Adult Mortality: 65 Years of Age and Over

Three-quarters of all deaths in the United States occur among persons 65 years of age and over (*Health, United States, 2003*, table 32). During the past 50 years overall death rates have declined by more than one-third for older persons, with chronic diseases causing most of the deaths throughout that period.

Among the elderly, the death rate for heart disease declined between 1950 and 2000 by more than 50 percent and for stroke by more than 60 percent (figure 30). Trends in the other leading causes of death among the elderly varied. The death rate for cancer, the second leading cause of death for the elderly in 2000, rose between 1950 and 1995 and has decreased slightly since 1995. The death rate for the fourth leading cause of death, chronic lower respiratory diseases, has generally increased since 1980 reflecting, in large part, the effects of cigarette smoking (1).

In 2000 the sixth leading cause of death for the elderly was diabetes. Diabetes was the underlying cause for more than 52,000 deaths in 2000. Diabetes was mentioned on the death certificates of more than twice as many additional deaths, contributing to deaths due to such underlying causes as heart disease, stroke, and kidney disease (2).

The large difference in the death rate due to influenza and pneumonia between 1998 and 1999 reflects, in large part, changes in the coding of this cause of death. A comparison of the comparability-modified 1998 rate with the 1999 rate indicates a decline of only 3 percent (see data table for figure 30 and Appendix II, Comparability ratio).

In 2000 deaths due to heart disease accounted for one-third of all deaths among the elderly (figure 31). The second leading cause of death, cancer, accounted for more than one-fifth of all deaths to this age group. Together the other leading causes of death, stroke, chronic lower respiratory diseases, influenza and pneumonia, and diabetes, accounted for more than one-fifth of deaths among the elderly.

References

1. Office of the Surgeon General, U.S. Public Health Service. The health consequences of smoking: Chronic obstructive lung disease. Rockville, Maryland: U.S. Department of Health and Human Services. 1984.

2. Centers for Disease Control and Prevention, National Center for Health Statistics, National Vital Statistics System, unpublished analysis.

Figure 31. Percent of deaths due to leading causes of death among persons 65 years of age and over: United States, 2000

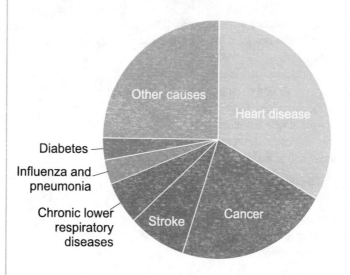

NOTE: See Data Table for data points graphed and additional notes.

SOURCE: Centers for Disease Control and Prevention, National Center for Health Statistics, National Vital Statistics System.

Special Feature: Diabetes

Prevalence

Diabetes, a group of diseases characterized by high levels of blood glucose (sugar), is a significant cause of illness, disability, and death in the United States. Complications of diabetes include heart disease, blindness, kidney disease, and damage to the peripheral nervous system. In 2000 diabetes was the fifth leading cause of death among women and the sixth leading cause of death among men. Type 1 diabetes usually strikes children and young adults. Type 2 diabetes, which accounts for 90–95 percent of diagnosed diabetes cases, is more common among individuals who are obese, physically inactive, older persons, and those with a family history of diabetes. Prevalence rates of type 2 diabetes are especially high among persons who are black, Hispanic, or American Indian (1). With increasing obesity (2,3), high levels of physical inactivity, and the aging of the population, diabetes is a critical public health concern for the 21st century.

Over the last half of the 20th century there was a steady increase in diabetes prevalence and rates have continued to rise in recent years (4). Between 1997 and 2002 the percent of adults with diagnosed diabetes increased for all age groups (figure 32). Concern about the rising prevalence of diabetes is not limited to just adults. Clinic-based reports and regional studies indicate that type 2 diabetes is becoming more common among American children and adolescents, particularly among racial and ethnic subgroups (5).

In 2002 more than 6 percent of the noninstitutionalized adult population reported they had diabetes. The percent of adults with diagnosed diabetes increased sharply with age from 2 percent among adults 18–44 years of age to 16 percent of adults 65 years of age and over (6).

Results from the National Health and Nutrition Examination Survey (NHANES) in 1988–94 demonstrated that a significant percentage of adults with diabetes were unaware of their disease and had not been diagnosed (7). Updated information from 1999–2000 NHANES shows that undiagnosed diabetes remains an important public health issue (8).

Screening high-risk individuals for diabetes in health care settings is important in order to minimize or prevent its serious health complications (9). Additional public health efforts focus on preventing diabetes. Results of a research study involving persons at high risk for developing diabetes suggest that lifestyle changes involving modest weight loss and moderate physical activity of at least 150 minutes per week or medication treatment prevent or delay the onset of diabetes. Lifestyle changes were more effective than medication in reducing the onset of diabetes during the study (10).

References

1. Centers for Disease Control and Prevention. 2002 National Diabetes Fact Sheet. Available from www.cdc.gov/diabetes/index.htm accessed on June 17, 2003.

2. Ogden CL, Flegal KM, Carroll MD, et al. Prevalence and trends in overweight among US children and adolescents, 1999–2000. JAMA 288:1728–32. 2002.

3. Flegal KM, Carroll MD, Ogden CL, et al. Prevalence and trends in obesity among US adults, 1999–2000. JAMA 288:1723–7. 2002.

4. National Diabetes Data Group. Diabetes in America, 2nd Edition. Bethesda, Maryland: National Institutes of Health (NIH publication no 95–1468). 1995.

5. Fagot-Campagna A, et al. Type 2 diabetes among North American children and adolescents: an epidemiologic review and a public health prospective. J Pediatr 136(5):664–72. 2000.

6. Ni H, Schiller J, Hao C, Cohen RA, Barnes P. Early release of selected estimates based on data from the 2002 National Health Interview Survey. Hyattsville, Maryland: National Center for Health Statistics. June 2003. Available from www.cdc.gov/nchs/nhis.htm.

7. Harris M, et al. Prevalence of diabetes, impaired fasting glucose, and impaired glucose tolerance in U.S. adults. Diabetes Care 21(4):518–24. 1998.

8. Centers for Disease Control and Prevention. Prevalence of diabetes and impaired fasting glucose in U.S. adults, 1999–2000. MMWR 52(35): 833–7. 2003.

9. Engelgau MM, Narayan KM, Herman WH. Screening for type 2 diabetes. Diabetes Care 23:1563–80. 2000.

10. Diabetes Prevention Program Research Group. Reduction in the incidence of type 2 diabetes with lifestyle intervention or metformin. N Engl J Med 346(6):393–403. 2002.

Figure 32. Diagnosed diabetes prevalence among adults 18 years of age and over by age: United States, 1997-2002

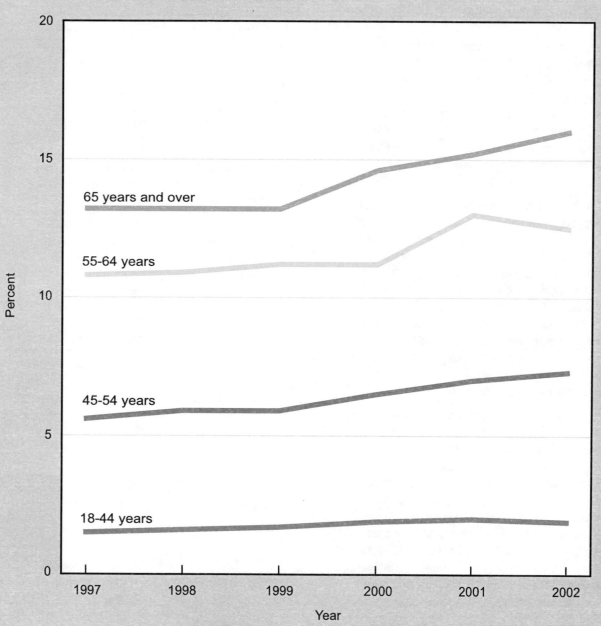

NOTES: Diabetes prevalence is based on self-reports of physician diagnosis. See Data Table for data points graphed, standard errors, and additional notes.

SOURCE: Centers for Disease Control and Prevention, National Center for Health Statistics, National Health Interview Survey.

Special Feature: Diabetes

Use Of Ambulatory Health Care Services

Persons with diabetes require frequent contact with the health care system in order to effectively manage this complex and chronic health condition. The hallmark of diabetes is abnormally high levels of blood sugar (glucose). Ambulatory care visits for diabetes focus on optimum management of blood sugar levels, treatment of complications, and provision of prevention-focused care such as eye, dental, and foot examinations. Tighter control of blood sugar levels has been shown to prevent some of the complications of diabetes (1,2).

Data from in-person health interview surveys indicate that adults with diagnosed diabetes are more likely than adults without diabetes to report frequent use of the health care system. In 2000–01, 37 percent of adults 18 years of age and over with diabetes reported 10 or more health care visits during the previous year compared with 14 percent of adults without diabetes. Adults with diabetes were more likely than adults without diabetes to report a recent podiatrist visit (22 percent compared with 5 percent), and eye doctor visit (57 percent compared with 34 percent) (3). However, use of preventive-care practices among persons with diabetes remains at less than desired levels (4).

Visits for diabetes have increased steadily between 1995–96 and 1999–2000 as measured by data from annual surveys of ambulatory care medical records (figure 33). A diabetes visit is defined as an ambulatory care visit to a physician office or hospital outpatient department with a diagnosis of diabetes recorded on the medical record. During this period the number of diabetes visits per 1,000 population increased for all age groups while the number of ambulatory care visits did not (*Health, United States, 2003*, table 82). In 1999–2000 ambulatory care visits for diabetes increased sharply with age with the rate among persons 65 years of age and over 12 times the rate among adults 18–44 years of age.

The upward trend in diabetes visit rates during this relatively short time period may reflect rising prevalence of diagnosed diabetes as shown in figure 32. Additional factors that may be contributing to the upward trend in diabetes visit rates include changes in diagnostic and clinical management practices. In 1997 the American Diabetes Association changed the standard for diagnosing diabetes to a more readily available blood test (5). The rise in diabetes visit rates may reflect increasing emphasis on tighter control of blood pressure and glucose levels to prevent complications among persons with diabetes (6). New information on the effectiveness of diet and exercise for glucose and blood pressure control and new medications provide practitioners with a wider array of management tools.

References

1. Stratton I, et al. Association of glycaemia with macrovascular and microvascular complications of type 2 diabetes (UKPDS 35): Prospective observational study. BMJ 321(7258):405–12. 2000.

2. The Diabetes Control and Complications Trial Research Group. The effect of intensive treatment of diabetes on the development and progression of long-term complications in insulin-dependent diabetes mellitus. N Engl J Med 329:977–86. 1993.

3. Centers for Disease Control and Prevention, National Center for Health Statistics, National Health Interview Survey, unpublished analysis.

4. Centers for Disease Control and Prevention. Preventive-care practices among persons with diabetes—United States, 1995 and 2001. MMWR 51(43):965–9. 2002.

5. The Expert Committee on the Diagnosis and Classification of Diabetes Mellitus. Report of the expert committee on the diagnosis and classification of diabetes mellitus. Diabetes Care 20:1183–97. 1997.

6. Centers for Disease Control and Prevention. Diabetes: Disabling, deadly, and on the rise: At a glance, 2002. www.cdc.gov/diabetes/pubs/glance.htm accessed on December 19, 2002.

Figure 33. Ambulatory care visits for diabetes among adults 18 years of age and over by age: United States, 1995-2000

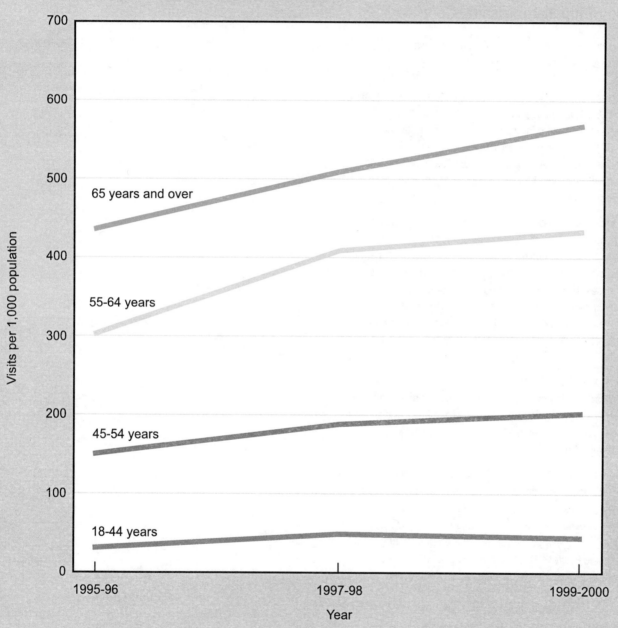

NOTES: Diabetes visits include any visit to a physician office or hospital outpatient department with a diagnosis of diabetes and are not limited to first-listed diagnosis. See Data Table for data points graphed, standard errors, and additional notes.

SOURCES: Centers for Disease Control and Prevention, National Center for Health Statistics, National Ambulatory Medical Care Survey and National Hospital Ambulatory Medical Care Survey.

Special Feature: Diabetes

Use of Inpatient Hospital Care

In addition to the human cost of diabetes— with its risk of complications, disability, and premature mortality— the medical costs of treating diabetes are substantial. Direct medical expenditures attributable to diabetes were estimated at $91.8 billion in 2002 with one-quarter of costs due to care for the complications of diabetes. Inpatient hospital care is one of the most expensive venues for diabetes care. In 2002 inpatient hospital care for diabetes was estimated at $40 billion and accounted for 44 percent of health care expenditures for diabetes (1).

Persons with diabetes are at increased risk of hospitalization for conditions such as heart disease, hypertension, and kidney disease. Examination of trends in hospital discharge rates with diabetes listed as any one of up to seven recorded diagnoses shows the increasing impact of diabetes on inpatient care. Hospital care for conditions unrelated to diabetes or its complications is more complex and expensive for persons with diabetes due to this chronic underlying condition.

Hospital discharges with any mention of diabetes represent a significant portion of inpatient care for middle-aged and elderly persons. In 2000–01, 22 percent of hospital discharges among persons 45 years of age and over included a diagnosis of diabetes (2).

Between 1990–91 and 2000–01 the number of discharges per 10,000 population with any mention of diabetes increased for all age groups (figure 34). In contrast, rates for discharges without mention of diabetes remained stable or declined slightly during this period (2). Discharge rates for any mention of diabetes increased with advancing age with the rate among the most elderly (75 years of age and over) five times the rate among persons 45–54 years of age. Diabetes discharge rates were similar for men and women of the same age (2).

Maintaining a healthy weight through diet and exercise decreases the risk of developing diabetes and is an important public health message for persons of all ages, and especially for younger persons. With the rising prevalence of obesity and inactivity among children, adolescents, and young adults (see related figures 13–15) there is a potential for further

increases in rates for diabetes, diabetic complications, and expensive hospital care.

References

1. American Diabetes Association. Economic costs of diabetes in the U.S. in 2002. Diabetes Care 26:917–32. 2003.

2. Centers for Disease Control and Prevention, National Center for Health Statistics, National Hospital Discharge Survey, unpublished analysis.

Figure 34. Hospital discharges for diabetes among adults 45 years of age and over by age: United States, 1990-2001

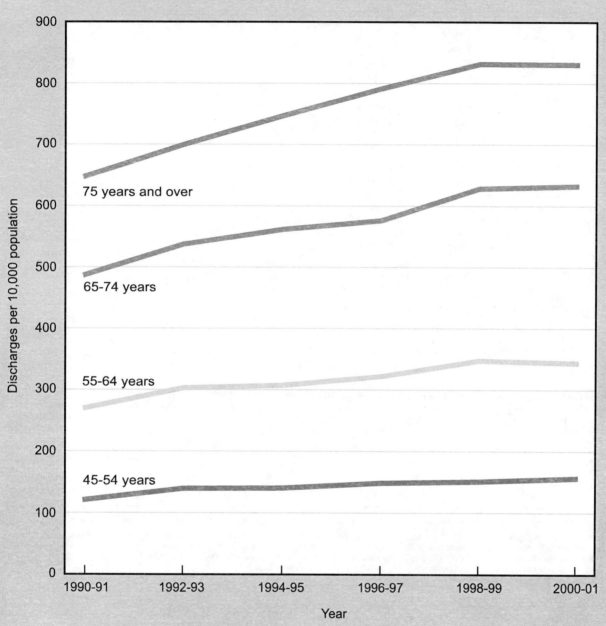

NOTES: Diabetes discharges include discharges with any listed diagnosis of diabetes. See Data Table for data points graphed, standard errors, and additional notes.

SOURCE: Centers for Disease Control and Prevention, National Center for Health Statistics, National Hospital Discharge Survey.

Data table for figure 1. Total and elderly population: United States, 1950–2050

Year	Total	65 years and over
1950	150,216,000	12,257,000
1960	179,326,000	16,207,000
1970	203,212,000	20,066,000
1980	226,546,000	25,549,000
1990	248,710,000	31,242,000
2000	281,422,000	34,992,000
2010	299,862,000	39,715,000
2020	324,927,000	53,733,000
2030	351,070,000	70,319,000
2040	377,350,000	77,177,000
2050	403,687,000	81,999,000

NOTES: Data are for the resident population. Data for 1950 exclude Alaska and Hawaii. Data for 2010–2050 are projected. See Appendix II, Population.

SOURCES: U.S. Census Bureau, 1980 Census of Population, General Population Characteristics, United States Summary (PC80-1-B1) [includes data for 1950–80]; 1990 Census of Population, General Population Characteristics, United States Summary (CO-1-1); 2000 Census of Population, Profiles of General Demographic Characteristics, United States, www.census.gov/prod/cen2000/dp1/2kh00.pdf accessed on September 27, 2001; Projections of the Total Resident Population by 5-Year Age Groups, and Sex with Special Age Categories: Middle Series, 2006 to 2010 through 2050 to 2070, www.census.gov/population/projections/nation/summary/np-t3-c.txt to np-t3-g.txt accessed on September 27, 2001.

Data table for figure 2. Percent of population in 3 age groups: United States, 1950, 2000, and 2050

Year	All ages	Under 18 years	18–64 years	65 years and over
		Percent		
1950	100.0	31.3	60.6	8.2
2000	100.0	25.7	61.9	12.4
2050	100.0	23.7	56.0	20.3

NOTES: Data are for the resident population. Data for 1950 exclude Alaska and Hawaii. Data for 2050 are projected. See Appendix II, Population.

SOURCES: U.S. Census Bureau, 1980 Census of Population, General Population Characteristics, United States Summary (PC80-1-B1) [data for 1950]; 2000 Census of Population, Profiles of General Demographic Characteristics, United States, www.census.gov/prod/cen2000/dp1/2kh00.pdf accessed on September 27, 2001; Projections of the Total Resident Population by 5-Year Age Groups, and Sex with Special Age Categories: Middle Series, 2050 to 2070, www.census.gov/population/projections/nation/summary/np-t3-g.txt accessed on September 27, 2001.

Data table for figure 3. Percent of population in selected race and Hispanic origin groups by age: United States, 1980–2000

Race and Hispanic origin	All ages			Under 18 years			18 years and over		
	1980	1990	2000	1980	1990	2000	1980	1990	2000
	Percent								
Total	100.0	100.0	100.0	100.0	100.0	100.0	100.0	100.0	100.0
Hispanic or Latino	6.4	9.0	12.5	8.8	12.2	17.1	5.5	7.9	11.0
Not Hispanic or Latino:									
White	79.9	75.7	69.5	74.2	68.9	61.3	82.1	78.1	72.3
Black or African American	11.5	11.8	12.2	14.5	14.7	14.9	10.4	10.7	11.3
Asian or Pacific Islander	1.6	2.8	3.9	1.7	3.1	3.7	1.5	2.7	3.9
American Indian or Alaska Native	0.6	0.7	0.7	0.8	1.0	1.0	0.5	0.6	0.7
2 or more races	. . .	. . .	1.2	. . .	. . .	2.1	. . .	. . .	0.8

. . . Category not applicable.

NOTES: Data are for the resident population. Persons of Hispanic origin may be of any race. Race data for 2000 are not directly comparable with data from 1980 and 1990. Individuals could report only one race in 1980 and 1990, and more than one race in 2000. Persons who selected only one race in 2000 are shown in single-race categories; persons who selected more than one race in 2000 are shown as having 2 or more races and are not included in the single-race categories. In 2000 the category "Asian or Pacific Islander" includes Asian and Native Hawaiian or Other Pacific Islander. See Appendix II, Hispanic origin and Race.

SOURCES: U.S. Census Bureau: U.S. population estimates, by age, sex, race, and Hispanic origin: 1980 to 1991. Current population reports, series P-25, no 1095. Washington. U.S. Government Printing Office, February 1993; U.S. Census Bureau: Census 2000 Modified Race Data Summary File: 2000 Census of Population and Housing, September 2002.

Data table for figure 4. Poverty rates by age: United States, 1996–2001

Year	All ages	Under 18 years	18–64 years	65 years and over
	Percent of persons with family income below the poverty level			
1966	14.7	17.6	10.5	28.5
1967	14.2	16.6	10.0	29.5
1968	12.8	15.6	9.0	25.0
1969	12.1	14.0	8.7	25.3
1970	12.6	15.1	9.0	24.6
1971	12.5	15.3	9.3	21.6
1972	11.9	15.1	8.8	18.6
1973	11.1	14.4	8.3	16.3
1974	11.2	15.4	8.3	14.6
1975	12.3	17.1	9.2	15.3
1976	11.8	16.0	9.0	15.0
1977	11.6	16.2	8.8	14.1
1978	11.4	15.9	8.7	14.0
1979	11.7	16.4	8.9	15.2
1980	13.0	18.3	10.1	15.7
1981	14.0	20.0	11.1	15.3
1982	15.0	21.9	12.0	14.6
1983	15.2	22.3	12.4	13.8
1984	14.4	21.5	11.7	12.4
1985	14.0	20.7	11.3	12.6
1986	13.6	20.5	10.8	12.4
1987	13.4	20.3	10.6	12.5
1988	13.0	19.5	10.5	12.0
1989	12.8	19.6	10.2	11.4
1990	13.5	20.6	10.7	12.2
1991	14.2	21.8	11.4	12.4
1992	14.8	22.3	11.9	12.9
1993	15.1	22.7	12.4	12.2
1994	14.5	21.8	11.9	11.7
1995	13.8	20.8	11.4	10.5
1996	13.7	20.5	11.4	10.8
1997	13.3	19.9	10.9	10.5
1998	12.7	18.9	10.5	10.5
1999	11.8	16.9	10.0	9.7
2000[1]	11.3	16.2	9.6	9.9
2001[1]	11.7	16.3	10.1	10.1

[1]Estimates of poverty for 2000 and 2001 have been calculated based on an expanded household sample and Census 2000-based population weights. Implementation of these changes had no effect on the all ages poverty rate for 2000 and a 0.1 to 0.3 percent difference in the age specific poverty rates for 2000.

NOTES: Data are for the civilian noninstitutionalized population. See Appendix II, Poverty level. See related *Health, United States, 2003,* table 2.

SOURCES: U.S. Census Bureau, Current population survey, March 1967–2002. U.S. Bureau of the Census. Proctor B, Dalaker J. Poverty in the United States: 2001. Current population reports, series P-60, no 219. Washington, DC: U.S. Government Printing Office. 2002.

Data table for figure 5. Low income population by age, race, and Hispanic origin: United States, 2001

Age, race, and Hispanic origin	Percent		Number in millions	
	Poor	Near poor	Poor	Near poor
All ages				
All races and origins	11.7	18.5	32.9	52.0
Hispanic or Latino	21.4	30.4	8.0	11.3
Black or African American	22.7	24.3	8.1	8.7
Asian and Pacific Islander	10.2	16.6	1.3	2.1
White, not Hispanic or Latino	7.8	15.3	15.3	29.6
Under 18 years				
All races and origins	16.3	21.9	11.7	15.8
Hispanic or Latino	28.0	33.5	3.6	4.3
Black or African American	30.2	27.1	3.5	3.1
Asian and Pacific Islander	11.5	19.0	0.4	0.6
White, not Hispanic or Latino	9.5	17.2	4.2	7.6
18–64 years				
All races and origins	10.1	15.3	17.8	26.8
Hispanic or Latino	17.7	28.2	4.0	6.4
Black or African American	18.7	21.5	4.0	4.6
Asian and Pacific Islander	9.7	17.1	0.8	1.2
White, not Hispanic or Latino	7.2	11.8	8.8	14.5
65 years and over				
All races and origins	10.1	28.1	3.4	9.5
Hispanic or Latino	21.8	34.5	0.4	0.7
Black or African American	21.9	34.5	0.6	1.0
Asian and Pacific Islander	10.2	26.1	0.1	0.2
White, not Hispanic or Latino	8.1	27.1	2.3	7.6

NOTES: Data are for the civilian noninstitutionalized population. Poor is defined as family income less than 100 percent of the poverty level and near poor as 100–199 percent of the poverty level. See Appendix II, Poverty level. Persons of Hispanic origin may be of any race. Black, and Asian and Pacific Islander races include persons of both Hispanic and non-Hispanic origin. See related *Health, United States, 2003,* table 2.

SOURCES: Proctor B, Dalaker J. Poverty in the United States: 2001. Current population reports, series P-60 no 219. Washington, DC: U.S. Government Printing Office. 2002; Table 2. Age, sex, household relationship, race and hispanic origin by ratio of income to poverty level: 2001, ferret.bls.census.gov/macro/032002/pov/new02_000.htm accessed on March 10, 2003.

Data table for figure 6. Health insurance coverage among persons under 65 years of age: United States, 1984–2001

| Year | Health insurance coverage | | | | | |
| | Private | | Medicaid | | Uninsured | |
	Percent	SE	Percent	SE	Percent	SE
1984	77.1	0.6	6.7	0.3	14.3	0.4
1989	76.2	0.4	7.1	0.2	15.3	0.3
1994	70.3	0.4	11.0	0.3	17.3	0.3
1995	71.6	0.4	11.3	0.2	15.9	0.2
1996	71.5	0.5	10.9	0.3	16.5	0.3
1997	70.9	0.3	9.6	0.2	17.4	0.2
1998	72.3	0.4	8.8	0.2	16.5	0.2
1999	72.9	0.3	9.0	0.2	16.1	0.2
2000	71.7	0.3	9.4	0.2	16.8	0.2
2001	71.5	0.4	10.3	0.2	16.2	0.2

SE Standard error.

NOTES: Data are for the civilian noninstitutionalized population. Percents are age adjusted to the 2000 standard population using three age groups: under 18 years, 18–44 years, and 45–64 years. Medicaid includes other public assistance through 1996; includes State-sponsored health plans starting in 1997; and includes State Child Health Insurance Program (SCHIP) starting in 1999. Uninsured persons are not covered by private insurance, Medicaid, SCHIP, public assistance (through 1996), State-sponsored or other government-sponsored health plans (starting in 1997), Medicare, or military plans. Percents do not add to 100 because the percent of persons with Medicare, military plans, and other government-sponsored plans is not shown and because persons with both private insurance and Medicaid appear in both categories. See Appendix II, Age adjustment and Health insurance coverage. See related *Health, United States, 2003,* tables 127–129.

SOURCE: Centers for Disease Control and Prevention, National Center for Health Statistics, National Health Interview Survey.

Data table for figure 7. No health insurance coverage among persons under 65 years of age by selected characteristics: United States, 2001

Characteristic	Percent	SE
Age		
Under 65 years, age adjusted	16.2	0.2
Under 18 years	11.0	0.3
18–24 years	29.3	0.7
25–34 years	22.3	0.5
35–44 years	16.7	0.4
45–54 years	13.0	0.4
55–64 years	11.0	0.4
Percent of poverty level		
Below 100 percent	33.3	0.9
100–149 percent	32.4	0.9
150–199 percent	26.4	1.0
200 percent or more	8.4	0.2
Unknown poverty level	20.0	0.5
Race and Hispanic origin		
White only, not Hispanic or Latino	11.9	0.3
Asian only	17.1	1.3
Black or African American only, not Hispanic or Latino	19.2	0.6
American Indian and Alaska Native only	33.4	4.6
Hispanic or Latino	34.8	0.7
Mexican	39.0	0.9
Other Hispanic	33.1	1.2
Cuban	19.2	2.1
Puerto Rican	16.0	1.1

SE Standard error.

NOTES: Data are for the civilian noninstitutionalized population. Percents for the total, by poverty level, race, and Hispanic origin are age adjusted to the year 2000 standard population using three age groups: under 18 years, 18–44 years, and 45–64 years. Persons of Hispanic origin may be of any race. Asian only, and American Indian and Alaska Native only races include persons of Hispanic and non-Hispanic origin. Uninsured persons are not covered by private insurance, Medicaid, State Child Health Insurance Program (SCHIP), State-sponsored or other government-sponsored health plans, Medicare, Indian Health Service only, or military plans. Percent of poverty level was unknown for 26 percent of sample persons under 65 years of age in 2001. See Appendix II, Age adjustment, Health insurance coverage, Poverty, and Race. See related Health, United States, 2003, table 129.

SOURCE: Centers for Disease Control and Prevention, National Center for Health Statistics, National Health Interview Survey.

Data table for figure 8. Early prenatal care among mothers: United States, 1970–2001

Year	Percent
1970	68.0
1975	72.4
1980	76.3
1985	76.2
1990	75.8
1993	78.9
1994	80.2
1995	81.3
1996	81.9
1997	82.5
1998	82.8
1999	83.2
2000	83.2
2001	83.4

NOTES: Early prenatal care begins during the first trimester of pregnancy. See related Health, United States, 2003, table 6.

SOURCE: Centers for Disease Control and Prevention, National Center for Health Statistics, National Vital Statistics System.

Data table for figure 9. Early prenatal care by detailed race and Hispanic origin of mother: United States, 2001

Race and Hispanic origin of mother	Percent
White, not Hispanic or Latino	88.5
Black or African American, not Hispanic or Latino	74.5
Hispanic or Latino	75.7
Cuban	91.8
Puerto Rican	79.1
Central and South American	77.4
Other and unknown Hispanic or Latino	77.3
Mexican	74.6
Asian or Pacific Islander	84.0
Japanese	90.1
Chinese	87.0
Filipino	85.0
Other Asian or Pacific Islander	82.7
Hawaiian	79.1
American Indian or Alaska Native	69.3

NOTES: Early prenatal care begins during the first trimester of pregnancy. Persons of Hispanic origin may be of any race. The race groups, Asian or Pacific Islander and American Indian or Alaska Native, include persons of Hispanic and non-Hispanic origin. See related Health, United States, 2003, table 6.

SOURCE: Centers for Disease Control and Prevention, National Center for Health Statistics, National Vital Statistics System.

Data table for figure 10. Influenza and pneumococcal vaccination among adults 65 years of age and over: United States, 1989–2001

Year	Influenza vaccination during past 12 months		Pneumococcal vaccination ever	
	Percent	SE	Percent	SE
1989	31.0	0.5	14.3	0.4
1990	- - -	- - -	- - -	- - -
1991	42.3	0.7	21.5	0.6
1992	- - -	- - -	- - -	- - -
1993	52.3	0.9	28.5	0.8
1994	55.6	0.9	29.9	0.8
1995	58.8	0.9	34.5	0.9
1996	- - -	- - -	- - -	- - -
1997	63.5	0.7	42.6	0.7
1998	63.6	0.7	46.3	0.8
1999	65.9	0.8	49.9	0.8
2000	64.5	0.7	53.2	0.8
2001	63.1	0.7	54.0	0.8

SE Standard error.
- - - Data not available.

NOTES: Data are for the civilian noninstitutionalized population and are age adjusted to the 2000 standard population using two age groups: 65–74 years and 75 years and over. See Appendix II, Age adjustment.

SOURCE: Centers for Disease Control and Prevention, National Center for Health Statistics, National Health Interview Survey.

Data table for figure 11. Influenza and pneumococcal vaccination among adults 65 years of age and over by race and Hispanic origin: United States, 1999–2001

Race and Hispanic origin	Influenza vaccination during past 12 months		Pneumococcal vaccination ever	
	Percent	SE	Percent	SE
White only, not Hispanic or Latino	66.7	0.5	56.0	0.5
Asian only	62.6	3.6	36.4	3.8
Black or African American only, not Hispanic or Latino	48.8	1.4	32.4	1.3
Hispanic or Latino	54.8	1.6	30.8	1.5

SE Standard error.

NOTES: Data are for the civilian noninstitutionalized population and are age adjusted to the 2000 standard population using two age groups: 65–74 years and 75 years and over. Persons of Hispanic origin may be of any race. Asian only race includes persons of both Hispanic and non-Hispanic origin. See Appendix II, Age adjustment and Race.

SOURCE: Centers for Disease Control and Prevention, National Center for Health Statistics, National Health Interview Survey.

Data table for figure 12. Cigarette smoking among men, women, high school students, and mothers during pregnancy: United States, 1965–2001

Year	Men		Women		High school students		Mothers during pregnancy
	Percent	SE	Percent	SE	Percent	SE	Percent
1965	51.2	0.3	33.7	0.3	- - -	- - -	- - -
1974	42.8	0.5	32.2	0.4	- - -	- - -	- - -
1979	37.0	0.5	30.1	0.5	- - -	- - -	- - -
1983	34.8	0.6	29.4	0.4	- - -	- - -	- - -
1985	32.2	0.5	27.9	0.4	- - -	- - -	- - -
1987	30.9	0.4	26.5	0.4	- - -	- - -	- - -
1988	30.3	0.4	25.7	0.3	- - -	- - -	- - -
1989	- - -	- - -	- - -	- - -	- - -	- - -	19.5
1990	28.0	0.4	22.9	0.3	- - -	- - -	18.4
1991	27.6	0.4	23.5	0.3	27.5	1.4	17.8
1992	28.1	0.5	24.6	0.5	- - -	- - -	16.9
1993	27.3	0.6	22.6	0.4	30.5	1.0	15.8
1994	27.6	0.5	23.1	0.5	- - -	- - -	14.6
1995	26.5	0.6	22.7	0.5	34.8	1.1	13.9
1996	- - -	- - -	- - -	- - -	- - -	- - -	13.6
1997	27.1	0.4	22.2	0.4	36.4	1.2	13.2
1998	25.9	0.4	22.1	0.4	- - -	- - -	12.9
1999	25.2	0.5	21.6	0.4	34.8	1.3	12.6
2000	25.2	0.4	21.1	0.4	- - -	- - -	12.2
2001	24.7	0.4	20.8	0.4	28.5	1.0	12.0

SE Standard error.
- - - Data not available.

NOTES: Data for men and women are for the civilian noninstitutionalized population. Percents for men and women are age adjusted to the 2000 standard population using five age groups: 18–24 years, 25–34 years, 35–44 years, 45–64 years, and 65 years and over. (See Appendix II, Age adjustment). Cigarette smoking is defined as follows: among men and women 18 years and over, those who ever smoked 100 cigarettes in their lifetime and now smoke every day or some days; among high school students (grades 9–12), those who smoked cigarettes on 1 or more of the 30 days preceding the survey; and among mothers with a live birth, those who smoked during pregnancy. Data from States that did not require the reporting of mother's tobacco use during pregnancy on the birth certificate are not included (see Appendix II, Tobacco use). See related *Health, United States, 2003,* tables 11 and 59.

SOURCES: Centers for Disease Control and Prevention, National Center for Health Statistics, National Health Interview Survey (data for men and women); National Vital Statistics System (data for mothers during pregnancy); National Center for Chronic Disease Prevention and Health Promotion, Youth Risk Behavior Survey (data for high school students).

Data table for figure 13. High school students not engaging in recommended amounts of physical activity (neither moderate nor vigorous) by grade and sex: United States, 2001

Grade	All students		Male students		Female students	
	Percent	SE	Percent	SE	Percent	SE
Grade 9	24.3	1.4	20.1	1.6	28.1	1.9
Grade 10	29.6	0.9	23.6	1.1	35.6	1.7
Grade 11	34.4	1.2	24.4	1.3	44.2	1.6
Grade 12	38.9	1.4	29.5	2.1	47.9	1.2
All grades	31.2	0.7	24.2	0.8	37.9	1.2

SE Standard error.

NOTES: The recommended amount of physical activity for high school students is at least 30 minutes of moderate activity (does not cause sweating or hard breathing) on 5 or more of the past 7 days; or at least 20 minutes of vigorous activity (causes sweating and hard breathing) on 3 or more of the past 7 days. The recommended amounts of physical activity for high school students are based on the Healthy People 2010 objectives 22–6 and 22–7 (moderate and vigorous activity in adolescents).

SOURCE: Centers for Disease Control and Prevention, National Center for Chronic Disease Prevention and Health Promotion, Youth Risk Behavior Survey.

Data table for figure 14. Overall physical activity levels for adults by age and sex: United States, 2000

Sex and age	Overall physical activity level									
	Inactive		Low		Medium		Medium/high		High	
	Percent	SE	Percent	SE	Percent	SE	Percent	SE	Percent	SE
Men										
18 years and over, age adjusted	7.3	0.3	15.0	0.4	33.2	0.5	23.3	0.5	21.3	0.4
18 years and over, crude	6.9	0.3	14.9	0.4	33.3	0.5	23.5	0.5	21.5	0.4
18–24 years	2.3	0.5	12.6	1.2	27.5	1.4	27.0	1.4	30.5	1.5
25–44 years	3.4	0.3	13.7	0.5	35.3	0.8	25.0	0.7	22.5	0.7
45–64 years	8.7	0.6	16.9	0.6	34.9	0.8	22.1	0.8	17.5	0.7
65 years and over	17.7	1.0	16.4	0.9	29.2	1.1	18.5	0.9	18.2	1.0
Women										
18 years and over, age adjusted	11.6	0.3	16.5	0.4	31.3	0.4	23.8	0.4	16.9	0.3
18 years and over, crude	11.7	0.3	16.5	0.4	31.2	0.4	23.7	0.4	16.9	0.3
18–24 years	6.4	0.7	15.7	1.0	32.2	1.4	28.0	1.4	17.7	1.1
25–44 years	7.2	0.3	16.2	0.6	32.8	0.7	25.3	0.6	18.5	0.6
45–64 years	11.4	0.5	17.8	0.6	31.2	0.8	22.9	0.7	16.7	0.6
65 years and over	26.1	1.0	15.4	0.7	27.0	0.9	18.4	0.7	13.1	0.7

SE Standard error.

NOTES: Data are for the civilian noninstitutionalized population and the total is age adjusted to the 2000 standard population using four age groups: 18–24, 25–44, 45–64, and 65 years and over. Overall physical activity level is based on two series of questions: (1) questions on frequency, duration, and intensity of leisure-time physical activity; and (2) questions on usual daily activity (sitting, standing, walking during most of the day; lifting or carrying things). Responses from the two series of questions were combined into a continuum of overall physical activity ranging from inactive to high. Persons coded as: Inactive reported being inactive during usual daily activities and never or unable to engage in leisure-time physical activity; Low activity level reported being moderately active during usual daily activities and never or unable to engage in leisure-time physical activity or inactive during usual daily activity and engaged in some leisure-time physical activity but less than regular; Medium activity level reported being very active during usual daily activities and never or unable to engage in leisure-time physical activity or moderately active during usual daily activities and engaged in some leisure-time physical activity but less than regular or inactive during usual daily activities and engaged in regular leisure-time physical activity; Medium/high activity level reported being very active during usual daily activities and engaged in some leisure-time physical activity but less than regular or moderately active during usual daily activities and engaged in regular leisure-time physical activity; High activity level reported being very active during usual daily activity and engaged in regular leisure-time physical activity. For more information see: Barnes, PM Schoenborn, CA. Physical activity among adults: United States, 2000. Advance data from vital and health statistics; no 333 Hyattsville, Maryland. National Center for Health Statistics. 2003. Available on the NCHS website: www.cdc.gov/nchs/data/ad/ad333.pdf.

SOURCE: Centers for Disease Control and Prevention, National Center for Health Statistics, National Health Interview Survey.

Data table for figure 15. Overweight and obesity by age: United States, 1960–2000

| | Children, 6–11 years | | Adolescents, 12–19 years | | Adults, 20–74 years | | | |
| | Overweight | | Overweight | | Overweight | | Obesity | |
Year	Percent	SE	Percent	SE	Percent	SE	Percent	SE
1960–62	- - -	- - -	- - -	- - -	44.8	1.0	13.3	0.6
1963–65	4.2	0.4	- - -	- - -	- - -	- - -	- - -	- - -
1966–70	- - -	- - -	4.6	0.3	- - -	- - -	- - -	- - -
1971–74	4.0	0.5	6.1	0.7	47.7	0.7	14.6	0.5
1976–80	6.5	0.6	5.0	0.6	47.4	0.8	15.1	0.5
1988–94	11.3	1.0	10.5	0.9	56.0	0.9	23.3	0.7
1999–2000	15.3	1.7	15.5	1.2	64.5	1.5	30.9	1.6

SE Standard error.

- - - Data not available.

NOTES: Data are for the civilian noninstitutionalized population. Percents for adults are age adjusted to the 2000 standard population using five age groups (20–34 years, 35–44 years, 45–54 years, 55–64 years, and 65–74 years) except for the 1999–2000 estimates which are age adjusted using three age groups (20–39 years, 40–59 years, and 60–74 years) due to a smaller sample size; however use of three rather than five groups had virtually no effect on age-adjusted rates. Overweight for children is defined as a body mass index (BMI) at or above the sex- and age-specific 95th percentile BMI cut points from the 2000 CDC Growth Charts: United States (www.cdc.gov/growthcharts/). Overweight for adults is defined as a BMI greater than or equal to 25 and obesity as a BMI greater than or equal to 30. Data for 1966–70 are for adolescents 12–17 years, not 12–19 years. Pregnant adolescents were excluded beginning in 1971–74. Pregnant women 20 years of age and over were excluded in all years. Estimates for 1999–2000 are based on a smaller sample size than estimates for earlier time periods and therefore are subject to greater sampling error. See Appendix II, Age adjustment and Body mass index (BMI). See related *Health, United States, 2003,* tables 68 and 69.

SOURCES: Centers for Disease Control and Prevention, National Center for Health Statistics, National Health Examination Survey and National Health and Nutrition Examination Survey.

Data table for figure 16. Obesity among adults 20–74 years of age by sex, race, and Hispanic origin: United States, 1999–2000

Age, race, and Hispanic origin	Obesity	
	Percent	SE
All races and origins	30.9	1.6
Men ·.................	27.7	1.7
Women	34.0	2.0
White only, not Hispanic or Latino	28.9	1.7
Men	27.4	1.9
Women	30.4	2.3
Black or African American only, not Hispanic or Latino	40.4	2.1
Men	28.9	2.4
Women	50.4	2.8
Mexican	34.9	2.3
Men	29.4	2.5
Women	40.1	3.8

SE Standard error.

NOTES: Data are for the civilian noninstitutionalized population. Percents are age adjusted to the 2000 standard population using three age groups: 20–39 years, 40–59 years, and 60–74 years. Obesity is defined as having a body mass index (BMI) greater than or equal to 30. Pregnant women were excluded. See Appendix II, Age adjustment and Body mass index (BMI). Estimates by race and Hispanic origin are tabulated using the 1997 Standards for Federal data on race and ethnicity. See Appendix II, Race. Persons of Hispanic origin may be of any race. See related *Health, United States, 2003,* table 68.

SOURCES: Centers for Disease Control and Prevention, National Center for Health Statistics, National Health Examination Survey and National Health and Nutrition Examination Survey.

Data table for figure 17. Limitation of activity caused by 1 or more chronic health conditions among children by sex and age: United States, 1999–2001

Sex and age	Any limitation of activity		Limitation of activity indicated by participation in special education or early intervention services only		All other limitation of activity	
	Percent	SE	Percent	SE	Percent	SE
Boys						
Under 18 years	7.9	0.2	5.9	0.1	2.0	0.1
Under 5 years	4.0	0.2	2.4	0.2	1.6	0.1
5–11 years	9.1	0.2	6.9	0.2	2.2	0.1
12–17 years	9.7	0.3	7.5	0.3	2.2	0.1
Girls						
Under 18 years	4.5	0.1	3.1	0.1	1.4	0.1
Under 5 years	2.4	0.2	1.2	0.1	1.2	0.1
5–11 years	5.1	0.2	3.9	0.2	1.2	0.1
12–17 years	5.4	0.2	3.6	0.2	1.8	0.1

SE Standard error.

NOTES: Data are for noninstitutionalized children. Children with limitation of activity caused by chronic health conditions may be identified by enrollment in special programs (special education or early intervention services) or by some other activity limitation. The category "All other limitation of activity" may include children receiving special education or early intervention services. See Appendix II, Limitation of activity.

SOURCE: Centers for Disease Control and Prevention, National Center for Health Statistics, National Health Interview Survey.

Data table for figure 18. Limitation of activity caused by 1 or more chronic health conditions among working-age adults by selected characteristics: United States, 1999–2001

	Any limitation of activity	
Characteristic	Percent	SE
Age		
18–44 years	6.1	0.1
45–54 years	12.9	0.2
55–64 years	20.5	0.3
Sex		
Male	9.3	0.1
Female	9.9	0.1
Percent of poverty level		
Below 100 percent	24.1	0.5
100–199 percent	17.5	0.3
200 percent or more	7.2	0.1
Race and Hispanic origin		
Hispanic or Latino	7.8	0.2
Not Hispanic or Latino:		
White only	9.7	0.1
Black or African American only	12.1	0.3

SE Standard error.

NOTES: Data are for the civilian noninstitutionalized population. Percents by sex, race and Hispanic origin, and poverty level are age adjusted to the year 2000 standard population using three age groups: 18–44 years, 45–54 years, and 55–64 years. Persons of Hispanic origin may be of any race. Limitation of activity is assessed by asking respondents a series of questions about limitations in their ability to perform activities usual for their age group because of a physical, mental, or emotional problem. Respondents are asked about limitations in activities of daily living, instrumental activities of daily living, limitations in work, walking, memory, and other activities. For adults identified as having limitation of activity, the causal health conditions are determined and respondents are considered limited if 1 or more of these conditions is chronic. See Appendix II, Limitation of activity. See related *Health, United States, 2003,* table 56.

SOURCE: Centers for Disease Control and Prevention, National Center for Health Statistics, National Health Interview Survey.

Data table for figure 19. Selected chronic health conditions causing limitation of activity among working-age adults by age: United States, 1999–2001

| | Number of persons with limitation of activity caused by selected chronic health conditions per 1,000 population | | | | | |
| | 18–44 years | | 45–54 years | | 55–64 years | |
Type of chronic health condition	Rate	SE	Rate	SE	Rate	SE
Mental illness	10.9	0.4	20.1	0.8	19.1	1.0
Fractures/joint injury	6.8	0.3	13.3	0.6	19.6	1.0
Lung	5.0	0.2	10.0	0.6	25.1	1.2
Diabetes	2.9	0.2	13.8	0.7	27.7	1.2
Heart/other circulatory	6.0	0.3	29.8	1.0	69.3	2.1
Arthritis/other musculoskeletal	21.1	0.6	59.2	1.4	98.3	2.4

SE Standard error.

NOTES: Data are for the civilian noninstitutionalized population. Selected chronic health conditions include the four leading causes of activity limitation among adults in each age category. Conditions refer to response categories in the National Health Interview Survey; some conditions include several response categories. "Mental illness" includes depression, anxiety or emotional problem, and other mental conditions. "Heart/other circulatory" includes heart problem, stroke problem, hypertension or high blood pressure, and other circulatory system conditions. "Arthritis/other musculoskeletal" includes arthritis/rheumatism, back or neck problem, and other musculoskeletal system conditions. Persons who reported more than one chronic health condition as the cause of their activity limitation were counted in each reported category. See Appendix II, Limitation of activity.

SOURCE: Centers for Disease Control and Prevention, National Center for Health Statistics, National Health Interview Survey.

Data table for figure 20. Limitation in activities of daily living among Medicare beneficiaries 65 years of age and over: United States, 1992–2001

| | All beneficiaries | | Noninstitutionalized beneficiaries | |
Year	Percent	SE	Percent	SE
1992	16.2	0.4	12.2	0.5
1993	16.0	0.4	12.0	0.4
1994	15.4	0.4	11.3	0.4
1995	15.2	0.4	11.1	0.4
1996	14.5	0.4	10.5	0.4
1997	13.9	0.4	10.0	0.4
1998	14.0	0.4	10.6	0.4
1999	13.4	0.4	9.8	0.4
2000	13.6	0.4	10.0	0.4
2001	13.7	0.3	10.1	0.3

SE Standard error.

NOTES: Percents are age adjusted to the year 2000 standard population using three age groups: 65–74 years, 75–84 years, and 85 years and over. Limitation in activities of daily living is defined as having difficulty and receiving help or supervision with at least one of the following six activities: bathing or showering, dressing, eating, getting in or out of bed or chairs, walking, and using the toilet (See Appendix II, Activities of daily living). Institutions are defined as facilities with 3 or more beds and providing long-term care services throughout the facility or in a separate identifiable unit. Data on institutionalized beneficiaries are obtained from proxy respondents.

SOURCE: Centers for Medicare and Medicaid Services, Medicare Current Beneficiary Survey, Access to Care files.

Data table for figure 21. Life expectancy at birth and at 65 years of age by sex: United States, 1901–2000

Year	At birth		At 65 years	
	Male	Female	Male	Female
	Life expectancy in years			
1900–02	47.9	50.7	11.5	12.2
1909–11	49.9	53.2	11.2	12.0
1919–21	55.5	57.4	12.2	12.7
1929–31	57.7	60.9	11.7	12.8
1939–41	61.6	65.9	12.1	13.6
1949–51	65.5	71.0	12.7	15.0
1959–61	66.8	73.2	13.0	15.8
1969–71	67.0	74.6	13.0	16.8
1979–81	70.1	77.6	14.2	18.4
1989–91	71.8	78.8	15.1	19.0
1997	73.6	79.4	15.9	19.2
1998	73.8	79.5	16.0	19.2
1999	73.9	79.4	16.1	19.1
2000	74.1	79.5	16.3	19.2

NOTES: Death rates used to calculate life expectancies for 1997–2000 are based on postcensal 1990-based population estimates. See Appendix I, Population Census and Population Estimates. Life expectancies prior to 1997 are from decennial life tables based on census data and deaths for a 3-year period around the census year. Beginning in 1997, the annual life tables are complete life tables based on a methodology similar to that used for decennial life tables. Alaska and Hawaii were included beginning in 1959. For decennial periods prior to 1929–31, data are limited to death registration States: 1900–02 and 1909–11, 10 States and the District of Columbia; 1919–21, 34 States and the District of Columbia. Deaths to nonresidents were excluded beginning in 1970. See Appendix II, Life expectancy. See related *Health, United States, 2003,* table 27.

SOURCES: Anderson RN. United States life tables, 1997. National vital statistics reports; vol 47 no 28. Hyattsville, Maryland: National Center for Health Statistics. 1999 (data for 1900–97); Anderson RN. United States life tables, 1998. National vital statistics reports; vol 48 no 18. Hyattsville, Maryland: National Center for Health Statistics. 2001 (data for 1998); Anderson RN, DeTurk PB. United States life tables, 1999. National vital statistics reports; vol 50 no 6. Hyattsville, Maryland: National Center for Health Statistics. 2002 (data for 1999); Arias E. United States life tables, 2000. National vital statistics reports; vol 51 no 3. Hyattsville, Maryland: National Center for Health Statistics. 2002 (data for 2000).

Data table for figure 22. Infant, neonatal, and postneonatal mortality rates: United States, 1950–2000

Year	Infant	Neonatal	Postneonatal
	Deaths per 1,000 live births		
1950	29.2	20.5	8.7
1960	26.0	18.7	7.3
1970	20.0	15.1	4.9
1980	12.6	8.5	4.1
1985	10.6	7.0	3.7
1990	9.2	5.8	3.4
1995	7.6	4.9	2.7
1996	7.3	4.8	2.5
1997	7.2	4.8	2.5
1998	7.2	4.8	2.4
1999	7.1	4.7	2.3
2000	6.9	4.6	2.3

NOTES: Infant is defined as under 1 year of age, neonatal as under 28 days of age, and postneonatal as between 28 days and 1 year of age. See related *Health, United States, 2003,* table 22.

SOURCE: Centers for Disease Control and Prevention, National Center for Health Statistics, National Vital Statistics System.

Data table for figure 23. Infant mortality rates by detailed race and Hispanic origin of mother: United States, 1998–2000

Race and Hispanic origin of mother	Infant deaths per 1,000 live births
White, not Hispanic or Latino	5.8
Black or African American, not Hispanic or Latino	13.9
Hispanic or Latino	5.7
Puerto Rican	8.1
Other and unknown Hispanic or Latino	6.9
Mexican	5.5
Central and South American	4.9
Cuban	4.3
Asian or Pacific Islander	5.1
Hawaiian	8.7
Filipino	5.9
Other Asian or Pacific Islander	5.2
Japanese	3.8
Chinese	3.5
American Indian or Alaska Native	9.0

NOTES: Infant is defined as under 1 year of age. Persons of Hispanic origin may be of any race. Asian or Pacific Islander, and American Indian or Alaska Native races include persons of Hispanic and non-Hispanic origin. See related *Health, United States, 2003*, table 19.

SOURCE: Centers for Disease Control and Prevention, National Center for Health Statistics, National Vital Statistics System, National Linked Birth/ Infant Death Data Sets.

Data table for figure 24. Death rates for leading causes of death among persons 15–24 years of age: United States, 1950–2000

Year	All causes	Unintentional injuries	Homicide	Suicide	Cancer	Heart disease
	Deaths per 100,000 population					
1950	128.1	54.8	5.8	4.5	8.6	6.8
1960	106.3	56.0	5.6	5.2	8.3	4.0
1970	127.7	68.7	11.3	8.8	8.3	3.0
1980	115.4	61.5	15.4	12.3	6.3	2.9
1985	94.9	47.8	11.7	12.8	5.4	2.8
1990	99.2	43.8	19.7	13.2	4.9	2.5
1995	93.4	37.6	19.6	13.0	4.5	2.8
1996	88.2	37.4	17.6	11.8	4.4	2.6
1997	84.6	35.7	16.3	11.2	4.4	2.9
1998	80.6	35.0	14.3	10.9	4.5	2.8
1998 (Comparability-modified)	80.6	36.1	14.3	10.9	4.5	2.8
1999	79.3	35.3	12.9	10.1	4.5	2.8
2000	79.9	36.0	12.6	10.2	4.4	2.6

NOTES: Causes of death shown are the five leading causes of death among persons 15–24 years of age in 2000. 1950 death rates are based on the 6th revision of the International Classification of Diseases (ICD-6), 1960 death rates on the ICD-7, 1970 death rates on the ICDA-8, and 1980–98 death rates on the ICD-9. 1998 (Comparability-modified) death rates use comparability ratios to adjust the rate to be comparable to records classified according to ICD-10. Starting in 1999 death rates are based on ICD-10. Comparability ratios for selected ICD revisions are available at gov/nchs/data/statab/comp2.pdf. Homicide refers to deaths due to assault. Suicide refers to deaths from intentional self-harm. Cancer refers to malignant neoplasms. The population estimates used to co rates for 1991 through 2000 differ from those used previously. Starting with *Health, United States, 2003*, rates for 1991–99 were revised using intercensal population estimates based on Census 2000. Rates for 2000 were computed using Census 2000 counts. See Appendix I, Population Census and Population Estimates. See Appendix II, Age adjustment, Cause of death, and Comparability ratio. See related *Health, United States, 2003*, tables 35, 36, 38, 45, and 46.

SOURCE: Centers for Disease Control and Prevention, National Center for Health Statistics, National Vital Statistics System.

Data table for figure 25. Percent of deaths due to leading causes of death among persons 15–24 years of age: United States, 2000

Cause of death	Number	Percent
All causes	31,307	100.0
Unintentional injuries	14,113	45.1
Homicide	4,939	15.8
Suicide	3,994	12.8
Cancer	1,713	5.5
Heart disease	1,031	3.3
Other causes	5,517	17.6

NOTES: 2000 deaths are coded according to the 10th revision of the International Classification of Diseases (ICD-10). Homicide refers to deaths due to assault. Suicide refers to deaths from intentional self-harm. Cancer refers to malignant neoplasms. See Appendix II, Cause of death. See related *Health, United States, 2003*, tables 32, 36, 38, 45, and 46.

SOURCE: Centers for Disease Control and Prevention, National Center for Health Statistics, National Vital Statistics System.

Data table for figure 26. Death rates for leading causes of death among persons 25–44 years of age: United States, 1950–2000

Year	All causes	Unintentional injuries	Cancer	Heart disease	Suicide	Year	Human immunodeficiency virus (HIV) disease
	Deaths per 100,000 population					Deaths per 100,000 population	
1950	276.9	45.7	43.3	55.9	11.9	1987	13.0
1960	229.8	41.9	41.4	47.8	12.3	1988	16.0
1970	243.1	49.7	39.9	41.6	15.6	1989	21.0
1980	185.9	41.1	32.7	28.1	15.7	1990	23.9
1985	169.8	34.3	31.0	24.6	14.9	1991	27.0
1990	185.0	33.6	29.3	20.6	15.3	1992	30.4
1995	193.0	32.4	27.1	21.1	15.1	1993	33.3
1996	175.9	31.5	26.6	20.2	14.8	1994	36.9
1997	160.3	31.4	26.2	19.9	14.5	1995	37.0
1998	155.7	31.5	25.6	20.2	14.3	1996	25.8
1998 (Comparability-modified) ...	155.7	32.5	25.8	19.9	14.2	1997	13.1
1999	154.4	31.9	24.8	19.9	13.6	1998	10.2
2000	154.6	32.0	24.4	19.3	13.4	1998 (Comparability-modified)	11.7
						1999	10.6
						2000	9.9

NOTES: Death rates are age adjusted to the year 2000 standard population using two age groups: 25–34 years and 35–44 years. Causes of death shown are the five leading causes of death among persons 25–44 years of age in 2000. 1950 death rates are based on the 6th revision of the International Classification of Diseases (ICD-6), 1960 death rates on the ICD-7, 1970 death rates on the ICDA-8, and 1980–98 death rates on the ICD-9. 1998 (Comparability-modified) death rates use comparability ratios to adjust the rate to be comparable to records classified according to ICD-10. Starting in 1999 death rates are based on ICD-10. Comparability ratios for selected ICD revisions are available at www.cdc.gov/nchs/data/statab/comp2.pdf. Cancer refers to malignant neoplasms. Suicide refers to deaths from intentional self-harm. The population estimates used to compute rates for 1991 through 2000 differ from those used previously. Starting with *Health, United States, 2003*, rates for 1991–99 were revised using intercensal population estimates based on Census 2000. Rates for 2000 were computed using Census 2000 counts. See Appendix I, Population Census and Population Estimates. See Appendix II, Age adjustment, Cause of death, and Comparability ratio. See related *Health, United States, 2003*, tables 35, 36, 38, 42, and 46.

SOURCE: Centers for Disease Control and Prevention, National Center for Health Statistics, National Vital Statistics System.

Data table for figure 27. Percent of deaths due to leading causes of death among persons 25–44 years of age: United States, 2000

Cause of death	Number	Percent
All causes	130,249	100.0
Unintentional injuries	27,182	20.9
Cancer	20,436	15.7
Heart disease	16,139	12.4
Suicide	11,354	8.7
Human immunodeficiency virus (HIV) disease	8,356	6.4
Other causes	46,782	35.9

NOTES: 2000 deaths are coded according to the 10th revision of the International Classification of Diseases (ICD-10). Cancer refers to malignant neoplasms. Suicide refers to deaths from intentional self-harm. See Appendix II, Cause of death. See related *Health, United States, 2003*, tables 32, 36, 38, 42, and 46.

SOURCE: Centers for Disease Control and Prevention, National Center for Health Statistics, National Vital Statistics System.

Data table for figure 28. Death rates for leading causes of death among persons 45–64 years of age: United States, 1950–2000

Year	All causes	Cancer	Heart disease	Unintentional injuries	Stroke	Diabetes	Chronic lower respiratory diseases
	Deaths per 100,000 population						
1950	1,265.3	259.8	504.8	60.0	119.0	24.1	- - -
1960	1,140.7	263.4	454.9	53.4	87.7	22.2	- - -
1970	1,094.9	277.0	401.0	57.3	70.8	22.2	- - -
1980	883.5	280.6	303.5	39.2	40.9	16.3	22.7
1985	823.7	281.9	267.4	32.4	34.4	15.7	25.0
1990	757.6	273.1	217.5	30.3	30.2	19.8	24.7
1995	709.8	247.2	192.3	29.3	28.5	22.8	23.7
1996	692.5	240.6	187.4	29.7	28.3	23.2	23.4
1997	669.8	234.1	179.9	29.9	27.3	22.6	23.0
1998	651.5	227.4	171.5	30.2	26.3	22.4	22.2
1998 (Comparability-modified)	651.5	228.9	169.1	31.1	27.8	22.6	23.3
1999	648.7	224.6	164.1	31.3	25.2	22.9	23.8
2000	648.2	221.5	159.8	31.9	25.8	22.8	22.6

- - - Data not available.

NOTES: Death rates are age adjusted to the year 2000 standard population using two age groups: 45–54 years and 55–64 years. Causes of death shown are the six leading causes of death among persons 45–64 years of age in 2000. 1950 death rates are based on the 6th revision of the International Classification of Diseases (ICD-6), 1960 death rates on the ICD-7, 1970 death rates on the ICDA-8, and 1980–98 death rates on the ICD-9. 1998 (Comparability-modified) death rates use comparability ratios to adjust the rate to be comparable to records classified according to ICD-10. Starting in 1999 death rates are based on ICD-10. Comparability ratios for selected ICD revisions are available at www.cdc.gov/nchs/data/statab/comp2.pdf. Death rates for chronic lower respiratory diseases are available prior to 1980 because of changes in medical terminology and the classification of these terms in the relevant ICD revisions. Cancer refers to malignant neoplasms. Stroke refers to cerebrovascular diseases. The population estimates used to compute rates for 1991 through 2000 differ from those used previously. Starting with *Health, United States, 2003*, rates for 1991–99 were revised using intercensal population estimates based on Census 2000. Rates for 2000 were computed using Census 2000 counts. See Appendix I, Population Census and Population Estimates. See Appendix II, Age adjustment, Cause of death, and Comparability ratio. See related *Health, United States, 2003*, tables 35, 36, 37, 38, and 41.

SOURCE: Centers for Disease Control and Prevention, National Center for Health Statistics, National Vital Statistics System.

Data table for figure 29. Percent of deaths due to leading causes of death among persons 45–64 years of age: United States, 2000

Cause of death	Number	Percent
All causes	401,187	100.0
Cancer	137,039	34.2
Heart disease	98,879	24.6
Unintentional injuries	19,783	4.9
Stroke	15,967	4.0
Diabetes	14,140	3.5
Chronic lower respiratory diseases	13,990	3.5
Other causes	101,389	25.3

NOTES: 2000 deaths are coded according to the 10th revision of the International Classification of Diseases (ICD-10). Cancer refers to malignant neoplasms. Stroke refers to cerebrovascular diseases. See Appendix II, Cause of death. See related *Health, United States, 2003*, tables 32, 36, 37, 38, and 41.

SOURCE: Centers for Disease Control and Prevention, National Center for Health Statistics, National Vital Statistics System.

Data table for figure 30. Death rates due to leading causes of death among persons 65 years of age and over: United States, 1950–2000

Year	All causes	Heart disease	Cancer	Stroke	Chronic lower respiratory diseases	Influenza and pneumonia	Diabetes
			Deaths per 100,000 population				
1950	7,933.3	3,613.3	952.4	1,188.8	- - -	273.0	130.5
1960	7,536.4	3,503.6	950.9	1,225.9	- - -	317.7	129.2
1970	6,717.5	3,089.4	971.0	1,015.5	- - -	243.9	142.6
1980	5,900.2	2,652.9	1,060.2	673.8	180.6	215.8	107.7
1985	5,694.0	2,430.8	1,091.2	531.0	225.4	242.9	103.4
1990	5,395.9	2,108.8	1,149.3	451.9	246.7	260.7	121.3
1995	5,264.7	1,927.4	1,152.5	437.6	271.1	237.1	135.9
1996	5,221.7	1,877.6	1,140.8	433.1	275.5	233.5	139.4
1997	5,178.8	1,827.2	1,127.3	423.7	280.2	236.3	140.2
1998	5,168.0	1,791.5	1,119.2	411.8	286.7	247.4	143.4
1998 (Comparability-modified) . . .	5,168.0	1,766.1	1,126.8	436.0	300.4	172.7	144.6
1999	5,220.0	1,766.9	1,126.1	433.2	313.0	167.4	150.0
2000	5,168.9	1,706.6	1,123.6	425.9	305.1	168.6	150.3

NOTES: Death rates are age adjusted to the year 2000 standard population using three age groups: 65–74 years, 75–84 years, and 85 years and over. Causes of death shown are the six leading causes of death among persons 65 years of age and over in 2000. 1950 death rates are based on the 6th revision of the International Classification of Diseases (ICD-6), 1960 death rates on the ICD-7, 1970 death rates on the ICDA-8, and 1980–98 death rates on the ICD-9. 1998 (Comparability-modified) death rate use comparability ratios to adjust the rate to be comparable to records classified according to ICD-10. Starting in 1999 death rates are based on ICD-10. Comparability ratios for selected ICD revisions are available at www.cdc.gov/nchs/data/statab/comp2.pdf. Death rates for chronic lower respiratory diseases are not shown prior to 1980 because of changes in medical terminology and the classification of these terms in the relevant ICD revisions. Cancer refers to malignant neoplasms. Stroke refers to cerebrovascular diseases. The population estimates used to compute rates for 1991 through 2000 differ from those used previously. Starting with *Health, United States, 2003,* rates for 1991–99 were revised using intercensal population estimates based on Census 2000. Rates for 2000 were computed using Census 2000 counts. See Appendix I, Population Census and Population Estimates. See Appendix II, Age adjustment, Cause of death, and Comparability ratio. See related *Health, United States, 2003,* tables 35, 36, 37, 38, and 41.

SOURCE: Centers for Disease Control and Prevention, National Center for Health Statistics, National Vital Statistics System.

Data table for figure 31. Percent of deaths due to leading causes of death among persons 65 years of age and over: United States, 2000

Cause of death	Number	Percent
All causes	1,799,825	100.0
Heart disease	593,707	33.0
Cancer	392,366	21.8
Stroke	148,045	8.2
Chronic lower respiratory diseases	106,375	5.9
Influenza and pneumonia	58,557	3.3
Diabetes	52,414	2.9
Other causes	448,361	24.9

NOTES: 2000 deaths are coded according to the 10th revision of the International Classification of Diseases (ICD-10). Cancer refers to malignant neoplasms. Stroke refers to cerebrovascular diseases. See Appendix II, Cause of death. See related *Health, United States, 2003,* tables 32, 36, 37, 38, and 41.

SOURCE: Centers for Disease Control and Prevention, National Center for Health Statistics, National Vital Statistics System.

Data table for figure 32. Diagnosed diabetes prevalence among adults 18 years of age and over by age: United States, 1997–2002

Year	All adults, age adjusted		All adults, crude		18–44 years		45–54 years		55–64 years		65 years and over	
	Percent	SE	Percent	SE	Percent	SE	Percent	SE	Percent	SE	Percent	SE
1997	5.3	0.1	5.1	0.1	1.5	0.1	5.6	0.3	10.8	0.6	13.2	0.5
1998	5.4	0.1	5.3	0.1	1.6	0.1	5.9	0.4	10.9	0.6	13.2	0.5
1999	5.5	0.1	5.4	0.1	1.7	0.1	5.9	0.4	11.2	0.6	13.2	0.5
2000	6.0	0.1	5.9	0.2	1.9	0.1	6.5	0.4	11.2	0.6	14.6	0.5
2001	6.5	0.2	6.4	0.2	2.0	0.1	7.0	0.4	13.0	0.6	15.2	0.5
2002	6.5	0.2	6.5	0.2	1.9	0.1	7.3	0.4	12.5	0.6	16.0	0.5

SE Standard error.

NOTES: Data are for the civilian noninstitutionalized population. Percents are age adjusted to the 2000 standard population using four age groups: 18–44 years, 45–54 years, 55–64 years, and 65 years and over. Diabetes prevalence is based on self-report of physician diagnosis and excludes women reporting diabetes only during pregnancy. Persons reporting borderline diabetes were not coded as having diabetes in this analysis. See Appendix II, Age adjustment.

SOURCE: Centers for Disease Control and Prevention, National Center for Health Statistics, National Health Interview Survey (1997–2001 data). Ni H, Schiller J, Hao C, Cohen RA, Barnes P. Early release of selected estimates based on data from the 2002 National Health Interview Survey. National Center for Health Statistics. Available from www.cdc.gov/nchs/nhis.htm. June 2003.

Data table for figure 33. Ambulatory care visits for diabetes among adults 18 years of age and over by age: United States, 1995–96, 1997–98, and 1999–2000

Year	18–44 years		45–54 years		55–64 years		65 years and over	
	Rate	SE	Rate	SE	Rate	SE	Rate	SE
	Visits per 1,000 population							
1995–96	31.1	3.4	150.1	12.1	302.9	21.7	436.3	24.9
1997–98	48.8	4.0	188.2	13.1	409.0	30.1	509.2	28.7
1999–2000	44.5	4.8	202.3	18.1	433.3	33.2	567.9	41.5

SE Standard error.

NOTES: Population estimates are for the civilian noninstitutionalized population. Population estimates are 1990-based postcensal estimates as of July 1 and are adjusted for net underenumeration using the 1990 National Population Adjustment Matrix from the U.S. Bureau of the Census. See Appendix I, Population Census and Population Estimates. Diabetes visits include visits to physician offices and hospital outpatient department clinics with a diagnosis of diabetes (ICD–9–CM:250) and are not limited to first-listed diagnosis.

SOURCES: Centers for Disease Control and Prevention, National Center for Health Statistics, National Ambulatory Medical Care Survey, and National Hospital Ambulatory Medical Care Survey.

Data table for figure 34. Hospital discharges for diabetes among adults 45 years of age and over by age: United States, 1990–2001

	Age									
	45 years and over, age adjusted		45–54 years		55–64 years		65–74 years		75 years and over	
Year	Rate	SE	Rate	SE	Rate	SE	Rate	SE	Rate	SE
	Discharges per 10,000 population									
1990–91	319.1	11.9	121.0	4.8	270.3	9.4	487.3	16.9	648.0	25.9
1992–93	352.7	13.0	139.4	5.2	302.9	11.8	536.9	19.3	699.5	25.5
1994–95	367.0	13.8	140.3	5.2	307.3	11.7	561.6	21.6	746.6	27.3
1996–97	384.3	13.0	148.5	5.6	322.1	11.5	576.1	19.3	791.1	24.8
1998–99	408.5	14.2	151.1	5.5	347.8	12.8	628.0	20.1	831.3	29.4
2000–01	410.4	15.8	156.6	5.4	344.0	13.9	632.4	24.2	830.6	32.4

SE Standard error.

NOTES: Population estimates are for the civilian population. Data for 1990–99 were computed using 1990-based postcensal population estimates as of July 1 and are adjusted for net underenumeration using the 1990 National Population Adjustment Matrix from the U.S. Bureau of the Census. Data for 2000–01 were computed using 2000-based postcensal estimates and are not strictly comparable with estimates for earlier years (See Appendix I, Population Census and Population Estimates). Rates for adults 45 years of age and over are age adjusted to the 2000 standard population using four age groups: 45–54 years, 55–64 years, 65–74 years, and 75 years and over. Diabetes discharges include any discharge diagnosis of diabetes (ICD–9–CM: 250) recorded and are not limited to first-listed diagnosis.

SOURCE: Centers for Disease Control and Prevention, National Center for Health Statistics, National Hospital Discharge Survey.

List of Trend Tables

Health Status and Determinants

Population

Fertility and Natality

Mortality

Determinants and Measures of Health

Utilization of Health Resources

Ambulatory Care

Inpatient Care

Health Care Resources

Personnel

Facilities

Health Care Expenditures

National Health Expenditures

Health Care Coverage and Major Federal Programs

State Health Expenditures and Health Insurance

Table 1 (page 1 of 2). Resident population, according to age, sex, race, and Hispanic origin: United States, selected years 1950–2001

[Data are based on decennial census updated by data from multiple sources]

Sex, race, Hispanic origin, and year	Total resident population	Under 1 year	1–4 years	5–14 years	15–24 years	25–34 years	35–44 years	45–54 years	55–64 years	65–74 years	75–84 years	85 years and over
All persons					Number in thousands							
1950	150,697	3,147	13,017	24,319	22,098	23,759	21,450	17,343	13,370	8,340	3,278	577
1960	179,323	4,112	16,209	35,465	24,020	22,818	24,081	20,485	15,572	10,997	4,633	929
1970	203,212	3,485	13,669	40,746	35,441	24,907	23,088	23,220	18,590	12,435	6,119	1,511
1980	226,546	3,534	12,815	34,942	42,487	37,082	25,635	22,800	21,703	15,581	7,729	2,240
1990	248,710	3,946	14,812	35,095	37,013	43,161	37,435	25,057	21,113	18,045	10,012	3,021
2000	281,422	3,806	15,370	41,078	39,184	39,892	45,149	37,678	24,275	18,391	12,361	4,240
2001	284,797	4,034	15,336	41,065	39,948	39,607	45,019	39,188	25,309	18,313	12,574	4,404
Male												
1950	74,833	1,602	6,634	12,375	10,918	11,597	10,588	8,655	6,697	4,024	1,507	237
1960	88,331	2,090	8,240	18,029	11,906	11,179	11,755	10,093	7,537	5,116	2,025	362
1970	98,912	1,778	6,968	20,759	17,551	12,217	11,231	11,199	8,793	5,437	2,436	542
1980	110,053	1,806	6,556	17,855	21,419	18,382	12,570	11,009	10,152	6,757	2,867	682
1990	121,239	2,018	7,581	17,971	18,915	21,564	18,510	12,232	9,955	7,907	3,745	841
2000	138,054	1,949	7,862	21,043	20,079	20,121	22,448	18,497	11,645	8,303	4,879	1,227
2001	139,813	2,064	7,841	21,033	20,485	20,014	22,403	19,236	12,154	8,297	4,987	1,299
Female												
1950	75,864	1,545	6,383	11,944	11,181	12,162	10,863	8,688	6,672	4,316	1,771	340
1960	90,992	2,022	7,969	17,437	12,114	11,639	12,326	10,393	8,036	5,881	2,609	567
1970	104,300	1,707	6,701	19,986	17,890	12,690	11,857	12,021	9,797	6,998	3,683	969
1980	116,493	1,727	6,259	17,087	21,068	18,700	13,065	11,791	11,551	8,824	4,862	1,559
1990	127,471	1,928	7,231	17,124	18,098	21,596	18,925	12,824	11,158	10,139	6,267	2,180
2000	143,368	1,857	7,508	20,034	19,105	19,771	22,701	19,181	12,629	10,088	7,482	3,013
2001	144,984	1,969	7,495	20,033	19,463	19,594	22,616	19,952	13,155	10,016	7,587	3,105
White male												
1950	67,129	1,400	5,845	10,860	9,689	10,430	9,529	7,836	6,180	3,736	1,406	218
1960	78,367	1,784	7,065	15,659	10,483	9,940	10,564	9,114	6,850	4,702	1,875	331
1970	86,721	1,501	5,873	17,667	15,232	10,775	9,979	10,090	7,958	4,916	2,243	487
1980	94,976	1,487	5,402	14,773	18,123	15,940	11,010	9,774	9,151	6,096	2,600	621
1990	102,143	1,604	6,071	14,467	15,389	18,071	15,819	10,624	8,813	7,127	3,397	760
2000	113,445	1,524	6,143	16,428	15,942	16,232	18,568	15,670	10,067	7,343	4,419	1,109
2001	114,659	1,609	6,124	16,398	16,235	16,103	18,461	16,240	10,497	7,311	4,504	1,176
White female												
1950	67,813	1,341	5,599	10,431	9,821	10,851	9,719	7,868	6,168	4,031	1,669	314
1960	80,465	1,714	6,795	15,068	10,596	10,204	11,000	9,364	7,327	5,428	2,441	527
1970	91,028	1,434	5,615	16,912	15,420	11,004	10,349	10,756	8,853	6,366	3,429	890
1980	99,835	1,412	5,127	14,057	17,653	15,896	11,232	10,285	10,325	7,951	4,457	1,440
1990	106,561	1,524	5,762	13,706	14,599	17,757	15,834	10,946	9,698	9,048	5,687	2,001
2000	116,641	1,447	5,839	15,576	14,966	15,574	18,386	15,921	10,731	8,757	6,715	2,729
2001	117,693	1,536	5,826	15,554	15,238	15,385	18,245	16,493	11,162	8,659	6,784	2,809
Black or African American male												
1950	7,300	- - -	[1]944	1,442	1,162	1,105	1,003	772	459	299	[2]113	- - -
1960	9,114	281	1,082	2,185	1,305	1,120	1,086	891	617	382	137	29
1970	10,748	245	975	2,784	2,041	1,226	1,084	979	739	461	169	46
1980	12,585	269	967	2,614	2,807	1,967	1,235	1,024	854	567	228	53
1990	14,420	322	1,164	2,700	2,669	2,592	1,962	1,175	878	614	277	66
2000	17,407	313	1,271	3,454	2,932	2,586	2,705	1,957	1,090	683	330	87
2001	17,710	334	1,263	3,462	3,033	2,574	2,727	2,067	1,131	691	340	88
Black or African American female												
1950	7,745	- - -	[1]941	1,446	1,300	1,260	1,112	796	443	322	[2]125	- - -
1960	9,758	283	1,085	2,191	1,404	1,300	1,229	974	663	430	160	38
1970	11,832	243	970	2,773	2,196	1,456	1,309	1,134	868	582	230	71
1980	14,046	266	951	2,578	2,937	2,267	1,488	1,258	1,059	776	360	106
1990	16,063	316	1,137	2,641	2,700	2,905	2,279	1,416	1,135	884	495	156
2000	19,187	302	1,228	3,348	2,971	2,866	3,055	2,274	1,353	971	587	233
2001	19,486	317	1,221	3,356	3,040	2,846	3,076	2,405	1,404	979	605	238

See notes at end of table.

Table 1 (page 2 of 2). Resident population, according to age, sex, race, and Hispanic origin: United States, selected years 1950–2001

[Data are based on decennial census updated by data from multiple sources]

Sex, race, Hispanic origin, and year	Total resident population	Under 1 year	1–4 years	5–14 years	15–24 years	25–34 years	35–44 years	45–54 years	55–64 years	65–74 years	75–84 years	85 years and over
American Indian or Alaska Native male						Number in thousands						
1980	702	17	59	153	161	114	75	53	37	22	9	2
1990	1,024	24	88	206	192	183	140	86	55	32	13	3
2000	1,488	28	109	301	271	229	229	165	88	45	18	5
2001	1,524	29	109	298	280	232	232	175	95	49	21	5
American Indian or Alaska Native female												
1980	718	16	57	149	158	118	79	57	41	27	12	4
1990	1,041	24	85	200	178	186	148	92	61	41	21	6
2000	1,496	26	106	293	254	219	236	174	95	54	28	10
2001	1,530	28	105	290	263	220	238	185	102	58	30	11
Asian or Pacific Islander male												
1980	1,814	35	130	321	334	366	252	159	110	72	30	6
1990	3,652	68	258	598	665	718	588	347	208	133	57	12
2000	5,713	84	339	861	934	1,073	947	705	399	231	112	27
2001	5,919	92	344	875	937	1,104	983	754	431	247	122	30
Asian or Pacific Islander female												
1980	1,915	34	127	307	325	423	269	192	126	71	33	9
1990	3,805	65	247	578	621	749	664	371	264	166	65	17
2000	6,044	81	336	817	914	1,112	1,024	812	451	305	152	41
2001	6,275	88	342	833	922	1,143	1,057	869	486	321	167	47
Hispanic or Latino male												
1980	7,280	187	661	1,530	1,646	1,255	761	570	364	201	86	19
1990	11,388	279	980	2,128	2,376	2,310	1,471	818	551	312	131	32
2000	18,162	395	1,506	3,469	3,564	3,494	2,653	1,551	804	474	203	50
2001	19,018	417	1,533	3,606	3,606	3,699	2,828	1,684	869	501	224	53
Hispanic or Latino female												
1980	7,329	181	634	1,482	1,547	1,249	805	615	411	257	116	30
1990	10,966	268	939	2,039	2,028	2,073	1,448	868	632	403	209	59
2000	17,144	376	1,441	3,318	3,017	3,016	2,476	1,585	907	603	303	101
2001	17,955	401	1,467	3,450	3,085	3,163	2,624	1,714	978	635	331	107
White, not Hispanic or Latino male												
1980	88,035	1,308	4,773	13,318	16,555	14,739	10,285	9,229	8,802	5,906	2,519	603
1990	91,743	1,351	5,181	12,525	13,219	15,967	14,481	9,875	8,303	6,837	3,275	729
2000	96,551	1,163	4,761	13,238	12,628	12,958	16,088	14,223	9,312	6,894	4,225	1,062
2001	96,966	1,228	4,719	13,082	12,885	12,634	15,816	14,669	9,680	6,836	4,291	1,126
White, not Hispanic or Latino female												
1980	92,872	1,240	4,522	12,647	16,185	14,711	10,468	9,700	9,935	7,708	4,345	1,411
1990	96,557	1,280	4,909	11,846	12,749	15,872	14,520	10,153	9,116	8,674	5,491	1,945
2000	100,774	1,102	4,517	12,529	12,183	12,778	16,089	14,446	9,879	8,188	6,429	2,633
2001	101,070	1,169	4,482	12,385	12,393	12,449	15,810	14,900	10,244	8,059	6,471	2,707

- - - Data not available.
[1]Population for age group under 5 years.
[2]Population for age group 75 years and over.

NOTES: The race groups, white, black, American Indian or Alaska Native, and Asian or Pacific Islander, include persons of Hispanic and non-Hispanic origin. Persons of Hispanic origin may be of any race. Population estimates for 1991 through 2000 differ from those shown previously. Starting with *Health, United States, 2003,* intercensal population estimates based on Census 2000 and Census 2000 counts replace estimates projected from the 1990 Census. Population estimates for 2001 are 2000-based postcensal estimates. Population figures are census counts as of April 1 for 1950, 1960, 1970, 1980, 1990, and 2000; estimates as of July 1 for other years. See Appendix I, Population Census and Population Estimates. Populations for age groups may not sum to the total due to rounding. Although population figures are shown rounded to the nearest 1,000, calculations of birth rates and death rates shown in this volume are based on unrounded population figures for decennial years and for all years starting with 1991. See Appendix II, Rate. Unrounded population figures are available in the spreadsheet version of this table (see www.cdc.gov/nchs/hus.htm). Data for additional years are available (see Appendix III).

SOURCES: U.S. Bureau of the Census: 1950 Nonwhite Population by Race. Special Report P-E, No. 3B. Washington. U.S. Government Printing Office, 1951; U.S. Census of Population: 1960, Number of Inhabitants, PC(1)-A1, United States Summary, 1964; 1970, Number of Inhabitants, Final Report PC(1)-A1, United States Summary, 1971; U.S. population estimates, by age, sex, race, and Hispanic origin: 1980 to 1991. Current population reports, series P-25, no 1095. Washington. U.S. Government Printing Office, Feb. 1993; National Center for Health Statistics. Estimates of the July 1, 1991–July 1, 1999, April 1, 2000, and July 1, 2001 United States resident population by age, sex, race, and Hispanic origin, prepared under a collaborative arrangement with the U.S. Census Bureau. Available at www.cdc.gov/nchs/about/major/dvs/popbridge/popbridge.htm. 2003.

Table 2 (page 1 of 2). Persons and families below poverty level, according to selected characteristics, race, and Hispanic origin: United States, selected years 1973–2001

[Data are based on household interviews of the civilian noninstitutionalized population]

Selected characteristics, race, and Hispanic origin	1973	1980	1985	1990	1995	1997	1998	1999	2000[1]	2001[1]
All persons					Percent below poverty					
All races	11.1	13.0	14.0	13.5	13.8	13.3	12.7	11.8	11.3	11.7
White	8.4	10.2	11.4	10.7	11.2	11.0	10.5	9.8	9.5	9.9
Black or African American	31.4	32.5	31.3	31.9	29.3	26.5	26.1	23.6	22.5	22.7
Asian or Pacific Islander	- - -	- - -	- - -	12.2	14.6	14.0	12.5	10.7	9.9	10.2
Hispanic or Latino	21.9	25.7	29.0	28.1	30.3	27.1	25.6	22.8	21.5	21.4
Mexican	- - -	- - -	28.8	28.1	31.2	27.9	27.1	24.1	22.9	22.8
Puerto Rican	- - -	- - -	43.3	40.6	38.1	34.2	30.9	25.8	25.6	26.1
White, not Hispanic or Latino	7.5	9.1	9.7	8.8	8.5	8.6	8.2	7.7	7.4	7.8
Related children under 18 years of age in families										
All races	14.2	17.9	20.1	19.9	20.2	19.2	18.3	16.3	15.6	15.8
White	9.7	13.4	15.6	15.1	15.5	15.4	14.4	12.9	12.4	12.8
Black or African American	40.6	42.1	43.1	44.2	41.5	36.8	36.4	32.7	30.9	30.0
Asian or Pacific Islander	- - -	- - -	- - -	17.0	18.6	19.9	17.5	11.5	12.5	11.1
Hispanic or Latino	27.8	33.0	39.6	37.7	39.3	36.4	33.6	29.9	27.6	27.4
Mexican	- - -	- - -	37.4	35.5	39.3	35.8	34.6	31.2	29.5	28.8
Puerto Rican	- - -	- - -	58.6	56.7	53.2	49.1	43.2	37.6	32.1	33.0
White, not Hispanic or Latino	- - -	11.3	12.3	11.6	10.6	10.7	10.0	8.8	8.5	8.9
Related children under 18 years of age in families with female householder and no spouse present										
All races	- - -	50.8	53.6	53.4	50.3	49.0	46.1	41.9	40.1	39.3
White	- - -	41.6	45.2	45.9	42.5	44.3	40.0	35.5	33.9	34.7
Black or African American	- - -	64.8	66.9	64.7	61.6	55.3	54.7	51.7	49.3	46.6
Asian or Pacific Islander	- - -	- - -	- - -	32.2	42.4	58.3	49.8	32.8	38.0	26.7
Hispanic or Latino	- - -	65.0	72.4	68.4	65.7	62.8	59.6	52.4	49.8	49.3
Mexican	- - -	- - -	64.4	62.4	65.9	62.2	61.5	51.4	51.4	50.9
Puerto Rican	- - -	- - -	85.4	82.7	79.6	71.0	61.6	50.9	55.3	52.9
White, not Hispanic or Latino	- - -	- - -	- - -	39.6	33.5	37.2	32.8	29.0	28.0	29.0
All persons					Number below poverty in thousands					
All races	22,973	29,272	33,064	33,585	36,425	35,574	34,476	32,258	31,581	32,907
White	15,142	19,699	22,860	22,326	24,423	24,396	23,454	21,922	21,645	22,739
Black or African American	7,388	8,579	8,926	9,837	9,872	9,116	9,091	8,360	7,982	8,136
Asian or Pacific Islander	- - -	- - -	- - -	858	1,411	1,468	1,360	1,163	1,258	1,275
Hispanic or Latino	2,366	3,491	5,236	6,006	8,574	8,308	8,070	7,439	7,747	7,997
Mexican	- - -	- - -	3,220	3,764	5,608	5,509	5,566	5,214	5,460	5,698
Puerto Rican	- - -	- - -	1,011	966	1,183	1,059	929	760	814	839
White, not Hispanic or Latino	12,864	16,365	17,839	16,622	16,267	16,491	15,799	14,875	14,366	15,271
Related children under 18 years of age in families										
All races	9,453	11,114	12,483	12,715	13,999	13,422	12,845	11,510	11,005	11,175
White	5,462	6,817	7,838	7,696	8,474	8,441	7,935	7,123	6,834	7,086
Black or African American	3,822	3,906	4,057	4,412	4,644	4,116	4,073	3,644	3,495	3,423
Asian or Pacific Islander	- - -	- - -	- - -	356	532	608	542	348	407	353
Hispanic or Latino	1,364	1,718	2,512	2,750	3,938	3,865	3,670	3,382	3,342	3,433
Mexican	- - -	- - -	1,589	1,733	2,655	2,666	2,654	2,512	2,537	2,613
Puerto Rican	- - -	- - -	535	490	610	519	433	365	329	319
White, not Hispanic or Latino	- - -	5,174	5,421	5,106	4,745	4,759	4,458	3,921	3,715	3,887

See footnotes at end of table.

Table 2 (page 2 of 2). Persons and families below poverty level, according to selected characteristics, race, and Hispanic origin: United States, selected years 1973–2001

[Data are based on household interviews of the civilian noninstitutionalized population]

Selected characteristics, race, and Hispanic origin	1973	1980	1985	1990	1995	1997	1998	1999	2000[1]	2001[1]
Related children under 18 years of age in families with female householder and no spouse present				Number below poverty in thousands						
All races	- - -	5,866	6,716	7,363	8,364	7,928	7,627	6,602	6,300	6,341
White	- - -	2,813	3,372	3,597	4,051	4,186	3,875	3,266	3,090	3,291
Black or African American.	- - -	2,944	3,181	3,543	3,954	3,402	3,366	2,997	2,908	2,741
Asian or Pacific Islander.	- - -	- - -	- - -	80	145	200	231	134	162	105
Hispanic or Latino	- - -	809	1,247	1,314	1,872	1,758	1,739	1,471	1,407	1,508
Mexican.	- - -	- - -	553	615	1,056	991	1,092	897	938	1,001
Puerto Rican	- - -	- - -	449	382	459	392	298	461	242	236
White, not Hispanic or Latino . . .	- - -	- - -	- - -	2,411	2,299	2,551	2,294	1,931	1,832	1,953

- - - Data not available.

[1]Estimates of poverty for 2000 have been recalculated based on an expanded household sample and Census 2000-based population weights. 2001 estimates are also based on an expanded household sample and 2000-based postcensal population weights. The 2000 estimates differ from those in *Health, United States, 2002*, which did not incorporate the sample expansion and were based on 1990 weights. See Appendix I, Current Population Survey.

NOTES: Estimates of poverty for the 1990s are based on 1990 postcensal population estimates. The race groups white, black, and Asian or Pacific Islander include persons of Hispanic and non-Hispanic origin; persons of Hispanic origin may be of any race. Poverty status is based on family income and family size using Bureau of the Census poverty thresholds. See Appendix II, Poverty status. The Current Population Survey is not large enough to produce reliable annual estimates for American Indian or Alaska Native persons. The 1999–2001 average poverty rate for this group was 24.5 percent, representing 783,000 persons. Data for additional years are available (see Appendix III).

SOURCES: U.S. Bureau of the Census. Proctor B, Dalaker J. Poverty in the United States: 2001. Current population reports, series P–60, no 219. Washington: U.S. Government Printing Office. 2002; and Table 2. Age, sex, household relationship, race and Hispanic origin by ratio of income to poverty level: 2001 accessed at http://ferret.bls.census.gov/macro/032002/pov/new02_001.htm.

Table 3 (page 1 of 2). Crude birth rates, fertility rates, and birth rates by age of mother, according to race and Hispanic origin: United States, selected years 1950–2001

[Data are based on birth certificates]

Race, Hispanic origin, and year	Crude birth rate[1]	Fertility rate[2]	10–14 years	15–19 years Total	15–17 years	18–19 years	20–24 years	25–29 years	30–34 years	35–39 years	40–44 years	45–54 years[3]
All races					Live births per 1,000 women							
1950	24.1	106.2	1.0	81.6	40.7	132.7	196.6	166.1	103.7	52.9	15.1	1.2
1960	23.7	118.0	0.8	89.1	43.9	166.7	258.1	197.4	112.7	56.2	15.5	0.9
1970	18.4	87.9	1.2	68.3	38.8	114.7	167.8	145.1	73.3	31.7	8.1	0.5
1980	15.9	68.4	1.1	53.0	32.5	82.1	115.1	112.9	61.9	19.8	3.9	0.2
1985	15.8	66.3	1.2	51.0	31.0	79.6	108.3	111.0	69.1	24.0	4.0	0.2
1990	16.7	70.9	1.4	59.9	37.5	88.6	116.5	120.2	80.8	31.7	5.5	0.2
1995	14.6	64.6	1.3	56.0	35.5	87.7	107.5	108.8	81.1	34.0	6.6	0.3
1996	14.4	64.1	1.2	53.5	33.3	84.7	107.8	108.6	82.1	34.9	6.8	0.3
1997	14.2	63.6	1.1	51.3	31.4	82.1	107.3	108.3	83.0	35.7	7.1	0.4
1998	14.3	64.3	1.0	50.3	29.9	80.9	108.4	110.2	85.2	36.9	7.4	0.4
1999	14.2	64.4	0.9	48.8	28.2	79.1	107.9	111.2	87.1	37.8	7.4	0.4
2000	14.4	65.9	0.9	47.7	26.9	78.1	109.7	113.5	91.2	39.7	8.0	0.5
2001	14.1	65.3	0.8	45.3	24.7	76.1	106.2	113.4	91.9	40.6	8.1	0.5
Race of child:[4] White												
1950	23.0	102.3	0.4	70.0	31.3	120.5	190.4	165.1	102.6	51.4	14.5	1.0
1960	22.7	113.2	0.4	79.4	35.5	154.6	252.8	194.9	109.6	54.0	14.7	0.8
1970	17.4	84.1	0.5	57.4	29.2	101.5	163.4	145.9	71.9	30.0	7.5	0.4
1980	14.9	64.7	0.6	44.7	25.2	72.1	109.5	112.4	60.4	18.5	3.4	0.2
Race of mother:[5] White												
1980	15.1	65.6	0.6	45.4	25.5	73.2	111.1	113.8	61.2	18.8	3.5	0.2
1985	15.0	64.1	0.6	43.3	24.4	70.4	104.1	112.3	69.9	23.3	3.7	0.2
1990	15.8	68.3	0.7	50.8	29.5	78.0	109.8	120.7	81.7	31.5	5.2	0.2
1995	14.1	63.6	0.8	49.5	29.7	80.0	104.7	111.7	83.3	34.2	6.4	0.3
1996	13.9	63.3	0.7	47.5	28.0	77.4	105.3	111.7	84.6	35.3	6.7	0.3
1997	13.7	62.8	0.7	45.5	26.6	74.8	104.5	111.3	85.7	36.1	6.9	0.3
1998	13.8	63.6	0.6	44.9	25.6	73.9	105.4	113.6	88.5	37.5	7.3	0.4
1999	13.7	64.0	0.6	44.0	24.5	72.8	105.0	114.9	90.7	38.5	7.4	0.4
2000	13.9	65.3	0.6	43.2	23.3	72.3	106.6	116.7	94.6	40.2	7.9	0.4
2001	13.7	65.0	0.5	41.2	21.4	70.8	103.7	117.0	95.8	41.3	8.0	0.5
Race of child:[4] Black or African American												
1960	31.9	153.5	4.3	156.1	- - -	- - -	295.4	218.6	137.1	73.9	21.9	1.1
1970	25.3	115.4	5.2	140.7	101.4	204.9	202.7	136.3	79.6	41.9	12.5	1.0
1980	22.1	88.1	4.3	100.0	73.6	138.8	146.3	109.1	62.9	24.5	5.8	0.3
Race of mother:[5] Black or African American												
1980	21.3	84.9	4.3	97.8	72.5	135.1	140.0	103.9	59.9	23.5	5.6	0.3
1985	20.4	78.8	4.5	95.4	69.3	132.4	135.0	100.2	57.9	23.9	4.6	0.3
1990	22.4	86.8	4.9	112.8	82.3	152.9	160.2	115.5	68.7	28.1	5.5	0.3
1995	17.8	71.0	4.1	94.4	68.6	134.6	133.7	95.6	63.0	28.4	6.0	0.3
1996	17.3	69.2	3.5	89.6	63.4	130.1	133.2	94.3	62.0	28.7	6.1	0.3
1997	17.1	69.0	3.1	86.3	59.4	127.4	135.2	95.0	62.6	29.3	6.5	0.3
1998	17.1	69.4	2.8	83.5	55.5	124.3	138.4	97.5	63.2	30.0	6.6	0.3
1999	16.8	68.5	2.5	79.1	50.7	120.1	137.9	97.3	62.7	30.2	6.5	0.3
2000	17.0	70.0	2.3	77.4	49.0	118.8	141.3	100.3	65.4	31.5	7.2	0.4
2001	16.3	67.6	2.0	71.8	43.9	114.0	133.2	99.2	64.8	31.6	7.2	0.4
American Indian or Alaska Native mothers[5]												
1980	20.7	82.7	1.9	82.2	51.5	129.5	143.7	106.6	61.8	28.1	8.2	*
1985	19.8	78.6	1.7	79.2	47.7	124.1	139.1	109.6	62.6	27.4	6.0	*
1990	18.9	76.2	1.6	81.1	48.5	129.3	148.7	110.3	61.5	27.5	5.9	*
1995	15.3	63.0	1.6	72.9	44.7	121.8	123.1	91.6	56.5	24.3	5.5	*
1996	14.9	61.8	1.6	68.2	42.7	112.9	123.5	91.1	56.5	24.4	5.5	*
1997	14.7	60.8	1.5	65.2	41.1	106.8	122.5	91.6	56.0	24.4	5.4	0.3
1998	14.8	61.3	1.5	64.7	39.8	106.5	125.1	92.0	56.8	24.6	5.3	*
1999	14.2	59.0	1.4	59.9	36.5	97.9	120.7	90.6	53.8	24.3	5.7	0.3
2000	14.0	58.7	1.1	58.3	34.1	97.1	117.2	91.8	55.5	24.6	5.7	0.3
2001	13.7	58.1	1.0	56.3	31.4	94.8	115.0	90.4	55.9	24.7	5.7	0.3

See footnotes at end of table.

Table 3 (page 2 of 2). Crude birth rates, fertility rates, and birth rates by age of mother, according to race and Hispanic origin: United States, selected years 1950–2001

[Data are based on birth certificates]

Race, Hispanic origin, and year	Crude birth rate[1]	Fertility rate[2]	10–14 years	15–19 years Total	15–17 years	18–19 years	20–24 years	25–29 years	30–34 years	35–39 years	40–44 years	45–54 years[3]
Asian or Pacific Islander mothers[5]						Live births per 1,000 women					
1980	19.9	73.2	0.3	26.2	12.0	46.2	93.3	127.4	96.0	38.3	8.5	0.7
1985	18.7	68.4	0.4	23.8	12.5	40.8	83.6	123.0	93.6	42.7	8.7	1.2
1990	19.0	69.6	0.7	26.4	16.0	40.2	79.2	126.3	106.5	49.6	10.7	1.1
1995	16.7	62.6	0.7	25.5	15.1	42.2	64.2	103.7	102.3	50.1	11.8	0.8
1996	16.5	62.3	0.6	23.5	14.3	38.6	63.5	102.8	104.1	50.2	11.9	0.8
1997	16.2	61.3	0.5	22.3	13.5	37.0	61.2	101.6	102.5	51.0	11.5	0.9
1998	15.9	60.1	0.5	22.2	13.2	36.9	59.2	98.7	101.6	51.4	11.8	0.9
1999	15.9	60.9	0.4	21.4	11.8	36.5	58.9	100.8	104.3	52.9	11.3	0.9
2000	17.1	65.8	0.3	20.5	11.6	32.6	60.3	108.4	116.5	59.0	12.6	0.8
2001	16.4	64.2	0.2	19.8	10.3	32.8	59.1	106.4	112.6	56.7	12.3	0.9
Hispanic or Latino mothers[5,6,7]												
1980	23.5	95.4	1.7	82.2	52.1	126.9	156.4	132.1	83.2	39.9	10.6	0.7
1990	26.7	107.7	2.4	100.3	65.9	147.7	181.0	153.0	98.3	45.3	10.9	0.7
1995	24.1	98.8	2.6	99.3	68.3	146.7	171.9	140.4	90.5	43.7	10.7	0.6
1996	23.8	97.5	2.4	94.6	64.1	140.5	170.2	140.7	91.3	43.9	10.7	0.6
1997	23.0	94.2	2.1	89.6	61.0	132.9	162.6	137.5	89.6	43.4	10.7	0.6
1998	22.7	93.2	1.9	87.9	58.4	131.7	159.3	136.1	90.5	43.4	10.8	0.6
1999	22.5	93.0	1.9	86.8	56.9	129.8	157.3	135.8	92.3	44.5	10.6	0.6
2000	23.1	95.9	1.7	87.3	55.5	132.6	161.3	139.9	97.1	46.6	11.5	0.6
2001	23.0	96.0	1.6	86.4	52.8	135.5	163.5	140.4	97.6	47.9	11.6	0.7
White, not Hispanic or Latino mothers[5,6,7]												
1980	14.2	62.4	0.4	41.2	22.4	67.7	105.5	110.6	59.9	17.7	3.0	0.1
1990	14.4	62.8	0.5	42.5	23.2	66.6	97.5	115.3	79.4	30.0	4.7	0.2
1995	12.5	57.5	0.4	39.3	22.0	65.9	90.2	105.1	81.5	32.8	5.9	0.3
1996	12.3	57.1	0.4	37.6	20.6	63.8	90.1	104.9	82.8	33.9	6.2	0.3
1997	12.2	56.8	0.4	36.0	19.4	61.9	90.0	104.8	84.3	34.8	6.5	0.3
1998	12.2	57.6	0.3	35.3	18.4	60.8	91.2	107.4	87.2	36.4	6.8	0.4
1999	12.1	57.7	0.3	34.1	17.1	59.3	90.6	108.6	89.5	37.3	6.9	0.4
2000	12.2	58.5	0.3	32.6	15.8	57.5	91.2	109.4	93.2	38.8	7.3	0.4
2001	11.8	57.7	0.3	30.3	14.0	54.8	87.1	108.9	94.3	39.8	7.5	0.4
Black or African American, not Hispanic or Latino mothers[5,6,7]												
1980	22.9	90.7	4.6	105.1	77.2	146.5	152.2	111.7	65.2	25.8	5.8	0.3
1990	23.0	89.0	5.0	116.2	84.9	157.5	165.1	118.4	70.2	28.7	5.6	0.3
1995	18.2	72.8	4.2	97.2	70.6	138.5	137.8	98.5	64.4	28.8	6.1	0.3
1996	17.6	70.7	3.6	91.9	65.0	133.4	137.0	96.7	63.2	29.1	6.2	0.3
1997	17.4	70.3	3.2	88.3	60.9	130.4	138.8	97.2	63.6	29.6	6.5	0.3
1998	17.5	70.9	2.9	85.7	57.0	127.4	142.5	99.9	64.4	30.4	6.7	0.3
1999	17.1	69.9	2.6	81.0	52.0	123.1	142.1	99.8	63.9	30.6	6.5	0.3
2000	17.3	71.4	2.4	79.2	50.1	121.9	145.4	102.8	66.5	31.8	7.2	0.4
2001	16.6	69.1	2.1	73.5	44.9	116.7	137.2	102.1	66.2	32.1	7.3	0.4

- - - Data not available.   * Rates based on fewer than 20 births are considered unreliable and are not shown.   [1]Live births per 1,000 population.

[2]Total number of live births regardless of age of mother per 1,000 women 15–44 years of age.

[3]Prior to 1997 data are for live births to mothers 45–49 years of age per 1,000 women 45–49 years of age. Starting in 1997 data are for live births to mothers 45–54 years of age per 1,000 women 45–49 years of age (see Appendix II, Age).

[4]Live births are tabulated by race of child.   [5]Live births are tabulated by race and/or Hispanic origin of mother.

[6]Prior to 1993, data from States lacking an Hispanic-origin item on the birth certificate were excluded. Interpretation of trend data should take into consideration expansion of reporting areas and immigration. See Appendix II, Hispanic origin.

[7]Rates in 1985 were not calculated because estimates for the Hispanic and non-Hispanic populations were not available.

NOTES: Data are based on births adjusted for underregistration for 1950 and on registered births for all other years. Beginning in 1970, births to persons who were not residents of the 50 States and the District of Columbia are excluded. The population estimates used to compute rates for 1991 through 2000 differ from those used previously. Starting with *Health, United States, 2003*, rates for 1991–99 were revised using intercensal population estimates based on Census 2000. Rates for 2000 were computed using Census 2000 counts and rates for 2001 were computed using 2000-based postcensal estimates. Estimates of intercensal populations used to compute birth rates for teenagers 15–17 and 18–19 years are based on adjustments of the revised populations for the 5-year age group, 15–19 years. See Appendix I, Population Census and Population Estimates. The race groups, white, black, American Indian or Alaska Native, and Asian or Pacific Islander, include persons of Hispanic and non-Hispanic origin. Persons of Hispanic origin may be of any race. Data for additional years are available (see Appendix III).

SOURCES: Centers for Disease Control and Prevention, National Center for Health Statistics, National Vital Statistics System, Birth File. Hamilton BE, Sutton PD, Ventura SJ. Revised birth and fertility rates for the 1990s: United States, and new rates for Hispanic populations, 2000 and 2001. National vital statistics reports; vol 51, (In preparation). Hyattsville, Maryland: National Center for Health Statistics, 2003. National vital statistics reports; vol 51, no 4. Hyattsville, Maryland: National Center for Health Statistics, 2003; Ventura SJ, Hamilton BE, Sutton PD. Revised birth and fertility rates for the United States, 2000 and 2001. National vital statistics reports; vol 51, no 4. Hyattsville, Maryland: National Center for Health Statistics, 2003; Ventura SJ. Births of Hispanic parentage, 1980 and 1985. Monthly vital statistics report; vol 32, no 6 and vol 36, no 11, suppl. Public Health Service. Hyattsville, Maryland. 1983 and 1988; Internet release of *Vital statistics of the United States, 1999, vol 1, natality*, tables 1–1 and 1–7 at www.cdc.gov/nchs/datawh/statab/unpubd/natality/natab99.htm. *Vital statistics of the United States, 2000, vol 1, natality*. In preparation.

Table 4. Women 15–44 years of age who have not had at least 1 live birth, by age: United States, selected years 1960–2002

[Data are based on birth certificates]

Year[1]	15–19 years	20–24 years	25–29 years	30–34 years	35–39 years	40–44 years
	Percent of women					
1960	91.4	47.5	20.0	14.2	12.0	15.1
1965	92.7	51.4	19.7	11.7	11.4	11.0
1970	93.0	57.0	24.4	11.8	9.4	10.6
1975	92.6	62.5	31.1	15.2	9.6	8.8
1980	93.4	66.2	38.9	19.7	12.5	9.0
1985	93.7	67.7	41.5	24.6	15.4	11.7
1986	93.8	68.0	42.0	25.1	16.1	12.2
1987	93.8	68.2	42.5	25.5	16.9	12.6
1988	93.8	68.4	43.0	25.7	17.7	13.0
1989	93.7	68.4	43.3	25.9	18.2	13.5
1990	93.3	68.3	43.5	25.9	18.5	13.9
1991	93.0	67.9	43.6	26.0	18.7	14.5
1992	92.7	67.3	43.7	26.0	18.8	15.2
1993	92.6	66.7	43.8	26.1	18.8	15.8
1994	92.6	66.1	43.9	26.2	18.7	16.2
1995	92.5	65.5	44.0	26.2	18.6	16.5
1996	92.5	65.0	43.8	26.2	18.5	16.6
1997	92.8	64.9	43.5	26.2	18.4	16.6
1998	93.1	65.1	43.0	26.1	18.2	16.5
1999	93.4	65.5	42.5	26.1	18.1	16.4
2000	93.7	66.0	42.1	25.9	17.9	16.2
2001	94.0	66.5	41.6	25.4	17.6	16.0
2002	94.3	66.5	41.3	24.8	17.2	15.8

[1]As of January 1.

NOTES: Data are based on cohort fertility. See Appendix II, Cohort fertility. Percents are derived from the cumulative childbearing experience of cohorts of women, up to the ages specified. Data on births are adjusted for underregistration and population estimates are corrected for underregistration and misstatement of age. Beginning in 1970 births to persons who were not residents of the 50 States and the District of Columbia are excluded.

SOURCES: Centers for Disease Control and Prevention, National Center for Health Statistics, National Vital Statistics System, Birth File. Table 1–32 at www.cdc.gov/nchs/datawh/statab/unpubd/natality/natab99.htm; *Vital statistics of the United States, 2001, vol 1, natality.* In preparation, forthcoming on CD-ROM.

Table 5. Live births, according to detailed race and Hispanic origin of mother: United States, selected years 1970–2001

[Data are based on birth certificates]

Race and Hispanic origin of mother	1970	1975	1980	1985	1990	1995	1999	2000	2001
	Total number of live births								
All races.	3,731,386	3,144,198	3,612,258	3,760,561	4,158,212	3,899,589	3,959,417	4,058,814	4,025,933
White.	3,109,956	2,576,818	2,936,351	3,037,913	3,290,273	3,098,885	3,132,501	3,194,005	3,177,626
Black or African American	561,992	496,829	568,080	581,824	684,336	603,139	605,970	622,598	606,156
American Indian or Alaska Native	22,264	22,690	29,389	34,037	39,051	37,278	40,170	41,668	41,872
Asian or Pacific Islander	- - -	- - -	74,355	104,606	141,635	160,287	180,776	200,543	200,279
Chinese	7,044	7,778	11,671	16,405	22,737	27,380	28,853	34,271	31,401
Japanese	7,744	6,725	7,482	8,035	8,674	8,901	8,722	8,969	9,048
Filipino	8,066	10,359	13,968	20,058	25,770	30,551	30,677	32,107	32,468
Hawaiian.	- - -	- - -	4,669	4,938	6,099	5,787	6,093	6,608	6,411
Other Asian or Pacific Islander	- - -	- - -	36,565	55,170	78,355	87,668	106,431	118,588	120,951
Hispanic or Latino[1]	- - -	- - -	307,163	372,814	595,073	679,768	764,339	815,868	851,851
Mexican	- - -	- - -	215,439	242,976	385,640	469,615	540,674	581,915	611,000
Puerto Rican.	- - -	- - -	33,671	35,147	58,807	54,824	57,138	58,124	57,568
Cuban.	- - -	- - -	7,163	10,024	11,311	12,473	13,088	13,429	14,017
Central and South American	- - -	- - -	21,268	40,985	83,008	94,996	103,307	113,344	121,365
Other and unknown Hispanic or Latino.	- - -	- - -	29,622	43,682	56,307	47,860	50,132	49,056	47,901
Not Hispanic or Latino:[1]									
White	- - -	- - -	1,245,221	1,394,729	2,626,500	2,382,638	2,346,450	2,362,968	2,326,578
Black or African American.	- - -	- - -	299,646	336,029	661,701	587,781	588,981	604,346	589,917

- - - Data not available.

[1]Prior to 1993, data from States lacking an Hispanic-origin item on the birth certificate were excluded (see Appendix II, Hispanic origin).

NOTES: The race groups, white, black, American Indian or Alaska Native, and Asian or Pacific Islander, include persons of Hispanic and non-Hispanic origin. Persons of Hispanic origin may be of any race. Interpretation of trend data should take into consideration expansion of reporting areas and immigration. Data for additional years are available (see Appendix III).

SOURCES: Centers for Disease Control and Prevention, National Center for Health Statistics, National Vital Statistics System, Birth File. Martin JA, Hamilton BE, Ventura SJ, Menacker F, Park MM, Sutton PD. Births: Final Data for 2001. National vital statistics reports; vol 51, no 2. Hyattsville, Maryland: National Center for Health Statistics, 2002; Births: Final data for each data year 1997–2000. National vital statistics reports. Hyattsville, Maryland; Final natality statistics for each data year 1970–96. Monthly vital statistics report. Hyattsville, Maryland.

Table 6. Prenatal care for live births, according to detailed race and Hispanic origin of mother: United States, selected years 1970–2001

[Data are based on birth certificates]

Prenatal care, race, and Hispanic origin of mother	1970	1975	1980	1985	1990	1995	1996	1997	1998	1999	2000	2001
Prenatal care began during 1st trimester					Percent of live births[1]							
All races	68.0	72.4	76.3	76.2	75.8	81.3	81.9	82.5	82.8	83.2	83.2	83.4
White	72.3	75.8	79.2	79.3	79.2	83.6	84.0	84.7	84.8	85.1	85.0	85.2
Black or African American	44.2	55.5	62.4	61.5	60.6	70.4	71.4	72.3	73.3	74.1	74.3	74.5
American Indian or Alaska Native	38.2	45.4	55.8	57.5	57.9	66.7	67.7	68.1	68.8	69.5	69.3	69.3
Asian or Pacific Islander	- - -	- - -	73.7	74.1	75.1	79.9	81.2	82.1	83.1	83.7	84.0	84.0
Chinese	71.8	76.7	82.6	82.0	81.3	85.7	86.8	87.4	88.5	88.5	87.6	87.0
Japanese	78.1	82.7	86.1	84.7	87.0	89.7	89.3	89.3	90.2	90.7	91.0	90.1
Filipino	60.6	70.6	77.3	76.5	77.1	80.9	82.5	83.3	84.2	84.2	84.9	85.0
Hawaiian	- - -	- - -	68.8	67.7	65.8	75.9	78.5	78.0	78.8	79.6	79.9	79.1
Other Asian or Pacific Islander	- - -	- - -	67.4	69.9	71.9	77.0	78.4	79.7	80.9	81.8	82.5	82.7
Hispanic or Latino[2]	- - -	- - -	60.2	61.2	60.2	70.8	72.2	73.7	74.3	74.4	74.4	75.7
Mexican	- - -	- - -	59.6	60.0	57.8	69.1	70.7	72.1	72.8	73.1	72.9	74.6
Puerto Rican	- - -	- - -	55.1	58.3	63.5	74.0	75.0	76.5	76.9	77.7	78.5	79.1
Cuban	- - -	- - -	82.7	82.5	84.8	89.2	89.2	90.4	91.8	91.4	91.7	91.8
Central and South American	- - -	- - -	58.8	60.6	61.5	73.2	75.0	76.9	78.0	77.6	77.6	77.4
Other and unknown Hispanic or Latino	- - -	- - -	66.4	65.8	66.4	74.3	74.6	76.0	74.8	74.8	75.8	77.3
Not Hispanic or Latino:[2]												
White	- - -	- - -	81.2	81.4	83.3	87.1	87.4	87.9	87.9	88.4	88.5	88.5
Black or African American	- - -	- - -	60.7	60.1	60.7	70.4	71.5	72.3	73.3	74.1	74.3	74.5
Prenatal care began during 3d trimester or no prenatal care												
All races	7.9	6.0	5.1	5.7	6.1	4.2	4.0	3.9	3.9	3.8	3.9	3.7
White	6.3	5.0	4.3	4.8	4.9	3.5	3.3	3.2	3.3	3.2	3.3	3.2
Black or African American	16.6	10.5	8.9	10.2	11.3	7.6	7.3	7.3	7.0	6.6	6.7	6.5
American Indian or Alaska Native	28.9	22.4	15.2	12.9	12.9	9.5	8.6	8.6	8.5	8.2	8.6	8.2
Asian or Pacific Islander	- - -	- - -	6.5	6.5	5.8	4.3	3.9	3.8	3.6	3.5	3.3	3.4
Chinese	6.5	4.4	3.7	4.4	3.4	3.0	2.5	2.4	2.2	2.0	2.2	2.4
Japanese	4.1	2.7	2.1	3.1	2.9	2.3	2.2	2.7	2.1	2.1	1.8	2.0
Filipino	7.2	4.1	4.0	4.8	4.5	4.1	3.3	3.3	3.1	2.8	3.0	3.0
Hawaiian	- - -	- - -	6.7	7.4	8.7	5.1	5.0	5.4	4.7	4.0	4.2	4.8
Other Asian or Pacific Islander	- - -	- - -	9.3	8.2	7.1	5.0	4.6	4.4	4.2	4.1	3.8	3.8
Hispanic or Latino[2]	- - -	- - -	12.0	12.4	12.0	7.4	6.7	6.2	6.3	6.3	6.3	5.9
Mexican	- - -	- - -	11.8	12.9	13.2	8.1	7.2	6.7	6.8	6.7	6.9	6.2
Puerto Rican	- - -	- - -	16.2	15.5	10.6	5.5	5.7	5.4	5.1	5.0	4.5	4.6
Cuban	- - -	- - -	3.9	3.7	2.8	2.1	1.6	1.5	1.2	1.4	1.4	1.3
Central and South American	- - -	- - -	13.1	12.5	10.9	6.1	5.5	5.0	4.9	5.2	5.4	5.7
Other and unknown Hispanic or Latino	- - -	- - -	9.2	9.4	8.5	6.0	5.9	5.3	6.0	6.3	5.9	5.4
Not Hispanic or Latino:[2]												
White	- - -	- - -	3.5	4.0	3.4	2.5	2.4	2.4	2.4	2.3	2.3	2.2
Black or African American	- - -	- - -	9.7	10.9	11.2	7.6	7.3	7.3	7.0	6.6	6.7	6.5

- - - Data not available.

[1]Excludes live births for whom trimester when prenatal care began is unknown.

[2]Prior to 1993, data from States lacking an Hispanic-origin item on the birth certificate were excluded (see Appendix II, Hispanic origin).

NOTES: Data for 1970 and 1975 exclude births that occurred in States not reporting prenatal care. The race groups, white, black, American Indian or Alaska Native, and Asian or Pacific Islander, include persons of Hispanic and non-Hispanic origin. Persons of Hispanic origin may be of any race. Interpretation of trend data should take into consideration expansion of reporting areas and immigration. See Appendix II, Hispanic origin and Prenatal care. Data for additional years are available (see Appendix III).

SOURCES: Centers for Disease Control and Prevention, National Center for Health Statistics, National Vital Statistics System, Birth File. Martin JA, Hamilton BE, Ventura SJ, Menacker F, Park MM, Sutton PD. Births: Final Data for 2001. National vital statistics reports; vol 51, no 2. Hyattsville, Maryland: National Center for Health Statistics, 2002; Births: Final data for each data year 1997–2000. National vital statistics reports. Hyattsville, Maryland; Final natality statistics for each data year 1970–96. Monthly vital statistics report. Hyattsville, Maryland.

Table 7 (page 1 of 2). Early prenatal care according to race and Hispanic origin of mother, geographic division, and State: United States, average annual 1993–95, 1996–98, and 1999–2001

[Data are based on birth certificates]

	All races			Not Hispanic or Latino					
				White			Black or African American		
Geographic division and State	1993–95	1996–98	1999–2001	1993–95	1996–98	1999–2001	1993–95	1996–98	1999–2001
	Percent of live births with early prenatal care (beginning in the 1st trimester)								
United States	80.1	82.4	83.2	86.4	87.7	88.5	68.2	72.4	74.3
New England	88.6	88.1	89.5	91.1	90.6	92.0	76.5	77.8	80.7
Maine.	88.8	89.3	88.7	89.2	89.7	89.0	80.2	84.3	80.1
New Hampshire	89.0	89.5	90.8	89.6	89.9	91.6	77.2	77.2	75.7
Vermont	86.1	87.6	88.5	86.4	87.8	88.8	62.7	*73.6	78.3
Massachusetts	88.8	87.4	89.5	91.7	90.4	92.4	76.7	76.3	79.3
Rhode Island	89.4	89.6	91.1	92.3	92.0	93.5	77.3	80.0	84.7
Connecticut	88.1	88.4	89.1	92.1	91.9	92.9	76.1	79.4	82.1
Middle Atlantic	79.1	81.7	82.0	87.0	88.2	88.4	63.0	68.3	69.7
New York	76.0	80.3	80.8	86.0	87.7	88.0	62.6	69.7	70.9
New Jersey	82.2	81.6	80.6	90.0	89.5	89.3	65.2	64.5	63.8
Pennsylvania	82.0	84.3	85.3	86.5	87.9	88.4	61.7	68.7	72.4
East North Central	82.0	83.4	84.0	86.6	87.5	88.2	66.9	70.1	71.7
Ohio	84.1	85.3	86.8	87.1	87.8	89.0	69.2	72.7	76.3
Indiana.	80.2	80.1	80.6	82.5	82.6	83.6	64.8	65.4	68.2
Illinois	80.1	82.2	82.9	88.1	89.3	89.9	65.9	69.5	71.4
Michigan	82.6	84.2	84.2	87.1	88.3	88.8	68.1	71.0	69.7
Wisconsin.	83.0	84.3	84.0	87.2	88.0	87.8	63.1	67.5	69.5
West North Central	84.0	85.2	86.0	86.9	88.0	89.0	68.3	72.4	75.3
Minnesota	83.2	84.0	84.6	86.6	87.4	88.7	57.7	65.0	66.7
Iowa	87.1	87.3	88.1	88.2	88.7	89.5	72.0	74.1	77.2
Missouri	83.5	85.9	87.5	86.7	88.4	89.7	68.6	73.4	78.0
North Dakota	83.2	85.0	86.2	84.8	87.1	88.9	83.8	76.8	76.9
South Dakota	81.2	82.2	80.1	84.9	86.0	84.3	74.3	70.5	67.6
Nebraska	83.5	84.1	83.6	86.3	87.0	87.0	68.9	72.0	69.9
Kansas.	84.7	85.6	86.5	88.0	89.1	90.0	73.1	76.0	78.5
South Atlantic.	81.5	84.3	84.6	87.6	89.5	89.9	69.4	74.3	76.0
Delaware	83.5	83.2	85.4	88.5	88.2	89.9	70.9	73.0	78.2
Maryland	86.6	88.3	85.7	92.1	92.9	91.4	76.0	79.8	77.4
District of Columbia	57.2	67.6	73.9	86.4	89.4	90.7	52.3	62.7	68.6
Virginia.	83.2	84.9	85.2	88.6	90.0	90.3	70.9	73.4	75.7
West Virginia	80.4	82.6	85.8	81.0	83.2	86.5	64.1	67.1	72.5
North Carolina	82.0	84.0	84.7	88.4	90.0	91.0	68.7	73.4	75.9
South Carolina	76.0	80.4	79.7	84.4	87.5	86.4	62.6	69.0	70.4
Georgia	81.6	85.8	86.8	87.8	91.0	91.7	72.1	78.6	80.8
Florida	81.3	83.6	83.9	86.7	88.6	89.1	69.3	72.6	74.0
East South Central	80.8	83.0	83.7	85.9	87.9	88.5	67.8	70.7	73.1
Kentucky	82.8	85.6	86.7	84.4	86.8	87.9	68.9	75.9	78.7
Tennessee	81.9	83.7	83.4	85.9	87.7	87.7	69.5	72.0	73.0
Alabama.	81.1	82.1	82.8	87.7	88.7	89.7	68.7	69.7	71.7
Mississippi	76.0	79.8	81.8	86.0	89.0	89.4	65.2	69.3	73.3
West South Central	75.7	78.9	79.9	83.6	85.8	86.9	67.9	72.1	74.5
Arkansas	75.2	76.1	79.5	80.0	80.7	83.6	60.6	63.8	69.5
Louisiana.	79.0	81.5	83.1	87.2	89.1	90.4	68.3	71.2	73.4
Oklahoma.	76.1	78.6	78.9	79.9	81.9	82.7	62.7	68.0	71.0
Texas.	74.9	78.6	79.5	84.2	86.8	87.6	69.6	74.8	76.7
Mountain	76.5	78.1	77.7	83.5	84.8	85.2	67.1	71.3	71.8
Montana.	81.2	82.5	83.2	83.7	84.9	86.1	79.1	75.9	86.5
Idaho	78.9	78.7	81.1	81.8	81.6	83.5	78.7	72.2	75.9
Wyoming	82.2	81.9	82.9	84.3	83.8	84.4	69.8	69.7	78.3
Colorado	80.2	82.2	80.7	85.4	87.5	87.8	70.1	76.4	74.3
New Mexico	66.7	69.2	68.1	76.8	77.8	75.7	59.6	62.3	64.6
Arizona	71.2	74.7	76.4	81.0	84.4	86.9	67.7	71.5	74.6
Utah	85.2	83.2	79.7	87.5	86.4	83.7	71.4	67.2	60.0
Nevada	74.7	76.1	75.1	81.0	83.3	84.5	63.2	66.8	67.6
Pacific.	78.4	81.7	84.0	85.1	86.8	88.1	75.4	79.0	81.4
Washington	82.0	83.2	82.9	85.1	86.0	86.0	73.9	77.0	75.8
Oregon.	79.1	80.4	81.2	81.7	83.1	84.2	70.8	78.4	76.4
California	77.7	81.6	84.5	85.6	87.7	89.7	75.4	79.0	81.8
Alaska	83.7	80.9	80.0	86.2	83.4	83.6	85.1	82.3	83.1
Hawaii	80.9	84.3	85.1	85.5	90.1	90.3	82.5	89.5	91.2

See footnotes at end of table.

Table 7 (page 2 of 2). Early prenatal care according to race and Hispanic origin of mother, geographic division, and State: United States, average annual 1993–95, 1996–98, and 1999–2001

[Data are based on birth certificates]

Geographic division and State	Hispanic or Latino[1]			American Indian or Alaska Native[2]			Asian or Pacific Islander[2]		
	1993–95	1996–98	1999–2001	1993–95	1996–98	1999–2001	1993–95	1996–98	1999–2001
	Percent of live births with early prenatal care (beginning in the 1st trimester)								
United States	68.8	73.4	74.9	65.1	68.2	69.4	79.1	82.2	83.9
New England	78.3	77.4	80.4	76.1	75.8	81.0	82.3	82.2	85.4
Maine.	77.5	80.2	80.6	77.2	72.9	76.2	79.7	81.5	86.8
New Hampshire	83.4	77.3	80.4	76.1	86.2	81.9	87.6	84.6	85.3
Vermont	78.2	82.8	82.2	*66.7	*79.3	*82.4	74.5	75.7	85.6
Massachusetts	78.7	75.9	80.2	77.0	71.1	82.3	81.7	81.0	84.7
Rhode Island	82.2	82.6	86.7	77.6	81.5	81.9	78.3	81.5	83.8
Connecticut	76.2	78.2	78.8	73.4	75.2	82.1	85.9	85.9	87.5
Middle Atlantic	63.8	70.7	71.6	71.5	74.2	77.1	74.5	77.8	78.5
New York	61.1	70.5	72.6	68.1	73.2	75.1	71.1	75.0	75.6
New Jersey	69.8	71.0	68.6	79.3	71.8	73.8	83.1	83.2	83.3
Pennsylvania	67.7	71.5	73.5	68.3	78.2	82.4	74.3	78.5	81.1
East North Central	69.7	72.4	72.6	70.3	72.6	75.2	77.7	82.1	83.4
Ohio	75.3	76.8	76.7	77.3	79.4	80.4	85.9	86.0	88.7
Indiana.	68.1	65.9	63.1	72.3	68.1	74.2	81.5	81.8	81.0
Illinois	69.1	72.6	74.0	68.9	75.1	77.8	81.0	85.2	85.0
Michigan	71.7	73.2	71.6	74.3	73.9	75.6	82.7	85.6	87.0
Wisconsin.	68.6	71.3	69.6	64.7	69.3	72.7	53.4	62.3	65.8
West North Central.	66.5	67.8	69.7	64.4	66.9	66.3	69.7	73.2	78.2
Minnesota	60.7	61.7	63.2	57.2	62.1	62.2	56.1	61.2	69.5
Iowa	71.9	71.0	73.3	69.3	69.9	74.7	82.6	82.0	83.7
Missouri	77.2	76.8	78.2	73.4	76.9	77.3	83.4	84.2	87.8
North Dakota	77.9	73.8	77.5	69.4	70.1	66.8	73.6	78.4	86.3
South Dakota	71.7	72.2	68.5	62.2	64.3	61.8	74.4	74.8	80.1
Nebraska	65.3	67.6	68.1	66.6	67.5	68.3	76.3	82.1	80.7
Kansas.	63.1	65.9	69.4	75.5	77.7	80.4	78.7	82.5	85.4
South Atlantic.	76.0	78.1	77.3	73.6	73.9	73.7	81.3	85.4	86.6
Delaware	68.2	68.7	72.3	80.9	*76.2	78.1	86.2	84.0	89.2
Maryland	80.6	81.4	77.3	80.9	84.0	82.6	87.4	89.5	87.0
District of Columbia	51.5	64.1	70.8	*	*	*	44.8	73.2	77.9
Virginia.	69.4	72.8	71.6	79.4	81.0	80.2	79.5	83.7	85.7
West Virginia	76.2	76.5	67.4	*64.1	*84.2	*74.4	79.9	82.2	80.4
North Carolina	68.2	68.5	69.1	74.5	72.5	76.5	80.1	81.9	83.5
South Carolina	66.0	65.9	61.7	65.9	76.1	77.4	76.8	76.0	79.5
Georgia	72.5	76.0	77.9	78.0	82.9	81.7	81.3	87.3	90.2
Florida	78.6	81.4	81.4	66.8	69.4	64.2	83.3	87.1	87.8
East South Central	71.4	66.7	60.8	73.8	75.7	78.6	80.7	83.4	84.6
Kentucky	76.1	74.0	68.6	78.2	79.4	85.2	81.1	84.6	87.2
Tennessee	69.9	64.5	58.5	69.6	73.8	78.2	81.9	84.0	83.1
Alabama.	69.1	62.5	55.7	75.7	80.0	79.4	81.9	83.4	86.7
Mississippi	74.8	77.1	73.4	74.6	72.8	75.8	74.6	80.1	83.0
West South Central	66.3	71.3	72.5	66.8	70.4	70.9	81.9	85.6	87.3
Arkansas	61.0	59.8	66.2	69.5	68.4	74.0	74.7	73.4	78.6
Louisiana	80.3	83.8	85.0	78.3	78.0	80.7	79.6	83.7	85.7
Oklahoma.	65.8	68.6	66.7	65.6	69.3	69.4	77.2	81.7	80.7
Texas.	66.2	71.4	72.6	69.1	74.1	74.6	82.9	86.6	88.4
Mountain	61.9	65.3	65.0	56.3	60.9	63.8	75.7	78.0	78.9
Montana.	72.6	76.7	79.3	63.1	66.4	65.6	76.1	79.7	80.4
Idaho.	59.0	61.2	66.9	57.6	59.3	67.5	79.7	78.2	80.4
Wyoming	67.2	71.1	73.5	65.6	65.1	71.8	80.5	84.4	82.2
Colorado	65.2	68.3	65.5	65.7	71.9	68.3	75.5	80.0	82.6
New Mexico	63.2	66.2	66.5	50.9	55.6	58.8	72.7	74.3	75.0
Arizona	59.2	64.1	65.7	56.0	61.0	65.9	78.3	82.4	84.5
Utah	68.0	64.5	61.3	60.7	59.0	55.3	71.7	69.8	64.7
Nevada	61.0	64.0	61.8	63.7	70.3	67.4	76.9	78.5	79.2
Pacific.	70.9	76.6	80.3	71.0	72.7	72.5	80.5	83.5	85.5
Washington	66.1	70.8	71.8	69.5	72.1	72.0	77.4	80.5	81.6
Oregon.	62.6	66.6	69.2	64.4	66.2	68.7	77.7	80.2	81.8
California	71.1	77.0	81.0	68.2	71.8	73.9	81.1	84.2	86.5
Alaska	82.5	78.1	80.8	76.9	75.7	71.3	81.3	75.2	76.4
Hawaii	78.3	83.0	83.7	81.3	82.9	83.4	79.2	82.3	83.4

* Percents preceded by an asterisk are based on fewer than 50 events. Percents not shown are based on fewer than 20 events.
[1] Persons of Hispanic origin may be of any race.
[2] Includes persons of Hispanic and non-Hispanic origin.

SOURCE: Centers for Disease Control and Prevention, National Center for Health Statistics, National Vital Statistics System, Birth File.

Table 8. Teenage childbearing, according to detailed race and Hispanic origin of mother: United States, selected years 1970–2001

[Data are based on birth certificates]

Maternal age, race, and Hispanic origin of mother	1970	1975	1980	1985	1990	1995	1996	1997	1998	1999	2000	2001
Age of mother under 18 years						Percent of live births						
All races	6.3	7.6	5.8	4.7	4.7	5.3	5.1	4.9	4.6	4.4	4.1	3.8
White	4.8	6.0	4.5	3.7	3.6	4.3	4.2	4.1	3.9	3.7	3.5	3.3
Black or African American	14.8	16.3	12.5	10.6	10.1	10.8	10.3	9.7	8.9	8.2	7.8	7.3
American Indian or Alaska Native	7.5	11.2	9.4	7.6	7.2	8.7	8.7	8.6	8.4	7.9	7.3	6.8
Asian or Pacific Islander	---	---	1.5	1.6	2.1	2.2	2.1	2.0	2.0	1.8	1.5	1.3
Chinese	1.1	0.4	0.3	0.3	0.4	0.3	0.3	0.3	0.3	0.2	0.2	0.2
Japanese	2.0	1.7	1.0	0.9	0.8	0.8	0.9	0.8	0.8	0.7	0.6	0.5
Filipino	3.7	2.4	1.6	1.6	2.0	2.2	2.1	2.1	2.1	1.8	1.6	1.5
Hawaiian	---	---	6.6	5.7	6.5	7.6	6.8	6.7	7.8	6.2	5.7	4.9
Other Asian or Pacific Islander	---	---	1.2	1.8	2.4	2.5	2.5	2.3	2.3	2.0	1.7	1.5
Hispanic or Latino[1]	---	---	7.4	6.4	6.6	7.6	7.3	7.2	6.9	6.7	6.3	5.8
Mexican	---	---	7.7	6.9	6.9	8.0	7.7	7.6	7.2	7.0	6.6	6.2
Puerto Rican	---	---	10.0	8.5	9.1	10.8	10.2	9.5	9.2	8.5	7.8	7.4
Cuban	---	---	3.8	2.2	2.7	2.8	2.8	2.7	2.9	2.9	3.1	2.7
Central and South American	---	---	2.4	2.4	3.2	4.1	4.0	3.9	3.6	3.5	3.3	3.1
Other and unknown Hispanic or Latino	---	---	6.5	7.0	8.0	9.0	8.8	8.9	8.8	8.1	7.6	6.8
Not Hispanic or Latino:[1]												
White	---	---	4.0	3.2	3.0	3.4	3.3	3.2	3.0	2.8	2.6	2.3
Black or African American	---	---	12.7	10.7	10.2	10.8	10.4	9.8	9.0	8.3	7.8	7.3
Age of mother 18–19 years												
All races	11.3	11.3	9.8	8.0	8.1	7.9	7.9	7.8	7.9	7.9	7.7	7.5
White	10.4	10.3	9.0	7.1	7.3	7.2	7.2	7.1	7.2	7.2	7.1	6.9
Black or African American	16.6	16.9	14.5	12.9	13.0	12.4	12.5	12.5	12.6	12.4	11.9	11.5
American Indian or Alaska Native	12.8	15.2	14.6	12.4	12.3	12.7	12.3	12.2	12.5	12.3	12.4	12.5
Asian or Pacific Islander	---	---	3.9	3.4	3.7	3.5	3.2	3.2	3.3	3.3	3.0	3.0
Chinese	3.9	1.7	1.0	0.6	0.8	0.6	0.6	0.6	0.6	0.7	0.7	0.8
Japanese	4.1	3.3	2.3	1.9	2.0	1.7	1.6	1.5	1.6	1.4	1.4	1.2
Filipino	7.1	5.0	4.0	3.7	4.1	4.1	4.0	3.8	4.1	4.0	3.7	3.6
Hawaiian	---	---	13.3	12.3	11.9	11.5	11.6	11.9	11.0	11.9	11.7	11.3
Other Asian or Pacific Islander	---	---	3.8	3.5	3.9	3.8	3.4	3.3	3.5	3.5	3.2	3.1
Hispanic or Latino[1]	---	---	11.6	10.1	10.2	10.3	10.1	9.8	10.0	10.0	9.9	9.7
Mexican	---	---	12.0	10.6	10.7	10.8	10.5	10.2	10.3	10.4	10.4	10.3
Puerto Rican	---	---	13.3	12.4	12.6	12.7	13.0	12.7	12.7	12.6	12.2	11.8
Cuban	---	---	9.2	4.9	5.0	4.9	4.9	4.7	4.0	4.8	4.4	4.8
Central and South American	---	---	6.0	5.8	5.9	6.5	6.5	6.5	6.6	6.5	6.5	6.3
Other and unknown Hispanic or Latino	---	---	10.8	10.5	11.1	11.1	11.1	10.9	11.4	11.4	11.3	10.5
Not Hispanic or Latino:[1]												
White	---	---	8.5	6.6	6.6	6.4	6.4	6.3	6.4	6.4	6.1	5.9
Black or African American	---	---	14.7	12.9	13.0	12.4	12.6	12.6	12.7	12.5	12.0	11.6

\- - - Data not available.

[1]Prior to 1993, data from States lacking an Hispanic-origin item on the birth certificate were excluded (see Appendix II, Hispanic origin).

NOTES: The race groups, white, black, American Indian or Alaska Native, and Asian or Pacific Islander, include persons of Hispanic and non-Hispanic origin. Persons of Hispanic origin may be of any race. Interpretation of trend data should take into consideration expansion of reporting areas and immigration. Data for additional years are available (see Appendix III).

SOURCES: Centers for Disease Control and Prevention, National Center for Health Statistics, National Vital Statistics System, Birth File. Martin JA, Hamilton BE, Ventura SJ, Menacker F, Park MM, Sutton PD. Births: Final Data for 2001. National vital statistics reports; vol 51, no 2. Hyattsville, Maryland: National Center for Health Statistics, 2002; Births: Final data for each data year 1997–2000. National vital statistics reports. Hyattsville, Maryland; Final natality statistics for each data year 1970–96. Monthly vital statistics report. Hyattsville, Maryland.

Table 9. Nonmarital childbearing according to detailed race and Hispanic origin of mother, and maternal age: United States, selected years 1970–2001

[Data are based on birth certificates]

Race, Hispanic origin of mother, and maternal age	1970	1975	1980	1985	1990	1995	1996	1997	1998	1999	2000	2001
	Live births per 1,000 unmarried women 15–44 years of age[1]											
All races and origins	26.4	24.5	29.4	32.8	43.8	45.1	44.8	44.0	44.3	44.4	45.2	45.0
White[2]	13.9	12.4	18.1	22.5	32.9	37.5	37.6	37.0	37.5	38.1	38.9	39.2
Black or African American[2]	95.5	84.2	81.1	77.0	90.5	75.9	74.4	73.4	73.3	71.5	72.5	70.1
Hispanic or Latino[3]	- - -	- - -	- - -	- - -	89.6	95.0	93.2	91.4	90.1	93.4	97.3	98.0
White, not Hispanic or Latino	- - -	- - -	- - -	- - -	- - -	28.2	28.3	27.0	27.4	27.9	27.9	27.7
	Percent of live births to unmarried mothers											
All races	10.7	14.3	18.4	22.0	28.0	32.2	32.4	32.4	32.8	33.0	33.2	33.5
White.	5.5	7.1	11.2	14.7	20.4	25.3	25.7	25.8	26.3	26.8	27.1	27.7
Black or African American	37.5	49.5	56.1	61.2	66.5	69.9	69.8	69.2	69.1	68.9	68.5	68.4
American Indian or Alaska Native	22.4	32.7	39.2	46.8	53.6	57.2	58.0	58.7	59.3	58.9	58.4	59.7
Asian or Pacific Islander	- - -	- - -	7.3	9.5	13.2	16.3	16.7	15.6	15.6	15.4	14.8	14.9
Chinese	3.0	1.6	2.7	3.0	5.0	7.9	9.2	6.5	6.4	6.9	7.6	8.4
Japanese	4.6	4.6	5.2	7.9	9.6	10.8	11.4	10.1	9.7	9.9	9.5	9.2
Filipino	9.1	6.9	8.6	11.4	15.9	19.5	19.4	19.5	19.7	21.1	20.3	20.4
Hawaiian	- - -	- - -	32.9	37.3	45.0	49.0	49.9	49.1	51.1	50.4	50.0	50.6
Other Asian or Pacific Islander	- - -	- - -	5.4	8.5	12.6	16.2	16.5	15.6	15.2	14.5	13.8	13.7
Hispanic or Latino[3]	- - -	- - -	23.6	29.5	36.7	40.8	40.7	40.9	41.6	42.2	42.7	42.5
Mexican.	- - -	- - -	20.3	25.7	33.3	38.1	37.9	38.9	39.6	40.1	40.7	40.8
Puerto Rican.	- - -	- - -	46.3	51.1	55.9	60.0	60.7	59.4	59.5	59.6	59.6	58.9
Cuban	- - -	- - -	10.0	16.1	18.2	23.8	24.7	24.4	24.8	26.4	27.3	27.2
Central and South American	- - -	- - -	27.1	34.9	41.2	44.1	44.1	41.8	42.0	43.7	44.7	44.3
Other and unknown Hispanic or Latino	- - -	- - -	22.4	31.1	37.2	44.0	43.5	43.6	45.3	45.8	46.2	44.2
Not Hispanic or Latino:[3]												
White.	- - -	- - -	9.6	12.4	16.9	21.2	21.5	21.5	21.9	22.1	22.1	22.5
Black or African American.	- - -	- - -	57.3	62.1	66.7	70.0	70.0	69.4	69.3	69.1	68.7	68.6
	Number of live births, in thousands											
Live births to unmarried mothers	399	448	666	828	1,165	1,254	1,260	1,257	1,294	1,309	1,347	1,349
Maternal age	Percent distribution of live births to unmarried mothers											
Under 20 years.	50.1	52.1	40.8	33.8	30.9	30.9	30.4	30.7	30.1	29.3	28.0	26.6
20–24 years.	31.8	29.9	35.6	36.3	34.7	34.5	34.2	34.9	35.6	36.4	37.4	38.2
25 years and over.	18.1	18.0	23.5	29.9	34.4	34.7	35.3	34.4	34.3	34.3	34.6	35.2

- - - Data not available.

[1]Rates computed by relating births to unmarried mothers, regardless of age of mother, to unmarried women 15–44 years of age. Population data for American Indian or Alaska Native and Asian or Pacific Islander women not available for rate calculations.

[2]For 1970 and 1975, birth rates are by race of child.

[3]Prior to 1993, data from States lacking an Hispanic-origin item on the birth certificate were excluded (see Appendix II, Hispanic origin).

NOTES: National estimates for 1970 and 1975 for unmarried mothers based on births occurring in States reporting marital status of mother (see Appendix II, Marital status). The race groups, white, black, American Indian or Alaska Native, and Asian or Pacific Islander, include persons of Hispanic and non-Hispanic origin. Persons of Hispanic origin may be of any race. Changes in reporting procedures for marital status have occurred in some States during the 1990s. Interpretation of trend data should also take into consideration expansion of reporting areas and immigration. Data for additional years are available (see Appendix III).

SOURCES: Centers for Disease Control and Prevention, National Center for Health Statistics, National Vital Statistics System, Birth File. Martin JA, Hamilton BE, Ventura SJ, Menacker F, Park MM, Sutton PD. Births: Final Data for 2001. National vital statistics reports; vol 51, no 2. Hyattsville, Maryland: National Center for Health Statistics, 2002; Births: Final data for each data year 1997–2000. National vital statistics reports. Hyattsville, Maryland; Final natality statistics for each data year 1993–96. Monthly vital statistics report. Hyattsville, Maryland; Ventura SJ. Births to unmarried mothers: United States, 1980–92. Vital Health Stat 21(53). 1995.

Table 10. Maternal education for live births, according to detailed race and Hispanic origin of mother: United States, selected years 1970–2001

[Data are based on birth certificates]

Education, race, and Hispanic origin of mother	1970	1975	1980	1985	1990	1995	1996	1997	1998	1999	2000	2001
Less than 12 years of education					Percent of live births[1]							
All races	30.8	28.6	23.7	20.6	23.8	22.6	22.4	22.1	21.9	21.7	21.7	21.7
White	27.1	25.1	20.8	17.8	22.4	21.6	21.6	21.3	21.2	21.3	21.4	21.7
Black or African American	51.2	45.3	36.4	32.6	30.2	28.7	28.2	27.6	26.9	26.0	25.5	24.9
American Indian or Alaska Native	60.5	52.7	44.2	39.0	36.4	33.0	33.0	32.8	32.7	32.2	31.6	31.0
Asian or Pacific Islander	- - -	- - -	21.0	19.4	20.0	16.1	15.0	14.0	12.9	12.4	11.6	10.8
Chinese	23.0	16.5	15.2	15.5	15.8	12.9	12.8	12.3	11.4	12.0	11.7	11.9
Japanese	11.8	9.1	5.0	4.8	3.5	2.6	2.7	2.3	2.4	2.0	2.1	1.8
Filipino	26.4	22.3	16.4	13.9	10.3	8.0	7.4	7.3	6.9	6.3	6.2	6.0
Hawaiian	- - -	- - -	20.7	18.7	19.3	17.6	16.9	16.8	18.5	16.8	16.7	15.4
Other Asian or Pacific Islander	- - -	- - -	27.6	24.3	26.8	21.2	19.4	17.8	15.9	14.8	13.5	12.2
Hispanic or Latino[2]	- - -	- - -	51.1	44.5	53.9	52.1	51.4	50.3	49.3	49.1	48.9	48.8
Mexican	- - -	- - -	62.8	59.0	61.4	58.6	57.7	56.3	55.2	55.2	55.0	55.0
Puerto Rican	- - -	- - -	55.3	46.6	42.7	38.6	38.1	37.1	35.9	34.4	33.4	32.3
Cuban	- - -	- - -	24.1	21.1	17.8	14.4	14.5	13.7	13.0	12.3	11.9	11.8
Central and South American	- - -	- - -	41.2	37.0	44.2	41.7	40.8	39.6	38.5	37.9	37.2	36.5
Other and unknown Hispanic or Latino	- - -	- - -	40.1	36.5	33.3	33.8	33.0	32.8	33.6	32.5	31.4	30.4
Not Hispanic or Latino:[2]												
White	- - -	- - -	18.3	15.8	15.2	13.3	13.0	12.9	12.8	12.6	12.2	12.0
Black or African American	- - -	- - -	37.4	33.5	30.0	28.6	28.0	27.5	26.7	25.9	25.3	24.8
16 years or more of education												
All races	8.6	11.4	14.0	16.7	17.5	21.4	22.1	22.8	23.4	24.1	24.7	25.2
White	9.6	12.7	15.5	18.6	19.3	23.1	23.9	24.6	25.1	25.7	26.3	26.7
Black or African American	2.8	4.3	6.2	7.0	7.2	9.5	10.0	10.5	11.0	11.4	11.7	12.1
American Indian or Alaska Native	2.7	2.2	3.5	3.7	4.4	6.2	6.3	6.8	6.8	7.2	7.8	8.2
Asian or Pacific Islander	- - -	- - -	30.8	30.3	31.0	35.0	36.2	38.0	39.7	40.9	42.8	44.0
Chinese	34.0	37.8	41.5	35.2	40.3	49.0	49.1	51.1	53.8	54.3	55.6	55.9
Japanese	20.7	30.6	36.8	38.1	44.1	46.2	46.8	48.3	49.1	49.5	51.1	52.0
Filipino	28.1	36.6	37.1	35.2	34.5	36.7	38.0	38.6	39.2	39.6	40.5	41.8
Hawaiian	- - -	- - -	7.9	6.5	6.8	9.7	11.3	11.0	11.0	12.7	13.5	13.2
Other Asian or Pacific Islander	- - -	- - -	29.2	30.2	27.3	30.5	32.2	34.4	36.7	38.5	40.7	42.6
Hispanic or Latino[2]	- - -	- - -	4.2	6.0	5.1	6.1	6.4	6.7	7.0	7.4	7.6	7.9
Mexican	- - -	- - -	2.2	3.0	3.3	4.0	4.2	4.5	4.7	5.0	5.1	5.3
Puerto Rican	- - -	- - -	3.0	4.6	6.5	8.7	8.9	9.2	9.5	10.3	10.4	11.1
Cuban	- - -	- - -	11.6	15.0	20.4	26.5	27.0	27.8	28.6	29.9	31.0	30.8
Central and South American	- - -	- - -	6.1	8.1	8.6	10.3	11.2	11.9	12.5	13.2	14.1	14.8
Other and unknown Hispanic or Latino	- - -	- - -	5.5	7.2	8.5	10.5	11.1	11.7	11.5	12.0	12.5	13.2
Not Hispanic or Latino:[2]												
White	- - -	- - -	16.4	19.3	22.6	27.7	28.8	29.7	30.4	31.4	32.5	33.3
Black or African American	- - -	- - -	5.7	6.7	7.3	9.5	10.0	10.6	11.0	11.4	11.7	12.2

- - - Data not available.

[1] Excludes live births for whom education of mother is unknown.

[2] Prior to 1993, data shown only for States with an Hispanic-origin item and education of mother item on the birth certificate (see Appendix II, Education; Hispanic origin).

NOTES: Starting in 1992, education of mother was reported on the birth certificate by all 50 States and the District of Columbia. Prior to 1992, data from States lacking an education of mother item were excluded (see Appendix II, Education). The race groups, white, black, American Indian or Alaska Native, and Asian or Pacific Islander, include persons of Hispanic and non-Hispanic origin. Persons of Hispanic origin may be of any race. Maternal education groups shown in this table generally represent the group at highest risk for unfavorable birth outcomes (less than 12 years of education) and the group at lowest risk (16 years or more of education). Interpretation of trend data should take into consideration expansion of reporting areas and immigration. Data for additional years are available (see Appendix III).

SOURCE: Centers for Disease Control and Prevention, National Center for Health Statistics, National Vital Statistics System, Birth File.

Table 11. Mothers who smoked cigarettes during pregnancy, according to mother's detailed race, Hispanic origin, age, and education: Selected States, 1989–2001

[Data are based on birth certificates]

Characteristic of mother	1989	1990	1995	1996	1997	1998	1999	2000	2001
Race of mother[1]	Percent of mothers who smoked[2]								
All races	19.5	18.4	13.9	13.6	13.2	12.9	12.6	12.2	12.0
White	20.4	19.4	15.0	14.7	14.3	14.0	13.6	13.2	13.0
Black or African American	17.1	15.9	10.6	10.2	9.7	9.5	9.3	9.1	9.0
American Indian or Alaska Native	23.0	22.4	20.9	21.3	20.8	20.2	20.2	20.0	19.9
Asian or Pacific Islander[3]	5.7	5.5	3.4	3.3	3.2	3.1	2.9	2.8	2.8
Chinese	2.7	2.0	0.8	0.7	1.0	0.8	0.5	0.6	0.7
Japanese	8.2	8.0	5.2	4.8	4.7	4.8	4.5	4.2	3.8
Filipino	5.1	5.3	3.4	3.5	3.4	3.3	3.3	3.2	3.2
Hawaiian	19.3	21.0	15.9	15.3	15.8	16.8	14.7	14.4	14.8
Other Asian or Pacific Islander	4.2	3.8	2.7	2.7	2.5	2.4	2.3	2.3	2.3
Hispanic origin and race of mother[4]									
Hispanic or Latino	8.0	6.7	4.3	4.3	4.1	4.0	3.7	3.5	3.2
Mexican	6.3	5.3	3.1	3.1	2.9	2.8	2.6	2.4	2.4
Puerto Rican	14.5	13.6	10.4	11.0	11.0	10.7	10.5	10.3	9.7
Cuban	6.9	6.4	4.1	4.7	4.2	3.7	3.3	3.3	3.0
Central and South American	3.6	3.0	1.8	1.8	1.8	1.5	1.4	1.5	1.3
Other and unknown Hispanic or Latino . .	12.1	10.8	8.2	9.1	8.5	8.0	7.7	7.4	6.8
Not Hispanic or Latino:									
White	21.7	21.0	17.1	16.9	16.5	16.2	15.9	15.6	15.5
Black or African American	17.2	15.9	10.6	10.3	9.8	9.6	9.4	9.2	9.1
Age of mother[1]									
Under 15 years	7.7	7.5	7.3	7.7	8.1	7.7	7.8	7.1	6.0
15–19 years	22.2	20.8	16.8	17.2	17.6	17.8	18.1	17.8	17.5
15–17 years	19.0	17.6	14.6	15.4	15.5	15.5	15.5	15.0	14.4
18–19 years	23.9	22.5	18.1	18.3	18.8	19.2	19.5	19.2	19.0
20–24 years	23.5	22.1	17.1	16.8	16.6	16.5	16.7	16.8	17.0
25–29 years	19.0	18.0	12.8	12.3	11.8	11.4	11.0	10.5	10.3
30–34 years	15.7	15.3	11.4	10.9	10.0	9.3	8.6	8.0	7.6
35–39 years	13.6	13.3	12.0	11.7	11.1	10.6	9.9	9.1	8.6
40–54 years[5]	13.2	12.3	10.1	10.1	10.1	10.0	9.5	9.5	9.3
Education of mother[6]	Percent of mothers 20 years of age and over who smoked[2]								
0–8 years	18.9	17.5	11.0	10.3	9.9	9.5	8.9	7.9	7.2
9–11 years	42.2	40.5	32.0	31.1	30.2	29.3	29.0	28.2	27.6
12 years	22.8	21.9	18.3	18.0	17.5	17.1	16.9	16.6	16.5
13–15 years	13.7	12.8	10.6	10.4	9.9	9.6	9.4	9.1	9.2
16 years or more	5.0	4.5	2.7	2.6	2.4	2.2	2.1	2.0	1.9

[1]Data from States that did not require the reporting of mother's tobacco use during pregnancy on the birth certificate are not included. Reporting area for tobacco use increased from 43 States and the District of Columbia (DC) in 1989 to 49 States and DC in 2000–01 (see Appendix II, Tobacco use).
[2]Excludes live births for whom smoking status of mother is unknown.
[3]Maternal tobacco use during pregnancy was not reported on the birth certificates of California, which in 2000 accounted for 32 percent of the births to Asian or Pacific Islander mothers.
[4]Data from States that did not require the reporting of either Hispanic origin of mother or tobacco use during pregnancy on the birth certificate are not included. Reporting area for tobacco use and Hispanic origin of mother increased from 42 States and DC in 1989 to 49 States and DC in 2000–01. See Appendix II, Hispanic origin; Tobacco use.
[5]Prior to 1997 data are for live births to mothers 45–49 years of age.
[6]Data from States that did not require the reporting of either mother's education or tobacco use during pregnancy on the birth certificate are not included. Reporting area for tobacco use and education of mother increased from 42 States and DC in 1989 to 49 States and DC in 2000–01. See Appendix II, Education; Hispanic origin).

NOTES: The race groups, white, black, American Indian or Alaska Native, and Asian or Pacific Islander, include persons of Hispanic and non-Hispanic origin. Persons of Hispanic origin may be of any race. Interpretation of trend data should take into consideration expansion of reporting areas and immigration. Data for additional years are available (see Appendix III).

SOURCES: Centers for Disease Control and Prevention, National Center for Health Statistics, National Vital Statistics System, Birth File. Martin JA, Hamilton BE, Ventura SJ, Menacker F, Park MM, Sutton PD. Births: Final Data for 2001. National vital statistics reports; vol 51, no 2. Hyattsville, Maryland: National Center for Health Statistics, 2002; Births: Final data for each data year 1997–2000. National vital statistics reports. Hyattsville, Maryland; Final natality statistics for each data year 1989–96. Monthly vital statistics report. Hyattsville, Maryland.

Table 12. Low-birthweight live births, according to mother's detailed race, Hispanic origin, and smoking status: United States, selected years 1970–2001

[Data are based on birth certificates]

Birthweight, race, Hispanic origin of mother, and smoking status of mother	1970	1975	1980	1985	1990	1995	1996	1997	1998	1999	2000	2001
Low birthweight (less than 2,500 grams)					Percent of live births[1]							
All races	7.93	7.38	6.84	6.75	6.97	7.32	7.39	7.51	7.57	7.62	7.57	7.68
White	6.85	6.27	5.72	5.65	5.70	6.22	6.34	6.46	6.52	6.57	6.55	6.68
Black or African American	13.90	13.19	12.69	12.65	13.25	13.13	13.01	13.01	13.05	13.11	12.99	12.95
American Indian or Alaska Native	7.97	6.41	6.44	5.86	6.11	6.61	6.49	6.75	6.81	7.15	6.76	7.33
Asian or Pacific Islander	- - -	- - -	6.68	6.16	6.45	6.90	7.07	7.23	7.42	7.45	7.31	7.51
Chinese	6.67	5.29	5.21	4.98	4.69	5.29	5.03	5.06	5.34	5.19	5.10	5.33
Japanese	9.03	7.47	6.60	6.21	6.16	7.26	7.27	6.82	7.50	7.95	7.14	7.28
Filipino	10.02	8.08	7.40	6.95	7.30	7.83	7.92	8.33	8.23	8.30	8.46	8.66
Hawaiian	- - -	- - -	7.23	6.49	7.24	6.84	6.77	7.20	7.15	7.69	6.76	7.91
Other Asian or Pacific Islander	- - -	- - -	6.83	6.19	6.65	7.05	7.42	7.54	7.76	7.76	7.67	7.76
Hispanic or Latino[2]	- - -	- - -	6.12	6.16	6.06	6.29	6.28	6.42	6.44	6.38	6.41	6.47
Mexican	- - -	- - -	5.62	5.77	5.55	5.81	5.86	5.97	5.97	5.94	6.01	6.08
Puerto Rican	- - -	- - -	8.95	8.69	8.99	9.41	9.24	9.39	9.68	9.30	9.30	9.34
Cuban	- - -	- - -	5.62	6.02	5.67	6.50	6.46	6.78	6.50	6.80	6.49	6.49
Central and South American	- - -	- - -	5.76	5.68	5.84	6.20	6.03	6.26	6.47	6.38	6.34	6.49
Other and unknown Hispanic or Latino	- - -	- - -	6.96	6.83	6.87	7.55	7.68	7.93	7.59	7.63	7.84	7.96
Not Hispanic or Latino:[2]												
White	- - -	- - -	5.67	5.60	5.61	6.20	6.36	6.47	6.55	6.64	6.60	6.76
Black or African American	- - -	- - -	12.71	12.61	13.32	13.21	13.12	13.11	13.17	13.23	13.13	13.07
Cigarette smoker[3]	- - -	- - -	- - -	- - -	11.25	12.18	12.13	12.06	12.01	12.06	11.88	11.90
Nonsmoker[3]	- - -	- - -	- - -	- - -	6.14	6.79	6.91	7.07	7.18	7.21	7.19	7.32
Very low birthweight (less than 1,500 grams)												
All races	1.17	1.16	1.15	1.21	1.27	1.35	1.37	1.42	1.45	1.45	1.43	1.44
White	0.95	0.92	0.90	0.94	0.95	1.06	1.09	1.13	1.15	1.15	1.14	1.16
Black or African American	2.40	2.40	2.48	2.71	2.92	2.97	2.99	3.04	3.08	3.14	3.07	3.04
American Indian or Alaska Native	0.98	0.95	0.92	1.01	1.01	1.10	1.21	1.19	1.24	1.26	1.16	1.26
Asian or Pacific Islander	- - -	- - -	0.92	0.85	0.87	0.91	0.99	1.05	1.10	1.08	1.05	1.03
Chinese	0.80	0.52	0.66	0.57	0.51	0.67	0.64	0.74	0.75	0.68	0.77	0.69
Japanese	1.48	0.89	0.94	0.84	0.73	0.87	0.81	0.78	0.84	0.86	0.75	0.71
Filipino	1.08	0.93	0.99	0.86	1.05	1.13	1.20	1.29	1.35	1.41	1.38	1.23
Hawaiian	- - -	- - -	1.05	1.03	0.97	0.94	0.97	1.41	1.53	1.41	1.39	1.50
Other Asian or Pacific Islander	- - -	- - -	0.96	0.91	0.92	0.91	1.04	1.07	1.12	1.09	1.04	1.06
Hispanic or Latino[2]	- - -	- - -	0.98	1.01	1.03	1.11	1.12	1.13	1.15	1.14	1.14	1.14
Mexican	- - -	- - -	0.92	0.97	0.92	1.01	1.01	1.02	1.02	1.04	1.03	1.05
Puerto Rican	- - -	- - -	1.29	1.30	1.62	1.79	1.70	1.85	1.86	1.86	1.93	1.85
Cuban	- - -	- - -	1.02	1.18	1.20	1.19	1.35	1.36	1.33	1.49	1.21	1.27
Central and South American	- - -	- - -	0.99	1.01	1.05	1.13	1.14	1.17	1.23	1.15	1.20	1.19
Other and unknown Hispanic or Latino	- - -	- - -	1.01	0.96	1.09	1.28	1.48	1.35	1.38	1.32	1.42	1.27
Not Hispanic or Latino:[2]												
White	- - -	- - -	0.86	0.90	0.93	1.04	1.08	1.12	1.15	1.15	1.14	1.17
Black or African American	- - -	- - -	2.46	2.66	2.93	2.98	3.02	3.05	3.11	3.18	3.10	3.08
Cigarette smoker[3]	- - -	- - -	- - -	- - -	1.73	1.85	1.85	1.83	1.87	1.91	1.91	1.88
Nonsmoker[3]	- - -	- - -	- - -	- - -	1.18	1.31	1.35	1.40	1.44	1.43	1.40	1.42

- - - Data not available.

[1] Excludes live births with unknown birthweight. Percent based on live births with known birthweight.

[2] Prior to 1993, data from States lacking an Hispanic-origin item on the birth certificate were excluded (see Appendix II, Hispanic origin).

[3] Percent based on live births with known smoking status of mother and known birthweight. Data from States that did not require the reporting of mother's tobacco use during pregnancy on the birth certificate are not included. Reporting area for tobacco use increased from 43 States and the District of Columbia (DC) in 1989 to 49 States and DC in 2000–01 (see Appendix II, Tobacco use).

NOTES: The race groups, white, black, American Indian or Alaska Native, and Asian or Pacific Islander, include persons of Hispanic and non-Hispanic origin. Persons of Hispanic origin may be of any race. Interpretation of trend data should take into consideration expansion of reporting areas and immigration. Data for additional years are available (see Appendix III).

SOURCES: Centers for Disease Control and Prevention, National Center for Health Statistics, National Vital Statistics System, Birth File. Martin JA, Hamilton BE, Ventura SJ, Menacker F, Park MM, Sutton PD. Births: Final Data for 2001. National vital statistics reports; vol 51, no 2. Hyattsville, Maryland: National Center for Health Statistics, 2002; Births: Final data for each data year 1997–2000. National vital statistics reports. Hyattsville, Maryland; Final natality statistics for each data year 1970–96. Monthly vital statistics report. Hyattsville, Maryland.

Table 13. Low-birthweight live births among mothers 20 years of age and over, by mother's detailed race, Hispanic origin, and education: United States, selected years 1989–2001

[Data are based on birth certificates]

Education, race, and Hispanic origin of mother	1989	1990	1995	1996	1997	1998	1999	2000	2001
Less than 12 years of education	Percent of live births weighing less than 2,500 grams[1]								
All races	9.0	8.6	8.4	8.3	8.4	8.4	8.3	8.2	8.2
White	7.3	7.0	7.1	7.1	7.2	7.2	7.2	7.1	7.1
Black or African American	17.0	16.5	16.0	15.5	15.4	15.0	15.0	14.8	14.6
American Indian or Alaska Native	7.3	7.4	8.0	7.7	7.7	8.0	8.1	7.2	8.3
Asian or Pacific Islander	6.6	6.4	6.7	7.1	6.8	7.4	7.1	7.2	7.5
Chinese	5.4	5.2	5.3	5.0	5.1	5.9	5.2	5.3	4.9
Japanese	4.0	10.6	11.0	8.3	2.6	5.0	11.0	6.8	8.4
Filipino	6.9	7.2	7.5	8.0	7.8	7.9	8.4	8.6	8.5
Hawaiian	11.0	10.7	9.8	10.1	7.4	8.5	7.2	9.4	8.9
Other Asian or Pacific Islander	6.8	6.4	6.7	7.5	7.1	7.8	7.5	7.5	8.1
Hispanic or Latino[2]	6.0	5.7	5.8	5.8	5.9	5.9	5.9	6.0	6.0
Mexican	5.3	5.2	5.4	5.4	5.6	5.6	5.5	5.6	5.7
Puerto Rican	11.3	10.3	10.5	10.4	10.6	10.7	10.5	10.9	10.4
Cuban	9.4	7.9	9.2	8.0	9.5	7.4	6.7	8.4	6.7
Central and South American	5.8	5.8	6.2	6.0	5.8	6.2	6.0	6.2	6.4
Other and unknown Hispanic or Latino	8.2	8.0	7.7	8.0	8.3	7.7	8.0	8.6	8.2
Not Hispanic or Latino:[2]									
White	8.4	8.3	8.9	9.1	9.1	9.1	9.2	9.0	9.1
Black or African American	17.6	16.7	16.2	15.8	15.6	15.3	15.2	15.2	14.9
12 years of education									
All races	7.1	7.1	7.6	7.7	7.7	7.9	8.0	7.9	8.1
White	5.7	5.8	6.4	6.6	6.6	6.7	6.8	6.8	7.0
Black or African American	13.4	13.1	13.3	13.2	13.1	13.1	13.3	13.0	13.1
American Indian or Alaska Native	5.6	6.1	6.5	6.0	6.4	6.9	6.9	6.7	7.2
Asian or Pacific Islander	6.4	6.5	7.0	7.0	7.2	7.2	7.4	7.4	7.5
Chinese	5.1	4.9	5.7	4.9	5.2	4.7	5.8	5.6	5.4
Japanese	7.4	6.2	7.4	7.2	7.9	8.0	8.9	7.2	8.6
Filipino	6.8	7.6	7.7	7.8	8.2	8.0	8.0	8.1	9.2
Hawaiian	7.0	6.7	6.6	6.5	7.2	6.7	8.7	6.8	7.5
Other Asian or Pacific Islander	6.5	6.7	7.1	7.4	7.3	7.6	7.3	7.7	7.4
Hispanic or Latino[2]	5.9	6.0	6.1	6.2	6.2	6.4	6.2	6.2	6.4
Mexican	5.2	5.5	5.6	5.8	5.7	6.0	5.8	5.8	6.0
Puerto Rican	8.8	8.3	8.7	8.8	8.7	9.4	8.6	8.8	9.3
Cuban	5.3	5.2	6.7	6.0	6.9	6.0	6.5	6.5	5.8
Central and South American	5.7	5.8	5.9	5.9	6.3	6.2	6.2	6.0	6.3
Other and unknown Hispanic or Latino	6.1	6.6	7.1	7.5	7.4	7.3	7.1	7.3	7.7
Not Hispanic or Latino:[2]									
White	5.7	5.7	6.5	6.7	6.7	6.8	7.0	6.9	7.2
Black or African American	13.6	13.2	13.4	13.3	13.2	13.3	13.4	13.1	13.3
13 years or more of education									
All races	5.5	5.4	6.0	6.2	6.4	6.5	6.6	6.6	6.7
White	4.6	4.6	5.3	5.5	5.7	5.8	5.8	5.8	6.0
Black or African American	11.2	11.1	11.4	11.4	11.4	11.5	11.6	11.6	11.6
American Indian or Alaska Native	5.6	4.7	5.7	6.0	6.2	5.9	6.1	6.5	6.7
Asian or Pacific Islander	6.1	6.0	6.6	6.8	7.0	7.2	7.2	7.0	7.3
Chinese	4.5	4.4	5.1	5.0	4.9	5.3	4.9	4.8	5.3
Japanese	6.6	6.0	7.1	7.2	6.6	7.4	7.6	7.0	6.9
Filipino	7.2	7.0	7.6	7.8	8.1	8.0	8.0	8.3	8.3
Hawaiian	6.3	4.7	5.0	5.4	6.6	6.6	6.3	4.5	7.7
Other Asian or Pacific Islander	6.1	6.2	6.7	7.0	7.3	7.5	7.6	7.4	7.6
Hispanic or Latino[2]	5.5	5.5	5.9	6.0	6.2	6.3	6.2	6.2	6.4
Mexican	5.1	5.2	5.6	5.6	5.8	5.8	5.6	5.8	6.0
Puerto Rican	7.4	7.4	7.9	7.8	8.2	8.2	8.2	7.9	8.0
Cuban	4.9	5.0	5.6	6.4	6.0	6.3	6.9	5.9	6.7
Central and South American	5.2	5.6	5.8	5.7	6.1	6.5	6.3	6.3	6.3
Other and unknown Hispanic or Latino	5.4	5.2	6.1	6.6	6.7	6.8	6.4	6.6	7.0
Not Hispanic or Latino:[2]									
White	4.6	4.5	5.2	5.4	5.6	5.7	5.8	5.8	6.0
Black or African American	11.2	11.1	11.5	11.4	11.5	11.6	11.7	11.7	11.7

[1]Excludes live births with unknown birthweight. Percent based on live births with known birthweight.
[2]Prior to 1993, data shown only for States with an Hispanic-origin item and education of mother item on the birth certificate (see Appendix II, Education; Hispanic origin).

NOTES: Starting in 1992, education of mother was reported on the birth certificate by all 50 States and the District of Columbia. Prior to 1992, data from States lacking an education of mother item were excluded (see Appendix II, Education). The race groups, white, black, American Indian or Alaska Native, and Asian or Pacific Islander, include persons of Hispanic and non-Hispanic origin. Persons of Hispanic origin may be of any race. Interpretation of trend data should take into consideration expansion of reporting areas and immigration. Data for additional years are available (see Appendix III).

SOURCE: Centers for Disease Control and Prevention, National Center for Health Statistics, National Vital Statistics System, Birth File.

Table 14 (page 1 of 2). Low-birthweight live births, according to race and Hispanic origin of mother, geographic division, and State: United States, average annual 1993–95, 1996–98, and 1999–2001

[Data are based on birth certificates]

Geographic division and State	All races			Not Hispanic or Latino White			Not Hispanic or Latino Black or African American		
	1993–95	1996–98	1999–2001	1993–95	1996–98	1999–2001	1993–95	1996–98	1999–2001
	Percent of live births weighing less than 2,500 grams[1]								
United States	7.27	7.49	7.62	6.06	6.46	6.67	13.33	13.13	13.14
New England	6.32	6.78	7.02	5.55	6.06	6.30	11.84	11.79	11.93
Maine.	5.73	5.88	6.03	5.74	5.95	6.06	*	*13.27	*9.97
New Hampshire	5.20	5.44	6.36	5.04	5.31	6.04	*10.70	*	11.88
Vermont	5.69	6.32	5.90	5.63	6.22	5.79	*	*	*
Massachusetts	6.29	6.77	7.11	5.53	6.13	6.43	11.48	11.12	11.44
Rhode Island	6.57	7.28	7.27	5.91	6.46	6.52	11.30	11.35	12.55
Connecticut	6.96	7.43	7.47	5.60	6.16	6.33	12.50	12.82	12.53
Middle Atlantic	7.55	7.73	7.82	5.82	6.27	6.56	13.49	13.02	12.73
New York	7.64	7.77	7.75	5.68	6.19	6.47	12.96	12.32	11.97
New Jersey	7.57	7.84	7.94	5.80	6.26	6.54	13.78	13.86	13.45
Pennsylvania	7.39	7.57	7.84	5.99	6.36	6.68	14.43	13.86	13.87
East North Central	7.49	7.64	7.76	6.08	6.47	6.63	14.25	13.73	13.81
Ohio	7.53	7.66	7.93	6.36	6.64	6.95	13.82	13.34	13.36
Indiana.	7.10	7.76	7.62	6.42	7.06	7.04	12.73	13.68	12.85
Illinois.	7.94	7.96	7.99	5.98	6.44	6.59	14.92	14.22	14.03
Michigan	7.71	7.72	7.95	6.08	6.35	6.43	14.23	13.51	14.47
Wisconsin.	6.17	6.40	6.59	5.22	5.58	5.82	13.95	13.21	13.28
West North Central.	6.39	6.69	6.78	5.72	6.20	6.27	13.09	12.91	12.47
Minnesota	5.66	5.84	6.17	5.03	5.61	5.79	12.05	11.42	10.61
Iowa	5.86	6.38	6.23	5.60	6.11	5.97	12.33	12.66	12.58
Missouri	7.56	7.68	7.64	6.38	6.65	6.68	13.63	13.48	13.22
North Dakota	5.33	6.15	6.26	5.15	6.17	6.23	*9.91	*11.69	*
South Dakota	5.63	5.73	6.15	5.45	5.72	6.02	*10.08	*10.36	*11.42
Nebraska	6.11	6.60	6.73	5.67	6.32	6.37	12.36	11.58	12.81
Kansas.	6.49	6.96	6.99	5.96	6.49	6.66	12.53	13.20	12.36
South Atlantic.	8.27	8.45	8.57	6.37	6.75	7.00	13.15	13.09	13.07
Delaware	7.87	8.54	8.84	6.23	6.50	7.28	13.03	14.41	13.71
Maryland	8.49	8.68	8.88	6.08	6.39	6.70	13.52	13.37	13.12
District of Columbia	14.09	13.60	12.37	5.25	6.15	6.56	16.62	16.28	15.17
Virginia.	7.50	7.77	7.85	5.91	6.28	6.52	12.59	12.49	12.39
West Virginia	7.52	8.10	8.28	7.29	7.95	8.11	13.59	12.94	13.20
North Carolina	8.66	8.80	8.87	6.75	7.08	7.39	13.59	13.82	13.72
South Carolina	9.26	9.30	9.69	6.75	6.99	7.30	13.49	13.60	14.29
Georgia	8.70	8.62	8.72	6.40	6.58	6.85	12.98	12.83	12.82
Florida	7.65	7.98	8.10	6.26	6.77	6.92	12.33	12.30	12.42
East South Central	8.71	8.98	9.32	6.98	7.42	7.77	13.41	13.48	13.97
Kentucky	7.47	7.94	8.26	6.98	7.49	7.73	12.59	12.73	13.69
Tennessee	8.76	8.89	9.21	7.12	7.46	7.96	14.32	14.07	14.12
Alabama.	8.91	9.26	9.56	6.88	7.33	7.58	12.94	13.34	13.87
Mississippi	9.92	10.03	10.55	6.81	7.34	7.72	13.33	13.31	14.03
West South Central	7.50	7.77	7.90	6.27	6.73	6.95	13.10	13.29	13.42
Arkansas	8.20	8.57	8.66	6.89	7.31	7.48	12.80	13.41	13.60
Louisiana	9.55	10.05	10.25	6.43	6.98	7.36	13.86	14.49	14.40
Oklahoma.	6.89	7.27	7.55	6.37	6.80	7.23	12.34	12.63	12.93
Texas.	7.08	7.30	7.43	6.09	6.54	6.68	12.71	12.51	12.76
Mountain	7.06	7.34	7.34	6.70	7.08	7.08	14.07	13.70	13.37
Montana.	6.03	6.56	6.65	5.84	6.28	6.69	*	*	*
Idaho.	5.57	6.02	6.43	5.44	5.84	6.31	*	*	*
Wyoming	7.83	8.76	8.32	7.59	8.69	8.15	*13.98	*15.82	*14.29
Colorado	8.46	8.75	8.43	7.90	8.34	8.02	15.46	14.48	14.39
New Mexico	7.39	7.63	7.87	7.39	7.68	7.85	10.43	13.46	13.37
Arizona	6.74	6.80	6.95	6.52	6.63	6.73	13.30	12.88	13.19
Utah	6.04	6.65	6.60	5.89	6.44	6.43	11.25	15.06	12.49
Nevada	7.45	7.57	7.45	6.93	7.28	7.38	14.59	13.78	12.69
Pacific.	5.97	6.07	6.13	5.33	5.47	5.59	12.30	11.73	11.56
Washington	5.32	5.63	5.74	4.99	5.25	5.40	10.75	10.32	10.30
Oregon.	5.34	5.39	5.52	5.14	5.14	5.32	10.68	10.71	10.64
California	6.08	6.15	6.20	5.48	5.61	5.72	12.46	11.90	11.73
Alaska	5.26	5.78	5.70	4.80	5.30	5.03	10.77	12.00	10.64
Hawaii	7.01	7.34	7.74	5.35	5.35	5.60	11.82	9.79	10.77

See footnotes at end of table.

Table 14 (page 2 of 2). Low-birthweight live births, according to race and Hispanic origin of mother, geographic division, and State: United States, average annual 1993–95, 1996–98, and 1999–2001

[Data are based on birth certificates]

Geographic division and State	Hispanic or Latino[2]			American Indian or Alaska Native[3]			Asian or Pacific Islander[3]		
	1993–95	1996–98	1999–2001	1993–95	1996–98	1999–2001	1993–95	1996–98	1999–2001
	Percent of live births weighing less than 2,500 grams[1]								
United States	6.26	6.38	6.42	6.49	6.69	7.08	6.76	7.24	7.42
New England	8.02	8.28	8.17	7.95	8.17	7.54	6.97	7.19	7.39
Maine	*7.36	*5.74	*4.91	*	*	*	*7.33	*5.03	*5.42
New Hampshire	*5.60	*6.48	5.89	*	*	*	*7.59	*8.30	5.83
Vermont	*	*	*	*	*	*	*	*	*
Massachusetts	7.76	8.03	8.28	*6.86	*6.37	*6.84	6.46	6.95	7.38
Rhode Island	6.82	7.68	7.07	*10.21	*10.49	*10.67	7.76	8.30	8.78
Connecticut	8.88	8.94	8.60	*9.07	*10.94	*8.09	8.07	7.73	7.59
Middle Atlantic	7.79	7.71	7.49	8.96	8.21	8.96	6.93	7.32	7.38
New York	7.76	7.65	7.41	8.26	7.40	8.44	6.81	7.24	7.24
New Jersey	7.46	7.30	7.19	9.38	12.20	10.04	6.87	7.52	7.67
Pennsylvania	8.99	9.34	8.95	10.63	7.31	9.41	7.58	7.26 `	7.38
East North Central	6.16	6.33	6.40	6.70	6.51	7.04	7.04	7.52	7.85
Ohio	7.45	7.38	7.23	9.81	7.20	8.39	6.51	7.43	7.36
Indiana	6.40	7.00	6.10	*6.94	*10.98	*6.89	5.93	6.50	7.42
Illinois	5.98	6.11	6.38	8.08	7.70	9.05	7.65	8.02	8.37
Michigan	6.32	6.48	6.37	6.75	6.12	7.24	6.96	7.25	7.72
Wisconsin	6.36	6.56	6.29	5.39	5.71	5.97	6.26	6.81	7.02
West North Central	6.03	6.09	6.06	6.63	6.12	6.65	6.82	7.04	7.42
Minnesota	6.18	6.13	5.98	7.13	6.21	6.92	7.05	6.66	7.48
Iowa	6.08	6.21	5.83	*5.86	8.48	*7.36	7.44	7.63	7.72
Missouri	6.25	6.24	5.98	*6.64	7.87	8.95	7.19	7.18	6.89
North Dakota	*6.23	*5.88	*6.89	5.87	5.66	6.21	*8.89	*	*
South Dakota	*6.37	*6.14	*6.07	6.44	5.58	6.25	*	*	*9.37
Nebraska	6.30	6.08	6.49	6.11	6.36	6.32	6.38	7.94	7.91
Kansas	5.64	5.95	6.00	8.48	6.40	6.36	5.33	7.49	7.34
South Atlantic	6.22	6.37	6.30	8.42	9.00	9.22	7.05	7.54	7.75
Delaware	6.83	7.76	6.62	*	*	*	8.68	8.04	8.98
Maryland	6.01	6.29	6.80	*5.63	*8.48	9.95	7.01	7.15	7.37
District of Columbia	6.78	6.73	6.99	*	*	*	7.31	*8.43	*8.79
Virginia	5.70	6.68	5.96	*7.42	*6.94	*9.23	6.51	7.30	7.15
West Virginia	*9.03	*	*	*	*	*	*7.31	*6.58	*7.94
North Carolina	6.01	6.14	6.21	9.11	10.22	10.33	7.45	7.61	8.05
South Carolina	6.28	5.99	6.57	*8.75	*9.40	10.20	7.10	7.56	7.10
Georgia	6.03	5.36	5.66	*6.98	*7.21	9.79	6.63	7.51	7.67
Florida	6.32	6.55	6.49	7.35	7.35	7.08	7.53	7.98	8.51
East South Central	5.63	6.53	6.73	7.27	7.73	7.61	6.92	7.60	7.84
Kentucky	5.96	7.14	7.18	*	*10.38	*	5.27	6.78	7.68
Tennessee	5.85	6.56	6.57	*7.69	*7.88	*7.13	6.84	8.40	8.03
Alabama	4.99	6.51	6.68	*6.96	*7.60	*8.25	7.69	7.94	7.59
Mississippi	*5.89	5.26	6.92	*7.52	*6.59	8.42	7.96	6.00	7.75
West South Central	6.43	6.61	6.73	5.71	6.20	6.57	7.04	7.50	7.75
Arkansas	5.93	6.34	5.92	*7.68	*5.97	7.95	7.81	7.40	8.80
Louisiana	7.35	6.04	6.70	*5.76	8.02	8.41	6.45	8.37	7.92
Oklahoma	6.14	6.13	6.03	5.56	6.07	6.34	6.19	7.02	7.19
Texas	6.43	6.63	6.76	6.00	6.34	6.76	7.16	7.45	7.74
Mountain	7.15	7.22	7.21	6.30	6.72	7.14	8.03	8.57	8.33
Montana	7.76	7.69	7.02	6.07	7.43	6.77	*8.07	*8.97	*6.42
Idaho	6.21	6.95	6.78	6.53	7.07	7.82	*6.86	*5.97	7.62
Wyoming	9.96	8.33	7.86	*6.38	7.51	8.93	*	*	*17.06
Colorado	8.55	8.71	8.23	9.14	8.16	8.60	9.36	9.92	10.10
New Mexico	7.62	7.69	7.93	6.16	6.27	6.88	7.46	9.26	8.28
Arizona	6.51	6.52	6.67	6.12	6.57	7.12	7.14	7.54	7.69
Utah	7.27	7.55	7.33	5.75	7.44	6.58	7.01	7.50	7.18
Nevada	5.98	6.26	6.21	7.72	6.23	7.80	8.60	9.17	7.88
Pacific	5.48	5.55	5.59	6.01	6.10	6.38	6.46	6.95	7.10
Washington	5.05	5.53	5.31	5.31	7.09	7.14	5.84	6.12	6.41
Oregon	5.67	5.72	5.51	5.80	5.72	6.79	5.72	6.45	6.08
California	5.48	5.53	5.59	6.88	5.85	6.27	6.32	6.84	6.98
Alaska	5.49	6.48	6.09	5.10	5.73	5.83	6.57	6.43	7.05
Hawaii	6.89	7.08	7.63	*8.48	*7.37	*6.11	7.42	7.95	8.29

* Percents preceded by an asterisk are based on fewer than 50 events. Percents not shown are based on fewer than 20 events.
[1] Excludes live births with unknown birthweight.
[2] Persons of Hispanic origin may be of any race.
[3] Includes persons of Hispanic and non-Hispanic origin.

SOURCE: Centers for Disease Control and Prevention, National Center for Health Statistics, National Vital Statistics System, Birth File.

Table 15 (page 1 of 2). Very low-birthweight live births, according to race and Hispanic origin of mother, geographic division, and State: United States, average annual 1993–95, 1996–98, and 1999–2001

[Data are based on birth certificates]

Geographic division and State	All races 1993–95	All races 1996–98	All races 1999–2001	White 1993–95	White 1996–98	White 1999–2001	Black or African American 1993–95	Black or African American 1996–98	Black or African American 1999–2001
				Not Hispanic or Latino					

Percent of live births weighing less than 1,500 grams[1]

Geographic division and State	1993–95	1996–98	1999–2001	1993–95	1996–98	1999–2001	1993–95	1996–98	1999–2001
United States	1.34	1.41	1.44	1.01	1.11	1.15	2.99	3.06	3.12
New England	1.15	1.30	1.38	0.92	1.08	1.14	2.95	3.05	3.28
Maine	1.00	1.05	1.13	1.00	1.06	1.14	*	*	*
New Hampshire	0.83	1.02	1.20	0.81	0.97	1.08	*	*	*
Vermont	0.82	1.08	1.09	0.78	1.04	1.05	*	*	*
Massachusetts	1.15	1.26	1.35	0.94	1.06	1.13	2.79	2.75	3.13
Rhode Island	1.07	1.39	1.49	0.89	1.17	1.24	2.29	2.82	2.99
Connecticut	1.36	1.56	1.56	0.95	1.14	1.17	3.30	3.49	3.58
Middle Atlantic	1.45	1.52	1.54	1.00	1.09	1.16	3.17	3.20	3.13
New York	1.47	1.51	1.51	0.96	1.02	1.10	3.08	3.06	2.93
New Jersey	1.51	1.60	1.63	1.03	1.13	1.20	3.37	3.57	3.52
Pennsylvania	1.37	1.45	1.51	1.03	1.13	1.21	3.17	3.21	3.22
East North Central	1.41	1.46	1.51	1.06	1.15	1.18	3.07	3.08	3.25
Ohio	1.39	1.45	1.48	1.09	1.18	1.21	3.01	2.99	3.05
Indiana	1.28	1.38	1.41	1.11	1.19	1.23	2.68	2.93	2.92
Illinois	1.53	1.55	1.61	1.08	1.18	1.21	3.14	3.14	3.35
Michigan	1.49	1.52	1.60	1.07	1.13	1.17	3.20	3.16	3.46
Wisconsin	1.11	1.21	1.24	0.89	1.00	1.04	2.88	2.93	3.13
West North Central	1.13	1.23	1.26	0.96	1.10	1.11	2.75	2.93	2.93
Minnesota	1.06	1.08	1.13	0.91	1.03	1.01	2.54	2.65	2.59
Iowa	1.01	1.23	1.18	0.94	1.14	1.11	2.72	3.47	2.76
Missouri	1.30	1.35	1.45	1.03	1.06	1.16	2.74	2.93	3.13
North Dakota	0.97	1.11	1.08	0.89	1.10	1.03	*	*	*
South Dakota	0.93	1.06	1.01	0.81	1.00	0.95	*	*	*
Nebraska	1.03	1.27	1.24	0.98	1.22	1.16	2.20	2.88	2.82
Kansas	1.17	1.32	1.30	1.00	1.19	1.20	3.20	3.11	2.82
South Atlantic	1.64	1.72	1.73	1.09	1.19	1.24	3.07	3.14	3.15
Delaware	1.52	1.78	1.84	1.08	1.19	1.27	2.99	3.59	3.41
Maryland	1.80	1.89	1.90	1.09	1.09	1.19	3.35	3.52	3.36
District of Columbia	3.46	3.35	2.90	*0.73	*1.10	*1.03	4.27	4.15	3.74
Virginia	1.48	1.59	1.59	1.02	1.13	1.20	2.93	3.05	2.98
West Virginia	1.25	1.39	1.41	1.21	1.34	1.36	2.15	2.69	3.03
North Carolina	1.78	1.86	1.91	1.22	1.32	1.42	3.26	3.47	3.49
South Carolina	1.79	1.89	1.95	1.16	1.21	1.26	2.87	3.14	3.32
Georgia	1.74	1.75	1.73	1.07	1.15	1.16	3.00	2.98	2.96
Florida	1.45	1.53	1.57	1.04	1.18	1.18	2.81	2.77	2.94
East South Central	1.60	1.74	1.79	1.13	1.28	1.32	2.89	3.07	3.20
Kentucky	1.28	1.46	1.49	1.14	1.33	1.35	2.75	2.86	2.94
Tennessee	1.60	1.67	1.65	1.14	1.25	1.26	3.18	3.22	3.22
Alabama	1.75	1.92	1.99	1.16	1.30	1.35	2.90	3.22	3.38
Mississippi	1.81	1.97	2.12	1.04	1.23	1.36	2.65	2.86	3.06
West South Central	1.34	1.41	1.42	1.03	1.13	1.13	2.83	2.98	3.08
Arkansas	1.49	1.60	1.60	1.20	1.28	1.24	2.48	2.82	3.07
Louisiana	1.89	2.02	2.11	1.07	1.15	1.19	3.04	3.28	3.45
Oklahoma	1.16	1.23	1.28	1.02	1.11	1.16	2.65	2.72	2.80
Texas	1.24	1.30	1.29	0.99	1.10	1.09	2.77	2.84	2.86
Mountain	1.05	1.13	1.13	0.97	1.06	1.06	2.73	2.71	2.64
Montana	0.90	1.06	1.09	0.87	0.97	1.07	*	*	*
Idaho	0.82	0.89	1.03	0.78	0.83	0.98	*	*	*
Wyoming	1.16	1.14	1.06	1.12	1.10	1.04	*	*	*
Colorado	1.19	1.32	1.24	1.06	1.23	1.14	3.04	2.69	2.90
New Mexico	1.05	1.07	1.19	1.14	1.17	1.15	*1.74	*2.40	*2.89
Arizona	1.09	1.13	1.10	1.01	1.07	1.03	2.79	2.79	2.63
Utah	0.89	1.03	1.05	0.85	0.97	1.02	*	*3.43	*
Nevada	1.14	1.18	1.14	1.01	1.07	1.06	2.58	2.67	2.44
Pacific	1.03	1.09	1.11	0.87	0.94	0.96	2.69	2.62	2.74
Washington	0.82	1.02	0.97	0.78	0.93	0.88	2.11	2.52	2.17
Oregon	0.88	0.89	0.95	0.84	0.83	0.92	1.94	*1.79	1.98
California	1.07	1.11	1.14	0.90	0.96	1.00	2.73	2.65	2.83
Alaska	0.94	1.14	1.03	0.84	0.97	0.89	*2.90	*3.04	*2.18
Hawaii	1.01	1.17	1.22	0.83	1.03	0.99	3.40	*2.45	*2.21

See footnotes at end of table.

Table 15 (page 2 of 2). **Very low-birthweight live births, according to race and Hispanic origin of mother, geographic division, and State: United States, average annual 1993–95, 1996–98, and 1999–2001**

[Data are based on birth certificates]

Geographic division and State	Hispanic or Latino[2]			American Indian or Alaska Native[3]			Asian or Pacific Islander[3]		
	1993–95	1996–98	1999–2001	1993–95	1996–98	1999–2001	1993–95	1996–98	1999–2001
	Percent of live births weighing less than 1,500 grams[1]								
United States	1.08	1.13	1.14	1.09	1.21	1.23	0.90	1.05	1.05
New England	1.49	1.70	1.68	*1.28	*1.66	*1.58	0.90	1.04	1.09
Maine	*	*	*	*	*	*	*	*	*
New Hampshire	*	*	*	*	*	*	*	*	*
Vermont	*	*	*	*	*	*	*	*	*
Massachusetts	1.47	1.65	1.59	*	*	*	0.80	0.90	1.09
Rhode Island	1.18	1.38	1.53	*	*	*	*	*	*2.09
Connecticut	1.64	1.90	1.88	*	*	*	*1.20	1.35	*0.88
Middle Atlantic	1.42	1.43	1.49	*1.14	*1.45	1.52	0.91	1.01	0.95
New York	1.40	1.39	1.47	*0.96	*1.23	*1.66	0.93	1.01	0.97
New Jersey	1.40	1.41	1.47	*	*	*	0.83	1.03	0.97
Pennsylvania	1.65	1.82	1.72	*	*	*	1.02	1.01	0.86
East North Central	1.19	1.19	1.21	1.31	1.29	1.33	1.00	1.09	1.05
Ohio	1.53	1.51	1.22	*	*	*	0.98	0.90	0.79
Indiana	1.25	1.39	1.25	*	*	*	*0.84	*1.00	*0.86
Illinois	1.13	1.12	1.23	*	*	*	1.12	1.17	1.22
Michigan	1.19	1.18	1.14	*1.17	*1.65	*1.54	0.92	0.99	0.99
Wisconsin	1.45	1.43	1.18	*1.23	*0.88	*1.14	*0.84	1.21	0.97
West North Central	0.98	1.13	1.20	1.36	1.34	1.17	0.87	0.98	1.08
Minnesota	1.15	1.18	1.24	*1.32	*1.44	*1.32	0.88	0.97	1.11
Iowa	*1.18	1.16	1.22	*	*	*	*	*1.37	*1.30
Missouri	*1.15	1.22	1.18	*	*	*	*0.81	*0.83	*0.91
North Dakota	*	*	*	*1.08	*1.02	*1.25	*	*	*
South Dakota	*	*	*	1.58	1.37	1.13	*	*	*
Nebraska	*0.87	1.01	1.12	*	*	*	*	*	*
Kansas	0.76	1.12	1.20	*	*	*	*0.85	*0.94	*1.06
South Atlantic	1.09	1.17	1.11	1.72	1.92	1.66	0.97	1.11	1.14
Delaware	*1.39	*1.12	*1.65	*	*	*	*	*	*
Maryland	1.03	1.30	1.25	*	*	*	0.91	1.27	1.05
District of Columbia	*1.06	*1.23	*1.56	*	*	*	*	*	*
Virginia	1.08	1.39	1.06	*	*	*	0.96	1.12	1.07
West Virginia	*	*	*	*	*	*	*	*	*
North Carolina	0.83	0.96	1.15	2.19	2.48	2.29	*0.92	1.12	1.32
South Carolina	*1.29	*1.20	0.95	*	*	*	*	*	*
Georgia	1.02	0.96	0.90	*	*	*	1.09	0.99	1.04
Florida	1.13	1.20	1.14	*	*1.11	*0.81	0.94	1.07	1.23
East South Central	0.97	1.09	1.01	*1.36	*1.50	*1.34	0.91	0.96	1.19
Kentucky	*	*1.38	*1.24	*	*	*	*	*	*1.11
Tennessee	*0.94	*0.90	0.90	*	*	*	*0.83	*1.15	*1.10
Alabama	*	*1.23	1.05	*	*	*	*1.45	*	*1.42
Mississippi	*	*	*	*	*	*	*	*	*
West South Central	1.06	1.10	1.09	0.80	1.00	1.05	0.88	0.98	1.06
Arkansas	*1.27	1.14	1.09	*	*	*	*	*	*
Louisiana	*1.15	*1.04	1.10	*	*	*	*0.83	*1.10	*1.20
Oklahoma	0.92	0.94	0.94	0.80	0.90	1.04	*0.88	*	*1.11
Texas	1.06	1.10	1.10	*0.92	*1.50	*1.25	0.86	1.00	1.06
Mountain	1.07	1.12	1.12	0.92	1.07	1.16	1.03	1.15	1.03
Montana	*	*	*	*0.75	1.36	1.49	*	*	*
Idaho	0.92	1.13	1.25	*	*	*	*	*	*
Wyoming	*1.34	*1.22	*1.26	*	*	*	*	*	*
Colorado	1.15	1.32	1.23	*	*	*1.13	1.19	1.11	1.20
New Mexico	1.04	1.02	1.20	0.77	0.81	0.98	*	*	*
Arizona	1.07	1.09	1.05	0.92	1.07	1.17	*1.00	*1.00	0.88
Utah	1.10	1.23	1.19	*1.18	*1.68	*1.46	*0.88	*1.24	*0.97
Nevada	0.94	0.95	0.96	*1.93	*	*1.63	*0.91	1.38	0.97
Pacific	0.97	1.02	1.03	1.08	1.13	1.21	0.86	1.05	1.05
Washington	0.71	0.95	0.97	1.01	1.30	1.35	0.52	0.94	1.02
Oregon	0.93	1.02	0.96	*1.09	*	*1.35	*0.97	1.17	0.85
California	0.97	1.02	1.03	1.19	1.06	1.20	0.86	1.02	1.02
Alaska	*	*1.84	*1.20	0.93	1.20	1.08	*	*	*
Hawaii	1.12	0.93	1.04	*	*	*	0.96	1.20	1.26

* Percents preceded by an asterisk are based on fewer than 50 events. Percents not shown are based on fewer than 20 events.
[1]Excludes live births with unknown birthweight.
[2]Persons of Hispanic origin may be of any race.
[3]Includes persons of Hispanic and non-Hispanic origin.

SOURCE: Centers for Disease Control and Prevention, National Center for Health Statistics, National Vital Statistics System, Birth File.

Table 16. Legal abortions and legal abortion ratios, according to selected patient characteristics: United States, selected years 1973–99

[Data are based on reporting by State health departments and by hospitals and other medical facilities]

Characteristic	1973	1975	1980	1985	1990	1994	1995	1996	1997	1998[1]	1999[1]
	Number of legal abortions reported in thousands										
Centers for Disease Control and Prevention	616	855	1,298	1,329	1,429	1,267	1,211	1,226	1,186	884	862
Alan Guttmacher Institute[2]	745	1,034	1,554	1,589	1,609	1,423	1,359	1,360	1,335	1,319	1,315
	Abortions per 100 live births[3]										
Total	19.6	27.2	35.9	35.4	34.4	32.1	31.1	31.5	30.6	26.4	25.6
Age											
Under 15 years	123.7	119.3	139.7	137.6	81.8	70.3	66.4	72.6	72.9	75.0	70.9
15–19 years.	53.9	54.2	71.4	68.8	51.1	41.4	39.9	41.8	40.7	39.1	37.5
20–24 years.	29.4	28.9	39.5	38.6	37.8	36.4	34.8	35.7	34.5	32.9	31.6
25–29 years.	20.7	19.2	23.7	21.7	21.8	22.1	22.0	22.8	22.4	21.6	20.8
30–34 years.	28.0	25.0	23.7	19.9	19.0	17.1	16.4	16.5	16.1	15.7	15.2
35–39 years.	45.1	42.2	41.0	33.6	27.3	23.3	22.3	22.1	20.9	20.0	19.3
40 years and over	68.4	66.8	80.7	62.3	50.6	40.9	38.5	37.8	35.2	33.8	32.9
Race											
White[4].	32.6	27.7	33.2	27.7	25.8	21.6	20.3	20.3	19.4	18.9	17.7
Black or African American[5]	42.0	47.6	54.3	47.2	53.7	53.7	53.1	55.9	54.3	51.2	52.9
Hispanic origin[6]											
Hispanic or Latino	- - -	- - -	- - -	- - -	- - -	28.5	27.1	28.2	26.8	27.3	26.1
Not Hispanic or Latino	- - -	- - -	- - -	- - -	- - -	29.0	27.9	28.6	27.2	27.1	25.2
Marital status											
Married	7.6	9.6	10.5	8.0	8.7	7.8	7.6	7.9	7.4	7.1	7.0
Unmarried	139.8	161.0	147.6	117.4	86.3	66.5	64.5	65.9	65.9	62.7	60.4
Previous live births[7]											
0.	43.7	38.4	45.7	45.1	36.0	30.8	28.6	28.9	26.4	25.5	24.3
1.	23.5	22.0	20.2	21.6	22.7	22.3	22.0	22.4	22.3	21.4	20.6
2.	36.8	36.8	29.5	29.9	31.5	30.9	30.6	31.3	31.0	30.0	29.0
3.	46.9	47.7	29.8	18.2	30.1	30.9	30.7	31.7	31.1	30.5	29.8
4 or more[8]	44.7	43.5	24.3	21.5	26.6	23.5	23.7	25.0	24.5	24.3	24.2
	Percent distribution[9]										
Total	100.0	100.0	100.0	100.0	100.0	100.0	100.0	100.0	100.0	100.0	100.0
Period of gestation											
Under 9 weeks.	36.1	44.6	51.7	50.3	51.6	53.7	54.0	54.6	55.4	55.7	57.6
9–10 weeks.	29.4	28.4	26.2	26.6	25.3	23.5	23.1	22.6	22.0	21.5	20.2
11–12 weeks	17.9	14.9	12.2	12.5	11.7	10.9	10.9	11.0	10.7	10.9	10.2
13–15 weeks	6.9	5.0	5.1	5.9	6.4	6.3	6.3	6.0	6.2	6.4	6.2
16–20 weeks	8.0	6.1	3.9	3.9	4.0	4.3	4.3	4.3	4.3	4.1	4.3
21 weeks and over	1.7	1.0	0.9	0.8	1.0	1.3	1.4	1.5	1.4	1.4	1.5
Previous induced abortions											
0.	078	81.9	67.6	60.1	57.1	54.7	55.1	54.7	53.4	53.8	53.7
1.	078	14.9	23.5	25.7	26.9	27.2	26.9	26.9	27.5	27.0	27.1
2.	078	2.5	6.6	9.8	10.1	11.1	10.9	11.2	11.5	11.4	11.5
3 or more	078	0.7	2.3	4.4	5.9	7.0	7.1	7.2	7.6	7.8	7.7

- - - Data not available.

[1]In 1998 and 1999 California, Alaska, New Hampshire, and Oklahoma did not report abortion data to CDC. For comparison, in 1997 the 48 corresponding reporting areas reported about 900,000 legal abortions.

[2]No surveys were conducted in 1983, 1986, 1989, 1990, 1993, 1994, 1997, or 1998. Data for these years were estimated by interpolation. Some estimates for previous years have been revised and differ from the previous edition of *Health, United States*. AGI estimated about 1,313,000 reported abortions in 2000.

[3]For calculation of ratios by each characteristic, abortions with characteristic unknown were distributed in proportion to abortions with characteristic known.

[4]For 1989 and later years, white race includes women of Hispanic ethnicity.   [5]Before 1989 black race includes races other than white.

[6]Includes data for 20–22 States, the District of Columbia (DC), and New York City (NYC) in 1991–95, 22 States and NYC in 1996, and 23–26 States, DC, and NYC in 1997–99. States with large Hispanic populations that are not included are California, Florida, and Illinois.

[7]For 1973–75 data indicate number of living children.

[8]For 1975 data refer to four previous live births, not four or more. For five or more previous live births, the ratio is 47.3.

[9]Excludes cases for which selected characteristic is unknown.

NOTES: See Appendix I, Abortion Surveillance and Alan Guttmacher Institute Abortion Survey, for methodological differences between these two data sources. The number of areas reporting adequate data (less than or equal to 15 percent missing) for each characteristic varies from year to year. See Appendix I, Abortion Surveillance. Data for additional years are available (see Appendix III).

SOURCES: Centers for Disease Control and Prevention, National Center for Chronic Disease Prevention and Health Promotion: Abortion Surveillance, 1973, 1975, 1979–80. Public Health Service, DHHS, Atlanta, Ga., May 1975, April 1977, May 1983; CDC Surveillance Summaries. Abortion Surveillance, United States, 1984 and 1985, Vol. 38, No. SS–2, Public Health Service, DHHS, Atlanta, Ga., Sept. 1989; 1986 and 1987, Vol. 39, No. SS–2, June 1990; 1990, Vol. 42, No. SS–6, Dec. 1993; 1993 and 1994, Vol. 46, No. SS–4, Aug. 1997; 1995, Vol. 47, No. SS–2, July 1998; 1996, Vol. 48, No. SS–4, July 1999; 1997, Vol. 49, No. SS–11, Dec. 2000; 1998, Vol. 51, No. SS–3, June 2002; 1999, Vol. 51, No. SS–9, Nov. 2002. Alan Guttmacher Institute Abortion Survey. Finer LB and Henshaw SK: Abortion incidence and services in the United States in 2000. Perspectives on Sexual and Reproductive Health. 35(1), Jan.-Feb. 2003.

Table 17 (page 1 of 3). Contraceptive use among women 15–44 years of age, according to age, race, Hispanic origin, and method of contraception: United States, 1982, 1988, and 1995

[Data are based on household interviews of samples of women in the childbearing ages]

Race, Hispanic origin, and year	Age in years				
	15–44	15–19	20–24	25–34	35–44
	Number of women in population in thousands				
All women:					
1982	54,099	9,521	10,629	19,644	14,305
1988	57,900	9,179	9,413	21,726	17,582
1995	60,201	8,961	9,041	20,758	21,440
Not Hispanic or Latino:					
White:					
1982	41,279	7,010	8,081	14,945	11,243
1988	42,575	6,531	6,630	15,929	13,486
1995	42,522	5,962	6,062	14,565	15,933
Black or African American:					
1982	6,825	1,383	1,456	2,392	1,593
1988	7,408	1,362	1,322	2,760	1,965
1995	8,210	1,392	1,328	2,801	2,689
Hispanic or Latino:[1]					
1982	4,393	886	811	1,677	1,018
1988	5,557	999	1,003	2,104	1,451
1995	6,702	1,150	1,163	2,450	1,940
	Percent of women in population using contraception				
All women:					
1982	55.7	24.2	55.8	66.7	61.6
1988	60.3	32.1	59.0	66.3	68.3
1995	64.2	29.8	63.5	71.1	72.3
Not Hispanic or Latino:					
White:					
1982	57.3	23.6	58.7	67.8	63.5
1988	62.9	34.0	62.6	67.7	71.5
1995	66.1	30.5	65.3	72.9	73.6
Black or African American:					
1982	51.6	29.8	52.2	63.5	52.0
1988	56.8	35.7	61.8	63.5	58.7
1995	62.1	34.8	67.9	66.8	68.5
Hispanic or Latino:[1]					
1982	50.6	*	*36.8	67.2	59.0
1988	50.4	*18.3	40.8	67.4	54.3
1995	59.0	26.1	50.6	69.2	70.8

See footnotes at end of table.

[Data are based on household interviews of samples of women in the childbearing ages]

Method of contraception and year	Age in years				
	15–44	15–19	20–24	25–34	35–44
Female sterilization	Percent of contracepting women				
1982	23.2	0.0	*4.5	22.1	43.5
1988	27.5	*	*4.6	25.0	47.6
1995	27.8	*	4.0	23.8	45.0
Male sterilization					
1982	10.9	*	*3.6	10.1	19.9
1988	11.7	*	*	10.2	20.8
1995	10.9	–	*	7.8	19.4
Implant[2]					
1982	. . .	. . .	. . .	. . .	. . .
1988	. . .	. . .	. . .	. . .	. . .
1995	1.3	*	3.7	1.3	*
Injectable[2]					
1982	. . .	. . .	. . .	. . .	. . .
1988	. . .	. . .	. . .	. . .	. . .
1995	3.0	9.7	6.1	2.8	*0.8
Birth control pill					
1982	28.0	63.9	55.1	25.7	*3.7
1988	30.7	58.8	68.2	32.6	4.3
1995	26.9	43.8	52.1	33.3	8.7
Intrauterine device					
1982	7.1	*	*4.2	9.7	6.9
1988	2.0	0.0	*	2.1	3.1
1995	0.8	–	*	*0.8	*1.1
Diaphragm					
1982	8.1	*6.0	10.2	10.3	4.0
1988	5.7	*	*3.7	7.3	6.0
1995	1.9	*	*	1.7	2.8
Condom					
1982	12.0	20.8	10.7	11.4	11.3
1988	14.6	32.8	14.5	13.7	11.2
1995	20.4	36.7	26.4	21.1	14.7

See footnotes at end of table.

Table 17 (page 3 of 3). **Contraceptive use among women 15–44 years of age, according to age, race, Hispanic origin, and method of contraception: United States, 1982, 1988, and 1995**

[Data are based on household interviews of samples of women in the childbearing ages]

Method of contraception and year	Not Hispanic or Latino		Hispanic or Latino[1]
	White	Black or African American	
Female sterilization	Percent of contracepting women		
1982	23.0	21.9	30.0
1988	25.6	37.8	31.7
1995	24.6	40.1	36.6
Male sterilization			
1982	*	13.0	*1.5
1988	14.3	*0.9	*
1995	13.6	*1.7	4.0
Implant[2]			
1982	...	...	...
1988	...	...	...
1995	1.0	*2.3	*2.0
Injectable[2]			
1982	...	...	...
1988	...	...	...
1995	2.4	5.3	4.7
Birth control pill			
1982	30.2	26.8	37.8
1988	29.5	38.1	33.4
1995	28.5	23.8	23.0
Intrauterine device			
1982	19.2	5.8	9.3
1988	1.5	3.2	*5.0
1995	0.7	*	*1.5
Diaphragm			
1982	*	9.2	*3.2
1988	6.6	*2.0	*
1995	2.3	*	*
Condom			
1982	*6.9	13.1	6.3
1988	15.2	10.1	13.6
1995	19.7	20.2	20.5

0.0 Quantity more than zero but less than 0.05.
– Quantity zero.
* Estimates with relative standard error of 20–30 percent are preceded by an asterisk and may have low reliability; those with relative standard error greater than 30 percent are considered unreliable and are not shown.
. . . Data not applicable.
[1] Persons of Hispanic origin may be of any race.
[2] Data collected in 1995 survey only.

NOTES: Method of contraception used in the month of interview. If multiple methods were reported, only the most effective method is shown. Methods are listed in the table in order of effectiveness.

SOURCE: Centers for Disease Control and Prevention, National Center for Health Statistics, National Survey of Family Growth.

Table 18. Breastfeeding by mothers 15–44 years of age by year of baby's birth, according to selected characteristics of mother: United States, average annual 1972–74 to 1993–94

[Data are based on household interviews of samples of women in the childbearing ages]

Selected characteristics of mother	1972–74	1975–77	1978–80	1981–83	1984–86	1987–89	1990–92	1993–94
	Percent of babies breastfed							
Total	30.1	36.7	47.5	58.1	54.5	52.3	54.2	58.1
Race and Hispanic origin[1]								
Not Hispanic or Latino:								
White	32.5	38.9	53.2	64.3	59.7	58.3	59.1	61.2
Black or African American	12.5	16.8	19.6	26.0	22.9	21.0	22.9	27.5
Hispanic or Latino	33.1	42.9	46.3	52.8	58.9	51.3	58.8	67.4
Education[2]								
No high school diploma or GED[3]	14.0	19.4	27.6	31.4	36.8	30.0	38.6	43.0
High school diploma or GED[3]	25.0	33.6	40.2	54.3	46.7	46.6	46.0	51.2
Some college, no bachelor's degree	35.2	43.5	63.2	66.7	66.1	57.8	60.7	65.9
Bachelor's degree or higher	65.5	66.9	71.3	83.2	75.3	79.2	80.8	80.6
Geographic region								
Northeast	29.9	34.7	49.3	68.2	55.3	49.9	54.0	56.7
Midwest	22.3	30.9	34.4	46.0	50.9	50.4	51.6	49.7
South	30.6	33.1	49.5	57.9	45.3	42.5	43.6	49.7
West	47.1	54.5	66.6	69.9	70.9	69.1	70.5	79.3
Age at baby's birth								
Under 20 years	17.0	22.1	31.4	31.0	30.6	26.2	35.2	45.3
20–24 years	28.7	33.5	44.7	50.8	50.2	46.7	44.7	50.9
25–29 years	38.7	45.9	53.6	62.2	59.8	57.1	56.5	55.9
30–44 years	43.1	47.5	55.2	73.1	65.9	65.3	67.5	71.1
	Percent of breastfed babies who were breastfed 3 months or more[4]							
Total	62.3	66.2	64.7	68.3	63.2	61.5	61.0	56.2
Race and Hispanic origin[1]								
Not Hispanic or Latino:								
White	62.1	66.7	67.6	68.1	62.5	62.3	62.6	56.8
Black or African American	47.8	60.7	58.5	61.1	56.8	46.9	56.7	45.4
Hispanic or Latino	64.7	62.7	46.3	65.6	66.4	64.3	58.2	55.5
Education[2]								
No high school diploma or GED[3]	54.4	54.7	53.7	50.5	59.8	57.3	55.5	44.5
High school diploma or GED[3]	53.7	62.5	59.4	59.6	58.0	58.3	58.2	49.7
Some college, no bachelor's degree	69.5	77.2	63.8	73.3	63.4	60.7	53.8	60.2
Bachelor's degree or higher	69.2	65.3	79.8	80.9	72.2	68.1	73.8	68.1
Geographic region								
Northeast	64.6	68.2	71.2	75.0	64.8	59.7	72.7	58.7
Midwest	44.4	54.3	53.1	64.4	60.4	58.6	63.1	56.7
South	72.6	74.1	67.6	65.0	60.3	55.2	50.8	50.9
West	69.0	70.6	66.8	69.6	66.9	69.9	60.4	59.0
Age at baby's birth								
Under 20 years	50.0	61.0	48.2	49.1	62.5	56.3	31.9	22.6
20–24 years	57.7	59.4	60.0	63.7	51.9	51.6	54.0	50.6
25–29 years	68.3	71.5	65.1	70.8	65.6	58.3	59.7	63.7
30–44 years	79.4	72.8	81.5	72.8	73.2	73.5	71.8	62.3

[1]Persons of Hispanic origin may be of any race.
[2]For women 22–44 years of age. Education is as of year of interview. See NOTES below.
[3]General equivalency diploma.
[4]For mothers interviewed in the first 3 months of 1995, only babies age 3 months and over are included so they would be eligible for breastfeeding for 3 months or more.

NOTES: Data on breastfeeding during 1972–83 are based on responses to questions in the National Survey of Family Growth (NSFG) Cycle 4, conducted in 1988. Data for 1984–94 are based on the NSFG Cycle 5, conducted in 1995. Data are based on all births to mothers 15–44 years of age at interview, including those births that occurred when the mothers were younger than 15 years of age.

SOURCE: Centers for Disease Control and Prevention, National Center for Health Statistics, National Survey of Family Growth, Cycle 4 1988, Cycle 5 1995.

Table 19 (page 1 of 2). Infant, neonatal, and postneonatal mortality rates, according to detailed race and Hispanic origin of mother: United States, selected years 1983–2000

[Data are based on linked birth and death certificates for infants]

Race and Hispanic origin of mother	1983[1]	1985[1]	1990[1]	1995[2]	1997[2]	1998[2]	1999[2]	2000[2]
	Infant[3] deaths per 1,000 live births							
All mothers	10.9	10.4	8.9	7.6	7.2	7.2	7.0	6.9
White	9.3	8.9	7.3	6.3	6.0	6.0	5.8	5.7
Black or African American	19.2	18.6	16.9	14.6	13.7	13.8	14.0	13.5
American Indian or Alaska Native	15.2	13.1	13.1	9.0	8.7	9.3	9.3	8.3
Asian or Pacific Islander	8.3	7.8	6.6	5.3	5.0	5.5	4.8	4.9
Chinese	9.5	5.8	4.3	3.8	3.1	4.0	2.9	3.5
Japanese	*5.6	*6.0	*5.5	*5.3	*5.3	*3.5	*3.4	*4.6
Filipino	8.4	7.7	6.0	5.6	5.8	6.2	5.8	5.7
Hawaiian	11.2	*9.9	*8.0	*6.6	9.0	10.0	*7.1	9.1
Other Asian or Pacific Islander	8.1	8.5	7.4	5.5	5.0	5.7	5.1	4.8
Hispanic or Latino[4,5]	9.5	8.8	7.5	6.3	6.0	5.8	5.7	5.6
Mexican	9.1	8.5	7.2	6.0	5.8	5.6	5.5	5.4
Puerto Rican	12.9	11.2	9.9	8.9	7.9	7.8	8.3	8.2
Cuban	7.5	8.5	7.2	5.3	5.5	*3.6	4.7	4.5
Central and South American	8.5	8.0	6.8	5.5	5.5	5.3	4.7	4.6
Other and unknown Hispanic or Latino	10.6	9.5	8.0	7.4	6.2	6.5	7.2	6.9
Not Hispanic or Latino:								
White[5]	9.2	8.6	7.2	6.3	6.0	6.0	5.8	5.7
Black or African American[5]	19.1	18.3	16.9	14.7	13.7	13.9	14.1	13.6
	Neonatal[3] deaths per 1,000 live births							
All mothers	7.1	6.8	5.7	4.9	4.8	4.8	4.7	4.6
White	6.1	5.8	4.6	4.1	4.0	4.0	3.9	3.8
Black or African American	12.5	12.3	11.1	9.6	9.2	9.4	9.5	9.1
American Indian or Alaska Native	7.5	6.1	6.1	3.9	4.5	5.0	5.0	4.4
Asian or Pacific Islander	5.2	4.8	3.9	3.4	3.2	3.9	3.2	3.4
Chinese	5.5	3.3	2.3	2.3	2.1	2.7	1.8	2.5
Japanese	*3.7	*3.1	*3.5	*3.3	*3.0	*2.5	*2.8	*2.7
Filipino	5.6	5.1	3.5	3.4	3.6	4.6	3.9	4.1
Hawaiian	*7.0	*5.7	*4.3	*4.0	*6.3	*7.3	*4.9	*6.2
Other Asian or Pacific Islander	5.0	5.4	4.4	3.7	3.3	3.9	3.3	3.4
Hispanic or Latino[4,5]	6.2	5.7	4.8	4.1	4.0	3.9	3.9	3.8
Mexican	5.9	5.4	4.5	3.9	3.8	3.7	3.7	3.6
Puerto Rican	8.7	7.6	6.9	6.1	5.4	5.2	5.9	5.8
Cuban	*5.0	6.2	5.3	*3.6	4.0	*2.7	*3.5	*3.2
Central and South American	5.8	5.6	4.4	3.7	3.9	3.6	3.3	3.3
Other and unknown Hispanic or Latino	6.4	5.6	5.0	4.8	3.7	4.5	4.8	4.6
Not Hispanic or Latino:								
White[5]	5.9	5.6	4.5	4.0	3.9	3.9	3.8	3.8
Black or African American[5]	12.0	11.9	11.0	9.6	9.2	9.4	9.6	9.2
	Postneonatal[3] deaths per 1,000 live births							
All mothers	3.8	3.6	3.2	2.6	2.4	2.4	2.3	2.3
White	3.2	3.1	2.7	2.2	2.1	2.0	1.9	1.9
Black or African American	6.7	6.3	5.9	5.0	4.5	4.4	4.5	4.3
American Indian or Alaska Native	7.7	7.0	7.0	5.1	4.2	4.3	4.3	3.9
Asian or Pacific Islander	3.1	2.9	2.7	1.9	1.8	1.7	1.7	1.4
Chinese	4.0	*2.5	*2.0	*1.5	*1.0	*1.3	*1.2	*1.0
Japanese	*	*2.9	*	*	*2.2	*	*	*
Filipino	*2.8	2.7	2.5	2.2	2.3	1.6	1.9	1.6
Hawaiian	*4.2	*4.3	*3.8	*	*	*	*	*
Other Asian or Pacific Islander	3.0	3.0	3.0	1.9	1.7	1.8	1.8	1.4
Hispanic or Latino[4,5]	3.3	3.2	2.7	2.1	2.0	1.9	1.8	1.8
Mexican	3.2	3.2	2.7	2.1	2.0	1.9	1.8	1.8
Puerto Rican	4.2	3.5	3.0	2.8	2.5	2.6	2.4	2.4
Cuban	*2.5	*2.3	*1.9	*1.7	*	*	*	*
Central and South American	2.6	2.4	2.4	1.9	1.5	1.7	1.4	1.4
Other and unknown Hispanic or Latino	4.2	3.9	3.0	2.6	2.5	2.0	2.5	2.3
Not Hispanic or Latino:								
White[5]	3.2	3.0	2.7	2.2	2.1	2.0	1.9	1.9
Black or African American[5]	7.0	6.4	5.9	5.0	4.5	4.5	4.6	4.4

See footnotes at end of table.

Table 19 (page 2 of 2). **Table 19 (page 2 of 2). Infant, neonatal, and postneonatal mortality rates, according to detailed race and Hispanic origin of mother: United States, selected years 1983–2000**

[Data are based on linked birth and death certificates for infants]

Race and Hispanic origin of mother	1983–85[1]	1986–88[1]	1989–91[1]	1995–97[2]	1998–2000[2]
	Infant[3] deaths per 1,000 live births				
All mothers	10.6	9.8	9.0	7.4	7.0
White	9.0	8.2	7.4	6.1	5.8
Black or African American	18.7	17.9	17.1	14.1	13.8
American Indian or Alaska Native	13.9	13.2	12.6	9.2	9.0
Asian or Pacific Islander	8.3	7.3	6.6	5.1	5.1
Chinese	7.4	5.8	5.1	3.3	3.5
Japanese	6.0	6.9	5.3	4.9	3.8
Filipino	8.2	6.9	6.4	5.7	5.9
Hawaiian	11.3	11.1	9.0	7.0	8.7
Other Asian or Pacific Islander	8.6	7.6	7.0	5.4	5.2
Hispanic or Latino[4,5]	9.2	8.3	7.5	6.1	5.7
Mexican	8.8	7.9	7.2	5.9	5.5
Puerto Rican	12.3	11.1	10.4	8.5	8.1
Cuban	8.0	7.3	6.2	5.3	4.3
Central and South American	8.2	7.5	6.6	5.3	4.9
Other and unknown Hispanic or Latino	9.8	9.0	8.2	7.1	6.9
Not Hispanic or Latino:[5]					
White[5]	8.8	8.1	7.3	6.1	5.8
Black or African American[5]	18.5	17.9	17.2	14.2	13.9
	Neonatal[3] deaths per 1,000 live births				
All mothers	6.9	6.3	5.7	4.8	4.7
White	5.9	5.2	4.7	4.0	3.9
Black or African American	12.2	11.7	11.1	9.4	9.3
American Indian or Alaska Native	6.7	5.9	5.9	4.4	4.8
Asian or Pacific Islander	5.2	4.5	3.9	3.3	3.5
Chinese	4.3	3.3	2.7	2.1	2.4
Japanese	3.4	4.4	3.0	2.8	2.6
Filipino	5.3	4.5	4.0	3.7	4.2
Hawaiian	7.4	7.1	4.8	4.5	6.1
Other Asian or Pacific Islander	5.5	4.7	4.2	3.5	3.5
Hispanic or Latino[4,5]	6.0	5.3	4.8	4.0	3.8
Mexican	5.7	5.0	4.5	3.8	3.7
Puerto Rican	8.3	7.2	7.0	5.7	5.6
Cuban	5.9	5.3	4.6	3.7	3.1
Central and South American	5.7	4.9	4.4	3.7	3.4
Other and unknown Hispanic or Latino	6.1	5.8	5.2	4.6	4.6
Not Hispanic or Latino:[5]					
White[5]	5.7	5.1	4.6	4.0	3.8
Black or African American[5]	11.8	11.4	11.1	9.4	9.4
	Postneonatal[3] deaths per 1,000 live births				
All mothers	3.7	3.5	3.3	2.5	2.3
White	3.1	3.0	2.7	2.1	1.9
Black or African American	6.4	6.2	6.0	4.7	4.4
American Indian or Alaska Native	7.2	7.3	6.7	4.8	4.2
Asian or Pacific Islander	3.1	2.8	2.6	1.8	1.6
Chinese	3.1	2.5	2.4	1.2	1.1
Japanese	2.6	2.5	2.2	2.1	*1.2
Filipino	2.9	2.4	2.3	2.1	1.7
Hawaiian	3.9	4.0	4.1	*2.5	*2.6
Other Asian or Pacific Islander	3.1	2.9	2.8	1.9	1.7
Hispanic or Latino[4,5]	3.2	3.0	2.7	2.1	1.8
Mexican	3.2	2.9	2.7	2.1	1.8
Puerto Rican	4.0	3.9	3.4	2.8	2.5
Cuban	2.2	2.0	1.6	1.5	*1.1
Central and South American	2.5	2.6	2.2	1.7	1.5
Other and unknown Hispanic or Latino	3.7	3.2	3.0	2.5	2.3
Not Hispanic or Latino:[5]					
White[5]	3.1	3.0	2.7	2.2	2.0
Black or African American[5]	6.7	6.5	6.1	4.8	4.5

* Estimates are considered unreliable. Rates preceded by an asterisk are based on fewer than 50 events. Rates not shown are based on fewer than 20 events.
[1] Rates based on unweighted birth cohort data.
[2] Rates based on a period file using weighted data (see Appendix I, National Vital Statistics System, Linked Birth/Infant Death Data Set).
[3] Infant (under 1 year of age), neonatal (under 28 days), and postneonatal (28 days–11 months).
[4] Persons of Hispanic origin may be of any race.
[5] Prior to 1995, data shown only for States with an Hispanic-origin item on their birth certificates (see Appendix II, Hispanic origin).

NOTES: The race groups white, black, American Indian or Alaska Native, and Asian or Pacific Islander include persons of Hispanic and non-Hispanic origin. National linked files do not exist for 1992–94. Data for additional years are available (see Appendix III).

SOURCE: Centers for Disease Control and Prevention, National Center for Health Statistics, National Vital Statistics System, Linked Birth/Infant Death Data Set.

Table 20. Infant mortality rates for mothers 20 years of age and over, according to mother's education, detailed race, and Hispanic origin: United States, selected years 1983–2000

[Data are based on linked birth and death certificates for infants]

Education, race, and Hispanic origin of mother	1983[1]	1990[1]	1995[2]	1999[2]	2000[2]	1983–85[1]	1986–88[1]	1989–91[1]	1995–97[2]	1998–2000[2]
Less than 12 years of education					Infant deaths per 1,000 live births					
All mothers	15.0	10.8	8.9	8.0	7.9	14.6	13.8	11.1	8.6	8.0
White	12.5	9.0	7.6	6.9	6.8	12.4	11.4	9.2	7.3	6.9
Black or African American	23.4	19.5	17.0	14.8	14.7	21.8	21.1	20.3	16.0	14.8
American Indian or Alaska Native	14.5	14.3	12.7	11.0	10.1	15.2	16.8	13.8	11.4	10.2
Asian or Pacific Islander[3]	9.7	6.6	5.7	5.4	5.9	9.5	8.2	6.9	5.8	5.7
Hispanic or Latino[4,5]	10.9	7.3	6.0	5.6	5.4	10.6	9.9	7.5	5.8	5.5
Mexican	8.7	7.0	5.8	5.5	5.2	9.5	8.3	7.1	5.6	5.3
Puerto Rican	15.3	10.1	10.6	9.4	9.6	14.1	12.8	11.7	9.5	8.9
Cuban	*14.5	*	*	*	*	*10.5	*9.4	*8.2	*6.7	*
Central and South American	9.8	7.0	5.1	4.4	4.9	8.6	9.2	6.8	5.4	5.0
Other and unknown Hispanic or Latino	9.2	9.9	7.3	7.0	7.6	10.1	10.6	10.0	7.0	7.4
Not Hispanic or Latino:										
White[5]	12.8	10.9	9.9	8.9	9.2	12.6	11.8	11.0	9.6	9.1
Black or African American[5]	24.7	19.7	17.3	15.1	15.0	22.6	21.6	20.6	16.3	15.1
12 years of education										
All mothers	10.2	8.8	7.8	7.4	7.3	10.0	9.6	8.9	7.6	7.4
White	8.7	7.1	6.4	6.0	6.0	8.5	8.0	7.2	6.3	6.0
Black or African American	17.8	16.0	14.7	14.0	13.3	17.7	17.1	16.4	14.1	13.9
American Indian or Alaska Native	15.5	13.4	7.9	9.0	7.8	13.4	11.6	12.3	8.5	8.7
Asian or Pacific Islander[3]	10.0	7.5	5.5	5.6	5.0	9.3	7.9	7.5	5.6	5.5
Hispanic or Latino[4,5]	8.4	7.0	5.9	5.3	5.0	9.1	8.3	6.8	5.8	5.2
Mexican	6.9	6.8	5.7	5.0	4.9	7.8	8.2	6.5	5.6	5.0
Puerto Rican	9.5	8.5	6.5	8.0	7.2	10.8	10.1	8.6	7.6	7.5
Cuban	*6.9	*8.0	*	*	*	8.6	6.6	7.6	5.4	*3.7
Central and South American	8.7	6.5	6.1	4.8	4.2	8.7	7.4	6.3	5.5	4.8
Other and unknown Hispanic or Latino	8.8	7.4	6.5	6.7	5.8	8.8	7.7	7.0	6.6	6.1
Not Hispanic or Latino:										
White[5]	8.7	7.1	6.5	6.2	6.3	8.3	7.9	7.3	6.4	6.3
Black or African American[5]	17.8	16.1	14.8	14.1	13.5	17.9	17.4	16.5	14.2	14.0
13 years or more of education										
All mothers	8.1	6.4	5.4	5.1	5.0	7.8	7.2	6.4	5.3	5.1
White	7.2	5.4	4.7	4.3	4.2	6.9	6.2	5.5	4.5	4.4
Black or African American	15.3	13.7	11.9	11.4	11.4	15.3	14.9	13.7	11.6	11.3
American Indian or Alaska Native	12.5	6.8	5.9	7.4	6.7	10.4	8.4	8.1	6.6	7.0
Asian or Pacific Islander[3]	6.6	5.1	4.4	4.0	3.9	6.7	5.9	5.1	4.1	4.1
Hispanic or Latino[4,5]	9.0	5.7	5.0	4.7	4.5	7.4	7.0	5.8	5.0	4.6
Mexican	*8.3	5.5	5.2	4.8	4.5	7.6	6.4	5.7	5.1	4.7
Puerto Rican	10.9	7.3	6.3	6.3	6.5	8.1	6.9	7.8	6.4	6.2
Cuban	*	*5.3	*5.3	*4.5	*4.9	5.5	5.9	4.2	4.3	4.2
Central and South American	*7.1	5.6	3.7	3.9	3.7	7.2	7.6	5.4	4.0	3.9
Other and unknown Hispanic or Latino	11.6	5.4	5.2	4.5	4.2	7.9	7.5	5.6	5.3	4.1
Not Hispanic or Latino:										
White[5]	7.0	5.4	4.6	4.2	4.2	6.8	6.1	5.4	4.5	4.3
Black or African American[5]	14.8	13.7	12.0	11.5	11.5	14.7	14.9	13.8	11.7	11.4

* Estimates are considered unreliable. Rates preceded by an asterisk are based on fewer than 50 events. Rates not shown are based on fewer than 20 events.
[1] Rates based on unweighted birth cohort data.
[2] Rates based on a period file using weighted data (see Appendix I, National Vital Statistics System, Linked Birth/Infant Death Data Set).
[3] The States not reporting maternal education on the birth certificate accounted for 49–51 percent of the Asian or Pacific Islander births in the United States in 1983–87, 59 percent in 1988, and 12 percent in 1989–91. Starting in 1992 maternal education was reported by all 50 States and the District of Columbia (DC).
[4] Persons of Hispanic origin may be of any race.
[5] Prior to 1995, data shown only for States with an Hispanic-origin item and education of mother on their birth certificates (see Appendix II, Education; Hispanic origin). The Hispanic-reporting States that did not report maternal education on the birth certificate during 1983–88 together accounted for 28–85 percent of the births in each Hispanic subgroup (except Cuban, 11–16 percent, and Puerto Rican, 6–7 percent in 1983–87); and in 1989–91 accounted for 27–39 percent of Central and South American and Puerto Rican births and 2–9 percent of births in other Hispanic subgroups.

NOTES: Prior to 1995, data for all mothers and by race are shown only for states reporting education of mother on their birth certificates (see Appendix II, Education). The race groups white, black, American Indian or Alaska Native, and Asian or Pacific Islander include persons of Hispanic and non-Hispanic origin. Persons of Hispanic origin may be of any race. National linked files do not exist for 1992–94. Data for additional years are available (see Appendix III).

SOURCE: Centers for Disease Control and Prevention, National Center for Health Statistics, National Vital Statistics System, Linked Birth/Infant Death Data Set.

Table 21. Infant mortality rates according to birthweight: United States, selected years 1983–2000

[Data are based on linked birth and death certificates for infants]

Birthweight	1983[1]	1985[1]	1990[1]	1991[1]	1995[2]	1996[2]	1997[2]	1998[2]	1999[2]	2000[2]
	Infant deaths per 1,000 live births[3]									
All birthweights	10.9	10.4	8.9	8.6	7.6	7.3	7.2	7.2	7.0	6.9
Less than 2,500 grams	95.9	93.9	78.1	74.3	65.3	63.6	62.4	62.3	61.3	60.2
Less than 1,500 grams	400.6	387.7	317.6	305.4	270.7	261.5	255.0	252.4	249.5	246.9
Less than 500 grams	890.3	895.9	898.2	889.9	904.9	890.1	885.2	869.6	857.7	847.9
500–999 grams	584.2	559.2	440.1	422.6	351.0	336.9	324.4	319.4	318.6	313.8
1,000–1,499 grams	162.3	145.4	97.9	91.3	69.6	64.7	61.8	60.6	59.2	60.9
1,500–1,999 grams	58.4	54.0	43.8	40.4	33.5	30.6	30.6	29.0	29.1	28.7
2,000–2,499 grams	22.5	20.9	17.8	17.0	13.7	13.6	12.5	12.7	12.0	11.9
2,500 grams or more	4.7	4.3	3.7	3.6	3.0	2.8	2.7	2.7	2.6	2.5
2,500–2,999 grams	8.8	7.9	6.7	6.7	5.5	5.1	5.0	4.9	4.7	4.6
3,000–3,499 grams	4.4	4.3	3.7	3.5	2.9	2.7	2.6	2.6	2.5	2.4
3,500–3,999 grams	3.2	3.0	2.6	2.5	2.0	1.9	1.9	1.8	1.7	1.7
4,000 grams or more	3.3	3.2	2.4	2.4	2.0	1.8	1.8	1.7	1.8	1.6
4,000–4,499 grams	2.9	2.9	2.2	2.2	1.8	1.7	1.7	1.7	1.6	1.5
4,500–4,999 grams	3.9	3.8	2.5	3.0	2.2	2.1	2.0	2.0	1.9	2.1
5,000 grams or more[4]	14.4	14.7	9.8	8.2	8.5	*6.2	*4.2	*4.3	*7.9	*6.1

* Estimates are considered unreliable. Rates preceded by an asterisk are based on fewer than 50 events.
[1] Rates based on unweighted birth cohort data.
[2] Rates based on a period file using weighted data; not stated birthweight imputed when period of gestation is known and proportionately distributed when period of gestation is unknown (see Appendix I, National Vital Statistics System, Linked Birth/Infant Death Data Set).
[3] For calculation of birthweight-specific infant mortality rates, unknown birthweight has been distributed in proportion to known birthweight separately for live births (denominator) and infant deaths (numerator).
[4] In 1989 a birthweight-gestational age consistency check instituted for the natality file resulted in a decrease in the number of deaths to infants coded with birthweights of 5,000 grams or more and a discontinuity in the mortality trend for infants weighing 5,000 grams or more at birth. Starting with 1989 the rates are believed to be more accurate.

NOTES: National linked files do not exist for 1992–94. Data for additional years are available (see Appendix III).

SOURCE: Centers for Disease Control and Prevention, National Center for Health Statistics, National Vital Statistics System, Linked Birth/Infant Death Data Set.

Table 22. Infant mortality rates, fetal mortality rates, and perinatal mortality rates, according to race: United States, selected years 1950–2000

[Data are based on death certificates, fetal death records, and birth certificates]

Race and year	Infant[1]	Neonatal[1] Under 28 days	Neonatal[1] Under 7 days	Postneonatal[1]	Fetal mortality rate[2]	Late fetal mortality rate[3]	Perinatal mortality rate[4]
All races	Deaths per 1,000 live births						
1950[5]	29.2	20.5	17.8	8.7	18.4	14.9	32.5
1960[5]	26.0	18.7	16.7	7.3	15.8	12.1	28.6
1970	20.0	15.1	13.6	4.9	14.0	9.5	23.0
1980	12.6	8.5	7.1	4.1	9.1	6.2	13.2
1985	10.6	7.0	5.8	3.7	7.8	4.9	10.7
1990	9.2	5.8	4.8	3.4	7.5	4.3	9.1
1995	7.6	4.9	4.0	2.7	7.0	3.6	7.6
1996	7.3	4.8	3.8	2.5	6.9	3.6	7.4
1997	7.2	4.8	3.8	2.5	6.8	3.5	7.3
1998	7.2	4.8	3.8	2.4	6.7	3.4	7.2
1999	7.1	4.7	3.8	2.3	6.7	3.4	7.1
2000	6.9	4.6	3.7	2.3	6.6	3.3	7.0
Race of child:[6] White							
1950[5]	26.8	19.4	17.1	7.4	16.6	13.3	30.1
1960[5]	22.9	17.2	15.6	5.7	13.9	10.8	26.2
1970	17.8	13.8	12.5	4.0	12.3	8.6	21.0
1980	11.0	7.5	6.2	3.5	8.1	5.7	11.9
Race of mother:[7] White							
1980	10.9	7.4	6.1	3.5	8.1	5.7	11.8
1985	9.2	6.0	5.0	3.2	6.9	4.5	9.5
1990	7.6	4.8	3.9	2.8	6.4	3.8	7.7
1995	6.3	4.1	3.3	2.2	5.9	3.3	6.5
1996	6.1	4.0	3.2	2.1	5.9	3.3	6.4
1997	6.0	4.0	3.2	2.0	5.8	3.2	6.3
1998	6.0	4.0	3.1	2.0	5.7	3.1	6.2
1999	5.8	3.9	3.1	1.9	5.7	3.0	6.1
2000	5.7	3.8	3.0	1.9	5.6	2.9	5.9
Race of child:[6] Black or African American							
1950[5]	43.9	27.8	23.0	16.1	32.1	- - -	- - -
1960[5]	44.3	27.8	23.7	16.5	- - -	- - -	- - -
1970	32.6	22.8	20.3	9.9	23.2	- - -	34.5
1980	21.4	14.1	11.9	7.3	14.4	8.9	20.7
Race of mother:[7] Black or African American							
1980	22.2	14.6	12.3	7.6	14.7	9.1	21.3
1985	19.0	12.6	10.8	6.4	12.8	7.2	17.9
1990	18.0	11.6	9.7	6.4	13.3	6.7	16.4
1995	15.1	9.8	8.2	5.3	12.7	5.7	13.8
1996	14.7	9.6	7.8	5.1	12.5	5.5	13.3
1997	14.2	9.4	7.8	4.8	12.5	5.5	13.2
1998	14.3	9.5	7.8	4.8	12.3	5.3	13.1
1999	14.6	9.8	7.9	4.8	12.6	5.4	13.2
2000	14.1	9.4	7.6	4.7	12.4	5.4	13.0

- - - Data not available.

[1]Infant (under 1 year of age), neonatal (under 28 days), early neonatal (under 7 days), and postneonatal (28 days–11 months).
[2]Number of fetal deaths of 20 weeks or more gestation per 1,000 live births plus fetal deaths.
[3]Number of fetal deaths of 28 weeks or more gestation per 1,000 live births plus late fetal deaths.
[4]Number of late fetal deaths plus infant deaths within 7 days of birth per 1,000 live births plus late fetal deaths.
[5]Includes births and deaths of persons who were not residents of the 50 States and the District of Columbia.
[6]Infant deaths are tabulated by race of decedent; live births and fetal deaths are tabulated by race of child (see Appendix II, Race).
[7]Infant deaths are tabulated by race of decedent; fetal deaths and live births are tabulated by race of mother (see Appendix II, Race).

NOTES: Infant mortality rates in this table are based on infant deaths from the mortality file (numerator) and live births from the natality file (denominator). Inconsistencies in reporting race for the same infant between the birth and death certificate can result in underestimated infant mortality rates for races other than white or black. Infant mortality rates for minority population groups are available from the Linked Birth/Infant Death Data Set and are presented in tables 19–20 and 23–24. Data for additional years are available (see Appendix III).

SOURCE: Centers for Disease Control and Prevention, National Center for Health Statistics, National Vital Statistics System: Minino AM, Arias E, Kochanek KD, Murphy SL, Smith BL. Deaths: Final data for 2000. National vital statistics reports. vol 50 no 15. Hyattsville, Maryland: National Center for Health Statistics. 2002.

This table will be updated with 2001 data on the web. Go to www.cdc.gov/nchs/hus.htm.

Table 23 (page 1 of 2). Infant mortality rates, according to race, Hispanic origin, geographic division, and State: United States, average annual 1989–91, 1995–97, and 1998–2000

[Data are based on linked birth and death certificates for infants]

Geographic division and State	All races			Not Hispanic or Latino					
				White			Black or African American		
	1989–91[1]	1995–97[2]	1998–2000[2]	1989–91[1]	1995–97[2]	1998–2000[2]	1989–91[1]	1995–97[2]	1998–2000[2]
	Infant[3] deaths per 1,000 live births								
United States.................	9.0	7.4	7.0	7.3	6.1	5.8	17.2	14.2	13.9
New England[4]	7.3	5.7	5.6	6.2	4.8	4.6	15.1	11.5	12.2
Maine........................	6.6	5.3	5.4	6.2	5.1	5.4	*	*	*
New Hampshire[4]............	7.1	4.8	5.4	7.2	4.6	4.7	*	*	*
Vermont.....................	6.6	6.3	6.3	6.3	6.1	6.2	*	*	*
Massachusetts..............	7.0	5.1	5.0	5.9	4.3	4.2	14.2	10.6	11.2
Rhode Island	8.7	6.5	6.4	7.5	5.0	4.9	*13.6	*	*13.5
Connecticut	7.9	6.9	6.5	5.9	5.3	4.7	17.0	13.6	13.5
Middle Atlantic..............	9.2	7.2	6.6	6.6	5.3	5.0	18.5	14.3	13.1
New York	9.5	7.1	6.3	6.3	4.8	4.7	18.4	13.5	11.8
New Jersey	8.4	6.6	6.4	6.1	4.5	4.4	17.8	13.8	13.8
Pennsylvania	9.2	7.7	7.2	7.2	6.2	5.6	19.1	16.6	15.4
East North Central	9.8	8.2	8.0	7.7	6.6	6.3	19.1	16.5	16.1
Ohio	9.0	8.1	7.9	7.7	6.8	6.7	16.2	15.3	14.4
Indiana.....................	9.4	8.4	7.8	8.4	7.5	6.9	17.3	15.6	15.4
Illinois.....................	10.7	8.8	8.5	7.6	6.5	6.2	20.5	17.5	17.1
Michigan	10.5	8.2	8.1	7.7	6.3	6.0	20.7	16.3	16.4
Wisconsin...................	8.4	7.0	6.9	7.4	5.9	5.7	17.0	16.3	16.6
West North Central..........	8.5	7.1	6.8	7.4	6.3	6.0	17.5	14.7	14.7
Minnesota	7.3	6.2	5.9	6.4	5.6	5.2	18.5	13.4	13.0
Iowa	8.2	7.1	6.2	7.8	6.7	5.8	15.8	*16.5	17.3
Missouri	9.7	7.5	7.5	8.0	6.2	6.1	18.0	14.5	16.0
North Dakota	8.0	6.3	8.0	7.3	5.8	7.0	*	*	*
South Dakota	9.5	7.4	7.8	7.5	6.0	6.7	*	*	*
Nebraska	8.1	7.9	7.0	7.2	7.3	6.2	18.3	*13.5	16.2
Kansas.....................	8.5	7.5	7.0	7.8	6.7	7.1	15.4	17.0	10.5
South Atlantic...............	10.4	8.4	8.1	7.6	6.3	6.0	17.2	14.2	13.9
Delaware	11.2	7.7	8.8	8.2	6.2	6.5	20.1	12.9	15.8
Maryland	9.1	8.7	8.1	6.3	5.7	5.2	15.0	14.9	13.9
District of Columbia...........	20.3	14.9	13.5	*8.2	*	*	23.9	18.5	16.8
Virginia....................	9.9	7.7	7.2	7.4	6.0	5.6	18.0	13.6	12.8
West Virginia	9.1	8.2	7.6	8.8	7.9	7.6	*15.7	*17.9	*9.8
North Carolina	10.7	9.2	9.0	8.0	7.0	6.7	16.9	15.3	15.7
South Carolina	11.8	9.2	9.5	8.4	6.3	6.3	17.2	14.4	15.5
Georgia	11.9	9.1	8.3	8.4	6.4	5.9	17.9	14.4	13.5
Florida.....................	9.4	7.4	7.2	7.2	6.1	5.8	16.2	12.6	12.6
East South Central	10.4	9.1	8.8	8.1	7.1	6.7	16.5	14.7	15.0
Kentucky	8.7	7.3	7.4	8.1	7.0	6.9	14.4	11.2	12.7
Tennessee..................	10.2	8.7	8.4	7.8	6.7	6.4	18.2	16.1	15.6
Alabama....................	11.4	9.9	9.8	8.6	7.6	7.1	16.8	14.6	15.4
Mississippi	11.5	10.6	10.3	7.9	7.3	6.6	15.2	14.5	14.7
West South Central[4]	8.4	7.2	6.9	7.2	6.5	6.2	14.2	12.1	12.2
Arkansas...................	9.8	8.9	8.4	8.1	7.7	7.4	15.2	13.4	12.6
Louisiana[4]	10.2	9.4	9.1	7.5	6.7	6.2	14.3	13.5	13.5
Oklahoma[4]	8.0	8.1	8.5	7.3	7.5	8.2	12.7	14.3	13.5
Texas......................	7.9	6.4	6.0	6.9	6.0	5.5	14.1	10.6	11.0
Mountain...................	8.4	6.7	6.6	7.9	6.3	6.1	16.9	12.5	13.7
Montana....................	9.0	6.9	6.8	8.0	6.6	6.0	*	*	*
Idaho......................	8.9	6.6	7.2	8.9	6.4	6.8	*	*	*
Wyoming	8.4	6.8	7.0	8.0	6.1	6.8	*	*	*
Colorado	8.7	6.7	6.5	8.0	6.1	5.9	16.7	13.6	14.8
New Mexico	8.4	6.3	6.9	8.1	6.2	7.0	*17.2	*	*
Arizona....................	8.8	7.4	7.0	8.2	7.1	6.6	17.3	14.1	15.0
Utah	7.0	5.8	5.3	6.8	5.5	5.2	*	*	*
Nevada	8.6	6.2	6.7	7.8	6.3	6.1	16.9	10.9	12.1
Pacific.....................	7.7	6.0	5.6	7.0	5.5	4.9	15.4	12.7	11.7
Washington	8.0	5.8	5.3	7.4	5.4	4.8	15.1	12.9	10.1
Oregon.....................	8.0	5.8	5.6	7.4	5.6	5.3	21.3	*11.4	*8.5
California	7.6	6.0	5.5	6.9	5.5	4.8	15.4	12.8	12.0
Alaska	9.2	7.4	6.3	7.2	5.8	5.0	*	*	*
Hawaii	7.0	6.0	7.4	5.5	5.2	6.4	*13.6	*	*

See footnotes at end of table.

Table 23 (page 2 of 2). Infant mortality rates, according to race, Hispanic origin, geographic division, and State: United States, average annual 1989–91, 1995–97, and 1998–2000

[Data are based on linked birth and death certificates for infants]

Geographic division and State	Hispanic or Latino[5]			American Indian or Alaska Native[6]			Asian or Pacific Islander[6]		
	1989–91[1]	1995–97[2]	1998–2000[2]	1989–91[1]	1995–97[2]	1998–2000[2]	1989–91[1]	1995–97[2]	1998–2000[2]
	Infant[3] deaths per 1,000 live births								
United States	7.5	6.1	5.7	12.6	9.2	9.0	6.6	5.1	5.1
New England[7]	8.1	7.8	6.9	*	*	*	5.8	4.3	3.9
Maine	*	*	*	*	*	*	*	*	*
New Hampshire[7]	- - -	*	*	*	*	*	*	*	*
Vermont	*	*	*	*	*	*	*	*	*
Massachusetts	8.3	6.7	5.5	*	*	*	5.7	*3.7	3.9
Rhode Island	*7.2	*9.7	*6.4	*	*	*	*	*	*
Connecticut	7.9	8.8	8.6	*	*	*	*	*	*
Middle Atlantic	9.1	6.9	6.2	*11.6	*	*	6.4	4.1	4.2
New York	9.4	6.6	5.9	*15.2	*	*	6.4	4.1	4.0
New Jersey	7.5	7.0	6.2	*	*	*	5.6	4.0	4.6
Pennsylvania	10.9	8.9	8.5	*	*	*	7.8	*4.4	*3.8
East North Central	8.7	7.4	7.2	11.6	10.1	8.5	6.1	5.3	6.2
Ohio	8.0	7.6	8.7	*	*	*	*4.8	*6.2	*4.3
Indiana	*7.2	8.1	6.8	*	*	*	*	*8.3	*6.6
Illinois	9.2	7.2	7.2	*	*	*	6.0	5.6	6.7
Michigan	7.9	6.7	6.6	*10.7	*9.9	*	*6.1	*3.9	6.7
Wisconsin	*7.3	9.6	7.4	*11.9	*8.8	*8.3	*6.7	*3.7	*5.8
West North Central	9.3	6.8	6.4	17.1	13.9	11.4	7.4	6.8	6.0
Minnesota	*8.4	*6.0	6.9	17.3	16.2	*10.4	*5.1	7.0	6.8
Iowa	*11.9	*7.0	*6.1	*	*	*	*	*	*
Missouri	*9.1	*5.3	*6.5	*	*	*	*9.1	*	*
North Dakota	*	*	*	*13.8	*10.5	*15.1	*	*	*
South Dakota	*	*	*	19.9	15.0	13.3	*	*	*
Nebraska	*8.8	9.2	7.8	*18.2	*	*15.4	*	*	*
Kansas	8.7	6.9	5.2	*	*	*	*	*	*
South Atlantic	7.4	5.7	5.2	12.7	11.3	8.6	6.8	5.6	5.2
Delaware	*	*	*	*	*	*	*	*	*
Maryland	7.2	5.7	5.8	*	*	*	7.5	6.8	*4.8
District of Columbia	*8.8	*	*9.1	*	*	*	*	*	*
Virginia	7.6	6.6	4.7	*	*	*	6.0	4.8	5.4
West Virginia	*	*	*	*	*	*	*	*	*
North Carolina	*7.5	6.5	6.2	12.2	12.7	11.7	*6.3	*5.7	*6.2
South Carolina	*	*8.1	*5.9	*	*	*	*	*	*
Georgia	9.0	6.7	5.1	*	*	*	*8.2	*5.3	*4.5
Florida	7.1	5.1	4.9	*	*10.6	*	*6.2	5.5	5.2
East South Central	*5.9	6.7	6.1	*	*13.7	*	*7.7	*5.8	*5.9
Kentucky	*	*	*	*	*	*	*	*	*
Tennessee	*	*6.4	*5.4	*	*	*	*	*	*5.9
Alabama	*	*8.4	*7.3	*	*	*	*	*	*
Mississippi	*	*	*	*	*	*	*	*	*
West South Central[7]	7.0	5.7	5.2	8.4	7.6	7.9	6.7	5.1	4.3
Arkansas	*	*8.6	*5.7	*	*	*	*	*	*
Louisiana[7]	- - -	*	*4.9	*	*	*	*	*7.2	*
Oklahoma[7]	- - -	*5.5	5.4	7.8	8.2	8.2	*	*	*
Texas	7.0	5.7	5.2	*	*	*	6.8	5.0	4.2
Mountain	7.9	6.7	6.6	11.6	8.5	8.8	8.1	6.0	5.5
Montana	*	*	*	16.7	*8.6	*11.3	*	*	*
Idaho	*7.2	*6.5	8.7	*	*	*	*	*	*
Wyoming	*	*	*	*	*	*	*	*	*
Colorado	8.5	6.8	6.5	*16.5	*	*	*7.8	*6.6	*4.9
New Mexico	7.8	6.2	6.6	9.8	7.3	7.6	*	*	*
Arizona	8.0	7.4	6.7	11.4	8.6	8.7	*8.5	*5.3	*5.1
Utah	*7.0	6.9	5.7	*10.0	*	*	*10.7	*6.9	*6.2
Nevada	7.0	4.6	6.0	*	*	*	*	*	*6.0
Pacific	7.1	5.6	5.2	14.6	8.0	9.4	6.5	5.3	5.2
Washington	7.6	4.9	5.0	19.6	*7.0	9.2	6.2	4.7	5.3
Oregon	8.5	6.5	6.4	*15.7	*	*10.6	*8.4	*4.5	*4.2
California	7.0	5.6	5.2	11.0	7.5	9.3	6.4	5.1	4.8
Alaska	*	*	*	15.7	10.7	9.7	*	*	*
Hawaii	10.7	*5.8	7.5	*	*	*	7.1	6.2	7.6

* Estimates are considered unreliable. Rates preceded by an asterisk are based on fewer than 50 events. Rates not shown are based on fewer than 20 events.

- - - Data not available.   [1]Rates based on unweighted birth cohort data.

[2]Rates based on period file using weighted data (see Appendix I, National Vital Statistics System, Linked Birth/Infant Death Data Set).

[3]Under 1 year of age.

[4]Rates for white and black are substituted for non-Hispanic white and non-Hispanic black for Louisiana 1989, Oklahoma 1989–90, and New Hampshire 1989–91.

[5]Persons of Hispanic origin may be of any race.   [6]Includes persons of Hispanic origin.

[7]Rates for Hispanic origin exclude data from States not reporting Hispanic origin on the birth certificate for 1 or more years in a 3-year period.

NOTE: National linked files do not exist for 1992–94.

SOURCE: Centers for Disease Control and Prevention, National Center for Health Statistics, National Vital Statistics System, Linked Birth/Infant Death Data Set.

Table 24 (page 1 of 2). **Neonatal mortality rates, according to race, Hispanic origin, geographic division, and State: United States, average annual 1989–91, 1995–97, and 1998–2000**

[Data are based on linked birth and death certificates for infants]

Geographic division and State	All races			Not Hispanic or Latino					
				White			Black or African American		
	1989–91[1]	1995–97[2]	1998–2000[2]	1989–91[1]	1995–97[2]	1998–2000[2]	1989–91[1]	1995–97[2]	1998–2000[2]
	Neonatal[3] deaths per 1,000 live births								
United States..................	5.7	4.8	4.7	4.6	4.0	3.8	11.1	9.4	9.4
New England[4]	5.1	4.2	4.2	4.2	3.5	3.5	11.0	8.4	9.1
Maine.........................	4.5	3.7	3.9	4.2	3.7	3.9	*	*	*
New Hampshire[4].............	4.3	3.4	3.9	4.4	3.2	3.4	*	*	*
Vermont......................	4.1	4.2	4.3	3.9	4.0	4.4	*	*	*
Massachusetts...............	4.9	3.8	3.9	4.1	3.2	3.3	10.4	7.6	8.8
Rhode Island	6.4	5.1	4.8	5.3	3.8	3.8	*9.8	*	*9.3
Connecticut	5.7	5.1	4.9	4.2	4.0	3.6	12.5	10.2	9.7
Middle Atlantic..............	6.3	5.0	4.7	4.6	3.7	3.5	12.3	9.6	9.1
New York....................	6.5	5.0	4.5	4.3	3.3	3.3	12.6	9.1	8.4
New Jersey	5.8	4.6	4.6	4.5	3.3	3.2	11.4	9.0	9.5
Pennsylvania	6.2	5.4	5.0	4.9	4.3	4.0	12.5	11.4	10.3
East North Central	6.3	5.5	5.4	4.9	4.4	4.3	12.1	10.7	10.7
Ohio	5.5	5.4	5.4	4.8	4.6	4.6	9.8	10.2	9.8
Indiana......................	6.0	5.5	5.2	5.2	4.9	4.6	11.5	10.3	10.1
Illinois......................	7.0	5.9	5.8	5.1	4.6	4.3	12.7	11.2	11.1
Michigan	6.9	5.4	5.5	4.9	4.1	4.0	14.0	10.8	11.4
Wisconsin...................	5.1	4.5	4.6	4.6	3.8	3.8	9.1	10.1	10.8
West North Central..........	5.0	4.5	4.5	4.5	4.0	3.9	10.2	9.6	9.9
Minnesota	4.3	3.8	3.9	3.9	3.5	3.5	10.7	8.2	8.8
Iowa........................	4.8	4.7	4.0	4.5	4.4	3.7	*10.5	*11.5	*10.5
Missouri.....................	6.0	4.8	4.9	5.0	3.9	3.9	10.6	9.5	10.8
North Dakota	5.0	3.8	5.0	4.7	3.8	4.7	*	*	*
South Dakota	5.1	4.1	4.3	4.5	3.5	4.1	*	*	*
Nebraska	4.5	5.4	4.7	4.2	5.1	4.1	*9.8	*9.6	*10.7
Kansas......................	4.9	4.9	4.7	4.6	4.3	4.7	8.3	11.6	7.5
South Atlantic...............	6.9	5.7	5.6	4.9	4.1	4.0	11.7	9.9	9.8
Delaware	7.5	5.1	6.3	5.8	3.8	4.2	12.4	9.7	12.6
Maryland	5.9	6.1	5.9	3.9	3.7	3.6	10.2	10.9	10.3
District of Columbia...........	14.1	10.8	9.4	*5.2	*	*	16.7	13.5	11.9
Virginia......................	6.8	5.4	5.1	4.8	4.0	3.8	13.0	10.0	9.3
West Virginia	5.8	5.5	4.6	5.6	5.3	4.6	*9.7	*12.5	*
North Carolina	7.3	6.3	6.5	5.3	4.8	4.8	11.9	10.6	11.5
South Carolina	7.7	6.4	6.7	5.4	4.2	4.1	11.3	10.3	11.4
Georgia	7.9	6.1	5.7	5.5	4.1	3.8	12.0	10.0	9.4
Florida	6.2	4.7	4.7	4.7	3.8	3.8	10.5	8.2	8.2
East South Central	6.6	5.7	5.7	5.0	4.3	4.2	10.6	9.5	9.9
Kentucky	5.0	4.5	4.8	4.6	4.2	4.5	8.9	7.2	8.0
Tennessee	6.5	5.3	5.5	4.9	3.9	4.1	11.8	10.0	10.6
Alabama.....................	7.5	6.5	6.2	5.7	4.8	4.3	11.1	9.8	10.3
Mississippi	7.1	6.6	6.3	4.9	4.4	3.8	9.5	9.1	9.3
West South Central[4]	5.0	4.3	4.2	4.2	3.9	3.8	8.4	7.4	7.6
Arkansas....................	5.4	5.4	4.9	4.5	4.6	4.3	8.5	8.1	7.7
Louisiana[4]	6.3	6.1	5.9	4.8	4.4	4.0	8.5	8.6	8.8
Oklahoma[4]	4.4	4.8	5.2	4.1	4.5	5.2	6.3	8.8	8.1
Texas........................	4.7	3.8	3.7	4.1	3.5	3.3	8.5	6.2	6.8
Mountain.....................	4.8	4.2	4.2	4.4	3.9	3.8	10.1	7.9	9.0
Montana.....................	4.6	3.9	3.7	4.2	3.7	3.2	*	*	*
Idaho........................	5.3	4.1	4.8	5.2	3.8	4.5	*	*	*
Wyoming	3.9	3.6	4.4	3.8	3.1	4.1	*	*	*
Colorado	5.0	4.4	4.3	4.7	4.0	3.8	10.9	9.3	11.1
New Mexico	5.0	3.9	4.0	4.8	4.0	4.3	*	*	*
Arizona......................	5.3	4.8	4.5	4.9	4.6	4.2	11.0	9.0	9.7
Utah	3.7	3.6	3.5	3.6	3.4	3.4	*	*	*
Nevada	4.3	3.4	3.8	3.8	3.2	3.2	*8.3	*5.5	*6.1
Pacific.......................	4.6	3.8	3.7	4.0	3.3	3.2	9.2	8.0	7.2
Washington	4.3	3.5	3.3	3.8	3.3	2.9	9.7	8.2	6.4
Oregon......................	4.4	3.3	3.6	4.0	3.2	3.4	*11.6	*	*
California	4.6	3.9	3.7	4.1	3.4	3.2	9.2	8.0	7.4
Alaska	4.1	3.9	3.2	3.7	3.2	2.8	*	*	*
Hawaii.......................	4.3	3.9	5.4	3.5	*3.6	*4.7	*	*	*

See footnotes at end of table.

Table 24 (page 2 of 2). Neonatal mortality rates, according to race, Hispanic origin, geographic division, and State: United States, average annual 1989–91, 1995–97, and 1998–2000

[Data are based on linked birth and death certificates for infants]

Geographic division and State	Hispanic or Latino[5]			American Indian or Alaska Native[6]			Asian or Pacific Islander[6]		
	1989–91[1]	1995–97[2]	1998–2000[2]	1989–91[1]	1995–97[2]	1998–2000[2]	1989–91[1]	1995–97[2]	1998–2000[2]
	Neonatal[3] deaths per 1,000 live births								
United States	4.8	4.0	3.8	5.9	4.4	4.8	3.9	3.3	3.5
New England[7]	5.5	5.7	5.2	*	*	*	4.4	3.0	2.7
Maine.	*	*	*	*	*	*	*	*	*
New Hampshire[7]	- - -	*	*	*	*	*	*	*	*
Vermont	*	*	*	*	*	*	*	*	*
Massachusetts	5.8	5.0	4.4	*	*	*	*3.9	*2.6	*2.6
Rhode Island	*4.9	*7.6	*4.1	*	*	*	*	*	*
Connecticut	5.3	6.2	6.5	*	*	*	*	*	*
Middle Atlantic	6.2	4.9	4.3	*	*	*	4.1	2.8	3.0
New York	6.4	4.8	4.1	*	*	*	4.1	2.9	2.9
New Jersey	5.1	4.7	4.3	*	*	*	*3.4	2.6	3.3
Pennsylvania	7.3	6.2	5.7	*	*	*	*5.2	*2.7	*2.7
East North Central	5.9	4.8	5.1	*6.2	*5.8	*4.5	3.6	3.5	4.4
Ohio	*5.4	*5.0	6.6	*	*	*	*	*4.4	*2.6
Indiana.	*4.7	5.7	5.0	*	*	*	*	*	*
Illinois	6.4	4.5	5.0	*	*	*	3.9	3.8	4.9
Michigan	5.2	4.6	4.2	*	*	*	*	*	*4.3
Wisconsin.	*3.9	6.5	5.5	*	*	*	*	*	*4.4
West North Central	5.3	4.6	4.6	6.1	6.3	5.0	4.6	4.1	4.3
Minnesota	*	*4.4	*4.8	*4.9	*7.9	*	*3.2	*3.9	*5.0
Iowa	*	*	*4.6	*	*	*	*	*	*
Missouri	*	*	*4.7	*	*	*	*	*	*
North Dakota	*	*	*	*	*	*	*	*	*
South Dakota	*	*	*	*8.2	*7.4	*5.1	*	*	*
Nebraska	*	*6.6	*5.8	*	*	*	*	*	*
Kansas.	*5.4	*4.3	*3.5	*	*	*	*	*	*
South Atlantic.	5.2	3.7	3.7	7.4	6.9	6.3	4.6	3.6	3.8
Delaware	*	*	*	*	*	*	*	*	*
Maryland	*4.7	*3.7	4.8	*	*	*	*4.5	*5.0	*3.7
District of Columbia	*	*	*	*	*	*	*	*	*
Virginia	*4.8	5.1	3.5	*	*	*	*4.1	*3.5	4.1
West Virginia	*	*	*	*	*	*	*	*	*
North Carolina	*5.5	4.6	4.5	*7.7	*8.1	*9.1	*	*4.0	*4.0
South Carolina	*	*	*4.4	*	*	*	*	*	*
Georgia	*5.7	4.5	3.5	*	*	*	*5.3	*	*3.3
Florida	5.1	3.2	3.5	*	*	*	*4.4	*3.1	3.8
East South Central	*	*4.3	3.7	*	*	*	*	*3.3	*4.3
Kentucky	*	*	*	*	*	*	*	*	*
Tennessee	*	*	*3.8	*	*	*	*	*	*
Alabama.	*	*	*4.1	*	*	*	*	*	*
Mississippi	*	*	*	*	*	*	*	*	*
West South Central[7]	4.2	3.5	3.3	4.3	3.5	4.2	4.1	3.1	2.8
Arkansas	*	*	*4.2	*	*	*	*	*	*
Louisiana[7]	- - -	*	*	*	*	*	*	*	*
Oklahoma[7]	- - -	*3.0	*3.3	*3.7	3.8	4.3	*	*	*
Texas.	4.2	3.5	3.3	*	*	*	4.0	2.9	2.8
Mountain	4.7	4.4	4.3	5.8	3.8	4.8	4.6	4.1	3.4
Montana.	*	*	*	*7.6	*	*6.4	*	*	*
Idaho.	*	*4.8	*5.7	*	*	*	*	*	*
Wyoming	*	*	*	*	*	*	*	*	*
Colorado	4.4	4.4	4.6	*	*	*	*	*4.9	*
New Mexico	4.9	4.0	3.8	4.9	*3.0	*3.4	*	*	*
Arizona	5.0	5.0	4.5	5.4	3.7	5.0	*	*	*
Utah	*3.6	*4.4	3.7	*	*	*	*	*	*
Nevada	*4.1	2.9	3.9	*	*	*	*	*	*4.0
Pacific.	4.5	3.7	3.6	6.5	3.6	4.7	3.7	3.3	3.5
Washington	4.9	3.1	3.3	*8.5	*	*4.8	*2.7	*2.9	3.6
Oregon.	6.5	4.4	4.6	*	*	*	*5.3	*	*3.1
California	4.4	3.7	3.5	6.3	*3.8	*5.0	3.6	3.2	3.1
Alaska	*	*	*	*5.7	*4.8	*4.2	*	*	*
Hawaii	*6.6	*3.7	*5.3	*	*	*	4.2	3.9	5.4

* Estimates are considered unreliable. Rates preceded by an asterisk are based on fewer than 50 events. Rates not shown are based on fewer than 20 events.
- - - Data not available.   [1]Rates based on unweighted birth cohort data.
[2]Rates based on period file using weighted data (see Appendix I, National Vital Statistics System, Linked Birth/Infant Death Data Set).
[3]Infants under 28 days of age.
[4]Rates for white and black are substituted for non-Hispanic white and non-Hispanic black for Louisiana 1989, Oklahoma 1989–90, and New Hampshire 1989–91.
[5]Persons of Hispanic origin may be of any race.   [6]Includes persons of Hispanic origin.
[7]Rates for Hispanic origin exclude data from States not reporting Hispanic origin on the birth certificate for 1 or more years in a 3-year period.

NOTE: National linked files do not exist for 1992–94.

SOURCE: Centers for Disease Control and Prevention, National Center for Health Statistics, National Vital Statistics System, Linked Birth/Infant Death Data Set.

Table 25. Infant mortality rates and international rankings: Selected countries, selected years 1960–99

[Data are based on reporting by countries]

Country[2]	1960	1970	1980	1990	1995	1998	1999[3]	International rankings[1] 1960	1999
			Infant[4] deaths per 1,000 live births						
Australia	20.2	17.9	10.7	8.2	5.7	5.0	5.7	5	22
Austria	37.5	25.9	14.3	7.8	5.4	4.9	4.4	24	9
Belgium	31.2	21.1	12.1	8.0	6.1	5.6	4.9	20	14
Bulgaria	45.1	27.3	20.2	14.8	14.8	14.4	14.5	30	35
Canada	27.3	18.8	10.4	6.8	6.0	5.3	5.3	14	18
Chile	125.1	78.8	33.0	16.0	11.1	10.9	10.1	36	32
Costa Rica	67.8	65.4	20.3	15.3	13.3	12.6	11.8	33	34
Cuba	37.3	38.7	19.6	10.7	9.4	7.1	6.4	23	26
Czech Republic	20.0	20.2	16.9	10.8	7.7	5.2	4.6	4	12
Denmark	21.5	14.2	8.4	7.5	5.1	4.7	4.2	8	7
England and Wales	22.5	18.5	12.1	7.9	6.2	5.7	5.8	8	24
Finland	21.0	13.2	7.6	5.6	4.0	4.1	3.7	6	5
France	27.5	18.2	10.0	7.3	4.9	4.6	4.3	15	8
Germany[5]	35.0	22.5	12.4	7.0	5.3	4.7	4.5	22	10
Greece	40.1	29.6	17.9	9.7	8.1	6.7	6.2	25	25
Hong Kong	41.5	19.2	11.2	6.2	4.6	3.2	3.1	26	1
Hungary	47.6	35.9	23.2	14.8	10.7	9.7	8.4	31	30
Ireland	29.3	19.5	11.1	8.2	6.3	6.2	5.5	17	19
Israel[6]	31.0	18.9	15.2	9.9	6.8	5.7	5.7	19	22
Italy	43.9	29.6	14.6	8.2	6.2	5.4	5.1	29	16
Japan	30.7	13.1	7.5	4.6	4.3	3.6	3.4	18	2
Netherlands	17.9	12.7	8.6	7.1	5.5	5.2	5.2	2	17
New Zealand	22.6	16.7	13.0	8.4	6.7	5.5	5.5	10	19
Northern Ireland	27.2	22.9	13.4	7.5	7.1	5.6	6.4	13	26
Norway	18.9	12.7	8.1	7.0	4.1	4.0	3.9	3	6
Poland	54.8	36.7	25.5	19.3	13.6	9.5	8.9	32	31
Portugal	77.5	55.5	24.3	11.0	7.5	6.0	5.6	35	21
Puerto Rico	43.3	27.9	18.5	13.4	12.7	10.5	10.6	27	33
Romania	75.7	49.4	29.3	26.9	21.2	20.5	18.6	34	37
Russian Federation[7]	- - -	- - -	22.0	17.6	18.2	16.4	17.1	- - -	36
Scotland	26.4	19.6	12.1	7.7	6.2	5.5	5.0	12	15
Singapore	34.8	21.4	11.7	6.7	4.0	4.2	3.5	21	4
Slovakia	28.6	25.7	20.9	12.0	11.0	8.8	8.3	16	29
Spain	43.7	28.1	12.3	7.6	5.5	4.9	4.5	28	10
Sweden	16.6	11.0	6.9	6.0	4.1	3.5	3.4	1	2
Switzerland	21.1	15.1	9.1	6.8	5.0	4.8	4.6	7	12
United States	26.0	20.0	12.6	9.2	7.6	7.2	7.1	11	28

- - - Data not available.

[1]Rankings are from lowest to highest infant mortality rates (IMR). Countries with the same IMR receive the same rank. The country with the next highest IMR is assigned the rank it would have received had the lower-ranked countries not been tied, i.e., skip a rank. Some of the variation in infant mortality rates is due to differences among countries in distinguishing between fetal and infant deaths.

[2]Refers to countries, territories, cities, or geographic areas with at least 1 million population and with "complete" counts of live births and infant deaths as indicated in the United Nations Demographic Yearbook.

[3]Rates for Israel and New Zealand are from 1998.

[4]Under 1 year of age.

[5]Rates for 1990 and earlier years were calculated by combining information from the Federal Republic of Germany and the German Democratic Republic.

[6]Includes data for East Jerusalem and Israeli residents in certain other territories under occupation by Israel military forces since June 1967.

[7]Excludes infants born alive after less than 28 weeks' gestation, of less than 1,000 grams in weight and 35 centimeters in length, who die within 7 days of birth.

NOTE: Some rates were revised and differ from the previous edition of *Health, United States*.

SOURCES: Organization for Economic Cooperation and Development (OECD): OECD Health Data 2002, A Comparative Analysis of 30 Countries, www.oecd.org/els/health/; United Nations: Demographic Yearbook Historical Supplement 1948–1997, United Nations Publication, Sales No. E/F.99.XIII.12, New York, 2000; World Health Organization: World Health Statistics Annual. Vols. 1997–1999. Geneva; http://www.euro.who.int/; United States and Puerto Rico: Centers for Disease Control and Prevention, National Center for Health Statistics. Vital Statistics of the United States, vol. II, mortality part A (selected years). Public Health Service. Washington; Sweden: Statistics Sweden; Costa Rica: Dirección General de Estadísticas y Censos. Elaboración y estimación, Centro Centroamericano de Población, Universidad de Costa Rica, http://populi.eest.ucr.ac.cr/observa/index1.htm; Russian Federation: Goskomstat http://www.gks.ru/eng/.

Table 26 (page 1 of 2). Life expectancy at birth and at 65 years of age, according to sex: Selected countries, selected years 1980–1998

[Data are based on reporting by countries]

	Male						Female					
Country	1980	1990	1995	1997	1998	1998	1980	1990	1995	1997	1998	1998
At birth	Life expectancy in years					Rank	Life expectancy in years					Rank
Australia.	71.0	73.9	75.0	75.6	75.9	7	78.1	80.1	80.8	81.3	81.5	8
Austria.	69.0	72.3	73.5	74.3	74.7	19	76.1	78.9	80.1	80.6	80.9	11
Belgium	70.0	72.7	73.4	74.1	74.3	21	76.8	79.4	80.2	80.6	80.5	17
Bulgaria	68.5	68.3	67.4	67.0	67.4	34	73.9	75.0	74.9	73.8	74.7	35
Canada	71.7	74.4	75.1	75.8	76.0	6	78.9	80.8	81.1	81.3	81.5	8
Chile	- - -	71.1	71.8	72.1	72.3	28	- - -	76.9	77.8	78.1	78.3	28
Costa Rica	71.8	74.7	74.0	74.5	74.8	16	77.0	79.1	78.6	79.5	79.3	23
Cuba	72.2	74.6	75.4	75.7	75.8	9	- - -	76.9	77.7	78.0	78.2	29
Czech Republic[1]	66.8	67.6	69.7	70.5	71.1	31	73.9	75.4	76.6	77.5	78.1	30
Denmark	71.2	72.0	72.7	73.6	73.9	23	77.3	77.7	77.8	78.4	78.8	27
England and Wales	70.8	73.1	74.2	74.9	75.1	15	76.8	78.8	79.5	79.8	80.0	19
Finland.	69.2	70.9	72.8	73.4	73.5	25	77.6	78.9	80.2	80.5	80.8	12
France.	70.2	72.7	73.9	74.6	74.8	16	78.4	81.0	81.9	82.3	82.4	3
Germany[2].	69.6	72.0	73.3	74.0	74.5	20	76.1	78.4	79.7	80.3	80.6	14
Greece.	72.2	74.6	75.0	75.6	75.5	10	76.8	79.5	80.3	80.8	80.6	14
Hong Kong.	71.6	74.6	76.0	77.2	77.4	1	77.9	80.3	81.5	83.2	83.0	2
Hungary.	65.5	65.1	65.3	66.4	66.1	36	72.7	73.7	74.5	75.1	75.2	34
Ireland	70.1	72.1	72.9	73.4	73.5	25	75.6	80.3	78.4	78.6	79.1	25
Israel	72.2	75.1	75.5	76.1	76.2	5	75.8	78.5	79.5	80.4	80.6	14
Italy	71.1	73.8	75.0	75.9	75.9	7	77.7	80.5	81.6	82.1	82.2	5
Japan	73.4	75.9	76.4	77.2	77.2	2	78.8	81.9	82.9	83.8	84.0	1
Netherlands	72.5	73.8	74.6	75.2	75.2	13	79.2	80.1	80.4	80.6	80.7	13
New Zealand	70.0	72.4	74.2	74.9	75.2	13	76.3	78.3	79.5	80.1	80.4	18
Northern Ireland	68.3	72.2	73.3	74.3	74.3	21	75.0	77.9	78.8	79.5	79.8	20
Norway	72.3	73.4	74.8	75.4	75.5	10	79.2	79.8	80.8	81.0	81.3	10
Poland.	66.0	66.5	67.6	68.5	68.9	32	74.4	75.5	76.4	77.0	77.3	32
Portugal.	67.7	70.4	71.2	71.6	71.7	29	75.2	77.4	78.6	78.8	78.9	26
Puerto Rico	70.8	69.1	69.6	73.9	71.4	30	76.9	77.2	78.9	78.5	79.3	23
Romania	66.6	66.6	65.5	65.3	66.3	35	71.9	73.1	73.5	73.4	73.8	36
Russian Federation	61.4	63.8	58.3	61.0	61.4	37	73.0	74.4	71.7	73.0	73.3	37
Scotland.	69.0	71.2	72.1	72.6	72.6	27	75.2	76.9	77.6	78.0	78.1	30
Singapore.	69.8	73.1	74.2	74.9	75.3	12	74.7	77.6	78.6	79.1	79.4	22
Slovakia[1]	66.8	66.6	68.4	66.6	68.7	33	74.3	75.8	76.5	77.0	77.0	33
Spain	72.5	73.3	74.3	74.9	74.8	16	78.6	80.4	81.5	81.9	82.2	5
Sweden	72.8	74.8	75.9	76.7	76.9	3	78.8	80.4	81.3	81.8	81.9	7
Switzerland.	72.8	74.0	75.3	76.3	76.3	4	79.6	80.7	81.7	82.1	82.4	3
United States	70.0	71.8	72.5	73.6	73.8	24	77.4	78.8	78.9	79.4	79.5	21

See footnotes at end of table.

Table 26 (page 2 of 2). **Life expectancy at birth and at 65 years of age, according to sex: Selected countries, selected years 1980–1998**

[Data are based on reporting by countries]

Country	Male						Female					
	1980	1990	1995	1997	1998	1998	1980	1990	1995	1997	1998	1998
At 65 years	Life expectancy in years					Rank	Life expectancy in years					Rank
Australia....................	13.7	15.2	15.7	16.1	16.3	7	17.9	19.0	19.5	19.8	20.0	8
Austria......................	12.9	14.4	15.2	15.4	15.6	15	16.3	18.0	18.7	19.1	19.3	12
Belgium.....................	13.0	14.3	14.8	15.2	15.2	18	16.9	18.5	19.1	19.4	19.3	12
Bulgaria	12.7	12.9	12.8	12.4	12.5	32	14.7	15.4	15.4	14.9	15.1	34
Canada	14.5	15.7	16.0	16.2	16.3	7	18.9	19.9	20.0	20.0	20.1	7
Chile	- - -	14.6	14.9	15.1	15.1	20	- - -	17.6	18.1	18.3	18.4	22
Costa Rica	- - -	- - -	- - -	- - -	- - -	- - -	- - -	- - -	- - -	- - -	- - -	- - -
Cuba........................	- - -	- - -	- - -	- - -	- - -	- - -	- - -	- - -	- - -	- - -	- - -	- - -
Czech Republic[1]	11.2	11.6	12.7	13.2	13.4	28	14.3	15.2	16.1	16.6	16.9	29
Denmark	13.6	14.0	14.1	14.6	14.8	23	17.6	17.8	17.5	17.9	18.1	23
England and Wales	12.9	14.2	14.8	15.2	15.5	16	16.9	18.1	18.5	19.8	18.7	19
Finland......................	12.5	13.7	14.5	15.0	14.9	21	16.5	17.7	18.6	18.9	19.1	15
France	13.6	15.6	16.1	16.3	16.4	5	18.2	19.9	20.6	20.9	20.9	2
Germany[2]....................	13.0	14.0	14.7	15.2	15.3	17	16.7	17.6	18.5	18.9	19.0	16
Greece......................	14.6	15.7	16.1	16.5	16.4	5	16.8	18.0	18.4	18.9	18.7	19
Hong Kong...................	13.9	15.3	16.2	16.9	17.1	1	13.9	18.8	19.5	21.1	20.7	3
Hungary.....................	11.6	12.0	12.1	12.2	12.2	33	14.6	15.3	15.8	15.9	16.0	31
Ireland......................	12.6	13.3	13.6	14.1	14.2	26	15.7	16.9	17.3	17.5	17.7	25
Israel	14.4	15.9	16.0	16.6	16.6	3	15.8	17.8	18.0	18.9	18.9	17
Italy........................	13.9	15.1	16.0	16.3	16.1	11	17.4	19.1	20.0	20.3	20.4	5
Japan	14.6	16.2	16.5	17.0	17.1	1	17.7	20.0	20.9	21.8	22.0	1
Netherlands	13.7	14.1	14.4	14.7	14.7	24	18.7	18.6	18.7	18.8	18.8	18
New Zealand	13.2	14.7	15.4	15.9	16.1	11	17.0	18.3	19.0	19.4	19.5	11
Northern Ireland	11.9	13.4	14.5	14.8	14.9	21	15.8	17.5	18.0	18.3	18.5	21
Norway	14.3	14.6	15.5	15.5	15.7	14	18.0	18.6	19.1	19.4	19.6	10
Poland......................	12.0	12.4	12.9	13.1	13.4	28	15.5	16.1	16.6	16.8	17.0	28
Portugal.....................	12.9	13.9	14.3	14.4	14.3	25	16.5	17.0	17.7	17.9	17.9	24
Puerto Rico	- - -	- - -	- - -	- - -	- - -	- - -	- - -	- - -	- - -	- - -	- - -	- - -
Romania	12.6	13.3	12.9	12.7	13.0	30	14.2	15.3	15.4	15.3	15.5	32
Russian Federation	11.6	12.1	11.0	11.4	11.6	34	15.6	15.9	15.1	15.3	15.5	32
Scotland.....................	12.3	13.1	13.7	14.0	14.2	26	16.2	16.8	17.1	17.3	17.4	27
Singapore....................	12.6	14.5	14.6	15.0	15.2	18	15.4	16.9	17.3	17.5	17.7	25
Slovakia[1]...................	12.3	12.2	12.7	12.7	12.9	31	- - -	16.1	16.3	16.6	16.6	30
Spain.......................	14.8	15.4	16.0	16.1	16.3	7	17.9	19.1	19.8	20.0	20.3	6
Sweden	14.3	15.3	16.0	16.2	16.3	7	17.9	19.0	19.7	19.9	20.0	8
Switzerland..................	14.4	15.3	16.1	16.5	16.6	3	17.9	19.4	20.2	20.4	20.5	4
United States	14.1	15.1	15.6	15.9	16.0	13	18.3	18.9	18.9	19.2	19.2	14

- - - Data not available.

[1]In 1993 Czechoslovakia was divided into two Nations, the Czech Republic and Slovakia. Data for years prior to 1993 are from the Czech and Slovak regions of Czechoslovakia.
[2]Until 1990 estimates refer to the Federal Republic of Germany; from 1995 onwards data refer to Germany after reunification.

NOTES: Rankings are from highest to lowest life expectancy (LE) for the most recent year available. Since calculation of LE estimates varies among countries, comparisons among them and their interpretation should be made with caution. See Appendix II, Life expectancy. Countries with the same LE receive the same rank. The country with the next lower LE is assigned the rank it would have received had the higher-ranked countries not been tied, i.e., skip a rank. Some estimates for 1997 were revised and differ from the previous edition of *Health, United States*.

SOURCES: Organization for Economic Cooperation and Development (OECD) Health Data 2002, A Comparative Analysis of 30 Countries, www.oecd.org/els/health/; European health for all database, World Health Organization Regional Office for Europe, http://hfadb.who.dk/hfal; Centers for Disease Control and Prevention, National Center for Health Statistics. Vital statistics of the United States, (selected years). Public Health Service. Washington, DC. http://www.cdc.gov/nchs/fastats/lifexpec.htm; Puerto Rico: Commonwealth of Puerto Rico, Department of Health, Auxiliary Secretariat for Planning, Evaluation, Statistics, and Information Systems: Unpublished data; Singapore: Singapore Department of Statistics, Population Statistics Section, http://www.singstat.gov.sg/stats/singstat/internet.html; England and Wales, Northern Ireland, and Scotland: Government Actuary's Department, London http://www.gad.gov.uk; Hong Kong: Government of Hong Kong, Special Administrative Region, Department of Health, http://info.gov.hk/dh/index.htm; Costa Rica: Instituto Nacional de Estadística y Censos (INEC) y Centro Centroamericano de Población (CCP) http://ccp.ucr.ac.cr/observa/series/serie3.htm; Chile: Instituto Nacional de Estadísticas, Departamento de Demografía. Gobierno de Chile. Ministerio de Salud Departamento de Estadísticas e Información de Salud; Cuba: Pan American Health Organization, Special Program for Health Analysis. Regional Initiative for Health Basic Data, Technical Information Health System, Washington, DC 2001.

Table 27. Life expectancy at birth, at 65 years of age, and at 75 years of age, according to race and sex: United States, selected years 1900–2000

[Data are based on death certificates]

Specified age and year	All races Both sexes	All races Male	All races Female	White Both sexes	White Male	White Female	Black or African American[1] Both sexes	Black or African American[1] Male	Black or African American[1] Female
At birth			Remaining life expectancy in years						
1900[2,3]	47.3	46.3	48.3	47.6	46.6	48.7	33.0	32.5	33.5
1950[3]	68.2	65.6	71.1	69.1	66.5	72.2	60.8	59.1	62.9
1960[3]	69.7	66.6	73.1	70.6	67.4	74.1	63.6	61.1	66.3
1970	70.8	67.1	74.7	71.7	68.0	75.6	64.1	60.0	68.3
1980	73.7	70.0	77.4	74.4	70.7	78.1	68.1	63.8	72.5
1985	74.7	71.1	78.2	75.3	71.8	78.7	69.3	65.0	73.4
1990	75.4	71.8	78.8	76.1	72.7	79.4	69.1	64.5	73.6
1991	75.5	72.0	78.9	76.3	72.9	79.6	69.3	64.6	73.8
1992	75.8	72.3	79.1	76.5	73.2	79.8	69.6	65.0	73.9
1993	75.5	72.2	78.8	76.3	73.1	79.5	69.2	64.6	73.7
1994	75.7	72.4	79.0	76.5	73.3	79.6	69.5	64.9	73.9
1995	75.8	72.5	78.9	76.5	73.4	79.6	69.6	65.2	73.9
1996	76.1	73.1	79.1	76.8	73.9	79.7	70.2	66.1	74.2
1997	76.5	73.6	79.4	77.1	74.3	79.9	71.1	67.2	74.7
1998	76.7	73.8	79.5	77.3	74.5	80.0	71.3	67.6	74.8
1999	76.7	73.9	79.4	77.3	74.6	79.9	71.4	67.8	74.7
2000	76.9	74.1	79.5	77.4	74.8	80.0	71.7	68.2	74.9
At 65 years									
1950[2]	13.9	12.8	15.0	- - -	12.8	15.1	13.9	12.9	14.9
1960[2]	14.3	12.8	15.8	14.4	12.9	15.9	13.9	12.7	15.1
1970	15.2	13.1	17.0	15.2	13.1	17.1	14.2	12.5	15.7
1980	16.4	14.1	18.3	16.5	14.2	18.4	15.1	13.0	16.8
1985	16.7	14.5	18.5	16.8	14.5	18.7	15.2	13.0	16.9
1990	17.2	15.1	18.9	17.3	15.2	19.1	15.4	13.2	17.2
1991	17.4	15.3	19.1	17.5	15.4	19.2	15.5	13.4	17.2
1992	17.5	15.4	19.2	17.6	15.5	19.3	15.7	13.5	17.4
1993	17.3	15.3	18.9	17.4	15.4	19.0	15.5	13.4	17.1
1994	17.4	15.5	19.0	17.5	15.6	19.1	15.7	13.6	17.2
1995	17.4	15.6	18.9	17.6	15.7	19.1	15.6	13.6	17.1
1996	17.5	15.7	19.0	17.6	15.8	19.1	15.8	13.9	17.2
1997	17.7	15.9	19.2	17.8	16.0	19.3	16.1	14.2	17.6
1998	17.8	16.0	19.2	17.8	16.1	19.3	16.1	14.3	17.4
1999	17.7	16.1	19.1	17.8	16.1	19.2	16.0	14.3	17.3
2000	17.9	16.3	19.2	17.9	16.3	19.2	16.2	14.5	17.4
At 75 years									
1980	10.4	8.8	11.5	10.4	8.8	11.5	9.7	8.3	10.7
1985	10.6	9.0	11.7	10.6	9.0	11.7	10.1	8.7	11.1
1990	10.9	9.4	12.0	11.0	9.4	12.0	10.2	8.6	11.2
1991	11.1	9.5	12.1	11.1	9.5	12.1	10.2	8.7	11.2
1992	11.2	9.6	12.2	11.2	9.6	12.2	10.4	8.9	11.4
1993	10.9	9.5	11.9	11.0	9.5	12.0	10.2	8.7	11.1
1994	11.0	9.6	12.0	11.1	9.6	12.0	10.3	8.9	11.2
1995	11.0	9.7	11.9	11.1	9.7	12.0	10.2	8.8	11.1
1996	11.1	9.8	12.0	11.1	9.8	12.0	10.3	9.0	11.2
1997	11.2	9.9	12.1	11.2	9.9	12.1	10.7	9.3	11.5
1998	11.3	10.0	12.2	11.3	10.0	12.2	10.5	9.2	11.3
1999	11.2	10.0	12.1	11.2	10.0	12.1	10.4	9.2	11.1
2000	11.3	10.1	12.1	11.3	10.1	12.1	10.5	9.4	11.2

[1]Data shown for 1900–60 are for the nonwhite population.
[2]Death registration area only. The death registration area increased from 10 States and the District of Columbia in 1900 to the coterminous United States in 1933. See Appendix II, Registration area.
[3]Includes deaths of persons who were not residents of the 50 States and the District of Columbia. See Appendix II, Registration area.

NOTES: Populations used for computing life expectancy and other life table values for 1991–2000 are postcensal estimates of U.S. resident population, based on the 1990 census. See Appendix I, Population Census and Population Estimates.
Beginning in 1997 life table methodology was revised to construct complete life tables by single years of age that extend to age 100. (Anderson RN. Method for Constructing Complete Annual U.S. Life Tables. National Center for Health Statistics. Vital Health Stat 2(129). 1999.) Previously abridged life tables were constructed for 5-year age groups ending with the age group 85 years and over. Data for additional years are available (see Appendix III).

SOURCES: Centers for Disease Control and Prevention, National Center for Health Statistics, National Vital Statistics System; Grove RD, Hetzel AM. Vital statistics rates in the United States, 1940–1960. Washington: U.S. Government Printing Office, 1968; life expectancy trend data available at www.cdc.gov/nchs/about/major/dvs/mortdata.htm; Minino AM, Arias E, Kochanek KD, Murphy SL, Smith BL. Deaths: Final data for 2000. National vital statistics reports. vol 50 no 15. Hyattsville, Maryland: National Center for Health Statistics. 2002.

This table will be updated with 2001 data on the web. Go to www.cdc.gov/nchs/hus.htm.

Table 28 (page 1 of 2). Age-adjusted death rates, according to race, Hispanic origin, geographic division, and State: United States, average annual 1979–81, 1989–91, and 1998–2000

[Data are based on death certificates]

Geographic division and State	All persons			White	Black or African American	American Indian or Alaska Native	Asian or Pacific Islander	Hispanic or Latino	White, not Hispanic or Latino
	1979–81	1989–91	1998–2000	1998–2000	1998–2000	1998–2000	1998–2000	1998–2000	1998–2000

Age-adjusted death rate per 100,000 population[1]

Geographic division and State	All persons 1979–81	1989–91	1998–2000	White 1998–2000	Black or African American 1998–2000	American Indian or Alaska Native 1998–2000	Asian or Pacific Islander 1998–2000	Hispanic or Latino 1998–2000	White, not Hispanic or Latino 1998–2000
United States	1,022.8	942.2	870.4	849.8	1,126.6	770.2	516.5	670.1	855.1
New England	979.9	882.4	814.2	812.7	922.3	*	424.2	572.6	808.0
Maine.................	1,002.9	918.7	865.5	863.8	1,064.2	*	1,030.0	*	856.5
New Hampshire	982.3	891.7	818.6	820.3	784.3	*	500.2	490.5	801.9
Vermont	990.2	908.6	817.7	818.4	*	*	*	*	819.1
Massachusetts...........	982.6	884.8	815.6	818.1	884.0	*	417.5	587.9	816.8
Rhode Island	990.8	889.6	813.1	808.9	1,005.5	*	447.3	431.0	804.7
Connecticut..............	961.5	857.5	792.1	781.4	960.3	*	388.9	604.9	773.6
Middle Atlantic.............	1,059.1	967.8	851.5	837.7	1,009.5	*	427.0	624.8	835.6
New York................	1,051.8	973.7	824.6	819.6	912.1	*	440.3	638.0	808.8
New Jersey	1,047.5	956.0	847.7	827.7	1,084.2	*	380.3	548.0	838.2
Pennsylvania	1,076.4	963.4	889.1	865.4	1,177.8	*	446.1	768.1	864.3
East North Central.........	1,048.0	957.9	900.0	871.6	1,182.6	*	449.1	604.0	871.1
Ohio	1,070.6	967.4	925.3	904.2	1,148.8	*	427.8	673.2	900.7
Indiana	1,048.3	962.0	925.3	907.3	1,188.9	*	568.2	670.2	910.1
Illinois	1,063.7	973.8	889.1	850.6	1,204.0	*	424.5	563.9	855.0
Michigan	1,050.2	966.0	908.1	869.8	1,191.3	*	480.3	720.4	862.2
Wisconsin	956.4	879.1	826.0	812.6	1,117.4	*	566.6	456.4	815.0
West North Central	951.6	876.6	839.2	821.9	1,190.4	*	564.3	769.6	818.5
Minnesota	892.9	825.2	770.1	761.8	1,019.0	1,259.7	611.9	779.5	757.5
Iowa	919.9	848.2	803.0	798.5	1,174.0	*	713.5	831.4	798.5
Missouri...............	1,033.7	952.4	934.2	907.2	1,228.5	*	497.2	963.0	906.6
North Dakota............	922.4	818.4	779.9	763.6	*	1,595.3	*	*	740.8
South Dakota............	941.9	846.4	807.5	768.3	*	1,613.6	*	*	768.8
Nebraska..............	930.6	867.9	812.5	799.6	1,173.1	1,912.2	473.1	647.8	796.7
Kansas	940.1	867.2	845.1	832.7	1,157.8	*	463.1	662.6	825.2
South Atlantic	1,033.1	951.3	884.7	838.7	1,138.4	*	435.3	603.5	850.2
Delaware..............	1,069.7	1,001.9	888.5	856.9	1,095.2	*	427.3	769.7	856.2
Maryland	1,063.3	985.2	904.2	846.6	1,119.9	*	439.3	#	858.5
District of Columbia	1,243.1	1,255.3	1,079.3	696.0	1,298.6	*	525.3	#	733.4
Virginia	1,054.0	963.1	890.0	850.8	1,123.3	*	492.6	556.3	852.3
West Virginia	1,100.3	1,031.5	1,009.1	1,006.1	1,193.6	*	*	497.3	1,007.4
North Carolina	1,050.4	986.0	936.1	883.9	1,174.0	1,013.9	471.8	312.5	887.0
South Carolina..........	1,104.6	1,030.0	970.8	908.7	1,166.6	*	547.5	401.1	911.2
Georgia...............	1,094.3	1,037.4	965.7	915.3	1,148.6	*	530.8	441.6	919.1
Florida................	960.8	870.9	807.1	780.9	1,082.4	*	335.3	635.0	799.2
East South Central	1,079.3	1,031.6	1,002.1	964.2	1,210.8	*	592.6	566.8	965.4
Kentucky..............	1,088.9	1,024.5	992.7	981.8	1,201.3	*	586.7	1,298.3	980.3
Tennessee..............	1,045.5	1,011.8	986.9	950.0	1,259.3	*	592.9	454.0	952.2
Alabama	1,091.2	1,037.9	1,004.3	959.8	1,178.7	*	587.6	319.1	962.9
Mississippi	1,108.7	1,071.4	1,045.0	975.9	1,213.9	*	649.3	418.0	976.8
West South Central	1,036.8	974.9	923.2	895.7	1,184.4	*	493.4	756.5	912.5
Arkansas..............	1,017.0	996.3	974.2	942.0	1,241.6	*	819.1	493.3	946.2
Louisiana..............	1,132.6	1,074.6	1,012.5	937.9	1,227.1	*	563.3	613.6	941.7
Oklahoma	1,025.6	961.4	975.3	972.0	1,203.2	*	620.7	767.2	976.2
Texas	1,014.9	947.6	883.4	864.4	1,146.2	*	469.5	761.6	882.2
Mountain	961.8	878.2	821.3	815.3	1,035.5	961.5	541.6	775.9	813.2
Montana	1,013.6	890.2	851.6	832.0	*	1,350.2	*	887.0	827.8
Idaho	936.7	856.6	812.7	810.1	2,101.8	1,053.3	622.6	720.3	810.3
Wyoming..............	1,016.1	897.4	872.8	863.4	1,280.2	1,509.8	*	842.7	862.0
Colorado..............	941.1	856.1	798.7	796.1	1,040.5	602.4	529.0	781.0	792.4
New Mexico.............	967.1	891.9	820.8	812.7	921.5	900.3	709.5	816.9	796.6
Arizona...............	951.5	873.5	809.6	799.2	1,026.2	1,000.2	458.8	793.5	791.0
Utah	924.9	823.2	783.4	782.8	1,058.0	890.8	630.4	722.3	782.7
Nevada	1,077.4	1,017.4	926.0	933.7	1,050.7	736.0	548.4	547.3	962.4

See footnotes at end of table.

Table 28 (page 2 of 2). Age-adjusted death rates, according to race, Hispanic origin, geographic division, and State: United States, average annual 1979–81, 1989–91, and 1998–2000

[Data are based on death certificates]

Geographic division and State	All persons			White	Black or African American	American Indian or Alaska Native	Asian or Pacific Islander	Hispanic or Latino	White, not Hispanic or Latino
	1979–81	1989–91	1998–2000	1998–2000	1998–2000	1998–2000	1998–2000	1998–2000	1998–2000

Age-adjusted death rate per 100,000 population[1]

Pacific	966.5	900.1	800.8	815.2	1,067.9	*	556.3	641.8	832.6
Washington	947.7	869.4	808.1	811.6	1,025.3	1,008.1	516.0	574.8	814.3
Oregon	953.9	893.0	838.7	840.2	1,076.1	*	551.3	583.8	844.1
California	975.5	911.0	799.2	813.8	1,075.0	*	527.3	640.6	837.8
Alaska	1,087.4	944.6	841.6	802.5	902.5	1,107.7	567.7	871.1	802.0
Hawaii	801.2	752.2	684.8	727.8	622.1	*	671.8	1,042.5	718.8

* Data for States with population under 10,000 in the middle year of a 3-year period or fewer than 50 deaths for the 3-year period are considered unreliable and are not shown. Data for American Indian or Alaska Native in States with more than 10 percent misclassification of American Indian or Alaska Native deaths on death certificates or without information on misclassification are also not shown. (Support Services International, Inc. Methodology for adjusting IHS mortality data for miscoding race-ethnicity of American Indians and Alaska Natives on State death certificates. Report submitted to Indian Health Service. 1996.) Division death rates for American Indian or Alaska Native are not shown when any State within the division does not meet reliability criteria.

Estimates of Hispanic death rates in Maryland (176.4 deaths per 1,000 population) and the District of Columbia (DC) (163.4) are substantially lower than for other States and are likely to be underestimates of actual death rates, possibly due to misreporting of Hispanic origin on some death certificates and/or inaccurate Hispanic population estimates for Maryland and DC.

[1]Average annual death rates, age-adjusted using the year 2000 standard population. See Appendix II, Age adjustment. Denominators for age-specific death rates are resident population estimates for the middle year of each 3-year period, multiplied by 3. Rates 1998–2000 differ from those shown previously. The 1999 population estimates used to compute rates for 1998–2000 in Health, United States, 2003 are intercensal estimates based on Census 2000. Previously rates were based on post–1990 population estimates. See Appendix I, Population Census and Population Estimates.

NOTES: The race groups, white, black, American Indian or Alaska Native, and Asian or Pacific Islander, include persons of Hispanic and non-Hispanic origin. Persons of Hispanic origin may be of any race. Death rates for the American Indian or Alaska Native and Asian or Pacific Islander populations are known to be underestimated. See Appendix II, Race, for a discussion of sources of bias in death rates by race and Hispanic origin.

SOURCES: Centers for Disease Control and Prevention, National Center for Health Statistics, National Vital Statistics System; numerator data from annual mortality files; denominator data from State population estimates prepared by the U.S. Bureau of the Census: 1980 from April 1, 1980 MARS Census File; 1990 from April 1, 1990 MARS Census File; 1999 from bridged-race intercensal estimates of the July 1, 1991-July 1, 1999 resident populations of the United States by State and county, race, age, sex, and Hispanic origin, produced by the Population Estimates Program of the U.S. Census Bureau with support from the National Cancer Institute (NCI).

This table will be updated with 1999–2001 data on the web. Go to www.cdc.gov/nchs/hus.htm.

Table 29 (page 1 of 4). Age-adjusted death rates for selected causes of death, according to sex, race, and Hispanic origin: United States, selected years 1950–2000

[Data are based on death certificates]

Sex, race, Hispanic origin, and cause of death[1]	1950[2]	1960[2]	1970	1980	1990	1995	1999[3]	2000
All persons								

	1950[2]	1960[2]	1970	1980	1990	1995	1999[3]	2000
All persons			Age-adjusted death rate per 100,000 population[4]					
All causes	1,446.0	1,339.2	1,222.6	1,039.1	938.7	909.8	875.6	869.0
Diseases of heart	586.8	559.0	492.7	412.1	321.8	293.4	266.5	257.6
Ischemic heart disease	- - -	- - -	- - -	345.2	249.6	219.7	194.6	186.8
Cerebrovascular diseases	180.7	177.9	147.7	96.2	65.3	63.1	61.6	60.9
Malignant neoplasms	193.9	193.9	198.6	207.9	216.0	209.9	200.8	199.6
Trachea, bronchus, and lung	15.0	24.1	37.1	49.9	59.3	58.4	55.5	56.1
Colon, rectum, and anus	- - -	30.3	28.9	27.4	24.5	22.5	20.9	20.8
Prostate[5]	28.6	28.7	28.8	32.8	38.4	37.0	31.3	30.4
Breast[6]	31.9	31.7	32.1	31.9	33.3	30.5	26.6	26.8
Chronic lower respiratory diseases	- - -	- - -	- - -	28.3	37.2	40.1	45.4	44.2
Influenza and pneumonia	48.1	53.7	41.7	31.4	36.8	33.4	23.5	23.7
Chronic liver disease and cirrhosis	11.3	13.3	17.8	15.1	11.1	9.9	9.6	9.5
Diabetes mellitus	23.1	22.5	24.3	18.1	20.7	23.2	25.0	25.0
Human immunodeficiency virus (HIV) disease	- - -	- - -	- - -	- - -	10.2	16.2	5.3	5.2
Unintentional injuries	78.0	62.3	60.1	46.4	36.3	34.4	35.3	34.9
Motor vehicle-related injuries	24.6	23.1	27.6	22.3	18.5	16.3	15.2	15.4
Suicide	13.2	12.5	13.1	12.2	12.5	11.8	10.5	10.4
Homicide	5.1	5.0	8.8	10.4	9.4	8.3	6.0	5.9
Male								
All causes	1,674.2	1,609.0	1,542.1	1,348.1	1,202.8	1,143.9	1,067.0	1,053.8
Diseases of heart	697.0	687.6	634.0	538.9	412.4	371.0	331.0	320.0
Ischemic heart disease	- - -	- - -	- - -	459.7	328.2	286.5	251.2	241.4
Cerebrovascular diseases	186.4	186.1	157.4	102.2	68.5	65.9	63.2	62.4
Malignant neoplasms	208.1	225.1	247.6	271.2	280.4	267.5	251.9	248.9
Trachea, bronchus, and lung	24.6	43.6	67.5	85.2	91.1	84.2	76.9	76.7
Colon, rectum, and anus	- - -	31.8	32.3	32.8	30.4	27.4	25.3	25.1
Prostate	28.6	28.7	28.8	32.8	38.4	37.0	31.3	30.4
Chronic lower respiratory diseases	- - -	- - -	- - -	49.9	55.4	54.8	58.7	55.8
Influenza and pneumonia	55.0	65.8	54.0	42.1	47.8	42.8	28.5	28.9
Chronic liver disease and cirrhosis	15.0	18.5	24.8	21.3	15.9	14.2	13.5	13.4
Diabetes mellitus	18.8	19.9	23.0	18.1	21.7	25.0	27.8	27.8
Human immunodeficiency virus (HIV) disease	- - -	- - -	- - -	- - -	18.5	27.3	8.2 ·	7.9
Unintentional injuries	101.8	85.5	87.4	69.0	52.9	49.6	49.8	49.3
Motor vehicle-related injuries	38.5	35.4	41.5	33.6	26.5	22.8	21.3	21.7
Suicide	21.2	20.0	19.8	19.9	21.5	20.3	17.8	17.7
Homicide	7.9	7.5	14.3	16.6	14.8	12.8	9.1	9.0
Female								
All causes	1,236.0	1,105.3	971.4	817.9	750.9	739.4	734.0	731.4
Diseases of heart	484.7	447.0	381.6	320.8	257.0	236.6	218.1	210.9
Ischemic heart disease	- - -	- - -	- - -	263.1	193.9	171.3	152.9	146.5
Cerebrovascular diseases	175.8	170.7	140.0	91.7	62.6	60.5	59.8	59.1
Malignant neoplasms	182.3	168.7	163.2	166.7	175.7	173.6	167.6	167.6
Trachea, bronchus, and lung	5.8	7.5	13.1	24.4	37.1	40.4	40.2	41.3
Colon, rectum, and anus	- - -	29.1	26.5	23.8	20.6	19.1	17.8	17.7
Breast	31.9	31.7	32.1	31.9	33.3	30.5	26.6	26.8
Chronic lower respiratory diseases	- - -	- - -	- - -	14.9	26.6	31.8	37.7	37.4
Influenza and pneumonia	41.9	43.8	32.7	25.1	30.5	28.1	20.6	20.7
Chronic liver disease and cirrhosis	7.8	8.7	11.9	9.9	7.1	6.2	6.1	6.2
Diabetes mellitus	27.0	24.7	25.1	18.0	19.9	21.8	23.0	23.0
Human immunodeficiency virus (HIV) disease	- - -	- - -	- - -	- - -	2.2	5.3	2.5	2.5
Unintentional injuries	54.0	40.0	35.1	26.1	21.5	21.0	22.3	22.0
Motor vehicle-related injuries	11.5	11.7	14.9	11.8	11.0	10.3	9.6	9.5
Suicide	5.6	5.6	7.4	5.7	4.8	4.3	4.0	4.0
Homicide	2.4	2.6	3.7	4.4	4.0	3.7	2.9	2.8

See footnotes at end of table.

Table 29 (page 2 of 4).

Table 29 (page 2 of 4). Age-adjusted death rates for selected causes of death, according to sex, race, and Hispanic origin: United States, selected years 1950–2000

[Data are based on death certificates]

Sex, race, Hispanic origin, and cause of death[1]	1950[2]	1960[2]	1970	1980	1990	1995	1999[3]	2000
White[7]				Age-adjusted death rate per 100,000 population				
All causes.	1,410.8	1,311.3	1,193.3	1,012.7	909.8	882.3	854.6	849.8
Diseases of heart	584.8	559.0	492.2	409.4	317.0	288.6	261.9	253.4
Ischemic heart disease	- - -	- - -	- - -	347.6	249.7	219.1	193.4	185.6
Cerebrovascular diseases	175.5	172.7	143.5	93.2	62.8	60.7	59.6	58.8
Malignant neoplasms	194.6	193.1	196.7	204.2	211.6	206.2	197.9	197.2
Trachea, bronchus, and lung	15.2	24.0	36.7	49.2	58.6	58.1	55.4	56.2
Colon, rectum, and anus	- - -	30.9	29.2	27.4	24.1	22.0	20.4	20.3
Prostate[5]	28.4	27.7	27.4	30.5	35.5	34.2	28.7	27.8
Breast[6]	32.4	32.0	32.5	32.1	33.2	30.1	26.0	26.3
Chronic lower respiratory diseases	- - -	- - -	- - -	29.3	38.3	41.5	47.1	46.0
Influenza and pneumonia	44.8	50.4	39.8	30.9	36.4	33.0	23.3	23.5
Chronic liver disease and cirrhosis	11.5	13.2	16.6	13.9	10.5	9.7	9.6	9.6
Diabetes mellitus	22.9	21.7	22.9	16.7	18.8	20.9	22.6	22.8
Human immunodeficiency virus (HIV) disease . . .	- - -	- - -	- - -	- - -	8.3	11.4	2.9	2.8
Unintentional injuries	77.0	60.4	57.8	45.3	35.5	33.9	35.2	35.1
Motor vehicle-related injuries	24.4	22.9	27.1	22.6	18.5	16.3	15.3	15.6
Suicide	13.9	13.1	13.8	13.0	13.4	12.6	11.3	11.3
Homicide	2.6	2.7	4.7	6.7	5.5	5.0	3.8	3.6
Black or African American[7]								
All causes.	1,722.1	1,577.5	1,518.1	1,314.8	1,250.3	1,213.9	1,135.7	1,121.4
Diseases of heart	586.7	548.3	512.0	455.3	391.5	363.8	334.3	324.8
Ischemic heart disease	- - -	- - -	- - -	334.5	267.0	244.9	224.9	218.3
Cerebrovascular diseases	233.6	235.2	197.1	129.1	91.6	86.9	81.8	81.9
Malignant neoplasms	176.4	199.1	225.3	256.4	279.5	267.7	252.5	248.5
Trachea, bronchus, and lung	11.1	23.7	41.3	59.7	72.4	69.0	64.8	64.0
Colon, rectum, and anus	- - -	22.8	26.1	28.3	30.6	29.3	28.4	28.2
Prostate[5]	30.9	41.2	48.5	61.1	77.0	76.6	69.0	68.1
Breast[6]	25.3	27.9	28.9	31.7	38.1	38.0	35.1	34.5
Chronic lower respiratory diseases	- - -	- - -	- - -	19.2	28.1	30.1	33.5	31.6
Influenza and pneumonia	76.7	81.1	57.2	34.4	39.4	36.4	25.4	25.6
Chronic liver disease and cirrhosis	9.0	13.6	28.1	25.0	16.5	12.0	10.1	9.4
Diabetes mellitus	23.5	30.9	38.8	32.7	40.5	46.7	49.7	49.5
Human immunodeficiency virus (HIV) disease . . .	- - -	- - -	- - -	- - -	26.7	54.2	23.6	23.3
Unintentional injuries	79.9	74.0	78.3	57.6	43.8	41.0	40.1	37.7
Motor vehicle-related injuries	26.0	24.2	31.1	20.2	18.8	16.7	15.9	15.7
Suicide	4.5	5.0	6.2	6.5	7.1	6.8	5.6	5.5
Homicide	28.3	26.0	44.0	39.0	36.3	29.7	20.1	20.5
American Indian or Alaska Native[7]								
All causes.	- - -	- - -	- - -	867.0	716.3	771.2	780.9	709.3
Diseases of heart	- - -	- - -	- - -	240.6	200.6	204.6	198.7	178.2
Ischemic heart disease	- - -	- - -	- - -	173.6	139.1	141.4	143.3	129.1
Cerebrovascular diseases	- - -	- - -	- - -	57.8	40.7	48.6	48.3	45.0
Malignant neoplasms	- - -	- - -	- - -	113.7	121.8	138.2	134.8	127.8
Trachea, bronchus, and lung	- - -	- - -	- - -	20.7	30.9	37.4	36.3	32.3
Colon, rectum, and anus	- - -	- - -	- - -	9.5	12.0	14.9	13.4	13.4
Prostate[5]	- - -	- - -	- - -	20.7	17.8	21.7	16.7	19.6
Breast[6]	- - -	- - -	- - -	10.8	13.7	15.0	15.5	13.6
Chronic lower respiratory diseases	- - -	- - -	- - -	14.2	25.4	27.6	34.7	32.8
Influenza and pneumonia	- - -	- - -	- - -	44.4	36.1	36.1	28.0	22.3
Chronic liver disease and cirrhosis	- - -	- - -	- - -	45.3	24.1	27.4	24.8	24.3
Diabetes mellitus	- - -	- - -	- - -	29.6	34.1	45.9	54.2	41.5
Human immunodeficiency virus (HIV) disease . . .	- - -	- - -	- - -	- - -	1.8	6.5	2.6	2.2
Unintentional injuries	- - -	- - -	- - -	99.0	62.6	55.3	55.8	51.3
Motor vehicle-related injuries	- - -	- - -	- - -	54.5	32.5	29.1	27.9	27.3
Suicide	- - -	- - -	- - -	11.9	11.7	10.6	10.1	9.8
Homicide	- - -	- - -	- - -	15.5	10.4	9.9	9.1	6.8

See footnotes at end of table.

Table 29 (page 3 of 4). Age-adjusted death rates for selected causes of death, according to sex, race, and Hispanic origin: United States, selected years 1950–2000

[Data are based on death certificates]

Sex, race, Hispanic origin, and cause of death[1]	1950[2]	1960[2]	1970	1980	1990	1995	1999[3]	2000
Asian or Pacific Islander[7]				Age-adjusted death rate per 100,000 population				
All causes	---	---	---	589.9	582.0	554.8	519.7	506.4
Diseases of heart	---	---	---	202.1	181.7	171.3	156.4	146.0
Ischemic heart disease	---	---	---	168.2	139.6	128.0	117.3	109.6
Cerebrovascular diseases	---	---	---	66.1	56.9	55.2	53.2	52.9
Malignant neoplasms	---	---	---	126.1	134.2	131.8	123.0	121.9
Trachea, bronchus, and lung	---	---	---	28.4	30.2	29.9	27.9	28.1
Colon, rectum, and anus	---	---	---	16.4	14.4	14.0	12.0	12.7
Prostate[5]	---	---	---	10.2	16.8	18.0	13.9	12.5
Breast[6]	---	---	---	11.9	13.7	13.9	12.7	12.3
Chronic lower respiratory diseases	---	---	---	12.9	19.4	19.3	19.4	18.6
Influenza and pneumonia	---	---	---	24.0	31.4	29.1	16.2	19.7
Chronic liver disease and cirrhosis	---	---	---	6.1	5.2	3.9	3.7	3.5
Diabetes mellitus	---	---	---	12.6	14.6	16.8	18.3	16.4
Human immunodeficiency virus (HIV) disease	---	---	---	---	2.2	3.2	0.8	0.6
Unintentional injuries	---	---	---	27.0	23.9	20.2	17.2	17.9
Motor vehicle-related injuries	---	---	---	13.9	14.0	11.4	8.3	8.6
Suicide	---	---	---	7.8	6.7	6.7	6.0	5.5
Homicide	---	---	---	5.9	5.0	4.7	3.0	3.0
Hispanic or Latino[7,8]								
All causes	---	---	---	---	692.0	700.2	676.4	665.7
Diseases of heart	---	---	---	---	217.1	211.0	205.8	196.0
Ischemic heart disease	---	---	---	---	173.3	166.4	162.2	153.2
Cerebrovascular diseases	---	---	---	---	45.2	46.3	46.6	46.4
Malignant neoplasms	---	---	---	---	136.8	138.5	134.8	134.9
Trachea, bronchus, and lung	---	---	---	---	26.5	25.9	25.0	24.8
Colon, rectum, and anus	---	---	---	---	14.7	14.1	14.3	14.1
Prostate[5]	---	---	---	---	23.3	27.4	23.0	21.6
Breast[6]	---	---	---	---	19.5	18.7	16.4	16.9
Chronic lower respiratory diseases	---	---	---	---	19.3	22.6	23.4	21.1
Influenza and pneumonia	---	---	---	---	29.7	26.2	18.8	20.6
Chronic liver disease and cirrhosis	---	---	---	---	18.3	17.4	16.1	16.5
Diabetes mellitus	---	---	---	---	28.2	35.7	37.8	36.9
Human immunodeficiency virus (HIV) disease	---	---	---	---	16.3	24.9	6.9	6.7
Unintentional injuries	---	---	---	---	34.6	32.2	30.6	30.1
Motor vehicle-related injuries	---	---	---	---	19.5	16.4	14.2	14.7
Suicide	---	---	---	---	7.8	7.2	5.9	5.9
Homicide	---	---	---	---	16.2	12.5	7.6	7.5

See footnotes at end of table.

Table 29 (page 4 of 4). Age-adjusted death rates for selected causes of death, according to sex, race, and Hispanic origin: United States, selected years 1950–2000

[Data are based on death certificates]

Sex, race, Hispanic origin, and cause of death[1]	1950[2]	1960[2]	1970	1980	1990	1995	1999[3]	2000
White, not Hispanic or Latino[8]				Age-adjusted death rate per 100,000 population				
All causes.	- - -	- - -	- - -	- - -	914.5	882.3	859.8	855.5
Diseases of heart	- - -	- - -	- - -	- - -	319.7	289.9	263.8	255.5
Ischemic heart disease	- - -	- - -	- - -	- - -	251.9	219.9	194.3	186.6
Cerebrovascular diseases	- - -	- - -	- - -	- - -	63.5	60.8	59.8	59.0
Malignant neoplasms.	- - -	- - -	- - -	- - -	215.4	208.9	201.2	200.6
Trachea, bronchus, and lung	- - -	- - -	- - -	- - -	60.3	59.6	57.2	58.2
Colon, rectum, and anus	- - -	- - -	- - -	- - -	24.6	22.3	20.7	20.5
Prostate[5]	- - -	- - -	- - -	- - -	36.1	34.4	28.9	28.0
Breast[6]	- - -	- - -	- - -	- - -	33.9	30.6	26.6	26.8
Chronic lower respiratory diseases	- - -	- - -	- - -	- - -	39.2	42.1	48.3	47.2
Influenza and pneumonia	- - -	- - -	- - -	- - -	36.5	33.0	23.4	23.5
Chronic liver disease and cirrhosis	- - -	- - -	- - -	- - -	9.9	9.0	9.0	9.0
Diabetes mellitus.	- - -	- - -	- - -	- - -	18.3	20.1	21.6	21.8
Human immunodeficiency virus (HIV) disease . . .	- - -	- - -	- - -	- - -	7.4	9.8	2.3	2.2
Unintentional injuries	- - -	- - -	- - -	- - -	35.0	33.4	35.3.	35.3
Motor vehicle-related injuries	- - -	- - -	- - -	- - -	18.2	16.1	15.3	15.6
Suicide	- - -	- - -	- - -	- - -	13.8	13.1	12.0	12.0
Homicide	- - -	- - -	- - -	- - -	4.0	3.6	2.9	2.8

- - - Data not available.

[1]Underlying cause of death code numbers are based on the applicable revision of the *International Classification of Diseases* (ICD) for data years shown. For the period 1980–98, causes were coded using ICD–9 codes that are most nearly comparable with the 113 cause list for ICD–10. See Appendix II, tables IV and V.
[2]Includes deaths of persons who were not residents of the 50 States and the District of Columbia.
[3]Starting with 1999 data, cause of death is coded according to ICD–10. To estimate change between 1998 and 1999, compare the 1999 rate with the comparability-modified rate for 1998. See Appendix II, Comparability ratio and tables V and VI.
[4]Age-adjusted rates are calculated using the year 2000 standard population starting with *Health, United States, 2001.* See Appendix II, Age adjustment.
[5]Rate for male population only.
[6]Rate for female population only.
[7]The race groups, white, black, Asian or Pacific Islander, and American Indian or Alaska Native, include persons of Hispanic and non-Hispanic origin. Persons of Hispanic origin may be of any race. Death rates for the American Indian or Alaska Native and Asian or Pacific Islander populations are known to be underestimated. See Appendix II, Race, for a discussion of sources of bias in death rates by race and Hispanic origin.
[8]Prior to 1997, excludes data from States lacking an Hispanic-origin item on the death certificate. See Appendix II, Hispanic origin.

NOTES: Population estimates used to compute rates for 1991–2000 differ from those used previously. Starting with *Health, United States, 2003*, rates for 1991–99 were revised using intercensal population estimates based on Census 2000. Rates for 2000 were revised based on Census 2000 counts. See Appendix I, Population Census and Population Estimates. Data for additional years are available (see Appendix III).

SOURCES: Centers for Disease Control and Prevention, National Center for Health Statistics, National Vital Statistics System; Grove RD, Hetzel AM. Vital statistics rates in the United States, 1940–1960. Washington: U.S. Government Printing Office. 1968; numerator data from National Vital Statistics System, annual mortality files; denominator data from national population estimates for race groups from table 1 and unpublished Hispanic population estimates for 1985–96 prepared by the Housing and Household Economic Statistics Division, U.S. Bureau of the Census; additional mortality tables available at www.cdc.gov/nchs/datawh/statab/unpubd/mortabs.htm; Anderson RN, Arias E. The effect of revised populations on mortality statistics for the U.S., 2000. National vital statistics reports. Vol 51 no 9. Hyattsville, Maryland: National Center for Health Statistics. 2003.

This table will be updated with 2001 data on the web. Go to www.cdc.gov/nchs/hus.htm.

Table 30 (page 1 of 4). Years of potential life lost before age 75 for selected causes of death, according to sex, race, and Hispanic origin: United States, selected years 1980–2000

[Data are based on death certificates]

Sex, race, Hispanic origin, and cause of death[2]	Crude 2000	Age adjusted[1] 1980	1990	1995	1999[3]	2000
All persons		Years lost before age 75 per 100,000 population under 75 years of age				
All causes	7,529.4	10,448.4	9,085.5	8,626.2	7,599.4	7,578.1
Diseases of heart	1,241.5	2,238.7	1,617.7	1,475.4	1,294.7	1,253.0
Ischemic heart disease	832.9	1,729.3	1,153.6	1,013.2	874.6	841.8
Cerebrovascular diseases	221.2	357.5	259.6	246.5	218.9	223.3
Malignant neoplasms	1,659.1	2,108.8	2,003.8	1,841.6	1,694.4	1,674.1
Trachea, bronchus, and lung	438.1	548.5	561.4	497.3	441.4	443.1
Colorectal	140.5	190.0	164.7	152.0	142.6	141.9
Prostate[4]	58.9	84.9	96.8	83.5	67.4	63.6
Breast[5]	337.6	463.2	451.6	398.6	328.9	332.6
Chronic lower respiratory diseases	186.3	169.1	187.4	190.4	195.9	188.1
Influenza and pneumonia	86.4	160.2	141.5	126.9	86.0	87.1
Chronic liver disease and cirrhosis	162.6	300.3	196.9	173.7	162.1	164.1
Diabetes mellitus	176.9	134.4	155.9	174.7	178.3	178.4
Human immunodeficiency virus (HIV) disease	174.7	- - -	383.8	595.3	183.3	174.6
Unintentional injuries	1,030.0	1,543.5	1,162.1	1,057.2	1,021.3	1,026.5
Motor vehicle-related injuries	577.4	912.9	716.4	616.3	561.6	574.3
Suicide	336.2	392.0	393.1	384.7	334.0	334.5
Homicide	268.7	425.5	417.4	378.6	271.0	266.5
Male						
All causes	9,386.0	13,777.2	11,973.5	11,289.2	9,606.8	9,572.2
Diseases of heart	1,691.9	3,352.1	2,356.0	2,117.4	1,823.0	1,766.0
Ischemic heart disease	1,196.3	2,715.1	1,766.3	1,531.5	1,302.5	1,255.4
Cerebrovascular diseases	234.1	396.7	286.6	276.9	241.0	244.6
Malignant neoplasms	1,732.0	2,360.8	2,214.6	2,008.5	1,844.4	1,810.8
Trachea, bronchus, and lung	524.9	821.1	764.8	645.6	557.2	554.9
Colorectal	159.6	214.9	194.3	179.4	165.9	167.3
Prostate	58.9	84.9	96.8	83.5	67.4	63.6
Chronic lower respiratory diseases	194.3	235.1	224.8	213.1	216.8	206.0
Influenza and pneumonia	99.8	202.5	180.0	155.7	100.1	102.8
Chronic liver disease and cirrhosis	230.1	415.0	283.9	254.8	236.9	236.9
Diabetes mellitus	195.8	140.4	170.4	194.6	202.7	203.8
Human immunodeficiency virus (HIV) disease	257.7	- - -	686.2	991.2	275.5	258.9
Unintentional injuries	1,494.7	2,342.7	1,715.1	1,531.6	1,463.9	1,475.6
Motor vehicle-related injuries	811.0	1,359.7	1,018.4	851.1	771.1	796.4
Suicide	544.6	605.6	634.8	628.4	537.5	539.1
Homicide	420.6	675.0	658.0	589.6	411.1	410.5
Female						
All causes	5,685.8	7,350.3	6,333.1	6,057.5	5,659.2	5,644.6
Diseases of heart	794.2	1,246.0	948.5	883.9	803.4	774.6
Ischemic heart disease	472.1	852.1	600.3	537.8	478.3	457.6
Cerebrovascular diseases	208.5	324.0	235.9	218.7	198.8	203.9
Malignant neoplasms	1,586.6	1,896.8	1,826.6	1,698.9	1,564.0	1,555.3
Trachea, bronchus, and lung	352.0	310.4	382.2	365.2	337.2	342.1
Colorectal	121.6	168.7	138.7	127.5	121.5	118.7
Breast	337.6	463.2	451.6	398.6	328.9	332.6
Chronic lower respiratory diseases	178.2	114.0	155.9	171.0	177.9	172.3
Influenza and pneumonia	73.1	122.0	106.2	100.2	73.0	72.3
Chronic liver disease and cirrhosis	95.5	194.5	115.1	96.6	90.9	94.5
Diabetes mellitus	158.3	128.5	142.3	155.9	155.3	154.4
Human immunodeficiency virus (HIV) disease	92.4	- - -	87.8	205.7	92.8	92.0
Unintentional injuries	568.5	755.3	607.4	580.1	575.4	573.2
Motor vehicle-related injuries	345.4	470.4	411.6	378.4	349.0	348.5
Suicide	129.3	184.2	153.3	140.8	130.0	129.1
Homicide	117.9	181.3	174.3	163.2	127.6	118.9

See footnotes at end of table.

Table 30 (page 2 of 4). Years of potential life lost before age 75 for selected causes of death, according to sex, race, and Hispanic origin: United States, selected years 1980–2000

[Data are based on death certificates]

Sex, race, Hispanic origin, and cause of death[2]	Crude 2000	Age adjusted[1] 1980	1990	1995	1999[3]	2000
		Years lost before age 75 per 100,000 population under 75 years of age				
White[6]						
All causes	7,034.8	9,554.1	8,159.5	7,744.9	6,937.2	6,949.5
Diseases of heart	1,185.5	2,100.8	1,490.3	1,353.0	1,186.1	1,149.4
Ischemic heart disease	833.7	1,682.7	1,113.4	975.2	836.4	805.3
Cerebrovascular diseases	192.8	300.7	213.1	205.2	183.1	187.1
Malignant neoplasms.	1,677.3	2,035.9	1,929.3	1,780.5	1,644.6	1,627.8
Trachea, bronchus, and lung.	453.2	529.9	544.2	487.1	434.0	436.3
Colorectal	138.7	186.8	157.8	145.0	135.5	134.1
Prostate[4]	53.6	74.8	86.6	73.0	57.9	54.3
Breast[5]	331.2	460.2	441.7	381.5	309.8	315.6
Chronic lower respiratory diseases	193.0	165.4	182.3	185.7	193.6	185.3
Influenza and pneumonia.	79.0	130.8	116.9	108.3	74.2	77.7
Chronic liver disease and cirrhosis	166.2	257.3	175.8	164.6	159.5	162.7
Diabetes mellitus.	160.5	115.7	133.7	149.4	153.3	155.6
Human immunodeficiency virus (HIV) disease	95.5	- - -	309.0	422.6	101.5	94.7
Unintentional injuries	1,026.1	1,520.4	1,139.7	1,040.9	1,020.2	1,031.8
Motor vehicle-related injuries.	581.5	939.9	726.7	623.6	571.0	586.1
Suicide.	363.2	414.5	417.7	411.6	359.8	362.0
Homicide	155.3	271.7	234.9	220.2	163.2	156.6
Black or African American[6]						
All causes	11,869.4	17,873.4	16,593.0	15,809.7	13,112.4	12,897.1
Diseases of heart	1,865.3	3,619.9	2,891.8	2,681.8	2,360.8	2,275.2
Ischemic heart disease	1,022.7	2,305.1	1,676.1	1,510.2	1,345.7	1,300.1
Cerebrovascular diseases	416.7	883.2	656.4	583.6	500.3	507.0
Malignant neoplasms.	1,864.7	2,946.1	2,894.8	2,597.1	2,344.9	2,294.7
Trachea, bronchus, and lung.	462.1	776.0	811.3	683.0	595.1	593.0
Colorectal	177.3	232.3	241.8	226.9	220.2	222.4
Prostate[4]	110.8	200.3	223.5	210.0	179.4	171.0
Breast[5]	438.0	524.2	592.9	577.4	516.5	500.0
Chronic lower respiratory diseases	196.5	203.7	240.6	244.0	239.4	232.7
Influenza and pneumonia.	144.0	384.9	330.8	269.8	172.9	161.2
Chronic liver disease and cirrhosis	157.2	644.0	371.8	250.3	193.2	185.6
Diabetes mellitus.	310.3	305.3	361.5	400.8	396.5	383.4
Human immunodeficiency virus (HIV) disease	715.9	- - -	1,014.7	1,945.4	786.1	763.3
Unintentional injuries	1,179.5	1,751.5	1,392.7	1,272.1	1,185.0	1,152.8
Motor vehicle-related injuries.	604.0	750.2	699.5	621.8	580.0	580.8
Suicide.	213.9	238.0	261.4	254.2	207.7	208.7
Homicide	1,003.9	1,580.8	1,612.9	1,352.8	924.9	941.6
American Indian or Alaska Native[6]						
All causes	7,003.8	13,390.9	9,506.2	9,332.5	8,277.2	7,758.2
Diseases of heart	767.3	1,819.9	1,391.0	1,296.3	1,076.0	1,030.1
Ischemic heart disease	507.4	1,208.2	901.8	877.3	729.2	709.3
Cerebrovascular diseases	146.5	269.3	223.3	255.3	210.3	198.1
Malignant neoplasms.	737.5	1,101.3	1,141.1	1,099.5	1,020.7	995.7
Trachea, bronchus, and lung.	152.0	181.1	268.1	267.7	254.8	227.8
Colorectal	68.0	78.8	82.4	103.5	84.4	93.8
Prostate[4]	24.6	66.7	42.0	51.1	*	44.5
Breast[5]	137.9	205.5	213.4	195.9	167.3	174.1
Chronic lower respiratory diseases	107.0	89.3	129.0	145.3	146.6	151.8
Influenza and pneumonia.	107.3	307.9	206.3	199.7	144.5	124.0
Chronic liver disease and cirrhosis	435.4	1,190.3	535.1	604.8	532.8	519.4
Diabetes mellitus.	216.7	305.5	292.3	360.6	385.2	305.6
Human immunodeficiency virus (HIV) disease	63.0	- - -	70.1	246.9	90.5	68.4
Unintentional injuries	1,786.6	3,541.0	2,183.9	1,980.9	1,708.0	1,700.1
Motor vehicle-related injuries.	1,110.2	2,102.4	1,301.5	1,210.3	995.4	1,032.2
Suicide.	424.9	515.0	495.9	445.2	415.6	403.1
Homicide	297.7	628.9	434.2	432.7	359.9	278.5

See footnotes at end of table.

Table 30 (page 3 of 4). Years of potential life lost before age 75 for selected causes of death, according to sex, race, and Hispanic origin: United States, selected years 1980–2000

[Data are based on death certificates]

Sex, race, Hispanic origin, and cause of death[2]	Crude 2000	Age adjusted[1] 1980	1990	1995	1999[3]	2000
Asian or Pacific Islander[6]		Years lost before age 75 per 100,000 population under 75 years of age				
All causes	3,545.8	5,378.4	4,705.2	4,333.2	3,828.8	3,811.1
Diseases of heart	485.7	952.8	702.2	664.9	587.9	567.9
Ischemic heart disease.	314.8	697.7	486.6	440.6	405.8	381.1
Cerebrovascular diseases	170.6	266.9	233.5	220.0	203.9	199.4
Malignant neoplasms.	915.3	1,218.6	1,166.4	1,122.1	1,042.2	1,033.8
Trachea, bronchus, and lung.	154.6	238.2	204.7	197.0	181.7	185.8
Colorectal	79.5	115.9	105.1	99.5	87.2	91.6
Prostate[4].	13.0	17.0	32.4	25.3	18.8	18.8
Breast[5]	190.7	222.2	216.5	237.8	183.5	200.8
Chronic lower respiratory diseases	48.3	56.4	72.8	65.8	57.5	56.5
Influenza and pneumonia.	42.2	79.3	74.0	64.3	43.7	48.6
Chronic liver disease and cirrhosis	40.6	85.6	72.4	48.4	44.1	44.8
Diabetes mellitus.	63.8	83.1	74.0	83.5	80.3	77.0
Human immunodeficiency virus (HIV) disease	20.5	- - -	77.0	110.4	25.5	19.9
Unintentional injuries	447.3	742.7	636.6	525.7	420.5	425.7
Motor vehicle-related injuries.	280.5	472.6	445.5	351.9	257.8	263.4
Suicide.	183.9	217.1	200.6	211.1	189.0	168.6
Homicide	120.6	201.1	205.8	202.3	126.7	113.1
Hispanic or Latino[6,7]						
All causes	5,325.5	- - -	7,963.3	7,426.7	6,067.1	6,037.6
Diseases of heart	522.1	- - -	1,082.0	962.0	871.7	821.3
Ischemic heart disease.	323.3	- - -	756.6	665.8	604.7	564.6
Cerebrovascular diseases	137.6	- - -	238.0	232.0	206.3	207.8
Malignant neoplasms.	742.9	- - -	1,232.2	1,172.0	1,108.4	1,098.2
Trachea, bronchus, and lung.	86.1	- - -	193.7	173.9	159.7	152.1
Colorectal	63.1	- - -	100.2	97.9	97.0	101.4
Prostate[4].	19.2	- - -	47.7	60.8	48.7	42.9
Breast[5]	162.3	- - -	299.3	257.7	220.9	230.7
Chronic lower respiratory diseases	44.7	- - -	78.8	82.1	79.3	68.5
Influenza and pneumonia.	62.2	- - -	130.1	108.5	67.1	76.0
Chronic liver disease and cirrhosis	169.2	- - -	329.1	281.4	248.9	252.1
Diabetes mellitus.	127.3	- - -	177.8	228.8	216.8	215.6
Human immunodeficiency virus (HIV) disease	178.5	- - -	600.1	865.0	225.8	209.4
Unintentional injuries	992.9	- - -	1,190.6	1,017.9	938.1	920.1
Motor vehicle-related injuries.	603.0	- - -	740.8	593.0	515.0	540.2
Suicide.	195.7	- - -	256.2	245.1	183.8	188.5
Homicide	389.6	- - -	720.8	575.4	343.2	335.1

See footnotes at end of table.

[Data are based on death certificates]

Sex, race, Hispanic origin, and cause of death[2]	Crude	Age adjusted[1]				
	2000	1980	1990	1995	1999[3]	2000
White, not Hispanic or Latino[7]	Years lost before age 75 per 100,000 population under 75 years of age					
All causes	7,247.9	- - -	8,022.5	7,607.5	6,943.3	6,960.5
Diseases of heart	1,291.1	- - -	1,504.0	1,368.2	1,209.3	1,175.1
Ischemic heart disease.	915.8	- - -	1,127.2	988.7	854.2	824.7
Cerebrovascular diseases	200.6	- - -	210.1	199.6	178.9	183.0
Malignant neoplasms.	1,829.4	- - -	1,974.1	1,814.2	1,685.3	1,668.4
Trachea, bronchus, and lung.	515.6	- - -	566.8	507.0	456.5	460.3
Colorectal	150.9	- - -	162.1	147.8	138.6	136.2
Prostate[4].	59.6	- - -	89.2	73.6	58.3	54.9
Breast[5]	357.3	- - -	451.5	389.3	316.6	322.3
Chronic lower respiratory diseases	217.6	- - -	188.1	190.6	201.5	193.8
Influenza and pneumonia.	80.7	- - -	112.3	105.8	73.8	76.4
Chronic liver disease and cirrhosis	162.8	- - -	162.4	151.4	148.0	150.9
Diabetes mellitus.	164.5	- - -	131.2	142.8	148.0	150.2
Human immunodeficiency virus (HIV) disease	78.1	- - -	271.2	362.1	81.2	76.0
Unintentional injuries	1,016.8	- - -	1,114.7	1,026.1	1,023.6	1,041.4
Motor vehicle-related injuries.	569.4	- - -	715.7	618.0	575.7	588.8
Suicide.	389.0	- - -	433.0	427.7	386.8	389.2
Homicide	109.7	- - -	162.0	148.6	120.5	113.2

- - - Data not available.

* Rate based on fewer than 20 deaths is considered unreliable and is not shown.

[1]Age-adjusted rates are calculated using the year 2000 standard population starting with *Health, United States, 2001*. See Appendix II, Age adjustment.

[2]Underlying cause of death code numbers are based on the applicable revision of the *International Classification of Diseases* (ICD) for data years shown. For the period 1980–98, causes were coded using ICD–9 codes that are most nearly comparable with the 113 cause list for ICD–10. See Appendix II, tables IV and V.

[3]Starting with 1999 data, cause of death is coded according to ICD–10. To estimate change between 1998 and 1999, compare the 1999 rate with the comparability-modified rate for 1998. See Appendix II, Comparability ratio and tables V and VI.

[4]Rate for male population only.

[5]Rate for female population only.

[6]The race groups, white, black, Asian or Pacific Islander, and American Indian or Alaska Native, include persons of Hispanic and non-Hispanic origin. Persons of Hispanic origin may be of any race. Death rates for the American Indian or Alaska Native and Asian or Pacific Islander populations are known to be underestimated. See Appendix II, Race, for a discussion of sources of bias in death rates by race and Hispanic origin.

[7]Prior to 1997, excludes data from States lacking an Hispanic-origin item on the death certificate. See Appendix II, Hispanic origin.

NOTES: Population estimates used to compute rates for 1991–2000 differ from those used previously. Starting with *Health, United States, 2003*, rates for 1991–99 were revised using intercensal population estimates based on Census 2000. Rates for 2000 were revised based on Census 2000 counts. See Appendix I, Population Census and Population Estimates. See Appendix II for definition of years of potential life lost (YPLL) and method of calculation. Data for additional years are available (see Appendix III).

SOURCES: Centers for Disease Control and Prevention, National Center for Health Statistics, National vital statistics system; numerator data from annual mortality files; denominator data from national population estimates for race groups from table 1 and unpublished Hispanic population estimates for 1990–96 prepared by the Housing and Household Economic Statistics Division, U.S. Bureau of the Census.

This table will be updated with 2001 data on the web. Go to www.cdc.gov/nchs/hus.htm.

Table 31 (page 1 of 4). Leading causes of death and numbers of deaths, according to sex, race, and Hispanic origin: United States, 1980 and 2000

[Data are based on death certificates]

Sex, race, Hispanic origin, and rank order	1980 Cause of death	Deaths	2000 Cause of death	Deaths
All persons				
. . .	All causes	1,989,841	All causes	2,403,351
1.	Diseases of heart	761,085	Diseases of heart	710,760
2.	Malignant neoplasms	416,509	Malignant neoplasms	553,091
3.	Cerebrovascular diseases	170,225	Cerebrovascular diseases	167,661
4.	Unintentional injuries	105,718	Chronic lower respiratory diseases	122,009
5.	Chronic obstructive pulmonary diseases	56,050	Unintentional injuries	97,900
6.	Pneumonia and influenza	54,619	Diabetes mellitus	69,301
7.	Diabetes mellitus	34,851	Influenza and pneumonia	65,313
8.	Chronic liver disease and cirrhosis	30,583	Alzheimer's disease	49,558
9.	Atherosclerosis	29,449	Nephritis, nephrotic syndrome and nephrosis	37,251
10.	Suicide	26,869	Septicemia	31,224
Male				
. . .	All causes	1,075,078	All causes	1,177,578
1.	Diseases of heart	405,661	Diseases of heart	344,807
2.	Malignant neoplasms	225,948	Malignant neoplasms	286,082
3.	Unintentional injuries	74,180	Cerebrovascular diseases	64,769
4.	Cerebrovascular diseases	69,973	Unintentional injuries	63,817
5.	Chronic obstructive pulmonary diseases	38,625	Chronic lower respiratory diseases	60,004
6.	Pneumonia and influenza	27,574	Diabetes mellitus	31,602
7.	Suicide	20,505	Influenza and pneumonia	28,658
8.	Chronic liver disease and cirrhosis	19,768	Suicide	23,618
9.	Homicide	18,779	Nephritis, nephrotic syndrome and nephrosis	17,811
10.	Diabetes mellitus	14,325	Chronic liver disease and cirrhosis	17,214
Female				
. . .	All causes	914,763	All causes	1,225,773
1.	Diseases of heart	355,424	Diseases of heart	365,953
2.	Malignant neoplasms	190,561	Malignant neoplasms	267,009
3.	Cerebrovascular diseases	100,252	Cerebrovascular diseases	102,892
4.	Unintentional injuries	31,538	Chronic lower respiratory diseases	62,005
5.	Pneumonia and influenza	27,045	Diabetes mellitus	37,699
6.	Diabetes mellitus	20,526	Influenza and pneumonia	36,655
7.	Atherosclerosis	17,848	Alzheimer's disease	35,120
8.	Chronic obstructive pulmonary diseases	17,425	Unintentional injuries	34,083
9.	Chronic liver disease and cirrhosis	10,815	Nephritis, nephrotic syndrome and nephrosis	19,440
10.	Certain conditions originating in the perinatal period	9,815	Septicemia	17,687
White				
. . .	All causes	1,738,607	All causes	2,071,287
1.	Diseases of heart	683,347	Diseases of heart	621,719
2.	Malignant neoplasms	368,162	Malignant neoplasms	480,011
3.	Cerebrovascular diseases	148,734	Cerebrovascular diseases	144,580
4.	Unintentional injuries	90,122	Chronic lower respiratory diseases	112,840
5.	Chronic obstructive pulmonary diseases	52,375	Unintentional injuries	82,592
6.	Pneumonia and influenza	48,369	Influenza and pneumonia	57,914
7.	Diabetes mellitus	28,868	Diabetes mellitus	55,561
8.	Atherosclerosis	27,069	Alzheimer's disease	46,460
9.	Chronic liver disease and cirrhosis	25,240	Nephritis, nephrotic syndrome and nephrosis	29,598
10.	Suicide	24,829	Suicide	26,475
Black or African American				
. . .	All causes	233,135	All causes	285,826
1.	Diseases of heart	72,956	Diseases of heart	77,523
2.	Malignant neoplasms	45,037	Malignant neoplasms	61,945
3.	Cerebrovascular diseases	20,135	Cerebrovascular diseases	19,221
4.	Unintentional injuries	13,480	Unintentional injuries	12,277
5.	Homicide	10,172	Diabetes mellitus	12,021
6.	Certain conditions originating in the perinatal period	6,961	Homicide	7,867
7.	Pneumonia and influenza	5,648	Human immunodeficiency virus (HIV) disease	7,848
8.	Diabetes mellitus	5,544	Chronic lower respiratory diseases	7,607
9.	Chronic liver disease and cirrhosis	4,790	Nephritis, nephrotic syndrome and nephrosis	6,911
10.	Nephritis, nephrotic syndrome, and nephrosis	3,416	Influenza and pneumonia	5,990

See footnotes at end of table.

Table 31 (page 2 of 4). Leading causes of death and numbers of deaths, according to sex, race, and Hispanic origin: United States, 1980 and 2000

[Data are based on death certificates]

Sex, race, Hispanic origin, and rank order	1980 Cause of death	1980 Deaths	2000 Cause of death	2000 Deaths
American Indian or Alaska Native				
. . .	All causes	6,923	All causes	11,363
1	Diseases of heart	1,494	Diseases of heart	2,417
2	Unintentional injuries	1,290	Malignant neoplasms	1,914
3	Malignant neoplasms	770	Unintentional injuries	1,353
4	Chronic liver disease and cirrhosis	410	Diabetes mellitus	616
5	Cerebrovascular diseases	322	Cerebrovascular diseases	572
6	Pneumonia and influenza	257	Chronic liver disease and cirrhosis	534
7	Homicide	217	Chronic lower respiratory diseases	429
8	Diabetes mellitus	210	Suicide	297
9	Certain conditions originating in the perinatal period	199	Influenza and pneumonia	289
10	Suicide	181	Nephritis, nephrotic syndrome and nephrosis	215
Asian or Pacific Islander				
. . .	All causes	11,071	All causes	34,875
1	Diseases of heart	3,265	Malignant neoplasms	9,221
2	Malignant neoplasms	2,522	Diseases of heart	9,101
3	Cerebrovascular diseases	1,028	Cerebrovascular diseases	3,288
4	Unintentional injuries	810	Unintentional injuries	1,678
5	Pneumonia and influenza	342	Chronic lower respiratory diseases	1,133
6	Suicide	249	Influenza and pneumonia	1,120
7	Certain conditions originating in the perinatal period	246	Diabetes mellitus	1,103
8	Diabetes mellitus	227	Suicide	616
9	Homicide	211	Nephritis, nephrotic syndrome and nephrosis	527
10	Chronic obstructive pulmonary diseases	207	Certain conditions originating in the perinatal period	392
Hispanic or Latino				
. . .	- - -	- - -	All causes	107,254
1	- - -	- - -	Diseases of heart	25,819
2	- - -	- - -	Malignant neoplasms	21,160
3	- - -	- - -	Unintentional injuries	8,830
4	- - -	- - -	Cerebrovascular diseases	6,187
5	- - -	- - -	Diabetes mellitus	5,328
6	- - -	- - -	Chronic liver disease and cirrhosis	3,187
7	- - -	- - -	Homicide	2,917
8	- - -	- - -	Chronic lower respiratory diseases	2,689
9	- - -	- - -	Influenza and pneumonia	2,625
10	- - -	- - -	Certain conditions originating in the perinatal period	2,145
White male				
. . .	All causes	933,878	All causes	1,007,191
1	Diseases of heart	364,679	Diseases of heart	301,551
2	Malignant neoplasms	198,188	Malignant neoplasms	247,403
3	Unintentional injuries	62,963	Cerebrovascular diseases	54,938
4	Cerebrovascular diseases	60,095	Chronic lower respiratory diseases	54,816
5	Chronic obstructive pulmonary diseases	35,977	Unintentional injuries	53,329
6	Pneumonia and influenza	23,810	Diabetes mellitus	26,009
7	Suicide	18,901	Influenza and pneumonia	25,002
8	Chronic liver disease and cirrhosis	16,407	Suicide	21,293
9	Diabetes mellitus	12,125	Chronic liver disease and cirrhosis	15,002
10	Atherosclerosis	10,543	Nephritis, nephrotic syndrome and nephrosis	14,385
Black or African American male				
. . .	All causes	130,138	All causes	145,184
1	Diseases of heart	37,877	Diseases of heart	36,740
2	Malignant neoplasms	25,861	Malignant neoplasms	32,817
3	Unintentional injuries	9,701	Unintentional injuries	8,531
4	Cerebrovascular diseases	9,194	Cerebrovascular diseases	8,026
5	Homicide	8,274	Homicide	6,482
6	Certain conditions originating in the perinatal period	3,869	Human immunodeficiency virus (HIV) disease	5,400
7	Pneumonia and influenza	3,386	Diabetes mellitus	4,771
8	Chronic liver disease and cirrhosis	3,020	Chronic lower respiratory diseases	4,238
9	Chronic obstructive pulmonary diseases	2,429	Nephritis, nephrotic syndrome and nephrosis	3,074
10	Diabetes mellitus	2,010	Influenza and pneumonia	2,915

See footnotes at end of table.

Table 31 (page 3 of 4). Leading causes of death and numbers of deaths, according to sex, race, and Hispanic origin: United States, 1980 and 2000

[Data are based on death certificates]

Sex, race, Hispanic origin, and rank order	1980 Cause of death	Deaths	2000 Cause of death	Deaths
American Indian or Alaska Native male				
...	All causes	4,193	All causes	6,185
1.............	Unintentional injuries	946	Diseases of heart	1,341
2.............	Diseases of heart	917	Malignant neoplasms	997
3.............	Malignant neoplasms	408	Unintentional injuries	900
4.............	Chronic liver disease and cirrhosis	239	Chronic liver disease and cirrhosis	298
5.............	Cerebrovascular diseases	163	Diabetes mellitus	275
6.............	Homicide	162	Cerebrovascular diseases	250
7.............	Pneumonia and influenza	148	Suicide	237
8.............	Suicide	147	Chronic lower respiratory diseases	228
9.............	Certain conditions originating in the perinatal period	107	Homicide	159
10.............	Diabetes mellitus	86	Influenza and pneumonia	149
Asian or Pacific Islander male				
...	All causes	6,809	All causes	19,018
1.............	Diseases of heart	2,174	Diseases of heart	5,175
2.............	Malignant neoplasms	1,485	Malignant neoplasms	4,865
3.............	Unintentional injuries	556	Cerebrovascular diseases	1,555
4.............	Cerebrovascular diseases	521	Unintentional injuries	1,057
5.............	Pneumonia and influenza	227	Chronic lower respiratory diseases	722
6.............	Suicide	159	Influenza and pneumonia	592
7.............	Chronic obstructive pulmonary diseases	158	Diabetes mellitus	547
8.............	Homicide	151	Suicide	452
9.............	Certain conditions originating in the perinatal period	128	Nephritis, nephrotic syndrome and nephrosis	254
9.............	...	...	Homicide	254
10.............	Diabetes mellitus	103	...	...
Hispanic or Latino male				
...	---	---	All causes	60,172
1.............	---	---	Diseases of heart	13,566
2.............	---	---	Malignant neoplasms	11,138
3.............	---	---	Unintentional injuries	6,696
4.............	---	---	Cerebrovascular diseases	2,865
5.............	---	---	Diabetes mellitus	2,507
6.............	---	---	Homicide	2,431
7.............	---	---	Chronic liver disease and cirrhosis	2,312
8.............	---	---	Suicide	1,525
9.............	---	---	Human immunodeficiency virus (HIV) disease	1,493
10.............	---	---	Chronic lower respiratory diseases	1,451
White female				
...	All causes	804,729	All causes	1,064,096
1.............	Diseases of heart	318,668	Diseases of heart	320,168
2.............	Malignant neoplasms	169,974	Malignant neoplasms	232,608
3.............	Cerebrovascular diseases	88,639	Cerebrovascular diseases	89,642
4.............	Unintentional injuries	27,159	Chronic lower respiratory diseases	58,024
5.............	Pneumonia and influenza	24,559	Alzheimer's disease	32,936
6.............	Diabetes mellitus	16,743	Influenza and pneumonia	32,912
7.............	Atherosclerosis	16,526	Diabetes mellitus	29,552
8.............	Chronic obstructive pulmonary diseases	16,398	Unintentional injuries	29,263
9.............	Chronic liver disease and cirrhosis	8,833	Nephritis, nephrotic syndrome and nephrosis	15,213
10.............	Certain conditions originating in the perinatal period	6,512	Septicemia	14,088
Black or African American female				
...	All causes	102,997	All causes	140,642
1.............	Diseases of heart	35,079	Diseases of heart	40,783
2.............	Malignant neoplasms	19,176	Malignant neoplasms	29,128
3.............	Cerebrovascular diseases	10,941	Cerebrovascular diseases	11,195
4.............	Unintentional injuries	3,779	Diabetes mellitus	7,250
5.............	Diabetes mellitus	3,534	Nephritis, nephrotic syndrome and nephrosis	3,837
6.............	Certain conditions originating in the perinatal period	3,092	Unintentional injuries	3,746
7.............	Pneumonia and influenza	2,262	Chronic lower respiratory diseases	3,369
8.............	Homicide	1,898	Septicemia	3,341
9.............	Chronic liver disease and cirrhosis	1,770	Influenza and pneumonia	3,075
10.............	Nephritis, nephrotic syndrome, and nephrosis	1,722	Human immunodeficiency virus (HIV) disease	2,448

See footnotes at end of table.

Table 31 (page 4 of 4). Leading causes of death and numbers of deaths, according to sex, race, and Hispanic origin: United States, 1980 and 2000

[Data are based on death certificates]

Sex, race, Hispanic origin, and rank order	1980		2000	
	Cause of death	Deaths	Cause of death	Deaths
American Indian or Alaska Native female				
. . .	All causes	2,730	All causes	5,178
1.	Diseases of heart	577	Diseases of heart	1,076
2.	Malignant neoplasms	362	Malignant neoplasms	917
3.	Unintentional injuries	344	Unintentional injuries	453
4.	Chronic liver disease and cirrhosis	171	Diabetes mellitus	341
5.	Cerebrovascular diseases	159	Cerebrovascular diseases	322
6.	Diabetes mellitus	124	Chronic liver disease and cirrhosis	236
7.	Pneumonia and influenza	109	Chronic lower respiratory diseases	201
8.	Certain conditions originating in the perinatal period	92	Influenza and pneumonia	140
9.	Nephritis, nephrotic syndrome, and nephrosis	56	Nephritis, nephrotic syndrome and nephrosis	117
10.	Homicide	55	Septicemia	88
Asian or Pacific Islander female				
. . .	All causes	4,262	All causes	15,857
1.	Diseases of heart	1,091	Malignant neoplasms	4,356
2.	Malignant neoplasms	1,037	Diseases of heart	3,926
3.	Cerebrovascular diseases	507	Cerebrovascular diseases	1,733
4.	Unintentional injuries	254	Unintentional injuries	621
5.	Diabetes mellitus	124	Diabetes mellitus	556
6.	Certain conditions originating in the perinatal period	118	Influenza and pneumonia	528
7.	Pneumonia and influenza	115	Chronic lower respiratory diseases	411
8.	Congenital anomalies	104	Nephritis, nephrotic syndrome and nephrosis	273
9.	Suicide	90	Essential (primary) hypertension and hypertensive renal disease	179
10.	Homicide	60	Septicemia	170
Hispanic or Latino female				
. . .	- - -	- - -	All causes	47,082
1.	- - -	- - -	Diseases of heart	12,253
2.	- - -	- - -	Malignant neoplasms	10,022
3.	- - -	- - -	Cerebrovascular diseases	3,322
4.	- - -	- - -	Diabetes mellitus	2,821
5.	- - -	- - -	Unintentional injuries	2,134
6.	- - -	- - -	Influenza and pneumonia	1,322
7.	- - -	- - -	Chronic lower respiratory diseases	1,238
8.	- - -	- - -	Certain conditions originating in the perinatal period	951
9.	- - -	- - -	Chronic liver disease and cirrhosis	875
10.	- - -	- - -	Nephritis, nephrotic syndrome and nephrosis	841

. . . Category not applicable.
- - - Data not available.

NOTES: For cause of death code numbers based on the *International Classification of Diseases, 9th Revision* (ICD–9) in 1980 and ICD–10 in 2000, see Appendix II, tables IV and V.

SOURCES: Centers for Disease Control and Prevention, National Center for Health Statistics, National Vital Statistics System; *Vital statistics of the United States, vol II, mortality, part A*, 1980. Washington: Public Health Service. 1985; Anderson RN. Deaths: Leading causes for 2000. National vital statistics reports. vol 50 no 16. Hyattsville, Maryland: National Center for Health Statistics. 2002.

This table will be updated with 2001 data on the web. Go to www.cdc.gov/nchs/hus.htm.

Table 32 (page 1 of 2). Leading causes of death and numbers of deaths, according to age: United States, 1980 and 2000

[Data are based on death certificates]

Age and rank order	1980 Cause of death	Deaths	2000 Cause of death	Deaths
Under 1 year				
...	All causes	45,526	All causes	28,035
1.............	Congenital anomalies	9,220	Congenital malformations, deformations and chromosomal abnormalities	5,743
2.............	Sudden infant death syndrome	5,510	Disorders related to short gestation and low birthweight, not elsewhere classified	4,397
3.............	Respiratory distress syndrome	4,989	Sudden infant death syndrome	2,523
4.............	Disorders relating to short gestation and unspecified low birthweight	3,648	Newborn affected by maternal complications of pregnancy	1,404
5.............	Newborn affected by maternal complications of pregnancy	1,572	Newborn affected by complications of placenta, cord and membranes	1,062
6.............	Intrauterine hypoxia and birth asphyxia	1,497	Respiratory distress of newborn	999
7.............	Unintentional injuries	1,166	Unintentional injuries	881
8.............	Birth trauma	1,058	Bacterial sepsis of newborn	768
9.............	Pneumonia and influenza	1,012	Diseases of circulatory system	663
10.............	Newborn affected by complications of placenta, cord, and membranes	985	Intrauterine hypoxia and birth asphyxia	630
1–4 years				
...	All causes	8,187	All causes	4,979
1.............	Unintentional injuries	3,313	Unintentional injuries	1,826
2.............	Congenital anomalies	1,026	Congenital malformations, deformations and chromosomal abnormalities	495
3.............	Malignant neoplasms	573	Malignant neoplasms	420
4.............	Diseases of heart	338	Homicide	356
5.............	Homicide	319	Diseases of heart	181
6.............	Pneumonia and influenza	267	Influenza and pneumonia	103
7.............	Meningitis	223	Septicemia	99
8.............	Meningococcal infection	110	Certain conditions originating in the perinatal period	79
9.............	Certain conditions originating in the perinatal period	84	In situ neoplasms, benign neoplasms and neoplasms of uncertain or unknown behavior	53
10.............	Septicemia	71	Chronic lower respiratory diseases	51
5–14 years				
...	All causes	10,689	All causes	7,413
1.............	Unintentional injuries	5,224	Unintentional injuries	2,979
2.............	Malignant neoplasms	1,497	Malignant neoplasms	1,014
3.............	Congenital anomalies	561	Congenital malformations, deformations and chromosomal abnormalities	399
4.............	Homicide	415	Homicide	371
5.............	Diseases of heart	330	Suicide	307
6.............	Pneumonia and influenza	194	Diseases of heart	271
7.............	Suicide	142	Chronic lower respiratory diseases	139
8.............	Benign neoplasms	104	In situ neoplasms, benign neoplasms and neoplasms of uncertain or unknown behavior	99
9.............	Cerebrovascular diseases	95	Influenza and pneumonia	87
10.............	Chronic obstructive pulmonary diseases	85	Cerebrovascular diseases	76
15–24 years				
...	All causes	49,027	All causes	31,307
1.............	Unintentional injuries	26,206	Unintentional injuries	14,113
2.............	Homicide	6,537	Homicide	4,939
3.............	Suicide	5,239	Suicide	3,994
4.............	Malignant neoplasms	2,683	Malignant neoplasms	1,713
5.............	Diseases of heart	1,223	Diseases of heart	1,031
6.............	Congenital anomalies	600	Congenital malformations, deformations and chromosomal abnormalities	441
7.............	Cerebrovascular diseases	418	Cerebrovascular diseases	199
8.............	Pneumonia and influenza	348	Chronic lower respiratory diseases	190
9.............	Chronic obstructive pulmonary diseases	141	Influenza and pneumonia	189
10.............	Anemias	133	Human immunodeficiency virus (HIV) disease	179

See footnotes at end of table.

Table 32 (page 2 of 2). Leading causes of death and numbers of deaths, according to age: United States, 1980 and 2000

[Data are based on death certificates]

Age and rank order	1980		2000	
	Cause of death	Deaths	Cause of death	Deaths
25–44 years				
. . .	All causes	108,658	All causes	130,249
1.	Unintentional injuries	26,722	Unintentional injuries	27,182
2.	Malignant neoplasms	17,551	Malignant neoplasms	20,436
3.	Diseases of heart	14,513	Diseases of heart	16,139
4.	Homicide	10,983	Suicide	11,354
5.	Suicide	9,855	Human immunodeficiency virus (HIV) disease	8,356
6.	Chronic liver disease and cirrhosis	4,782	Homicide	7,383
7.	Cerebrovascular diseases	3,154	Chronic liver disease and cirrhosis	3,786
8.	Diabetes mellitus	1,472	Cerebrovascular diseases	3,201
9.	Pneumonia and influenza	1,467	Diabetes mellitus	2,549
10.	Congenital anomalies	817	Influenza and pneumonia	1,432
45–64 years				
. . .	All causes	425,338	All causes	401,187
1.	Diseases of heart	148,322	Malignant neoplasms	137,039
2.	Malignant neoplasms	135,675	Diseases of heart	98,879
3.	Cerebrovascular diseases	19,909	Unintentional injuries	19,783
4.	Unintentional injuries	18,140	Cerebrovascular diseases	15,967
5.	Chronic liver disease and cirrhosis	16,089	Diabetes mellitus	14,140
6.	Chronic obstructive pulmonary diseases	11,514	Chronic lower respiratory diseases	13,990
7.	Diabetes mellitus	7,977	Chronic liver disease and cirrhosis	12,428
8.	Suicide	7,079	Suicide	8,382
9.	Pneumonia and influenza	5,804	Human immunodeficiency virus (HIV) disease	5,381
10.	Homicide	4,019	Nephritis, nephrotic syndrome and nephrosis	4,751
65 years and over				
. . .	All causes	1,341,848	All causes	1,799,825
1.	Diseases of heart	595,406	Diseases of heart	593,707
2.	Malignant neoplasms	258,389	Malignant neoplasms	392,366
3.	Cerebrovascular diseases	146,417	Cerebrovascular diseases	148,045
4.	Pneumonia and influenza	45,512	Chronic lower respiratory diseases	106,375
5.	Chronic obstructive pulmonary diseases	43,587	Influenza and pneumonia	58,557
6.	Atherosclerosis	28,081	Diabetes mellitus	52,414
7.	Diabetes mellitus	25,216	Alzheimer's disease	48,993
8.	Unintentional injuries	24,844	Nephritis, nephrotic syndrome and nephrosis	31,225
9.	Nephritis, nephrotic syndrome, and nephrosis	12,968	Unintentional injuries	31,051
10.	Chronic liver disease and cirrhosis	9,519	Septicemia	24,786

. . . Category not applicable.

NOTES: For cause of death code numbers based on the *International Classification of Diseases, 9th Revision* (ICD–9) in 1980 and ICD–10 in 2000, see Appendix II, tables IV and V.

SOURCES: Centers for Disease Control and Prevention, National Center for Health Statistics, National Vital Statistics System; *Vital statistics of the United States, vol II, mortality, part A*, 1980. Washington: Public Health Service. 1985; Anderson RN. Deaths: Leading causes for 2000. National vital statistics reports. vol 50 no 16. Hyattsville, Maryland: National Center for Health Statistics. 2002.

This table will be updated with 2001 data on the web. Go to www.cdc.gov/nchs/hus.htm.

Table 33 (page 1 of 3). Age-adjusted death rates, according to race, sex, region, and urbanization level: United States, average annual 1984–86, 1989–91, and 1997–99

[Data are based on the National Vital Statistics System]

Sex, region, and urbanization level[1]	All races			White			Black or African American		
	1984–86	1989–91	1997–99	1984–86	1989–91	1997–99	1984–86	1989–91	1997–99
Both sexes	Age-adjusted death rate per 100,000 standard population[2]								
All regions:									
Metropolitan counties:									
Large central	1,013.9	977.1	870.3	975.1	929.4	831.5	1,277.5	1,292.7	1,157.9
Large fringe	953.9	894.8	831.0	946.1	884.3	823.9	1,170.3	1,144.0	1,049.7
Small	970.1	926.2	882.9	948.7	900.8	863.5	1,255.5	1,250.9	1,146.0
Nonmetropolitan counties:									
With a city of 10,000 or more . .	979.5	946.9	923.5	961.5	926.5	907.2	1,262.9	1,262.5	1,177.7
Without a city of 10,000 or more.	987.5	960.8	935.2	966.7	936.8	916.9	1,232.7	1,249.3	1,140.8
Northeast:									
Metropolitan counties:									
Large central	1,056.2	1,020.6	881.3	1,014.1	967.8	854.2	1,256.0	1,260.1	1,030.2
Large fringe	967.1	896.9	817.3	961.5	889.7	817.4	1,146.9	1,093.4	927.9
Small	973.5	907.7	855.5	965.3	896.9	848.5	1,220.9	1,186.9	1,040.6
Nonmetropolitan counties:									
With a city of 10,000 or more . .	1,003.6	932.3	895.1	1,003.7	932.4	897.5	1,192.9	1,064.3	885.8
Without a city of 10,000 or more.	996.1	939.7	886.7	995.8	939.3	886.8	1,250.2	1,135.9	1,076.2
Midwest:									
Metropolitan counties:									
Large central	1,055.6	1,018.7	942.1	997.6	943.3	871.3	1,296.5	1,311.9	1,211.2
Large fringe	970.2	908.4	858.0	961.0	896.6	845.8	1,243.0	1,209.9	1,200.3
Small	960.7	912.3	876.9	947.7	895.4	861.0	1,230.9	1,227.7	1,163.3
Nonmetropolitan counties:									
With a city of 10,000 or more . .	935.9	902.7	879.5	932.7	898.3	876.5	1,208.7	1,196.0	1,064.6
Without a city of 10,000 or more.	922.0	894.1	865.8	917.8	888.0	860.1	1,193.5	1,247.9	1,062.7
South:									
Metropolitan counties:									
Large central	1,021.1	999.1	915.9	945.6	908.3	824.7	1,318.4	1,343.8	1,299.8
Large fringe	944.0	899.6	850.5	927.6	879.2	833.9	1,163.7	1,154.2	1,075.2
Small	986.8	951.7	912.2	945.5	905.3	875.6	1,268.2	1,267.4	1,167.5
Nonmetropolitan counties:									
With a city of 10,000 or more . .	1,028.6	1,009.6	998.3	989.0	966.7	964.4	1,274.7	1,277.3	1,205.3
Without a city of 10,000 or more.	1,039.8	1,020.8	1,001.8	1,009.1	984.9	980.1	1,235.1	1,252.4	1,147.1
West:									
Metropolitan counties:									
Large central	942.7	904.2	792.4	944.9	905.7	799.0	1,198.3	1,219.4	1,050.5
Large fringe	896.7	851.5	775.3	901.1	853.3	779.8	1,130.9	1,144.6	1,037.2
Small	921.6	891.2	837.3	928.2	897.8	850.2	1,180.0	1,169.6	956.6
Nonmetropolitan counties:									
With a city of 10,000 or more . .	929.1	899.0	861.3	929.7	897.6	864.1	1,117.8	1,177.7	#
Without a city of 10,000 or more.	936.6	901.0	870.8	927.4	892.8	858.9	933.5	1,078.6	#

See footnotes at end of table.

Table 33 (page 2 of 3). Age-adjusted death rates, according to race, sex, region, and urbanization level: United States, average annual 1984–86, 1989–91, and 1997–99

[Data are based on the National Vital Statistics System]

Sex, region, and urbanization level[1]	All races			White			Black or African American		
	1984–86	1989–91	1997–99	1984–86	1989–91	1997–99	1984–86	1989–91	1997–99
Male	Age-adjusted death rate per 100,000 standard population[2]								
All regions:									
Metropolitan counties:									
Large central	1,309.4	1,255.2	1,062.2	1,261.1	1,192.6	1,015.2	1,675.8	1,714.5	1,434.4
Large fringe	1,218.9	1,129.0	992.4	1,210.7	1,116.3	984.7	1,490.6	1,458.2	1,264.8
Small	1,258.4	1,184.6	1,076.4	1,235.0	1,152.6	1,052.2	1,615.7	1,634.9	1,436.1
Nonmetropolitan counties:									
With a city of 10,000 or more . .	1,274.4	1,219.7	1,127.5	1,255.7	1,195.6	1,106.7	1,624.1	1,644.9	1,487.3
Without a city of 10,000 or more .	1,285.1	1,241.7	1,143.1	1,261.6	1,211.9	1,119.2	1,598.2	1,640.8	1,441.6
Northeast:									
Metropolitan counties:									
Large central	1,375.0	1,326.8	1,083.6	1,319.6	1,255.1	1,053.7	1,668.8	1,698.6	1,278.1
Large fringe	1,237.1	1,134.2	983.3	1,230.6	1,125.5	984.5	1,479.2	1,405.1	1,120.2
Small	1,269.7	1,169.2	1,048.5	1,259.8	1,154.8	1,040.7	1,584.1	1,575.1	1,272.5
Nonmetropolitan counties:									
With a city of 10,000 or more . .	1,297.3	1,202.5	1,089.9	1,299.0	1,203.3	1,094.0	1,409.3	1,331.9	1,020.2
Without a city of 10,000 or more .	1,284.0	1,200.6	1,068.7	1,284.6	1,201.0	1,070.4	1,516.9	1,392.4	1,156.1
Midwest:									
Metropolitan counties:									
Large central	1,379.4	1,322.4	1,169.7	1,309.7	1,225.0	1,086.8	1,690.4	1,730.8	1,510.6
Large fringe	1,250.3	1,151.3	1,031.4	1,241.0	1,137.8	1,018.1	1,560.7	1,523.6	1,429.8
Small	1,257.1	1,173.7	1,080.5	1,242.6	1,152.8	1,062.3	1,574.6	1,583.3	1,427.0
Nonmetropolitan counties:									
With a city of 10,000 or more . .	1,224.9	1,171.0	1,081.5	1,222.0	1,166.6	1,079.0	1,508.6	1,485.7	1,270.8
Without a city of 10,000 or more .	1,201.6	1,156.2	1,060.7	1,197.2	1,149.5	1,054.0	1,381.0	1,444.1	1,265.0
South:									
Metropolitan counties:									
Large central	1,322.2	1,300.0	1,127.4	1,223.7	1,179.1	1,015.1	1,734.3	1,796.7	1,640.0
Large fringe	1,209.2	1,140.4	1,016.2	1,190.3	1,114.4	996.3	1,488.7	1,485.8	1,308.9
Small	1,280.9	1,222.1	1,117.6	1,232.3	1,160.9	1,069.1	1,640.0	1,668.5	1,484.4
Nonmetropolitan counties:									
With a city of 10,000 or more . .	1,353.0	1,318.6	1,239.1	1,311.2	1,265.8	1,192.9	1,653.8	1,684.2	1,547.0
Without a city of 10,000 or more .	1,364.1	1,332.3	1,235.5	1,330.6	1,286.9	1,205.2	1,610.2	1,656.6	1,459.2
West:									
Metropolitan counties:									
Large central	1,199.8	1,134.8	950.3	1,205.6	1,138.3	955.6	1,544.1	1,554.7	1,236.5
Large fringe	1,123.6	1,050.9	899.3	1,132.1	1,055.9	904.8	1,364.3	1,330.9	1,161.6
Small	1,173.2	1,111.1	992.4	1,187.4	1,123.2	1,007.7	1,431.7	1,422.7	1,088.0
Nonmetropolitan counties:									
With a city of 10,000 or more . .	1,172.6	1,109.7	1,011.0	1,176.1	1,110.6	1,012.8	1,361.7	1,387.8	#
Without a city of 10,000 or more .	1,172.4	1,118.1	1,028.5	1,162.0	1,108.5	1,011.6	1,087.2	1,199.9	#

See footnotes at end of table.

[Data are based on the National Vital Statistics System]

Sex, region, and urbanization level[1]	All races			White			Black or African American		
	1984–86	1989–91	1997–99	1984–86	1989–91	1997–99	1984–86	1989–91	1997–99
Female	Age-adjusted death rate per 100,000 standard population[2]								
All regions:									
Metropolitan counties:									
Large central	810.1	779.4	727.4	780.5	743.6	694.9	999.8	1,000.9	958.0
Large fringe.	772.4	733.4	710.4	766.0	725.3	704.4	936.5	918.5	887.7
Small	769.7	744.4	737.5	751.2	724.7	721.6	999.0	983.2	941.2
Nonmetropolitan counties:									
With a city of 10,000 or more . .	769.0	752.9	767.0	752.9	736.0	753.8	1,003.2	996.6	961.1
Without a city of 10,000 or more.	762.0	749.8	767.3	743.9	730.3	752.4	960.1	967.1	923.6
Northeast:									
Metropolitan counties:									
Large central	842.2	808.5	736.2	810.5	769.4	711.5	983.7	972.0	858.3
Large fringe.	788.0	737.6	697.2	783.7	732.2	697.0	915.7	876.3	785.6
Small	778.6	734.7	717.7	772.3	726.9	711.7	961.5	917.8	866.3
Nonmetropolitan counties:									
With a city of 10,000 or more . .	802.8	748.3	748.3	802.1	748.2	749.8	1,016.6	856.5	749.7
Without a city of 10,000 or more.	787.3	751.7	744.2	786.9	751.2	744.0	1,044.1	917.1	977.4
Midwest:									
Metropolitan counties:									
Large central	840.8	814.9	781.4	797.4	760.6	724.2	1,015.2	1,018.8	992.7
Large fringe.	783.8	747.7	733.9	775.8	738.1	723.3	1,008.7	982.6	1,021.1
Small	764.6	737.8	732.9	753.6	724.5	719.7	982.4	976.9	962.6
Nonmetropolitan counties:									
With a city of 10,000 or more . .	737.1	718.3	730.4	734.1	714.4	727.3	973.9	975.1	901.4
Without a city of 10,000 or more.	712.0	699.0	708.7	708.4	693.7	704.4	1,030.4	1,097.8	878.7
South:									
Metropolitan counties:									
Large central	808.3	782.4	758.1	750.1	713.2	682.1	1,028.4	1,031.9	1,063.4
Large fringe.	753.5	726.6	722.4	739.7	710.7	708.2	923.3	917.6	903.7
Small	778.3	758.7	757.5	742.5	722.5	727.8	1,007.8	992.6	952.8
Nonmetropolitan counties:									
With a city of 10,000 or more . .	798.2	793.4	819.2	761.4	757.5	791.8	1,007.8	1,001.0	975.0
Without a city of 10,000 or more.	796.1	789.5	816.8	768.0	759.9	798.9	958.1	964.6	925.4
West:									
Metropolitan counties:									
Large central	759.1	731.4	668.5	760.9	732.2	674.8	942.5	964.5	898.1
Large fringe.	733.9	706.1	675.6	736.9	707.2	679.7	935.6	973.0	920.6
Small	730.6	720.7	707.1	735.2	725.7	718.6	953.8	946.5	825.1
Nonmetropolitan counties:									
With a city of 10,000 or more . .	734.7	728.7	730.6	735.8	727.9	735.2	889.6	995.7	#
Without a city of 10,000 or more.	738.1	719.0	727.3	731.6	713.6	720.0	*	*	#

Estimates of death rates for the black population in nonmetropolitan counties in the West in 1997–99 are substantially lower than expected, possibly due to anomalies in population estimates for the black population in nonmetropolitan counties in this region.
* Data for groups with population under 5,000 in the middle year of a 3-year period are considered unreliable and are not shown.
[1]Urbanization levels are for county of residence of decedent. See Appendix II, Urbanization for definition of urbanization levels.
[2]Average annual death rate.

NOTES: Age-adjusted rates are calculated using the year 2000 standard population starting with *Health, United States, 2001*. See Appendix II, Age adjustment. Denominators for rates are population estimates for the middle year of each 3-year period multiplied by 3. Age-adjusted death rates for 1997–99 were calculated using age-specific rates with 1990-based postcensal population estimates in the denominator. See Appendix I, Population Census and Population Estimates.

SOURCE: Centers for Disease Control and Prevention, National Center for Health Statistics, National Vital Statistics System, Compressed Mortality File.

This table will be updated with 2000 data on the web. Go to www.cdc.gov/nchs/hus.htm.

Table 34 (page 1 of 2). Age-adjusted death rates for persons 25–64 years of age for selected causes of death, according to sex and educational attainment: Selected States, 1994–2000

[Data are based on death certificates]

Cause of death[2] and year	Both sexes Years of educational attainment[1]			Male Years of educational attainment[1]			Female Years of educational attainment[1]		
	Less than 12	12	13 or more	Less than 12	12	13 or more	Less than 12	12	13 or more
All causes	Age-adjusted death rate per 100,000 population[3]								
1994	594.6	506.4	254.8	793.6	707.1	323.5	397.3	342.9	182.1
1995	604.7	512.5	251.9	801.1	713.2	316.8	408.6	348.1	183.5
1996	579.6	492.5	241.8	763.9	669.6	300.7	396.6	344.2	180.3
1997	554.1	473.4	232.7	719.7	634.4	283.4	387.2	337.5	180.2
1998	561.6	465.8	223.9	727.6	627.1	271.9	395.6	330.9	174.3
1999[5]	585.3	474.5	219.1	763.7	636.7	264.2	409.9	337.3	172.6
2000	591.0	484.5	216.7	780.2	641.8	260.8	409.0	347.7	171.9
Chronic and noncommunicable diseases									
1994	440.5	380.7	193.7	561.9	504.4	228.4	325.0	286.8	155.5
1995	445.1	384.0	192.1	563.4	507.3	224.4	332.1	290.0	156.3
1996	432.7	375.3	189.0	550.6	486.9	222.1	321.2	287.7	153.4
1997	419.0	368.8	187.4	527.0	474.1	219.0	316.0	284.6	153.8
1998	425.2	362.9	180.9	534.4	470.2	211.3	321.3	277.9	148.6
1998 comparability-modified[4]	429.5	366.5	182.7	539.7	474.9	213.4	324.5	280.7	150.1
1999[5]	447.0	369.8	177.2	563.0	477.6	205.5	337.2	283.6	147.4
2000	446.2	377.6	175.7	567.2	481.5	202.9	334.3	292.3	147.2
Injuries									
1994	95.8	73.4	31.9	149.4	119.2	45.7	38.9	31.7	17.9
1995	96.6	74.3	31.6	149.4	120.3	45.3	40.0	32.1	17.8
1996	92.3	73.0	32.0	139.8	116.2	45.7	40.6	32.7	18.4
1997	92.7	73.5	31.9	138.8	116.4	45.5	41.1	33.4	18.4
1998	93.9	73.8	31.2	139.4	116.6	44.4	43.8	33.7	18.3
1998 comparability-modified[4]	95.0	74.7	31.6	141.0	118.0	44.9	44.3	34.1	18.5
1999[5]	94.8	75.2	30.6	143.7	118.3	43.2	42.6	34.4	18.1
2000	99.8	76.4	30.3	153.9	118.6	43.1	43.7	35.2	17.9
Communicable diseases									
1994	57.5	51.6	28.9	81.5	82.8	49.1	32.5	23.7	8.4
1995	62.1	53.4	27.9	87.3	84.7	46.7	35.8	25.2	8.9
1996	53.7	43.3	20.2	72.5	65.6	32.6	33.8	23.0	8.0
1997	41.6	30.1	12.9	53.1	42.9	18.4	29.3	18.7	7.6
1998	41.5	28.2	11.4	52.8	39.4	15.7	29.6	18.4	7.0
1998 comparability-modified[4]	35.4	24.1	9.7	45.1	33.6	13.4	25.3	15.7	6.0
1999[5]	42.1	28.5	10.8	54.8	39.5	15.1	29.4	18.8	6.6
2000	43.5	29.4	10.3	56.9	40.4	14.3	30.3	19.5	6.4
HIV disease:									
1994	36.2	36.5	21.4	54.7	63.0	39.7	16.8	12.3	2.9
1995	39.7	38.0	20.6	59.0	64.4	37.8	19.0	13.7	3.5
1996	31.9	27.7	13.1	45.4	45.4	23.8	17.2	11.2	2.4
1997	19.4	14.3	5.8	26.3	23.0	10.1	11.8	6.2	1.6
1998	17.3	11.7	4.3	23.4	18.3	7.5	10.6	5.6	1.1
1998 comparability-modified[4]	19.8	13.4	4.9	26.8	20.9	8.6	12.1	6.4	1.3
1999[5]	19.0	13.1	4.6	26.1	20.1	7.9	11.7	6.6	1.4
2000	19.8	13.2	4.1	26.9	19.8	7.1	12.6	7.1	1.2

See notes at end of table.

Table 34 (page 2 of 2). Age-adjusted death rates for persons 25–64 years of age for selected causes of death, according to sex and educational attainment: Selected States, 1994–2000

[Data are based on death certificates]

Cause of death[2] and year	Both sexes Years of educational attainment[1]			Male Years of educational attainment[1]			Female Years of educational attainment[1]		
	Less than 12	12	13 or more	Less than 12	12	13 or more	Less than 12	12	13 or more
	Age-adjusted death rate per 100,000 population[3]								
Other communicable diseases:									
1994	21.2	15.1	7.5	26.8	19.7	9.4	15.7	11.4	5.5
1995	22.4	15.5	7.2	28.2	20.3	8.8	16.8	11.5	5.5
1996	21.8	15.7	7.2	27.2	20.2	8.8	16.7	11.9	5.6
1997	22.2	15.9	7.1	26.8	19.9	8.2	17.6	12.5	6.0
1998	24.2	16.5	7.1	29.4	21.1	8.2	19.0	12.8	5.9
1998 comparability-modified[4]	19.4	13.2	5.7	23.6	16.9	6.6	15.2	10.3	4.7
1999[5]	23.1	15.4	6.2	28.8	19.4	7.2	17.6	12.2	5.3
2000	23.7	16.2	6.2	30.0	20.6	7.2	17.7	12.4	5.1

[1]Educational attainment for the numerator is based on the death certificate item "highest grade completed." Educational attainment for the denominator is based on answers to the Current Population Survey question "What is the highest level of school completed or highest degree received?" (Kominski R, Adams A. Educational Attainment in the United States: March 1993 and 1992, U.S. Bureau of the Census, Current Population Reports, P20–476, Washington, DC. 1994.)
[2]Underlying cause of death code numbers are based on the applicable revision of the *International Classification of Diseases* (ICD) for data years shown. See Appendix II, tables IV and V.
[3]Age-adjusted rates are calculated using the year 2000 standard population starting with *Health, United States, 2001*. See Appendix II, Age adjustment. Death records that are missing information about decedent's education are not included. Percent with not stated education averages 3–9 percent of the deaths comprising the age-adjusted death rates for causes of death in this table. Age-adjusted death rates for 1994–2000 were calculated using age-specific rates with 1990-based postcensal population estimates in the denominator. See Appendix I, Population Census and Population Estimates.
[4]Calculated by multiplying the 1998 rate by its comparability ratio to adjust for differences between ICD–9 and ICD–10. See Appendix II, Comparability ratio and table VI.
[5]Starting with 1999 data, cause of death is coded according to ICD–10. To estimate change between 1998 and 1999, compare the 1999 rate with the comparability-modified rate for 1998. See Appendix II, Comparability ratio and tables V and VI.

NOTES: Based on data from 45–46 States and the District of Columbia. Death rates for age groups 65 years and over are not shown because reporting quality of educational attainment on the death certificate is poorer at older than younger ages. See Appendix II, Education, for information about reporting States and sources of bias in death rates by educational attainment.

SOURCES: Centers for Disease Control and Prevention, National Center for Health Statistics, National Vital Statistics System; numerator data from annual mortality files; denominator data from unpublished population estimates prepared by the Housing and Household Economic Statistics Division, U.S. Bureau of the Census.

This table will be updated with 2001 data on the web. Go to www.cdc.gov/nchs/hus.htm.

Table 35 (page 1 of 4). Death rates for all causes, according to sex, race, Hispanic origin, and age: United States, selected years 1950–2000

[Data are based on death certificates]

Sex, race, Hispanic origin, and age	1950[1]	1960[1]	1970	1980	1990	1995	1997	1998	1999	2000
All persons				Deaths per 100,000 resident population						
All ages, age adjusted[2]	1,446.0	1,339.2	1,222.6	1,039.1	938.7	909.8	878.1	870.6	875.6	869.0
All ages, crude	963.8	954.7	945.3	878.3	863.8	868.3	848.8	847.3	857.0	854.0
Under 1 year	3,299.2	2,696.4	2,142.4	1,288.3	971.9	780.3	747.6	754.0	736.0	736.7
1–4 years	139.4	109.1	84.5	63.9	46.8	40.4	35.5	34.1	34.2	32.4
5–14 years	60.1	46.6	41.3	30.6	24.0	22.2	20.2	19.3	18.6	18.0
15–24 years	128.1	106.3	127.7	115.4	99.2	93.4	84.6	80.6	79.3	79.9
25–34 years	178.7	146.4	157.4	135.5	139.2	137.3	110.1	104.3	102.2	101.4
35–44 years	358.7	299.4	314.5	227.9	223.2	239.4	202.2	198.6	198.0	198.9
45–54 years	853.9	756.0	730.0	584.0	473.4	454.3	423.9	415.8	418.2	425.6
55–64 years	1,901.0	1,735.1	1,658.8	1,346.3	1,196.9	1,104.7	1,049.8	1,015.7	1,005.0	992.2
65–74 years	4,104.3	3,822.1	3,582.7	2,994.9	2,648.6	2,549.0	2,484.9	2,471.6	2,457.3	2,399.1
75–84 years	9,331.1	8,745.2	8,004.4	6,692.6	6,007.2	5,811.3	5,676.6	5,672.8	5,714.5	5,666.5
85 years and over	20,196.9	19,857.5	16,344.9	15,980.3	15,327.4	15,248.6	15,211.2	15,190.8	15,554.6	15,524.4
Male										
All ages, age adjusted[2]	1,674.2	1,609.0	1,542.1	1,348.1	1,202.8	1,143.9	1,088.1	1,069.4	1,067.0	1,053.8
All ages, crude	1,106.1	1,104.5	1,090.3	976.9	918.4	900.8	864.6	856.4	859.2	853.0
Under 1 year	3,728.0	3,059.3	2,410.0	1,428.5	1,082.8	856.3	822.2	818.6	805.0	806.5
1–4 years	151.7	119.5	93.2	72.6	52.4	44.5	39.4	37.1	37.9	35.9
5–14 years	70.9	55.7	50.5	36.7	28.5	26.4	23.3	22.7	21.5	20.9
15–24 years	167.9	152.1	188.5	172.3	147.4	137.4	122.0	116.7	113.1	114.9
25–34 years	216.5	187.9	215.3	196.1	204.3	198.0	152.6	142.6	139.7	138.6
35–44 years	428.8	372.8	402.6	299.2	310.4	331.0	264.7	257.0	254.9	255.2
45–54 years	1,067.1	992.2	958.5	767.3	610.3	589.9	540.8	531.0	533.1	542.8
55–64 years	2,395.3	2,309.5	2,282.7	1,815.1	1,553.4	1,400.7	1,314.5	1,271.5	1,252.0	1,230.7
65–74 years	4,931.4	4,914.4	4,873.8	4,105.2	3,491.5	3,263.8	3,157.3	3,112.1	3,073.7	2,979.6
75–84 years	10,426.0	10,178.4	10,010.2	8,816.7	7,888.6	7,399.6	7,152.4	7,095.5	7,083.3	6,972.6
85 years and over	21,636.0	21,186.3	17,821.5	18,801.1	18,056.6	17,861.0	17,648.1	17,357.2	17,597.2	17,501.4
Female										
All ages, age adjusted[2]	1,236.0	1,105.3	971.4	817.9	750.9	739.4	725.6	724.7	734.0	731.4
All ages, crude	823.5	809.2	807.8	785.3	812.0	837.2	833.6	838.5	854.9	855.0
Under 1 year	2,854.6	2,321.3	1,863.7	1,141.7	855.7	700.5	669.4	686.0	663.6	663.4
1–4 years	126.7	98.4	75.4	54.7	41.0	36.0	31.5	31.0	30.3	28.7
5–14 years	48.9	37.3	31.8	24.2	19.3	17.9	17.0	15.8	15.6	15.0
15–24 years	89.1	61.3	68.1	57.5	49.0	47.3	45.2	42.7	43.7	43.1
25–34 years	142.7	106.6	101.6	75.9	74.2	76.1	67.2	65.6	64.1	63.5
35–44 years	290.3	229.4	231.1	159.3	137.9	149.3	140.4	140.9	141.8	143.2
45–54 years	641.5	526.7	517.2	412.9	342.7	324.1	311.5	304.9	307.6	312.5
55–64 years	1,404.8	1,196.4	1,098.9	934.3	878.8	835.2	807.3	780.6	777.6	772.2
65–74 years	3,333.2	2,871.8	2,579.7	2,144.7	1,991.2	1,975.8	1,940.7	1,950.2	1,952.3	1,921.2
75–84 years	8,399.6	7,633.1	6,677.6	5,440.1	4,883.1	4,818.6	4,733.5	4,755.6	4,825.4	4,814.7
85 years and over	19,194.7	19,008.4	15,518.0	14,746.9	14,274.3	14,242.3	14,255.4	14,329.9	14,731.3	14,719.2
White male[3]										
All ages, age adjusted[2]	1,642.5	1,586.0	1,513.7	1,317.6	1,165.9	1,107.5	1,059.1	1,042.0	1,040.0	1,029.4
All ages, crude	1,089.5	1,098.5	1,086.7	983.3	930.9	921.0	893.3	887.3	892.1	887.8
Under 1 year	3,400.5	2,694.1	2,113.2	1,230.3	896.1	720.7	690.6	678.3	667.0	667.6
1–4 years	135.5	104.9	83.6	66.1	45.9	39.0	35.3	32.6	33.9	32.6
5–14 years	67.2	52.7	48.0	35.0	26.4	24.3	21.7	20.7	19.7	19.8
15–24 years	152.4	143.7	170.8	167.0	131.3	120.1	107.9	105.7	102.8	105.8
25–34 years	185.3	163.2	176.6	171.3	176.1	171.9	133.9	125.8	125.4	124.1
35–44 years	380.9	332.6	343.5	257.4	268.2	286.8	235.4	232.1	230.8	233.6
45–54 years	984.5	932.2	882.9	698.9	548.7	528.3	489.2	481.3	484.6	496.9
55–64 years	2,304.4	2,225.2	2,202.6	1,728.5	1,467.2	1,319.3	1,236.2	1,196.5	1,179.7	1,163.3
65–74 years	4,864.9	4,848.4	4,810.1	4,035.7	3,397.7	3,173.3	3,081.7	3,041.8	2,998.7	2,905.7
75–84 years	10,526.3	10,299.6	10,098.8	8,829.8	7,844.9	7,347.3	7,117.2	7,053.4	7,040.1	6,933.1
85 years and over	22,116.3	21,750.0	18,551.7	19,097.3	18,268.3	18,050.7	17,833.2	17,534.2	17,752.9	17,716.4

See footnotes at end of table.

[Data are based on death certificates]

Sex, race, Hispanic origin, and age	1950[1]	1960[1]	1970	1980	1990	1995	1997	1998	1999	2000
Black or African American male[3]					Deaths per 100,000 resident population					
All ages, age adjusted[2]	1,909.1	1,811.1	1,873.9	1,697.8	1,644.5	1,585.7	1,458.8	1,430.5	1,432.6	1,403.5
All ages, crude	1,257.7	1,181.7	1,186.6	1,034.1	1,008.0	960.2	867.1	848.2	847.4	834.1
Under 1 year	- - -	5,306.8	4,298.9	2,586.7	2,112.4	1,664.7	1,594.2	1,629.3	1,592.8	1,567.6
1–4 years[4]	1,412.6	208.5	150.5	110.5	85.8	73.1	61.8	62.6	59.0	54.5
5–14 years	95.1	75.1	67.1	47.4	41.2	38.5	32.7	33.2	32.0	28.2
15–24 years	289.7	212.0	320.6	209.1	252.2	246.6	214.2	193.5	184.6	181.4
25–34 years	503.5	402.5	559.5	407.3	430.8	407.4	298.9	272.5	258.6	261.0
35–44 years	878.1	762.0	956.6	689.8	699.6	716.8	520.2	478.9	469.2	453.0
45–54 years	1,905.0	1,624.8	1,777.5	1,479.9	1,261.0	1,238.9	1,074.7	1,037.7	1,030.7	1,017.7
55–64 years	3,773.2	3,316.4	3,256.9	2,873.0	2,618.4	2,382.0	2,242.4	2,182.0	2,145.6	2,080.1
65–74 years	5,310.3	5,798.7	5,803.2	5,131.1	4,946.1	4,707.8	4,428.6	4,337.6	4,352.3	4,253.5
75–84 years[5]	10,101.9	8,605.1	9,454.9	9,231.6	9,129.5	8,862.0	8,433.8	8,526.7	8,559.1	8,486.0
85 years and over	- - -	14,844.8	12,222.3	16,098.8	16,954.9	17,016.0	16,935.0	16,700.2	17,304.5	16,791.0
American Indian or Alaska Native male[3]										
All ages, age adjusted[2]	- - -	- - -	- - -	1,111.5	916.2	932.0	974.8	943.9	925.9	841.5
All ages, crude	- - -	- - -	- - -	597.1	476.4	459.4	458.2	441.9	431.8	415.6
Under 1 year	- - -	- - -	- - -	1,598.1	1,056.6	696.0	833.8	883.9	721.8	700.2
1–4 years	- - -	- - -	- - -	82.7	77.4	73.3	43.4	52.5	46.6	44.9
5–14 years	- - -	- - -	- - -	43.7	33.4	27.0	24.4	24.5	18.8	20.2
15–24 years	- - -	- - -	- - -	311.1	219.8	182.1	158.9	143.0	154.2	136.2
25–34 years	- - -	- - -	- - -	360.6	256.1	263.6	223.6	208.5	189.6	179.1
35–44 years	- - -	- - -	- - -	556.8	365.4	377.4	335.9	314.2	296.5	295.2
45–54 years	- - -	- - -	- - -	871.3	619.9	601.0	579.6	555.1	554.8	520.0
55–64 years	- - -	- - -	- - -	1,547.5	1,211.3	1,276.0	1,255.5	1,200.0	1,122.4	1,090.4
65–74 years	- - -	- - -	- - -	2,968.4	2,461.7	2,660.8	2,849.8	2,687.1	2,786.2	2,478.3
75–84 years	- - -	- - -	- - -	5,607.0	5,389.2	5,787.7	6,078.4	5,828.4	6,157.2	5,351.2
85 years and over	- - -	- - -	- - -	12,635.2	11,243.9	10,604.7	13,018.1	13,391.2	11,769.3	10,725.8
Asian or Pacific Islander male[3]										
All ages, age adjusted[2]	- - -	- - -	- - -	786.5	716.4	693.4	660.2	646.9	641.2	624.2
All ages, crude	- - -	- - -	- - -	375.3	334.3	341.4	336.8	335.4	333.2	332.9
Under 1 year	- - -	- - -	- - -	816.5	605.3	468.3	477.9	444.0	451.0	529.4
1–4 years	- - -	- - -	- - -	50.9	45.0	28.0	27.4	18.9	28.9	23.3
5–14 years	- - -	- - -	- - -	23.4	20.7	19.6	17.7	18.3	13.5	12.9
15–24 years	- - -	- - -	- - -	80.8	76.0	73.0	60.1	53.4	51.6	55.2
25–34 years	- - -	- - -	- - -	83.5	79.6	75.4	65.3	65.8	57.3	55.0
35–44 years	- - -	- - -	- - -	128.3	130.8	124.9	110.3	105.2	108.2	104.9
45–54 years	- - -	- - -	- - -	342.3	287.1	273.0	263.8	265.1	240.1	249.7
55–64 years	- - -	- - -	- - -	881.1	789.1	714.2	718.5	676.7	661.0	642.4
65–74 years	- - -	- - -	- - -	2,236.1	2,041.4	1,894.8	1,785.8	1,745.9	1,689.5	1,661.0
75–84 years	- - -	- - -	- - -	5,389.5	5,008.6	4,729.9	4,536.3	4,466.3	4,457.0	4,328.2
85 years and over	- - -	- - -	- - -	13,753.6	12,446.3	13,252.0	12,559.3	12,462.8	12,732.5	12,125.3
Hispanic or Latino male[3,6]										
All ages, age adjusted[2]	- - -	- - -	- - -	- - -	886.4	897.6	840.5	833.6	830.5	818.1
All ages, crude	- - -	- - -	- - -	- - -	411.6	391.6	343.2	336.0	332.6	331.3
Under 1 year	- - -	- - -	- - -	- - -	921.8	684.6	645.6	662.1	623.4	637.1
1–4 years	- - -	- - -	- - -	- - -	53.8	39.3	33.5	32.0	32.9	31.5
5–14 years	- - -	- - -	- - -	- - -	26.0	24.6	17.4	18.8	17.8	17.9
15–24 years	- - -	- - -	- - -	- - -	159.3	147.3	117.1	109.9	104.1	107.7
25–34 years	- - -	- - -	- - -	- - -	234.0	196.7	138.1	121.5	120.6	120.2
35–44 years	- - -	- - -	- - -	- - -	341.8	333.6	235.4	217.7	215.1	211.0
45–54 years	- - -	- - -	- - -	- - -	533.9	528.5	460.6	440.8	444.4	439.0
55–64 years	- - -	- - -	- - -	- - -	1,123.7	1,076.9	983.9	980.9	974.8	965.7
65–74 years	- - -	- - -	- - -	- - -	2,368.2	2,429.3	2,382.7	2,432.6	2,368.9	2,287.9
75–84 years	- - -	- - -	- - -	- - -	5,369.1	5,557.4	5,369.3	5,362.8	5,379.2	5,395.3
85 years and over	- - -	- - -	- - -	- - -	12,272.1	13,295.9	13,406.3	13,329.3	13,485.9	13,086.2

See footnotes at end of table.

Table 35 (page 3 of 4). Death rates for all causes, according to sex, race, Hispanic origin, and age: United States, selected years 1950–2000

[Data are based on death certificates]

Sex, race, Hispanic origin, and age	1950[1]	1960[1]	1970	1980	1990	1995	1997	1998	1999	2000
White, not Hispanic or Latino male[6]					Deaths per 100,000 resident population					
All ages, age adjusted[2]	- - -	- - -	- - -	- - -	1,170.9	1,105.6	1,063.2	1,046.7	1,045.5	1,035.4
All ages, crude	- - -	- - -	- - -	- - -	985.9	984.8	970.6	969.2	979.6	978.5
Under 1 year	- - -	- - -	- - -	- - -	865.4	703.8	681.7	662.3	658.1	658.7
1–4 years	- - -	- - -	- - -	- - -	43.8	37.8	35.2	32.2	33.4	32.4
5–14 years	- - -	- - -	- - -	- - -	25.7	23.5	22.2	20.8	19.9	20.0
15–24 years	- - -	- - -	- - -	- - -	123.4	111.5	103.9	102.9	100.8	103.5
25–34 years	- - -	- - -	- - -	- - -	165.3	163.5	130.8	124.4	124.5	123.0
35–44 years	- - -	- - -	- - -	- - -	257.1	276.5	232.3	231.0	230.0	233.9
45–54 years	- - -	- - -	- - -	- - -	544.5	520.7	487.3	480.2	483.7	497.7
55–64 years	- - -	- - -	- - -	- - -	1,479.7	1,322.7	1,246.7	1,204.5	1,187.4	1,170.9
65–74 years	- - -	- - -	- - -	- - -	3,434.5	3,188.5	3,105.1	3,062.6	3,023.2	2,930.5
75–84 years	- - -	- - -	- - -	- - -	7,920.4	7,367.4	7,157.3	7,098.1	7,088.0	6,977.8
85 years and over	- - -	- - -	- - -	- - -	18,505.4	18,132.6	17,942.9	17,649.2	17,871.2	17,853.2
White female[3]										
All ages, age adjusted[2]	1,198.0	1,074.4	944.0	796.1	728.8	718.7	707.8	707.3	716.6	715.3
All ages, crude	803.3	800.9	812.6	806.1	846.9	883.2	885.0	891.6	910.4	912.3
Under 1 year	2,566.8	2,007.7	1,614.6	962.5	690.0	574.4	556.2	570.5	542.0	550.5
1–4 years	112.2	85.2	66.1	49.3	36.1	31.3	28.1	27.6	27.5	25.5
5–14 years	45.1	34.7	29.9	22.9	17.9	16.5	15.3	14.7	14.6	14.1
15–24 years	71.5	54.9	61.6	55.5	45.9	43.7	43.0	40.6	41.5	41.1
25–34 years	112.8	85.0	84.1	65.4	61.5	62.9	58.0	56.5	56.2	55.1
35–44 years	235.8	191.1	193.3	138.2	117.4	125.5	120.6	122.0	123.2	125.7
45–54 years	546.4	458.8	462.9	372.7	309.3	291.9	281.6	274.8	277.9	281.4
55–64 years	1,293.8	1,078.9	1,014.9	876.2	822.7	783.4	758.7	733.0	731.0	730.9
65–74 years	3,242.8	2,779.3	2,470.7	2,066.6	1,923.5	1,913.2	1,880.4	1,893.1	1,893.9	1,868.3
75–84 years	8,481.5	7,696.6	6,698.7	5,401.7	4,839.1	4,775.3	4,705.8	4,721.8	4,787.8	4,785.3
85 years and over	19,679.5	19,477.7	15,980.2	14,979.6	14,400.6	14,405.8	14,415.8	14,498.9	14,900.6	14,890.7
Black or African American female[3]										
All ages, age adjusted[2]	1,545.5	1,369.7	1,228.7	1,033.3	975.1	955.9	922.1	921.6	933.6	927.6
All ages, crude	1,002.0	905.0	829.2	733.3	747.9	743.2	720.1	722.6	734.3	733.0
Under 1 year	- - -	4,162.2	3,368.8	2,123.7	1,735.5	1,399.9	1,316.6	1,321.9	1,317.4	1,279.8
1–4 years[4]	1,139.3	173.3	129.4	84.4	67.6	59.5	46.9	48.8	46.1	45.3
5–14 years	72.8	53.8	43.8	30.5	27.5	25.4	25.5	21.5	20.9	20.0
15–24 years	213.1	107.5	111.9	70.5	68.7	68.9	60.4	56.7	58.6	58.3
25–34 years	393.3	273.2	231.0	150.0	159.5	162.8	129.9	125.7	117.6	121.8
35–44 years	758.1	568.5	533.0	323.9	298.6	324.9	284.0	281.9	279.4	271.9
45–54 years	1,576.4	1,177.0	1,043.9	768.2	639.4	612.1	581.8	572.5	569.8	588.3
55–64 years	3,089.4	2,510.9	1,986.2	1,561.0	1,452.6	1,354.3	1,313.0	1,279.8	1,262.7	1,227.2
65–74 years	4,000.2	4,064.2	3,860.9	3,057.4	2,865.7	2,837.5	2,756.1	2,744.2	2,751.5	2,689.6
75–84 years[5]	8,347.0	6,730.0	6,691.5	6,212.1	5,688.3	5,671.9	5,452.3	5,601.0	5,742.4	5,696.5
85 years and over	- - -	13,052.6	10,706.6	12,367.2	13,309.5	13,073.3	13,280.4	13,252.2	13,805.9	13,941.3
American Indian or Alaska Native female[3]										
All ages, age adjusted[2]	- - -	- - -	- - -	662.4	561.8	643.9	625.3	640.5	668.2	604.5
All ages, crude	- - -	- - -	- - -	380.1	330.4	360.1	347.7	354.2	367.1	346.1
Under 1 year	- - -	- - -	- - -	1,352.6	688.7	780.6	606.7	743.8	682.6	492.2
1–4 years	- - -	- - -	- - -	87.5	37.8	54.4	56.6	43.8	34.2	39.8
5–14 years	- - -	- - -	- - -	33.5	25.5	20.0	18.9	16.2	17.6	17.7
15–24 years	- - -	- - -	- - -	90.3	69.0	60.4	52.2	57.5	59.6	58.9
25–34 years	- - -	- - -	- - -	178.5	102.3	106.3	103.5	103.9	106.9	84.8
35–44 years	- - -	- - -	- - -	286.0	156.4	171.9	164.9	160.4	168.9	171.9
45–54 years	- - -	- - -	- - -	491.4	380.9	349.1	333.4	326.8	298.7	284.9
55–64 years	- - -	- - -	- - -	837.1	805.9	876.2	797.7	781.6	852.3	772.1
65–74 years	- - -	- - -	- - -	1,765.5	1,679.4	1,935.6	1,923.0	1,938.1	2,015.8	1,899.8
75–84 years	- - -	- - -	- - -	3,612.9	3,073.2	4,067.6	4,016.7	4,000.8	4,266.5	3,850.0
85 years and over	- - -	- - -	- - -	8,567.4	8,201.1	9,201.8	9,113.1	10,165.3	10,639.6	9,118.2

See footnotes at end of table.

Table 35 (page 4 of 4). Death rates for all causes, according to sex, race, Hispanic origin, and age: United States, selected years 1950–2000

[Data are based on death certificates]

Sex, race, Hispanic origin, and age	1950[1]	1960[1]	1970	1980	1990	1995	1997	1998	1999	2000
Asian or Pacific Islander female[3]				Deaths per 100,000 resident population						
All ages, age adjusted[2]	---	---	---	425.9	469.3	446.7	432.6	426.7	427.5	416.8
All ages, crude	---	---	---	222.5	234.3	250.4	253.9	254.9	262.5	262.3
Under 1 year	---	---	---	755.8	518.2	396.6	394.2	436.6	425.3	434.3
1–4 years	---	---	---	35.4	32.0	24.9	26.4	21.3	20.9	20.0
5–14 years	---	---	---	21.5	13.0	15.4	14.1	12.8	11.9	11.7
15–24 years	---	---	---	32.3	28.8	31.1	30.1	26.2	26.1	22.4
25–34 years	---	---	---	45.4	37.5	35.6	29.6	31.3	29.5	27.6
35–44 years	---	---	---	89.7	69.9	66.2	70.6	60.4	59.0	65.6
45–54 years	---	---	---	214.1	182.7	184.1	159.5	153.7	164.4	155.5
55–64 years	---	---	---	440.8	483.4	457.7	408.1	397.8	408.7	390.9
65–74 years	---	---	---	1,027.7	1,089.2	1,037.8	1,091.6	1,062.7	1,070.8	996.4
75–84 years	---	---	---	2,833.6	3,127.9	3,089.9	2,992.9	2,892.0	2,930.8	2,882.4
85 years and over	---	---	---	7,923.3	10,254.0	9,406.1	9,062.8	9,325.2	9,126.7	9,052.2
Hispanic or Latino female[3,6]										
All ages, age adjusted[2]	---	---	---	---	537.1	546.1	538.8	536.9	555.9	546.0
All ages, crude	---	---	---	---	285.4	281.9	272.9	270.0	277.2	274.6
Under 1 year	---	---	---	---	746.6	572.0	562.0	559.0	542.3	553.6
1–4 years	---	---	---	---	42.1	33.1	27.8	26.7	28.7	27.5
5–14 years	---	---	---	---	17.3	15.0	14.5	13.1	13.3	13.4
15–24 years	---	---	---	---	40.6	37.5	34.5	31.2	32.9	31.7
25–34 years	---	---	---	---	62.9	58.6	48.2	45.0	44.9	43.4
35–44 years	---	---	---	---	109.3	118.9	98.9	94.9	97.4	100.5
45–54 years	---	---	---	---	253.3	238.8	227.0	225.2	224.9	223.8
55–64 years	---	---	---	---	607.5	602.3	593.6	563.5	555.8	548.4
65–74 years	---	---	---	---	1,453.8	1,457.2	1,442.5	1,465.5	1,448.8	1,423.2
75–84 years	---	---	---	---	3,351.3	3,506.4	3,524.7	3,530.2	3,675.7	3,624.5
85 years and over	---	---	---	---	10,098.7	10,540.5	10,594.7	10,662.6	11,547.3	11,202.8
White, non-Hispanic or Latino female[6]										
All ages, age adjusted[2]	---	---	---	---	734.6	721.1	712.5	712.8	722.3	721.5
All ages, crude	---	---	---	---	903.6	951.7	964.3	976.5	1,001.3	1,007.3
Under 1 year	---	---	---	---	655.3	553.9	535.6	556.7	524.6	530.9
1–4 years	---	---	---	---	34.0	30.3	27.7	27.4	26.7	24.4
5–14 years	---	---	---	---	17.6	16.4	15.2	14.8	14.7	13.9
15–24 years	---	---	---	---	46.0	44.0	44.1	42.0	42.9	42.6
25–34 years	---	---	---	---	60.6	62.2	59.0	57.9	57.8	56.8
35–44 years	---	---	---	---	116.8	124.1	122.0	124.3	125.6	128.1
45–54 years	---	---	---	---	312.1	293.0	284.3	277.4	281.0	285.0
55–64 years	---	---	---	---	834.5	789.8	767.5	742.5	741.6	742.1
65–74 years	---	---	---	---	1,940.2	1,925.9	1,896.8	1,910.9	1,915.1	1,891.0
75–84 years	---	---	---	---	4,887.3	4,794.9	4,732.7	4,753.6	4,817.7	4,819.3
85 years and over	---	---	---	---	14,533.1	14,450.9	14,484.9	14,576.7	14,967.5	14,971.7

- - - Data not available.

[1]Includes deaths of persons who were not residents of the 50 States and the District of Columbia.

[2]Age-adjusted rates are calculated using the year 2000 standard population starting with *Health, United States, 2001*. See Appendix II, Age adjustment.

[3]The race groups, white, black, Asian or Pacific Islander, and American Indian or Alaska Native, include persons of Hispanic and non-Hispanic origin. Persons of Hispanic origin may be of any race. Death rates for the American Indian or Alaska Native and Asian or Pacific Islander populations are known to be underestimated. See Appendix II, Race, for a discussion of sources of bias in death rates by race and Hispanic origin.

[4]In 1950 rate is for the age group under 5 years.

[5]In 1950 rate is for the age group 75 years and over.

[6]Prior to 1997, excludes data from States lacking an Hispanic-origin item on the death certificate. See Appendix I, Hispanic origin.

NOTES: Population estimates used to compute rates for 1991–2000 differ from those used previously. Starting with *Health, United States, 2003*, rates for 1991–99 were revised using intercensal population estimates based on Census 2000. Rates for 2000 were revised based on Census 2000 counts. See Appendix I, Population Census and Population Estimates. Data for additional years are available (see Appendix III).

SOURCES: Centers for Disease Control and Prevention, National Center for Health Statistics, National Vital Statistics System; Grove RD, Hetzel AM. *Vital statistics rates in the United States, 1940–60*. Washington: U.S. Government Printing Office, 1968; numerator data from National Vital Statistics System, annual mortality files; denominator data from national population estimates for race groups from table 1 and unpublished Hispanic population estimates for 1985–96 prepared by the Housing and Household Economic Statistics Division, U.S. Bureau of the Census; additional mortality tables are available at www.cdc.gov/nchs/datawh/statab/unpubd/mortabs.htm; Anderson RN, Arias E. The effect of revised populations on mortality statistics for the U.S., 2000. National vital statistics reports. Vol 51 no 9. Hyattsville, Maryland: National Center for Health Statistics. 2003.

This table will be updated with 2001 data on the web. Go to www.cdc.gov/nchs/hus.htm.

Table 36 (page 1 of 3). Death rates for diseases of heart, according to sex, race, Hispanic origin, and age: United States, selected years 1950–2000

[Data are based on death certificates]

Sex, race, Hispanic origin, and age	1950[1]	1960[1]	1970	1980	1990	1995	1999[2]	2000
All persons	Deaths per 100,000 resident population							
All ages, age adjusted[3]	586.8	559.0	492.7	412.1	321.8	293.4	266.5	257.6
All ages, crude	355.5	369.0	362.0	336.0	289.5	277.0	259.9	252.6
Under 1 year.	3.5	6.6	13.1	22.8	20.1	17.4	13.8	13.0
1–4 years	1.3	1.3	1.7	2.6	1.9	1.6	1.2	1.2
5–14 years	2.1	1.3	0.8	0.9	0.9	0.8	0.7	0.7
15–24 years	6.8	4.0	3.0	2.9	2.5	2.8	2.8	2.6
25–34 years	19.4	15.6	11.4	8.3	7.6	8.2	7.6	7.4
35–44 years	86.4	74.6	66.7	44.6	31.4	31.8	30.2	29.2
45–54 years	308.6	271.8	238.4	180.2	120.5	109.6	95.7	94.2
55–64 years	808.1	737.9	652.3	494.1	367.3	320.1	269.9	261.2
65–74 years	1,839.8	1,740.5	1,558.2	1,218.6	894.3	795.4	701.7	665.6
75–84 years	4,310.1	4,089.4	3,683.8	2,993.1	2,295.7	2,050.5	1,849.9	1,780.3
85 years and over	9,150.6	9,317.8	7,891.3	7,777.1	6,739.9	6,391.5	6,063.0	5,926.1
Male								
All ages, age adjusted[3]	697.0	687.6	634.0	538.9	412.4	371.0	331.0	320.0
All ages, crude	423.4	439.5	422.5	368.6	297.6	278.5	257.0	249.8
Under 1 year.	4.0	7.8	15.1	25.5	21.9	17.7	13.9	13.3
1–4 years	1.4	1.4	1.9	2.8	1.9	1.7	1.3	1.4
5–14 years	2.0	1.4	0.9	1.0	0.9	0.8	0.8	0.8
15–24 years	6.8	4.2	3.7	3.7	3.1	3.5	3.4	3.2
25–34 years	22.9	20.1	15.2	11.4	10.3	11.0	9.8	9.6
35–44 years	118.4	112.7	103.2	68.7	48.1	46.9	43.0	41.4
45–54 years	440.5	420.4	376.4	282.6	183.0	166.1	142.0	140.2
55–64 years	1,104.5	1,066.9	987.2	746.8	537.3	460.1	383.0	371.7
65–74 years	2,292.3	2,291.3	2,170.3	1,728.0	1,250.0	1,095.3	950.6	898.3
75–84 years	4,825.0	4,742.4	4,534.8	3,834.3	2,968.2	2,622.9	2,336.4	2,248.1
85 years and over	9,659.8	9,788.9	8,426.2	8,752.7	7,418.4	6,993.5	6,561.6	6,430.0
Female								
All ages, age adjusted[3]	484.7	447.0	381.6	320.8	257.0	236.6	218.1	210.9
All ages, crude	288.4	300.6	304.5	305.1	281.8	275.5	262.6	255.3
Under 1 year.	2.9	5.4	10.9	20.0	18.3	17.0	13.7	12.5
1–4 years	1.2	1.1	1.6	2.5	1.9	1.5	1.1	1.0
5–14 years	2.2	1.2	0.8	0.9	0.8	0.7	0.6	0.5
15–24 years	6.7	3.7	2.3	2.1	1.8	2.1	2.1	2.1
25–34 years	16.2	11.3	7.7	5.3	5.0	5.4	5.4	5.2
35–44 years	55.1	38.2	32.2	21.4	15.1	17.0	17.5	17.2
45–54 years	177.2	127.5	109.9	84.5	61.0	55.4	51.0	49.8
55–64 years	510.0	429.4	351.6	272.1	215.7	192.6	165.6	159.3
65–74 years	1,419.3	1,261.3	1,082.7	828.6	616.8	554.9	497.9	474.0
75–84 years	3,872.0	3,582.7	3,120.8	2,497.0	1,893.8	1,692.7	1,533.9	1,475.1
85 years and over	8,796.1	9,016.8	7,591.8	7,350.5	6,478.1	6,159.6	5,862.1	5,720.9
White male[4]								
All ages, age adjusted[3]	700.2	694.5	640.2	539.6	409.2	367.0	327.1	316.7
All ages, crude	433.0	454.6	438.3	384.0	312.7	294.4	272.9	265.8
45–54 years	423.6	413.2	365.7	269.8	170.6	153.9	132.1	130.7
55–64 years	1,081.7	1,056.0	979.3	730.6	516.7	439.2	361.4	351.8
65–74 years	2,308.3	2,297.9	2,177.2	1,729.7	1,230.5	1,071.8	928.4	877.8
75–84 years	4,907.3	4,839.9	4,617.6	3,883.2	2,983.4	2,625.6	2,338.8	2,247.0
85 years and over	9,950.5	10,135.8	8,818.0	8,958.0	7,558.7	7,125.1	6,669.0	6,560.8
Black or African American male[4]								
All ages, age adjusted[3]	639.4	615.2	607.3	561.4	485.4	451.3	407.2	392.5
All ages, crude	346.2	330.6	330.3	301.0	256.8	239.1	218.5	211.1
45–54 years	622.5	514.0	512.8	433.4	328.9	308.6	255.0	247.2
55–64 years	1,433.1	1,236.8	1,135.4	987.2	824.0	740.5	660.0	631.2
65–74 years	2,139.1	2,281.4	2,237.8	1,847.2	1,632.9	1,514.1	1,346.4	1,268.8
75–84 years[5]	4,106.1	3,533.6	3,783.4	3,578.8	3,107.1	2,908.7	2,623.5	2,597.6
85 years and over	- - -	6,037.9	5,367.6	6,819.5	6,479.6	6,088.5	5,858.8	5,633.5

See footnotes at end of table.

[Data are based on death certificates]

Sex, race, Hispanic origin, and age	1950[1]	1960[1]	1970	1980	1990	1995	1999[2]	2000
American Indian or Alaska Native male[4]				Deaths per 100,000 resident population				
All ages, age adjusted[3]	---	---	---	320.5	264.1	256.4	245.8	222.2
All ages, crude	---	---	---	130.6	108.0	101.0	92.3	90.1
45–54 years	---	---	---	238.1	173.8	136.2	107.0	108.5
55–64 years	---	---	---	496.3	411.0	375.7	294.0	285.0
65–74 years	---	---	---	1,009.4	839.1	938.2	856.7	748.2
75–84 years	---	---	---	2,062.2	1,788.8	1,858.5	1,890.2	1,655.7
85 years and over	---	---	---	4,413.7	3,860.3	3,306.5	3,695.9	3,318.3
Asian or Pacific Islander male[4]								
All ages, age adjusted[3]	---	---	---	286.9	220.7	214.5	198.9	185.5
All ages, crude	---	---	---	119.8	88.7	93.2	93.7	90.6
45–54 years	---	---	---	112.0	70.4	69.8	60.9	61.1
55–64 years	---	---	---	306.7	226.1	205.4	191.0	182.6
65–74 years	---	---	---	852.4	623.5	581.0	488.9	482.5
75–84 years	---	---	---	2,010.9	1,642.2	1,533.8	1,419.5	1,354.7
85 years and over	---	---	---	5,923.0	4,617.8	4,888.9	4,747.5	4,154.2
Hispanic or Latino male[4,6]								
All ages, age adjusted[3]	---	---	---	---	270.0	260.8	249.2	238.2
All ages, crude	---	---	---	---	91.0	83.1	77.7	74.7
45–54 years	---	---	---	---	116.4	102.0	92.2	84.3
55–64 years	---	---	---	---	363.0	311.2	272.1	264.8
65–74 years	---	---	---	---	829.9	784.6	737.0	684.8
75–84 years	---	---	---	---	1,971.3	1,854.0	1,816.0	1,733.2
85 years and over	---	---	---	---	4,711.9	5,104.0	5,012.2	4,897.5
White, not Hispanic or Latino male[6]								
All ages, age adjusted[3]	---	---	---	---	413.6	369.1	330.0	319.9
All ages, crude	---	---	---	---	336.5	320.6	304.0	297.5
45–54 years	---	---	---	---	172.8	155.9	135.0	134.3
55–64 years	---	---	---	---	521.3	443.2	365.6	356.3
65–74 years	---	---	---	---	1,243.4	1,077.0	935.2	885.1
75–84 years	---	---	---	---	3,007.7	2,635.3	2,352.6	2,261.9
85 years and over	---	---	---	---	7,663.4	7,156.4	6,713.7	6,606.6
White female[4]								
All ages, age adjusted[3]	478.0	441.7	376.7	315.9	250.9	230.8	212.8	205.6
All ages, crude	289.4	306.5	313.8	319.2	298.4	294.7	282.4	274.5
45–54 years	141.9	103.4	91.4	71.2	50.2	45.5	42.2	40.9
55–64 years	460.2	383.0	317.7	248.1	192.4	172.0	147.8	141.3
65–74 years	1,400.9	1,229.8	1,044.0	796.7	583.6	523.2	468.7	445.2
75–84 years	3,925.2	3,629.7	3,143.5	2,493.6	1,874.3	1,670.3	1,509.0	1,452.4
85 years and over	9,084.7	9,280.8	7,839.9	7,501.6	6,563.4	6,251.3	5,945.3	5,801.4
Black or African American female[4]								
All ages, age adjusted[3]	536.9	488.9	435.6	378.6	327.5	304.0	283.7	277.6
All ages, crude	287.6	268.5	261.0	249.7	237.0	226.3	216.0	212.6
45–54 years	525.3	360.7	290.9	202.4	155.3	141.5	125.8	125.0
55–64 years	1,210.2	952.3	710.5	530.1	442.0	386.0	337.9	332.8
65–74 years	1,659.4	1,680.5	1,553.2	1,210.3	1,017.5	938.2	838.6	815.2
75–84 years[5]	3,499.3	2,926.9	2,964.1	2,707.2	2,250.9	2,100.7	1,980.3	1,913.1
85 years and over	---	5,650.0	5,003.8	5,796.5	5,766.1	5,448.5	5,348.5	5,298.7

See footnotes at end of table.

[Data are based on death certificates]

Sex, race, Hispanic origin, and age	1950[1]	1960[1]	1970	1980	1990	1995	1999[2]	2000
American Indian or Alaska Native female[4]			Deaths per 100,000 resident population					
All ages, age adjusted[3]	- - -	- - -	- - -	175.4	153.1	164.8	163.0	143.6
All ages, crude	- - -	- - -	- - -	80.3	77.5	80.2	77.5	71.9
45–54 years	- - -	- - -	- - -	65.2	62.0	62.4	42.1	40.2
55–64 years	- - -	- - -	- - -	193.5	197.0	200.7	162.8	149.4
65–74 years	- - -	- - -	- - -	577.2	492.8	514.2	458.3	391.8
75–84 years	- - -	- - -	- - -	1,364.3	1,050.3	1,184.3	1,239.9	1,044.1
85 years and over	- - -	- - -	- - -	2,893.3	2,868.7	3,118.1	3,442.9	3,146.3
Asian or Pacific Islander female[4]								
All ages, age adjusted[3]	- - -	- - -	- - -	132.3	149.2	137.6	124.2	115.7
All ages, crude	- - -	- - -	- - -	57.0	62.0	66.3	67.4	65.0
45–54 years	- - -	- - -	- - -	28.6	17.5	20.8	17.8	15.9
55–64 years	- - -	- - -	- - -	92.9	99.0	89.5	72.7	68.8
65–74 years	- - -	- - -	- - -	313.3	323.9	288.3	262.5	229.6
75–84 years	- - -	- - -	- - -	1,053.2	1,130.9	1,001.8	927.6	866.2
85 years and over	- - -	- - -	- - -	3,211.0	4,161.2	3,942.4	3,558.5	3,367.2
Hispanic or Latino female[4,6]								
All ages, age adjusted[3]	- - -	- - -	- - -	- - -	177.2	173.8	172.3	163.7
All ages, crude	- - -	- - -	- - -	- - -	79.4	76.5	74.6	71.5
45–54 years	- - -	- - -	- - -	- - -	43.5	32.0	30.5	28.2
55–64 years	- - -	- - -	- - -	- - -	153.2	141.0	122.5	111.2
65–74 years	- - -	- - -	- - -	- - -	460.4	419.0	379.0	366.3
75–84 years	- - -	- - -	- - -	- - -	1,259.7	1,231.3	1,236.1	1,169.4
85 years and over	- - -	- - -	- - -	- - -	4,440.3	4,653.1	4,828.9	4,605.8
White, not Hispanic or Latino female[6]								
All ages, age adjusted[3]	- - -	- - -	- - -	- - -	252.6	231.5	213.9	206.8
All ages, crude	- - -	- - -	- - -	- - -	320.0	319.7	312.3	304.9
45–54 years	- - -	- - -	- - -	- - -	50.2	46.1	43.1	41.9
55–64 years	- - -	- - -	- - -	- - -	193.6	172.0	149.0	142.9
65–74 years	- - -	- - -	- - -	- - -	584.7	525.2	472.3	448.5
75–84 years	- - -	- - -	- - -	- - -	1,890.2	1,674.9	1,514.5	1,458.9
85 years and over	- - -	- - -	- - -	- - -	6,615.2	6,265.8	5,962.4	5,822.7

- - - Data not available.

[1]Includes deaths of persons who were not residents of the 50 States and the District of Columbia.

[2]Starting with 1999 data, cause of death is coded according to ICD–10. To estimate change between 1998 and 1999, compare the 1999 rate with the comparability-modified rate for 1998. See Appendix II, Comparability ratio and tables V and VI.

[3]Age-adjusted rates are calculated using the year 2000 standard population starting with Health, United States, 2001. See Appendix II, Age adjustment.

[4]The race groups, white, black, Asian or Pacific Islander, and American Indian or Alaska Native, include persons of Hispanic and non-Hispanic origin. Persons of Hispanic origin may be of any race. Death rates for the American Indian or Alaska Native and Asian or Pacific Islander populations are known to be underestimated. See Appendix II, Race, for a discussion of sources of bias in death rates by race and Hispanic origin.

[5]In 1950 rate is for the age group 75 years and over.

[6]Prior to 1997, excludes data from States lacking an Hispanic-origin item on the death certificate. See Appendix II, Hispanic origin.

NOTES: Population estimates used to compute rates for 1991–2000 differ from those used previously. Starting with Health, United States, 2003, rates for 1991–99 were revised using intercensal population estimates based on Census 2000. Rates for 2000 were revised based on Census 2000 counts. See Appendix I, Population Census and Population Estimates. Underlying cause of death code numbers are based on the applicable revision of the International Classification of Diseases (ICD) for data years shown. For the period 1980–98, causes were coded using ICD–9 codes that are most nearly comparable with the 113 cause list for ICD–10. See Appendix II, tables IV and V. Age groups were selected to minimize the presentation of unstable age-specific death rates based on small numbers of deaths and for consistency among comparison groups. Data for additional years are available (see Appendix III).

SOURCES: Centers for Disease Control and Prevention, National Center for Health Statistics, National Vital Statistics System; numerator data from annual mortality files; denominator data from national population estimates for race groups from table 1 and unpublished Hispanic population estimates for 1985–96 prepared by the Housing and Household Economic Statistics Division, U.S. Bureau of the Census; additional mortality tables are available at www.cdc.gov/nchs/datawh/statab/unpubd/mortabs.htm; Anderson RN, Arias E. The effect of revised populations on mortality statistics for the U.S., 2000. National vital statistics reports. Vol 51 no 9. Hyattsville, Maryland: National Center for Health Statistics. 2003.

This table will be updated with 2001 data on the web. Go to www.cdc.gov/nchs/hus.htm.

Table 37 (page 1 of 3). Death rates for cerebrovascular diseases, according to sex, race, Hispanic origin, and age: United States, selected years 1950–2000

[Data are based on death certificates]

Sex, race, Hispanic origin, and age	1950[1]	1960[1]	1970	1980	1990	1995	1999[2]	2000
All persons			Deaths per 100,000 resident population					
All ages, age adjusted[3]	180.7	177.9	147.7	96.2	65.3	63.1	61.6	60.9
All ages, crude	104.0	108.0	101.9	75.0	57.8	59.2	60.0	59.6
Under 1 year.	5.1	4.1	5.0	4.4	3.8	5.9	2.7	3.3
1–4 years	0.9	0.8	1.0	0.5	0.3	0.4	0.3	0.3
5–14 years	0.5	0.7	0.7	0.3	0.2	0.2	0.2	0.2
15–24 years	1.6	1.8	1.6	1.0	0.6	0.5	0.5	0.5
25–34 years	4.2	4.7	4.5	2.6	2.2	1.7	1.4	1.5
35–44 years	18.7	14.7	15.6	8.5	6.4	6.5	5.7	5.8
45–54 years	70.4	49.2	41.6	25.2	18.7	17.4	15.2	16.0
55–64 years	194.2	147.3	115.8	65.1	47.9	45.6	40.6	41.0
65–74 years	554.7	469.2	384.1	219.0	144.2	136.2	130.8	128.6
75–84 years	1,499.6	1,491.3	1,254.2	786.9	498.0	477.1	469.8	461.3
85 years and over	2,990.1	3,680.5	3,014.3	2,283.7	1,628.9	1,607.2	1,614.8	1,589.2
Male								
All ages, age adjusted[3]	186.4	186.1	157.4	102.2	68.5	65.9	63.2	62.4
All ages, crude	102.5	104.5	94.5	63.4	46.7	47.2	47.1	46.9
Under 1 year.	6.4	5.0	5.8	5.0	4.4	6.4	3.3	3.8
1–4 years	1.1	0.9	1.2	0.4	0.3	0.4	0.3	*
5–14 years	0.5	0.7	0.8	0.3	0.2	0.2	0.2	0.2
15–24 years	1.8	1.9	1.8	1.1	0.7	0.5	0.5	0.5
25–34 years	4.2	4.5	4.4	2.6	2.1	1.8	1.5	1.5
35–44 years	17.5	14.6	15.7	8.7	6.8	7.0	5.8	5.8
45–54 years	67.9	52.2	44.4	27.2	20.5	19.5	16.7	17.5
55–64 years	205.2	163.8	138.7	74.6	54.3	52.7	46.5	47.2
65–74 years	589.6	530.7	449.5	258.6	166.6	154.7	147.3	145.0
75–84 years	1,543.6	1,555.9	1,361.6	866.3	551.1	517.7	500.4	490.8
85 years and over	3,048.6	3,643.1	2,895.2	2,193.6	1,528.5	1,522.1	1,512.8	1,484.3
Female								
All ages, age adjusted[3]	175.8	170.7	140.0	91.7	62.6	60.5	59.8	59.1
All ages, crude	105.6	111.4	109.0	85.9	68.4	70.7	72.3	71.8
Under 1 year.	3.7	3.2	4.0	3.8	3.1	5.3	2.1	2.7
1–4 years	0.7	0.7	0.7	0.5	0.3	0.3	0.3	0.4
5–14 years	0.4	0.6	0.6	0.3	0.2	0.1	0.2	0.2
15–24 years	1.5	1.6	1.4	0.8	0.6	0.4	0.5	0.5
25–34 years	4.3	4.9	4.7	2.6	2.2	1.6	1.4	1.5
35–44 years	19.9	14.8	15.6	8.4	6.1	6.0	5.6	5.7
45–54 years	72.9	46.3	39.0	23.3	17.0	15.3	13.8	14.5
55–64 years	183.1	131.8	95.3	56.8	42.2	39.1	35.1	35.3
65–74 years	522.1	415.7	333.3	188.7	126.7	121.4	117.2	115.1
75–84 years	1,462.2	1,441.1	1,183.1	740.1	466.2	451.8	449.8	442.1
85 years and over	2,949.4	3,704.4	3,081.0	2,323.1	1,667.6	1,640.0	1,656.0	1,632.0
White male[4]								
All ages, age adjusted[3]	182.1	181.6	153.7	98.7	65.5	62.9	60.8	59.8
All ages, crude	100.5	102.7	93.5	63.1	46.9	48.0	48.7	48.4
45–54 years	53.7	40.9	35.6	21.7	15.4	14.7	12.8	13.6
55–64 years	182.2	139.0	119.9	64.0	45.7	44.2	38.9	39.7
65–74 years	569.7	501.0	420.0	239.8	152.9	142.1	136.0	133.8
75–84 years	1,556.3	1,564.8	1,361.6	852.7	539.2	503.8	490.3	480.0
85 years and over	3,127.1	3,734.8	3,018.1	2,230.8	1,545.4	1,536.0	1,522.7	1,490.7
Black or African American male[4]								
All ages, age adjusted[3]	228.8	238.5	206.4	142.0	102.2	97.0	89.6	89.6
All ages, crude	122.0	122.9	108.8	73.0	53.0	49.8	45.9	46.1
45–54 years	211.9	166.1	136.1	82.1	68.4	62.3	48.6	49.5
55–64 years	522.8	439.9	343.4	189.7	141.7	130.8	117.9	115.4
65–74 years	783.6	899.2	780.1	472.3	326.9	297.0	274.7	268.5
75–84 years[5]	1,504.9	1,475.2	1,445.7	1,066.3	721.5	705.9	650.6	659.2
85 years and over	- - -	2,700.0	1,963.1	1,873.2	1,421.5	1,410.1	1,448.3	1,458.8

See footnotes at end of table.

Table 37 (page 2 of 3). Death rates for cerebrovascular diseases, according to sex, race, Hispanic origin, and age: United States, selected years 1950–2000

[Data are based on death certificates]

Sex, race, Hispanic origin, and age	1950[1]	1960[1]	1970	1980	1990	1995	1999[2]	2000
American Indian or Alaska Native male[4]				Deaths per 100,000 resident population				
All ages, age adjusted[3]	- - -	- - -	- - -	66.4	44.3	51.7	50.0	46.1
All ages, crude	- - -	- - -	- - -	23.1	16.0	18.4	16.7	16.8
45–54 years	- - -	- - -	- - -	*	*	25.5	13.8	13.3
55–64 years	- - -	- - -	- - -	72.0	39.8	42.6	31.7	48.6
65–74 years	- - -	- - -	- - -	170.5	120.3	156.4	143.2	144.7
75–84 years	- - -	- - -	- - -	523.9	325.9	351.2	467.9	373.3
85 years and over	- - -	- - -	- - -	1,384.7	949.8	1,072.4	865.0	834.9
Asian or Pacific Islander male[4]								
All ages, age adjusted[3]	- - -	- - -	- - -	71.4	59.1	64.0	58.7	58.0
All ages, crude	- - -	- - -	- - -	28.7	23.3	27.5	27.0	27.2
45–54 years	- - -	- - -	- - -	17.0	15.6	16.5	17.3	15.0
55–64 years	- - -	- - -	- - -	59.9	51.8	59.6	49.0	49.3
65–74 years	- - -	- - -	- - -	197.9	167.9	155.6	132.5	135.6
75–84 years	- - -	- - -	- - -	619.5	483.9	521.9	459.6	438.7
85 years and over	- - -	- - -	- - -	1,399.0	1,196.6	1,382.1	1,401.3	1,415.6
Hispanic or Latino male[4,6]								
All ages, age adjusted[3]	- - -	- - -	- - -	- - -	46.5	51.2	52.6	50.5
All ages, crude	- - -	- - -	- - -	- - -	15.6	16.2	16.1	15.8
45–54 years	- - -	- - -	- - -	- - -	20.0	20.3	19.5	18.1
55–64 years	- - -	- - -	- - -	- - -	49.2	46.9	46.1	48.8
65–74 years	- - -	- - -	- - -	- - -	126.4	138.1	140.8	136.1
75–84 years	- - -	- - -	- - -	- - -	356.6	373.3	395.2	392.9
85 years and over	- - -	- - -	- - -	- - -	866.3	1,079.5	1,136.6	1,029.9
White, not Hispanic or Latino male[6]								
All ages, age adjusted[3]	- - -	- - -	- - -	- - -	66.3	62.8	60.8	59.9
All ages, crude	- - -	- - -	- - -	- - -	50.6	51.9	53.9	53.9
45–54 years	- - -	- - -	- - -	- - -	14.9	13.9	12.0	13.0
55–64 years	- - -	- - -	- - -	- - -	45.1	43.3	38.0	38.7
65–74 years	- - -	- - -	- - -	- - -	154.5	141.4	135.0	133.1
75–84 years	- - -	- - -	- - -	- - -	547.3	506.2	492.8	482.3
85 years and over	- - -	- - -	- - -	- - -	1,578.7	1,544.8	1,535.1	1,505.9
White female[4]								
All ages, age adjusted[3]	169.7	165.0	135.5	89.0	60.3	58.6	58.0	57.3
All ages, crude	103.3	110.1	109.8	88.6	71.6	75.1	77.6	76.9
45–54 years	55.0	33.8	30.5	18.6	13.5	12.6	10.7	11.2
55–64 years	156.9	103.0	78.1	48.6	35.8	33.3	29.4	30.2
65–74 years	498.1	383.3	303.2	172.5	116.1	111.7	108.6	107.3
75–84 years	1,471.3	1,444.7	1,176.8	728.8	456.5	443.4	442.8	434.2
85 years and over	3,017.9	3,795.7	3,167.6	2,362.7	1,685.9	1,656.7	1,675.4	1,646.7
Black or African American female[4]								
All ages, age adjusted[3]	238.4	232.5	189.3	119.6	84.0	79.4	76.2	76.2
All ages, crude	128.3	127.7	112.2	77.8	60.7	59.1	57.9	58.3
45–54 years	248.9	166.2	119.4	61.8	44.1	36.0	35.3	38.1
55–64 years	567.7	452.0	272.4	138.4	96.9	85.6	78.9	76.4
65–74 years	754.4	830.5	673.5	361.7	236.7	222.3	201.7	190.9
75–84 years[5]	1,496.7	1,413.1	1,338.3	917.5	595.0	565.1	556.8	549.2
85 years and over	- - -	2,578.9	2,210.5	1,891.6	1,495.2	1,518.4	1,509.1	1,556.5

See footnotes at end of table.

Table 37 (page 3 of 3). Death rates for cerebrovascular diseases, according to sex, race, Hispanic origin, and age: United States, selected years 1950–2000

[Data are based on death certificates]

Sex, race, Hispanic origin, and age	1950[1]	1960[1]	1970	1980	1990	1995	1999[2]	2000
American Indian or Alaska Native female[4]				Deaths per 100,000 resident population				
All ages, age adjusted[3]	- - -	- - -	- - -	51.2	38.4	46.3	46.4	43.7
All ages, crude	- - -	- - -	- - -	22.0	19.3	22.0	21.8	21.5
45–54 years	- - -	- - -	- - -	*	*	*	*	14.4
55–64 years	- - -	- - -	- - -	*	40.7	41.5	41.8	37.9
65–74 years	- - -	- - -	- - -	128.3	100.5	114.8	91.3	79.5
75–84 years	- - -	- - -	- - -	404.2	282.0	364.4	360.5	391.1
85 years and over	- - -	- - -	- - -	1,095.5	776.2	983.9	1,123.7	931.5
Asian or Pacific Islander female[4]								
All ages, age adjusted[3]	- - -	- - -	- - -	60.8	54.9	48.3	49.0	49.1
All ages, crude	- - -	- - -	- - -	26.4	24.3	24.2	27.7	28.7
45–54 years	- - -	- - -	- - -	20.3	19.7	15.6	14.9	13.3
55–64 years	- - -	- - -	- - -	43.7	42.1	37.6	39.5	33.3
65–74 years	- - -	- - -	- - -	136.1	124.0	101.0	103.6	102.8
75–84 years	- - -	- - -	- - -	446.6	396.6	381.8	360.2	386.0
85 years and over	- - -	- - -	- - -	1,545.2	1,395.0	1,197.0	1,275.5	1,246.6
Hispanic or Latino female[4,6]								
All ages, age adjusted[3]	- - -	- - -	- - -	- - -	43.7	42.7	42.2	43.0
All ages, crude	- - -	- - -	- - -	- - -	20.1	19.4	18.8	19.4
45–54 years	- - -	- - -	- - -	- - -	15.2	15.1	11.9	12.4
55–64 years	- - -	- - -	- - -	- - -	38.5	36.5	30.3	31.9
65–74 years	- - -	- - -	- - -	- - -	102.6	102.3	98.1	95.2
75–84 years	- - -	- - -	- - -	- - -	308.5	307.3	317.1	311.3
85 years and over	- - -	- - -	- - -	- - -	1,055.3	1,021.0	1,049.2	1,108.9
White, not Hispanic or Latino female[6]								
All ages, age adjusted[3]	- - -	- - -	- - -	- - -	61.0	58.7	58.4	57.6
All ages, crude	- - -	- - -	- - -	- - -	77.2	81.5	86.1	85.5
45–54 years	- - -	- - -	- - -	- - -	13.2	12.3	10.5	10.9
55–64 years	- - -	- - -	- - -	- - -	35.7	32.6	29.1	29.9
65–74 years	- - -	- - -	- - -	- - -	116.9	111.4	108.8	107.6
75–84 years	- - -	- - -	- - -	- - -	461.9	445.9	447.0	438.3
85 years and over	- - -	- - -	- - -	- - -	1,714.7	1,666.8	1,693.0	1,661.6

- - - Data not available.

[1]Includes deaths of persons who were not residents of the 50 States and the District of Columbia.
[2]Starting with 1999 data, cause of death is coded according to ICD–10. To estimate change between 1998 and 1999, compare the 1999 rate with the comparability-modified rate for 1998. See Appendix II, Comparability ratio and tables V and VI.
[3]Age-adjusted rates are calculated using the year 2000 standard population starting with *Health, United States, 2001*. See Appendix II, Age adjustment.
[4]The race groups, white, black, Asian or Pacific Islander, and American Indian or Alaska Native, include persons of Hispanic and non-Hispanic origin. Persons of Hispanic origin may be of any race. Death rates for the American Indian or Alaska Native and Asian or Pacific Islander populations are known to be underestimated. See Appendix II, Race, for a discussion of sources of bias in death rates by race and Hispanic origin.
[5]In 1950 rate is for the age group 75 years and over.
[6]Prior to 1997, excludes data from States lacking an Hispanic-origin item on the death certificate. See Appendix II, Hispanic origin.

NOTES: Population estimates used to compute rates for 1991–2000 differ from those used previously. Starting with *Health, United States, 2003*, rates for 1991–99 were revised using intercensal population estimates based on Census 2000. Rates for 2000 were revised based on Census 2000 counts. See Appendix I, Population Census and Population Estimates. Underlying cause of death code numbers are based on the applicable revision of the *International Classification of Diseases* (ICD) for data years shown. For the period 1980–98, causes were coded using ICD–9 codes that are most nearly comparable with the 113 cause list for ICD–10. See Appendix II, tables IV and V. Age groups were selected to minimize the presentation of unstable age-specific death rates based on small numbers of deaths and for consistency among comparison groups. Data for additional years are available (see Appendix III).

SOURCES: Centers for Disease Control and Prevention, National Center for Health Statistics, National Vital Statistics System; Grove RD, Hetzel AM. Vital statistics rates in the United States, 1940–1960. Washington: U.S. Government Printing Office. 1968; numerator data from National Vital Statistics System, annual mortality files; denominator data from national population estimates for race groups from table 1 and unpublished Hispanic population estimates for 1985–96 prepared by the Housing and Household Economic Statistics Division, U.S. Bureau of the Census; additional mortality tables are available at www.cdc.gov/nchs/datawh/statab/unpubd/mortabs.htm; Anderson RN, Arias E. The effect of revised populations on mortality statistics for the U.S., 2000. National vital statistics reports. Vol 51 no 9. Hyattsville, Maryland: National Center for Health Statistics. 2003.

This table will be updated with 2001 data on the web. Go to www.cdc.gov/nchs/hus.htm.

Table 38 (page 1 of 4). Death rates for malignant neoplasms, according to sex, race, Hispanic origin, and age: United States, selected years 1950–2000

[Data are based on death certificates]

Sex, race, Hispanic origin, and age	1950[1]	1960[1]	1970	1980	1990	1995	1999[2]	2000
All persons				Deaths per 100,000 resident population				
All ages, age adjusted[3]	193.9	193.9	198.6	207.9	216.0	209.9	200.8	199.6
All ages, crude	139.8	149.2	162.8	183.9	203.2	202.2	197.0	196.5
Under 1 year	8.7	7.2	4.7	3.2	2.3	1.8	1.8	2.4
1–4 years	11.7	10.9	7.5	4.5	3.5	3.1	2.7	2.7
5–14 years	6.7	6.8	6.0	4.3	3.1	2.7	2.5	2.5
15–24 years	8.6	8.3	8.3	6.3	4.9	4.5	4.5	4.4
25–34 years	20.0	19.5	16.5	13.7	12.6	11.6	10.0	9.8
35–44 years	62.7	59.7	59.5	48.6	43.3	40.1	37.1	36.6
45–54 years	175.1	177.0	182.5	180.0	158.9	140.4	127.6	127.5
55–64 years	390.7	396.8	423.0	436.1	449.6	412.3	374.6	366.7
65–74 years	698.8	713.9	754.2	817.9	872.3	863.3	827.1	816.3
75–84 years	1,153.3	1,127.4	1,169.2	1,232.3	1,348.5	1,355.4	1,331.5	1,335.6
85 years and over	1,451.0	1,450.0	1,320.7	1,594.6	1,752.9	1,797.7	1,805.8	1,819.4
Male								
All ages, age adjusted[3]	208.1	225.1	247.6	271.2	280.4	267.5	251.9	248.9
All ages, crude	142.9	162.5	182.1	205.3	221.3	216.3	208.9	207.2
Under 1 year	9.7	7.7	4.4	3.7	2.4	1.9	1.9	2.6
1–4 years	12.5	12.4	8.3	5.2	3.7	3.6	2.9	3.0
5–14 years	7.4	7.6	6.7	4.9	3.5	3.0	2.7	2.7
15–24 years	9.7	10.2	10.4	7.8	5.7	5.4	5.2	5.1
25–34 years	17.7	18.8	16.3	13.4	12.6	11.3	9.7	9.2
35–44 years	45.6	48.9	53.0	44.0	38.5	36.3	33.3	32.7
45–54 years	156.2	170.8	183.5	188.7	162.5	141.5	131.7	130.9
55–64 years	413.1	459.9	511.8	520.8	532.9	475.1	428.4	415.8
65–74 years	791.5	890.5	1,006.8	1,093.2	1,122.2	1,083.0	1,019.4	1,001.9
75–84 years	1,332.6	1,389.4	1,588.3	1,790.5	1,914.4	1,847.9	1,767.0	1,760.6
85 years and over	1,668.3	1,741.2	1,720.8	2,369.5	2,739.9	2,818.7	2,722.2	2,710.7
Female								
All ages, age adjusted[3]	182.3	168.7	163.2	166.7	175.7	173.6	167.6	167.6
All ages, crude	136.8	136.4	144.4	163.6	186.0	188.8	185.6	186.2
Under 1 year	7.6	6.8	5.0	2.7	2.2	1.8	1.7	2.3
1–4 years	10.8	9.3	6.7	3.7	3.2	2.6	2.5	2.5
5–14 years	6.0	6.0	5.2	3.6	2.8	2.3	2.3	2.2
15–24 years	7.6	6.5	6.2	4.8	4.1	3.5	3.7	3.6
25–34 years	22.2	20.1	16.7	14.0	12.6	11.9	10.3	10.4
35–44 years	79.3	70.0	65.6	53.1	48.1	43.8	40.9	40.4
45–54 years	194.0	183.0	181.5	171.8	155.5	139.3	123.7	124.2
55–64 years	368.2	337.7	343.2	361.7	375.2	355.1	325.0	321.3
65–74 years	612.3	560.2 ·	557.9	607.1	677.4	687.1	669.5	663.6
75–84 years	1,000.7	924.1	891.9	903.1	1,010.3	1,047.5	1,048.5	1,058.5
85 years and over	1,299.7	1,263.9	1,096.7	1,255.7	1,372.1	1,404.4	1,436.5	1,456.4
White male[4]								
All ages, age adjusted[3]	210.0	224.7	244.8	265.1	272.2	260.6	246.5	243.9
All ages, crude	147.2	166.1	185.1	208.7	227.7	225.3	219.5	218.1
25–34 years	17.7	18.8	16.2	13.6	12.3	11.0	9.5	9.2
35–44 years	44.5	46.3	50.1	41.1	35.8	34.1	31.9	30.9
45–54 years	150.8	164.1	172.0	175.4	149.9	132.7	123.5	123.5
55–64 years	409.4	450.9	498.1	497.4	508.2	456.0	412.7	401.9
65–74 years	798.7	887.3	997.0	1,070.7	1,090.7	1,056.1	1,002.3	984.3
75–84 years	1,367.6	1,413.7	1,592.7	1,779.7	1,883.2	1,817.4	1,741.8	1,736.0
85 years and over	1,732.7	1,791.4	1,772.2	2,375.6	2,715.1	2,789.4	2,696.3	2,693.7
Black or African American male[4]								
All ages, age adjusted[3]	178.9	227.6	291.9	353.4	397.9	374.3	346.1	340.3
All ages, crude	106.6	136.7	171.6	205.5	221.9	204.8	191.0	188.5
25–34 years	18.0	18.4	18.8	14.1	15.7	14.8	11.4	10.1
35–44 years	55.7	72.9	81.3	73.8	64.3	57.2	47.3	48.4
45–54 years	211.7	244.7	311.2	333.0	302.6	243.9	221.3	214.2
55–64 years	490.8	579.7	689.2	812.5	859.2	738.1	659.0	626.4
65–74 years	636.5	938.5	1,168.9	1,417.2	1,613.9	1,541.4	1,369.8	1,363.8
75–84 years[5]	853.5	1,053.3	1,624.8	2,029.6	2,478.3	2,449.8	2,359.4	2,351.8
85 years and over	- - -	1,155.2	1,387.0	2,393.9	3,238.3	3,395.5	3,340.7	3,264.8

See footnotes at end of table.

Table 38 (page 2 of 4). **Death rates for malignant neoplasms, according to sex, race, Hispanic origin, and age: United States, selected years 1950–2000**

[Data are based on death certificates]

Sex, race, Hispanic origin, and age	1950[1]	1960[1]	1970	1980	1990	1995	1999[2]	2000
American Indian or Alaska Native male[4]				Deaths per 100,000 resident population				
All ages, age adjusted[3]	---	---	---	140.5	145.8	169.0	169.0	155.8
All ages, crude	---	---	---	58.1	61.4	67.8	67.3	67.0
25–34 years	---	---	---	*	*	*	*	*
35–44 years	---	---	---	*	22.8	14.3	16.1	21.4
45–54 years	---	---	---	86.9	86.9	79.2	74.2	70.3
55–64 years	---	---	---	213.4	246.2	279.8	250.1	255.6
65–74 years	---	---	---	613.0	530.6	684.7	708.7	648.0
75–84 years	---	---	---	936.4	1,038.4	1,346.3	1,297.6	1,152.5
85 years and over	---	---	---	1,471.2	1,654.4	1,549.0	1,808.7	1,584.2
Asian or Pacific Islander male[4]								
All ages, age adjusted[3]	---	---	---	165.2	172.5	164.3	151.2	150.8
All ages, crude	---	---	---	81.9	82.7	83.7	84.3	85.2
25–34 years	---	---	---	6.3	9.2	8.2	8.5	7.4
35–44 years	---	---	---	29.4	27.7	26.1	25.6	26.1
45–54 years	---	---	---	108.2	92.6	82.4	80.3	78.5
55–64 years	---	---	---	298.5	274.6	244.8	229.4	229.2
65–74 years	---	---	---	581.2	687.2	614.3	569.4	559.4
75–84 years	---	---	---	1,147.6	1,229.9	1,167.2	1,055.9	1,086.1
85 years and over	---	---	---	1,798.7	1,837.0	2,081.3	1,860.4	1,823.2
Hispanic or Latino male[4,6]								
All ages, age adjusted[3]	---	---	---	---	174.7	180.9	170.6	171.7
All ages, crude	---	---	---	---	65.5	65.4	61.2	61.3
25–34 years	---	---	---	---	8.0	8.4	6.6	6.9
35–44 years	---	---	---	---	22.5	24.7	19.8	20.1
45–54 years	---	---	---	---	96.6	85.0	84.6	79.4
55–64 years	---	---	---	---	294.0	281.6	268.1	253.1
65–74 years	---	---	---	---	655.5	697.9	668.9	651.2
75–84 years	---	---	---	---	1,233.4	1,359.8	1,252.9	1,306.4
85 years and over	---	---	---	---	2,019.4	2,018.6	1,945.3	2,049.7
White, not Hispanic or Latino male[6]								
All ages, age adjusted[3]	---	---	---	---	276.7	263.5	250.4	247.7
All ages, crude	---	---	---	---	246.2	246.0	245.1	244.4
25–34 years	---	---	---	---	12.8	11.2	10.1	9.7
35–44 years	---	---	---	---	36.8	34.8	33.5	32.3
45–54 years	---	---	---	---	153.9	135.6	126.7	127.2
55–64 years	---	---	---	---	520.6	464.9	422.3	412.0
65–74 years	---	---	---	---	1,109.0	1,069.9	1,019.3	1,002.1
75–84 years	---	---	---	---	1,906.6	1,825.4	1,757.7	1,750.2
85 years and over	---	---	---	---	2,744.4	2,810.8	2,721.3	2,714.1
White female[4]								
All ages, age adjusted[3]	182.0	167.7	162.5	165.2	174.0	172.1	166.4	166.9
All ages, crude	139.9	139.8	149.4	170.3	196.1	200.6	198.2	199.4
25–34 years	20.9	18.8	16.3	13.5	11.9	11.2	10.1	10.1
35–44 years	74.5	66.6	62.4	50.9	46.2	41.9	38.7	38.2
45–54 years	185.8	175.7	177.3	166.4	150.9	135.0	120.2	120.1
55–64 years	362.5	329.0	338.6	355.5	368.5	350.3	320.7	319.7
65–74 years	616.5	562.1	554.7	605.2	675.1	685.6	669.4	665.6
75–84 years	1,026.6	939.3	903.5	905.4	1,011.8	1,047.9	1,049.6	1,063.4
85 years and over	1,348.3	1,304.9	1,126.6	1,266.8	1,372.3	1,405.4	1,438.2	1,459.1

See footnotes at end of table.

Table 38 (page 3 of 4). Death rates for malignant neoplasms, according to sex, race, Hispanic origin, and age: United States, selected years 1950–2000

[Data are based on death certificates]

Sex, race, Hispanic origin, and age	1950[1]	1960[1]	1970	1980	1990	1995	1999[2]	2000
Black or African American female[4]				Deaths per 100,000 resident population				
All ages, age adjusted[3]	174.1	174.3	173.4	189.5	205.9	203.8	196.9	193.8
All ages, crude	111.8	113.8	117.3	136.5	156.1	155.8	153.3	151.8
25–34 years	34.3	31.0	20.9	18.3	18.7	16.5	13.0	13.5
35–44 years	119.8	102.4	94.6	73.5	67.4	61.7	59.8	58.9
45–54 years	277.0	254.8	228.6	230.2	209.9	190.6	168.5	173.9
55–64 years	484.6	442.7	404.8	450.4	482.4	444.9	411.1	391.0
65–74 years	477.3	541.6	615.8	662.4	773.2	803.5	772.7	753.1
75–84 years[5]	605.3	696.3	763.3	923.9	1,059.9	1,120.8	1,142.6	1,124.0
85 years and over	- - -	728.9	791.5	1,159.9	1,431.3	1,446.2	1,510.4	1,527.7
American Indian or Alaska Native female[4]								
All ages, age adjusted[3]	- - -	- - -	- - -	94.0	106.9	117.7	113.1	108.3
All ages, crude	- - -	- - -	- - -	50.4	62.1	64.5	62.4	61.3
25–34 years	- - -	- - -	- - -	*	*	10.2	*	*
35–44 years	- - -	- - -	- - -	36.9	31.0	29.7	22.1	23.7
45–54 years	- - -	- - -	- - -	96.9	104.5	76.9	64.3	59.7
55–64 years	- - -	- - -	- - -	198.4	213.3	213.2	227.2	200.9
65–74 years	- - -	- - -	- - -	350.8	438.9	437.0	482.1	458.3
75–84 years	- - -	- - -	- - -	446.4	554.3	819.9	780.4	714.0
85 years and over	- - -	- - -	- - -	786.5	843.7	1,039.4	824.9	983.2
Asian or Pacific Islander female[4]								
All ages, age adjusted[3]	- - -	- - -	- - -	93.0	103.0	107.4	102.3	100.7
All ages, crude	- - -	- - -	- - -	54.1	60.5	69.5	71.4	72.1
25–34 years	- - -	- - -	- - -	9.5	7.3	9.9	6.8	8.1
35–44 years	- - -	- - -	- - -	38.7	29.8	27.6	27.3	28.9
45–54 years	- - -	- - -	- - -	99.8	93.9	94.4	78.7	78.2
55–64 years	- - -	- - -	- - -	174.7	196.2	203.5	185.3	176.5
65–74 years	- - -	- - -	- - -	301.9	346.2	343.3	367.2	357.4
75–84 years	- - -	- - -	- - -	522.1	641.4	681.0	659.5	650.1
85 years and over	- - -	- - -	- - -	800.0	971.7	1,092.7	999.5	988.5
Hispanic or Latino female[4,6]								
All ages, age adjusted[3]	- - -	- - -	- - -	- - -	111.9	110.8	110.9	110.8
All ages, crude	- - -	- - -	- - -	- - -	60.7	58.7	58.0	58.5
25–34 years	- - -	- - -	- - -	- - -	9.7	8.5	8.3	7.8
35–44 years	- - -	- - -	- - -	- - -	34.8	30.7	29.4	30.7
45–54 years	- - -	- - -	- - -	- - -	100.5	89.7	85.1	84.7
55–64 years	- - -	- - -	- - -	- - -	205.4	203.0	187.2	192.5
65–74 years	- - -	- - -	- - -	- - -	404.8	398.0	404.3	410.0
75–84 years	- - -	- - -	- - -	- - -	663.0	706.2	709.8	716.5
85 years and over	- - -	- - -	- - -	- - -	1,022.7	1,028.6	1,136.5	1,056.5

See footnotes at end of table.

Table 38 (page 4 of 4). Death rates for malignant neoplasms, according to sex, race, Hispanic origin, and age: United States, selected years 1950–2000

[Data are based on death certificates]

Sex, race, Hispanic origin, and age	1950[1]	1960[1]	1970	1980	1990	1995	1999[2]	2000
White, not Hispanic or Latino female[6]				Deaths per 100,000 resident population				
All ages, age adjusted[3]	- - -	- - -	- - -	- - -	177.5	174.7	169.4	170.0
All ages, crude	- - -	- - -	- - -	- - -	210.6	217.3	218.4	220.6
25–34 years	- - -	- - -	- - -	- - -	11.9	11.5	10.3	10.5
35–44 years	- - -	- - -	- - -	- - -	47.0	42.7	39.7	38.9
45–54 years	- - -	- - -	- - -	- - -	154.9	137.8	123.0	123.0
55–64 years	- - -	- - -	- - -	- - -	379.5	359.3	330.5	328.9
65–74 years	- - -	- - -	- - -	- - -	688.5	697.9	684.6	681.0
75–84 years	- - -	- - -	- - -	- - -	1,027.2	1,056.1	1,060.5	1,075.3
85 years and over	- - -	- - -	- - -	- - -	1,385.7	1,411.6	1,444.2	1,468.7

- - - Data not available.

* Rates based on fewer than 20 deaths are considered unreliable and are not shown.

[1]Includes deaths of persons who were not residents of the 50 States and the District of Columbia.

[2]Starting with 1999 data, cause of death is coded according to ICD–10. To estimate change between 1998 and 1999, compare the 1999 rate with the comparability-modified rate for 1998. See Appendix II, Comparability ratio and tables V and VI.

[3]Age-adjusted rates are calculated using the year 2000 standard population starting with *Health, United States, 2001*. See Appendix II, Age adjustment.

[4]The race groups, white, black, Asian or Pacific Islander, and American Indian or Alaska Native, include persons of Hispanic and non-Hispanic origin. Persons of Hispanic origin may be of any race. Death rates for the American Indian or Alaska Native and Asian or Pacific Islander populations are known to be underestimated. See Appendix II, Race, for a discussion of sources of bias in death rates by race and Hispanic origin.

[5]In 1950 rate is for the age group 75 years and over.

[6]Prior to 1997, excludes data from States lacking an Hispanic-origin item on the death certificate. See Appendix II, Hispanic origin.

NOTES: Population estimates used to compute rates for 1991–2000 differ from those used previously. Starting with *Health, United States, 2003*, rates for 1991–99 were revised using intercensal population estimates based on Census 2000. Rates for 2000 were revised based on Census 2000 counts. See Appendix I, Population Census and Population Estimates. Underlying cause of death code numbers are based on the applicable revision of the *International Classification of Diseases* (ICD) for data years shown. See Appendix II, tables IV and V. Age groups were selected to minimize the presentation of unstable age-specific death rates based on small numbers of deaths and for consistency among comparison groups. Data for additional years are available (see Appendix III).

SOURCES: Centers for Disease Control and Prevention, National Center for Health Statistics, National Vital Statistics System; Grove RD, Hetzel AM. Vital statistics rates in the United States, 1940–1960. Washington: U.S. Government Printing Office. 1968; numerator data from National Vital Statistics System, annual mortality files; denominator data from national population estimates for race groups from table 1 and unpublished Hispanic population estimates for 1985–96 prepared by the Housing and Household Economic Statistics Division, U.S. Bureau of the Census; additional mortality tables are available at www.cdc.gov/nchs/datawh/statab/unpubd/mortabs.htm; Anderson RN, Arias E. The effect of revised populations on mortality statistics for the U.S., 2000. National vital statistics reports. Vol 51 no 9. Hyattsville, Maryland: National Center for Health Statistics. 2003.

This table will be updated with 2001 data on the web. Go to www.cdc.gov/nchs/hus.htm.

Table 39 (page 1 of 3). Death rates for malignant neoplasms of trachea, bronchus, and lung, according to sex, race, Hispanic origin, and age: United States, selected years 1950–2000

[Data are based on death certificates]

Sex, race, Hispanic origin, and age	1950[1]	1960[1]	1970	1980	1990	1995	1999[2]	2000
All persons			Deaths per 100,000 resident population					
All ages, age adjusted[3]	15.0	24.1	37.1	49.9	59.3	58.4	55.5	56.1
All ages, crude	12.2	20.3	32.1	45.8	56.8	56.8	54.5	55.3
Under 25 years	0.1	0.0	0.1	0.0	0.0	0.0	0.0	0.0
25–34 years	0.8	1.0	0.9	0.6	0.7	0.6	0.4	0.5
35–44 years	4.5	6.8	11.0	9.2	6.8	6.0	6.0	6.1
45–54 years	20.4	29.6	43.4	54.1	46.8	37.5	31.3	31.6
55–64 years	48.7	75.3	109.1	138.2	160.6	141.6	123.4	122.4
65–74 years	59.7	108.1	164.5	233.3	288.4	295.4	281.5	284.2
75–84 years	55.8	91.5	163.2	240.5	333.3	358.9	362.1	370.8
85 years and over	42.3	65.6	101.7	176.0	242.5	279.9	297.0	302.1
Male								
All ages, age adjusted[3]	24.6	43.6	67.5	85.2	91.1	84.2	76.9	76.7
All ages, crude	19.9	35.4	53.4	68.6	75.1	70.5	65.4	65.5
Under 25 years	0.0	0.0	0.1	0.1	0.0	0.1	*	*
25–34 years	1.1	1.4	1.3	0.8	0.9	0.7	0.5	0.5
35–44 years	7.1	10.5	16.1	11.9	8.5	7.0	6.6	6.9
45–54 years	35.0	50.6	67.5	76.0	59.7	46.3	38.2	38.5
55–64 years	83.8	139.3	189.7	213.6	222.9	185.3	158.0	154.0
65–74 years	98.7	204.3	320.8	403.9	430.4	414.3	377.2	377.9
75–84 years	82.6	167.1	330.8	488.8	572.9	553.8	527.6	532.2
85 years and over	62.5	107.7	194.0	368.1	513.2	540.3	529.2	521.2
Female								
All ages, age adjusted[3]	5.8	7.5	13.1	24.4	37.1	40.4	40.2	41.3
All ages, crude	4.5	6.4	11.9	24.3	39.4	43.6	44.1	45.4
Under 25 years	0.1	0.0	0.0	*	*	*	*	*
25–34 years	0.5	5.4	0.5	0.5	0.5	0.6	0.4	0.5
35–44 years	1.9	3.2	6.1	6.5	5.2	5.0	5.5	5.3
45–54 years	5.8	9.2	21.0	33.7	34.5	29.1	24.6	25.0
55–64 years	13.6	15.4	36.8	72.0	105.0	101.9	91.5	93.3
65–74 years	23.3	24.4	43.1	102.7	177.6	200.0	203.1	206.9
75–84 years	32.9	32.8	52.4	94.1	190.1	237.2	254.5	265.6
85 years and over	28.2	38.8	50.0	91.9	138.1	179.6	203.5	212.8
White male[4]								
All ages, age adjusted[3]	25.1	43.6	67.1	83.8	89.0	82.6	75.6	75.7
All ages, crude	20.8	36.4	54.6	70.2	77.8	74.0	69.1	69.4
45–54 years	35.1	49.2	63.3	70.9	55.2	43.2	35.2	35.7
55–64 years	85.4	139.2	186.8	205.6	213.7	178.9	153.9	150.8
65–74 years	101.5	207.5	325.0	401.0	422.1	408.0	373.4	374.9
75–84 years	85.5	170.4	336.7	493.5	572.2	550.8	523.5	529.9
85 years and over	67.4	109.4	199.6	374.1	516.3	539.3	531.5	522.4
Black or African American male[4]								
All ages, age adjusted[3]	17.8	42.6	75.4	107.6	125.4	115.1	103.0	101.1
All ages, crude	12.1	28.1	47.7	66.6	73.7	65.6	58.9	58.3
45–54 years	34.4	68.4	115.4	133.8	114.9	85.2	72.6	70.7
55–64 years	68.3	146.8	234.3	321.1	358.6	288.5	237.6	223.5
65–74 years	53.8	168.3	300.5	472.3	585.4	559.5	484.4	488.8
75–84 years[5]	36.2	107.3	271.6	472.9	645.4	667.1	661.0	642.5
85 years and over	- - -	82.8	137.0	311.3	499.5	583.0	574.2	562.8
American Indian or Alaska Native male[4]								
All ages, age adjusted[3]	- - -	- - -	- - -	31.7	47.5	53.6	49.4	42.9
All ages, crude	- - -	- - -	- - -	14.2	20.0	21.8	20.2	18.1
45–54 years	- - -	- - -	- - -	*	26.6	23.8	16.4	14.5
55–64 years	- - -	- - -	- - -	72.0	97.8	98.9	96.4	86.0
65–74 years	- - -	- - -	- - -	202.8	194.3	261.5	264.5	184.8
75–84 years	- - -	- - -	- - -	*	356.2	409.7	343.1	367.9
85 years and over	- - -	- - -	- - -	*	*	*	*	*

See footnotes at end of table.

Table 39 (page 2 of 3). Death rates for malignant neoplasms of trachea, bronchus, and lung, according to sex, race, Hispanic origin, and age: United States, selected years 1950–2000

[Data are based on death certificates]

Sex, race, Hispanic origin, and age	1950[1]	1960[1]	1970	1980	1990	1995	1999[2]	2000
Asian or Pacific Islander male[4]				Deaths per 100,000 resident population				
All ages, age adjusted[3]	- - -	- - -	- - -	43.3	44.2	41.0	39.1	40.9
All ages, crude	- - -	- - -	- - -	22.1	20.7	20.7	21.6	22.7
45–54 years	- - -	- - -	- - -	33.3	18.8	18.6	15.2	17.2
55–64 years	- - -	- - -	- - -	94.4	74.4	64.4	56.1	61.4
65–74 years	- - -	- - -	- - -	174.3	215.8	184.0	196.3	183.2
75–84 years	- - -	- - -	- - -	301.3	307.5	296.6	311.4	323.2
85 years and over	- - -	- - -	- - -	*	421.3	439.0	298.0	378.0
Hispanic or Latino male[4,6]								
All ages, age adjusted[3]	- - -	- - -	- - -	- - -	44.1	42.2	39.6	39.0
All ages, crude	- - -	- - -	- - -	- - -	16.2	14.8	13.6	13.3
45–54 years	- - -	- - -	- - -	- - -	21.5	17.5	14.2	14.8
55–64 years	- - -	- - -	- - -	- - -	80.7	69.9	68.1	58.6
65–74 years	- - -	- - -	- - -	- - -	195.5	192.0	175.3	167.3
75–84 years	- - -	- - -	- - -	- - -	313.4	324.4	316.0	327.5
85 years and over	- - -	- - -	- - -	- - -	420.7	382.8	362.3	368.8
White, not Hispanic or Latino male[6]								
All ages, age adjusted[3]	- - -	- - -	- - -	- - -	91.1	84.1	77.6	77.9
All ages, crude	- - -	- - -	- - -	- - -	84.7	81.5	78.1	78.9
45–54 years	- - -	- - -	- - -	- - -	57.8	44.9	37.1	37.7
55–64 years	- - -	- - -	- - -	- - -	221.0	184.8	160.1	157.7
65–74 years	- - -	- - -	- - -	- - -	431.4	416.0	384.4	387.3
75–84 years	- - -	- - -	- - -	- - -	580.4	554.8	531.1	537.7
85 years and over	- - -	- - -	- - -	- - -	520.9	542.7	536.9	527.3
White female[4]								
All ages, age adjusted[3]	5.9	6.8	13.1	24.5	37.6	41.1	41.0	42.3
All ages, crude	4.7	5.9	12.3	25.6	42.4	47.5	48.2	49.9
45–54 years	5.7	9.0	20.9	33.0	34.6	29.3	24.4	24.8
55–64 years	13.7	15.1	37.2	71.9	105.7	104.0	93.8	96.1
65–74 years	23.7	24.8	42.9	104.6	181.3	203.8	208.6	213.2
75–84 years	34.0	32.7	52.6	95.2	194.6	243.3	259.1	272.7
85 years and over	29.3	39.1	50.6	92.4	138.3	181.0	205.3	215.9
Black or African American female[4]								
All ages, age adjusted[3]	4.5	6.8	13.7	24.8	36.8	38.8	39.9	39.8
All ages, crude	2.8	4.3	9.4	18.3	28.1	29.5	30.7	30.8
45–54 years	7.5	11.3	23.9	43.4	41.3	34.5	31.9	32.9
55–64 years	12.9	17.9	33.5	79.9	117.9	106.9	94.4	95.3
65–74 years	14.0	18.1	46.1	88.0	164.3	196.2	192.3	194.1
75–84 years[5]	*	31.3	49.1	79.4	148.1	183.2	234.9	224.3
85 years and over	- - -	34.2	44.8	85.8	134.9	158.9	184.4	185.9
American Indian or Alaska Native female[4]								
All ages, age adjusted[3]	- - -	- - -	- - -	11.7	19.3	25.9	27.3	24.8
All ages, crude	- - -	- - -	- - -	6.0	11.2	13.8	14.9	14.0
45–54 years	- - -	- - -	- - -	*	22.9	*	*	12.1
55–64 years	- - -	- - -	- - -	*	53.7	45.7	71.2	52.6
65–74 years	- - -	- - -	- - -	*	78.5	134.6	146.8	151.5
75–84 years	- - -	- - -	- - -	*	111.8	209.5	190.2	136.3
85 years and over	- - -	- - -	- - -	*	*	*	*	*

See footnotes at end of table.

Table 39 (page 3 of 3). Death rates for malignant neoplasms of trachea, bronchus, and lung, according to sex, race, Hispanic origin, and age: United States, selected years 1950–2000

[Data are based on death certificates]

Sex, race, Hispanic origin, and age	1950[1]	1960[1]	1970	1980	1990	1995	1999[2]	2000
Asian or Pacific Islander female[4]				Deaths per 100,000 resident population				
All ages, age adjusted[3]	- - -	- - -	- - -	15.4	18.9	21.4	19.3	18.4
All ages, crude	- - -	- - -	- - -	8.4	10.5	13.0	13.0	12.6
45–54 years	- - -	- - -	- - -	13.5	11.3	11.6	11.5	9.9
55–64 years	- - -	- - -	- - -	24.6	38.3	37.6	30.4	30.4
65–74 years	- - -	- - -	- - -	62.4	71.6	84.2	82.8	77.0
75–84 years	- - -	- - -	- - -	117.7	137.9	153.5	130.2	135.0
85 years and over	- - -	- - -	- - -	*	172.9	235.5	217.0	175.3
Hispanic or Latino female[4,6]								
All ages, age adjusted[3]	- - -	- - -	- - -	- - -	14.1	14.3	14.6	14.7
All ages, crude	- - -	- - -	- - -	- - -	7.2	7.1	7.1	7.2
45–54 years	- - -	- - -	- - -	- - -	8.7	7.1	6.7	7.1
55–64 years	- - -	- - -	- - -	- - -	25.1	25.5	23.1	22.2
65–74 years	- - -	- - -	- - -	- - -	66.8	59.2	64.0	66.0
75–84 years	- - -	- - -	- - -	- - -	94.3	111.0	102.3	112.3
85 years and over	- - -	- - -	- - -	- - -	118.2	128.3	162.2	137.5
White, not Hispanic or Latino female[6]								
All ages, age adjusted[3]	- - -	- - -	- - -	- - -	39.0	42.5	42.7	44.1
All ages, crude	- - -	- - -	- - -	- - -	46.2	52.3	54.3	56.4
45–54 years	- - -	- - -	- - -	- - -	36.6	31.0	26.1	26.4
55–64 years	- - -	- - -	- - -	- - -	111.3	109.4	99.5	102.2
65–74 years	- - -	- - -	- - -	- - -	186.4	210.4	217.5	222.9
75–84 years	- - -	- - -	- - -	- - -	199.1	247.2	265.0	279.2
85 years and over	- - -	- - -	- - -	- - -	139.0	181.6	206.2	218.0

0.0 Quantity more than zero but less than 0.05.

* Rates based on fewer than 20 deaths are considered unreliable and are not shown.

- - - Data not available.

[1]Includes deaths of persons who were not residents of the 50 States and the District of Columbia.

[2]Starting with 1999 data, cause of death is coded according to ICD–10. To estimate change between 1998 and 1999, compare the 1999 rate with the comparability-modified rate for 1998. See Appendix II, Comparability ratio and tables V and VI.

[3]Age-adjusted rates are calculated using the year 2000 standard population starting with *Health, United States, 2001*. See Appendix II, Age adjustment.

[4]The race groups, white, black, Asian or Pacific Islander, and American Indian or Alaska Native, include persons of Hispanic and non-Hispanic origin. Persons of Hispanic origin may be of any race. Death rates for the American Indian or Alaska Native and Asian or Pacific Islander populations are known to be underestimated. See Appendix II, Race, for a discussion of sources of bias in death rates by race and Hispanic origin.

[5]In 1950 rate is for the age group 75 years and over.

[6]Prior to 1997, excludes data from States lacking an Hispanic-origin item on the death certificate. See Appendix II, Hispanic origin.

NOTES: Population estimates used to compute rates for 1991–2000 differ from those used previously. Starting with *Health, United States, 2003*, rates for 1991–99 were revised using intercensal population estimates based on Census 2000. Rates for 2000 were revised based on Census 2000 counts. See Appendix I, Population Census and Population Estimates. Underlying cause of death code numbers are based on the applicable revision of the *International Classification of Diseases* (ICD) for data years shown. For the period 1980–98, causes were coded using ICD–9 codes that are most nearly comparable with the 113 cause list for ICD–10. See Appendix II, tables IV and V. Age groups were selected to minimize the presentation of unstable age-specific death rates based on small numbers of deaths and for consistency among comparison groups. Data for additional years are available (see Appendix III).

SOURCES: Centers for Disease Control and Prevention, National Center for Health Statistics, National Vital Statistics System; Grove RD, Hetzel AM. Vital statistics rates in the United States, 1940–1960. Washington: U.S. Government Printing Office. 1968; numerator data from National Vital Statistics System, annual mortality files; denominator data from national population estimates for race groups from table 1 and unpublished Hispanic population estimates for 1985–96 prepared by the Housing and Household Economic Statistics Division, U.S. Bureau of the Census; additional mortality tables are available at www.cdc.gov/nchs/datawh/statab/unpubd/mortabs.htm; Anderson RN, Arias E. The effect of revised populations on mortality statistics for the U.S., 2000. National vital statistics reports. Vol 51 no 9. Hyattsville, Maryland: National Center for Health Statistics. 2003.

This table will be updated with 2001 data on the web. Go to www.cdc.gov/nchs/hus.htm.

Table 40 (page 1 of 2). Death rates for malignant neoplasm of breast for females, according to race, Hispanic origin, and age: United States, selected years 1950–2000

[Data are based on death certificates]

Race, Hispanic origin, and age	1950[1]	1960[1]	1970	1980	1990	1995	1999[2]	2000
All persons				Deaths per 100,000 resident population				
All ages, age adjusted[3]	31.9	31.7	32.1	31.9	33.3	30.5	26.6	26.8
All ages, crude	24.7	26.1	28.4	30.6	34.0	32.2	28.9	29.2
Under 25 years	*	*	*	*	*	*	*	*
25–34 years	3.8	3.8	3.9	3.3	2.9	2.6	2.2	2.3
35–44 years	20.8	20.2	20.4	17.9	17.8	14.9	12.0	12.4
45–54 years	46.9	51.4	52.6	48.1	45.4	41.0	32.9	33.0
55–64 years	69.9	70.8	77.6	80.5	78.6	69.4	59.2	59.3
65–74 years	95.0	90.0	93.8	101.1	111.7	102.8	88.9	88.3
75–84 years	139.8	129.9	127.4	126.4	146.3	140.1	128.9	128.9
85 years and over	195.5	191.9	157.1	169.3	196.8	200.2	200.8	205.7
White[4]								
All ages, age adjusted[3]	32.4	32.0	32.5	32.1	33.2	30.1	26.0	26.3
All ages, crude	25.7	27.2	29.9	32.3	35.9	33.8	30.2	30.7
35–44 years	20.8	19.7	20.2	17.3	17.1	14.0	10.8	11.3
45–54 years	47.1	51.2	53.0	48.1	44.3	38.9	30.9	31.2
55–64 years	70.9	71.8	79.3	81.3	78.5	68.3	57.5	57.9
65–74 years	96.3	91.6	95.9	103.7	113.3	103.3	88.9	89.3
75–84 years	143.6	132.8	129.6	128.4	148.2	141.4	129.5	130.2
85 years and over	204.2	199.7	161.9	171.7	198.0	202.6	202.9	205.5
Black or African American[4]								
All ages, age adjusted[3]	25.3	27.9	28.9	31.7	38.1	38.0	35.1	34.5
All ages, crude	16.4	18.7	19.7	22.9	29.0	29.6	28.2	27.9
35–44 years	21.0	24.8	24.4	24.1	25.8	22.9	21.7	20.9
45–54 years	46.5	54.4	52.0	52.7	60.5	61.9	53.0	51.5
55–64 years	64.3	63.2	64.7	79.9	93.1	89.1	82.2	80.9
65–74 years	67.0	72.3	77.3	84.3	112.2	117.9	106.2	98.6
75–84 years[5]	81.0	87.5	101.8	114.1	140.5	147.2	145.4	139.8
85 years and over	- - -	92.1	112.1	149.9	201.5	192.7	199.3	238.7
American Indian or Alaska Native[4]								
All ages, age adjusted[3]	- - -	- - -	- - -	10.8	13.7	15.0	15.5	13.6
All ages, crude	- - -	- - -	- - -	6.1	8.6	9.0	9.1	8.7
35–44 years	- - -	- - -	- - -	*	*	*	*	*
45–54 years	- - -	- - -	- - -	*	23.9	21.6	16.1	14.4
55–64 years	- - -	- - -	- - -	*	*	37.4	31.6	40.0
65–74 years	- - -	- - -	- - -	*	*	46.3	69.4	42.5
75–84 years	- - -	- - -	- - -	*	*	*	*	71.8
85 years and over	- - -	- - -	- - -	*	*	*	*	*
Asian or Pacific Islander[4]								
All ages, age adjusted[3]	- - -	- - -	- - -	11.9	13.7	13.9	12.7	12.3
All ages, crude	- - -	- - -	- - -	8.2	9.3	10.8	10.0	10.2
35–44 years	- - -	- - -	- - -	10.4	8.4	8.0	6.4	8.1
45–54 years	- - -	- - -	- - -	23.4	26.4	29.1	19.8	22.3
55–64 years	- - -	- - -	- - -	35.7	33.8	37.9	36.7	31.3
65–74 years	- - -	- - -	- - -	*	38.5	36.6	37.5	34.7
75–84 years	- - -	- - -	- - -	*	48.0	42.3	44.6	37.5
85 years and over	- - -	- - -	- - -	*	*	*	77.7	68.2
Hispanic or Latino[4,6]								
All ages, age adjusted[3]	- - -	- - -	- - -	- - -	19.5	18.7	16.4	16.9
All ages, crude	- - -	- - -	- - -	- - -	11.5	10.6	9.3	9.7
35–44 years	- - -	- - -	- - -	- - -	11.7	9.5	8.3	8.7
45–54 years	- - -	- - -	- - -	- - -	32.8	27.7	23.9	23.9
55–64 years	- - -	- - -	- - -	- - -	45.8	45.0	36.6	39.1
65–74 years	- - -	- - -	- - -	- - -	64.8	58.0	49.1	54.9
75–84 years	- - -	- - -	- - -	- - -	67.2	80.9	71.8	74.9
85 years and over	- - -	- - -	- - -	- - -	102.8	115.6	127.9	105.8

See footnotes at end of table.

Table 40 (page 2 of 2). Death rates for malignant neoplasm of breast for females, according to race, Hispanic origin, and age: United States, selected years 1950–2000

[Data are based on death certificates]

Race, Hispanic origin, and age	1950[1]	1960[1]	1970	1980	1990	1995	1999[2]	2000
White, not Hispanic or Latino[6]				Deaths per 100,000 resident population				
All ages, age adjusted[3]	- - -	- - -	- - -	- - -	33.9	30.6	26.6	26.8
All ages, crude	- - -	- - -	- - -	- - -	38.5	36.6	33.3	33.8
35–44 years	- - -	- - -	- - -	- - -	17.5	14.4	11.1	11.6
45–54 years	- - -	- - -	- - -	- - -	45.2	39.5	31.5	31.7
55–64 years	- - -	- - -	- - -	- - -	80.6	69.5	58.9	59.2
65–74 years	- - -	- - -	- - -	- - -	115.7	105.4	91.2	91.4
75–84 years	- - -	- - -	- - -	- - -	151.4	143.2	131.5	132.2
85 years and over	- - -	- - -	- - -	- - -	201.5	204.4	204.9	208.3

* Rates based on fewer than 20 deaths are considered unreliable and are not shown.
0.0 Quantity more than zero but less than 0.05.
- - - Data not available.
[1]Includes deaths of persons who were not residents of the 50 States and the District of Columbia.
[2]Starting with 1999 data, cause of death is coded according to ICD–10. To estimate change between 1998 and 1999, compare the 1999 rate with the comparability-modified rate for 1998. See Appendix II, Comparability ratio and tables V and VI.
[3]Age-adjusted rates are calculated using the year 2000 standard population starting with *Health, United States, 2001.* See Appendix II, Age adjustment.
[4]The race groups, white, black, Asian or Pacific Islander, and American Indian or Alaska Native, include persons of Hispanic and non-Hispanic origin. Persons of Hispanic origin may be of any race. Death rates for the American Indian or Alaska Native and Asian or Pacific Islander populations are known to be underestimated. See Appendix II, Race, for a discussion of sources of bias in death rates by race and Hispanic origin.
[5]In 1950 rate is for the age group 75 years and over.
[6]Prior to 1997, excludes data from States lacking an Hispanic-origin item on the death certificate. See Appendix II, Hispanic origin.

NOTES: Population estimates used to compute rates for 1991–2000 differ from those used previously. Starting with *Health, United States, 2003*, rates for 1991–99 were revised using intercensal population estimates based on Census 2000. Rates for 2000 were revised based on Census 2000 counts. See Appendix I, Population Census and Population Estimates. Underlying cause of death code numbers are based on the applicable revision of the *International Classification of Diseases* (ICD) for data years shown. See Appendix II, tables IV and V. Age groups were selected to minimize the presentation of unstable age-specific death rates based on small numbers of deaths and for consistency among comparison groups. Data for additional years are available (see Appendix III).

SOURCES: Centers for Disease Control and Prevention, National Center for Health Statistics, National Vital Statistics System; numerator data from annual mortality files; denominator data from national population estimates for race groups from table 1 and unpublished Hispanic population estimates for 1985–96 prepared by the Housing and Household Economic Statistics Division, U.S. Bureau of the Census; additional mortality tables are available at www.cdc.gov/nchs/datawh/statab/unpubd/mortabs.htm; Anderson RN, Arias E. The effect of revised populations on mortality statistics for the U.S., 2000. National vital statistics reports. Vol 51 no 9. Hyattsville, Maryland: National Center for Health Statistics. 2003.

This table will be updated with 2001 data on the web. Go to www.cdc.gov/nchs/hus.htm.

Table 41 (page 1 of 3). Death rates for chronic lower respiratory diseases, according to sex, race, Hispanic origin, and age: United States, selected years 1980–2000

[Data are based on death certificates]

Sex, race, Hispanic origin, and age	1980	1990	1995	1997	1998	Comparability modified 1998[1]	1999[1]	2000
All persons				Deaths per 100,000 resident population				
All ages, age adjusted[2]	28.3	37.2	40.1	41.1	41.8	43.8	45.4	44.2
All ages, crude	24.7	34.9	38.6	40.0	40.8	42.8	44.5	43.4
Under 1 year	1.6	1.4	1.1	1.3	1.0	1.0	0.9	0.9
1–4 years	0.4	0.4	0.2	0.3	0.3	0.3	0.4	0.3
5–14 years	0.2	0.3	0.4	0.3	0.4	0.4	0.3	0.3
15–24 years	0.3	0.5	0.7	0.5	0.6	0.6	0.5	0.5
25–34 years	0.5	0.7	0.9	0.9	0.8	0.8	0.8	0.7
35–44 years	1.6	1.6	1.9	2.0	2.0	2.1	2.0	2.1
45–54 years	9.8	9.1	8.7	8.3	8.0	8.4	8.5	8.6
55–64 years	42.7	48.9	46.8	45.7	44.1	46.2	47.5	44.2
65–74 years	129.1	152.5	159.6	163.6	167.4	175.4	177.2	169.4
75–84 years	224.4	321.1	349.3	356.2	363.7	381.1	397.8	386.1
85 years and over	274.0	433.3	520.1	556.8	572.2	599.6	646.0	648.6
Male								
All ages, age adjusted[2]	49.9	55.5	54.8	54.6	54.4	57.0	58.7	55.8
All ages, crude	35.1	40.8	41.4	41.9	42.2	44.2	45.6	43.5
Under 1 year	1.9	1.6	1.4	1.7	1.2	1.3	*	1.2
1–4 years	0.5	0.5	0.2	0.3	0.4	0.4	0.4	0.4
5–14 years	0.2	0.4	0.5	0.3	0.4	0.4	0.4	0.4
15–24 years	0.4	0.5	0.7	0.7	0.8	0.8	0.6	0.6
25–34 years	0.6	0.7	0.9	0.9	0.9	0.9	0.8	0.8
35–44 years	1.7	1.7	1.7	1.9	1.9	2.0	1.8	1.9
45–54 years	12.1	9.4	8.8	8.6	8.0	8.4	8.6	9.0
55–64 years	59.9	58.6	52.3	49.6	48.6	50.9	52.3	47.8
65–74 years	210.0	204.0	195.6	199.1	199.1	208.6	210.7	195.2
75–84 years	437.4	500.0	483.8	471.9	476.4	499.2	513.2	488.5
85 years and over	583.4	815.1	889.8	912.0	900.6	943.6	996.7	967.9
Female								
All ages, age adjusted[2]	14.9	26.6	31.8	33.4	34.4	36.0	37.7	37.4
All ages, crude	15.0	29.2	36.0	38.1	39.5	41.4	43.4	43.2
Under 1 year	1.3	1.2	*	*	*	*	*	*
1–4 years	*	*	*	*	*	*	0.3	0.3
5–14 years	0.3	0.3	0.2	0.3	0.3	0.3	0.2	0.3
15–24 years	0.3	0.5	0.6	0.4	0.5	0.5	0.5	0.4
25–34 years	0.5	0.7	0.9	0.8	0.8	0.8	0.9	0.7
35–44 years	1.5	1.5	2.2	2.1	2.0	2.1	2.1	2.2
45–54 years	7.7	8.8	8.7	8.0	8.1	8.5	8.4	8.3
55–64 years	27.6	40.3	41.9	42.2	40.1	42.0	43.1	41.0
65–74 years	67.1	112.3	130.8	134.8	141.7	148.5	149.8	148.2
75–84 years	98.7	214.2	265.3	282.3	291.1	305.0	322.9	319.2
85 years and over	138.7	286.0	377.7	417.5	441.7	462.8	504.6	518.5
White male[3]								
All ages, age adjusted[2]	51.6	56.6	55.9	55.8	55.7	58.4	60.0	57.2
All ages, crude	37.9	44.3	45.5	46.3	46.7	48.9	50.6	48.3
35–44 years	1.2	1.3	1.4	1.5	1.5	1.6	1.5	1.6
45–54 years	11.4	8.6	8.1	8.1	7.4	7.8	8.1	8.4
55–64 years	60.0	58.7	52.7	50.3	49.2	51.6	53.1	48.6
65–74 years	218.4	208.1	200.0	204.7	205.7	215.5	217.3	201.4
75–84 years	459.8	513.5	497.9	483.4	489.8	513.2	525.4	503.6
85 years and over	611.2	847.0	918.3	943.1	930.5	975.0	1,029.4	997.4
Black or African American male[3]								
All ages, age adjusted[2]	34.0	47.6	47.4	46.7	46.4	48.6	51.5	47.5
All ages, crude	19.3	25.2	24.4	23.9	23.9	25.0	26.2	24.3
35–44 years	5.8	5.3	4.3	4.8	4.9	5.1	4.7	4.8
45–54 years	19.7	18.8	16.9	14.3	14.5	15.2	15.3	15.0
55–64 years	66.6	67.4	60.5	54.7	54.4	57.0	59.3	54.6
65–74 years	142.0	184.5	178.7	175.9	170.1	178.2	184.6	176.9
75–84 years	229.8	390.9	370.0	381.1	381.8	400.1	434.4	370.3
85 years and over	271.6	498.0	624.1	617.5	613.5	642.8	701.9	693.1

See footnotes at end of table.

Table 41 (page 2 of 3). **Death rates for chronic lower respiratory diseases, according to sex, race, Hispanic origin, and age: United States, selected years 1980–2000**

[Data are based on death certificates]

Sex, race, Hispanic origin, and age	1980	1990	1995	1997	1998	Comparability modified 1998[1]	1999[1]	2000
American Indian or Alaska Native male[3]				Deaths per 100,000 resident population				
All ages, age adjusted[2]	23.0	38.3	35.6	46.8	45.7	47.9	41.8	43.7
All ages, crude	8.4	13.8	12.3	15.8	15.3	16.0	14.0	15.3
35–44 years	*	*	*	*	*	*	*	*
45–54 years	*	*	*	*	*	*	*	*
55–64 years	*	*	36.5	48.1	41.4	43.4	34.2	46.4
65–74 years	*	135.7	132.1	127.9	140.0	146.7	165.0	111.3
75–84 years	*	363.8	307.3	430.8	413.5	433.3	393.0	416.6
85 years and over	*	*	*	806.7	789.3	827.0	576.7	770.7
Asian or Pacific Islander male[3]								
All ages, age adjusted[2]	21.5	29.8	28.9	28.8	26.0	27.2	29.6 `	28.3
All ages, crude	8.7	11.3	11.8	12.4	11.4	11.9	13.1	12.6
35–44 years	*	*	*	*	*	*	*	*
45–54 years	*	*	*	*	*	*	*	4.8
55–64 years	*	22.1	15.7	15.9	16.3	17.1	14.3	8.8
65–74 years	70.6	91.4	87.9	81.4	71.0	74.4	81.9	71.3
75–84 years	155.7	258.6	240.6	263.9	213.1	223.3	270.6	254.3
85 years and over	472.4	615.2	650.4	604.9	617.1	646.6	652.3	670.7
Hispanic or Latino male[3,4]								
All ages, age adjusted[2]	- - -	28.6	31.8	31.5	31.1	32.6	33.0	28.8
All ages, crude	- - -	8.4	8.9	8.6	8.5	8.9	8.9	8.0
35–44 years	- - -	*	1.1	1.5	1.2	1.3	1.4	0.9
45–54 years	- - -	4.1	3.9	3.5	3.7	3.9	3.6	3.4
55–64 years	- - -	17.2	19.1	18.0	17.9	18.8	17.6	18.2
65–74 years	- - -	81.0	82.4	81.4	77.7	81.4	81.9	72.4
75–84 years	- - -	252.4	292.0	248.9	272.2	285.2	272.7	250.3
85 years and over	- - -	613.9	689.0	810.9	725.9	760.6	836.8	671.1
White, not Hispanic or Latino male[4]								
All ages, age adjusted[2]	- - -	57.9	56.6	56.8	56.8	59.5	61.3	58.5
All ages, crude	- - -	48.5	50.2	51.8	52.6	55.1	57.3	55.1
35–44 years	- - -	1.4	1.4	1.5	1.5	1.6	1.5	1.7
45–54 years	- - -	9.0	8.4	8.5	7.7	8.1	8.5	8.9
55–64 years	- - -	61.3	54.6	52.6	51.4	53.9	55.6	50.8
65–74 years	- - -	213.4	204.3	210.8	212.4	222.6	224.9	208.8
75–84 years	- - -	523.7	501.7	491.0	497.4	521.2	534.9	513.6
85 years and over	- - -	860.6	922.6	944.2	935.4	980.1	1,033.5	1,008.6
White female[3]								
All ages, age adjusted[2]	15.5	27.8	33.3	35.0	36.1	37.8	39.7	39.5
All ages, crude	16.4	32.8	40.8	43.5	45.1	47.3	49.8	49.7
35–44 years	1.3	1.2	1.7	1.7	1.6	1.7	1.8	1.8
45–54 years	7.6	8.3	8.4	7.7	7.6	8.0	8.1	7.9
55–64 years	28.7	41.9	44.0	44.3	42.3	44.3	45.6	43.2
65–74 years	71.0	118.8	139.0	143.7	151.4	158.6	160.3	159.6
75–84 years	104.0	226.3	279.5	299.0	308.3	323.0	341.5	339.1
85 years and over	144.2	298.4	395.5	436.9	462.7	484.8	529.7	544.8
Black or African American female[3]								
All ages, age adjusted[2]	9.1	16.6	20.2	20.8	21.9	22.9	23.4	22.7
All ages, crude	6.8	12.6	15.5	16.0	16.9	17.7	18.0	17.6
35–44 years	3.4	3.8	5.4	5.0	5.2	5.4	4.6	4.7
45–54 years	9.3	14.0	12.8	12.0	14.0	14.7	12.6	13.4
55–64 years	20.8	33.4	34.7	35.9	34.0	35.6	34.9	35.3
65–74 years	32.7	64.7	78.7	81.9	85.5	89.6	88.9	82.9
75–84 years	41.1	96.0	132.7	131.6	143.4	150.3	166.4	158.4
85 years and over	63.2	133.0	185.8	214.1	225.6	236.4	254.5	255.0

See footnotes at end of table.

Table 41 (page 3 of 3). Death rates for chronic lower respiratory diseases, according to sex, race, Hispanic origin, and age: United States, selected years 1980–2000

[Data are based on death certificates]

Sex, race, Hispanic origin, and age	1980	1990	1995	1997	1998	Comparability modified 1998[1]	1999[1]	2000
American Indian or Alaska Native female[3]			Deaths per 100,000 resident population					
All ages, age adjusted[2]	7.7	16.8	22.8	21.2	24.0	25.1	30.4	26.2
All ages, crude	3.8	8.7	11.5	10.8	11.8	12.4	14.7	13.4
35–44 years	*	*	*	*	*	*	*	*
45–54 years	*	*	*	*	*	*	*	*
55–64 years	*	*	38.8	32.8	28.6	30.0	39.6	31.6
65–74 years	*	56.4	79.5	88.2	118.6	124.3	109.1	136.8
75–84 years	*	116.7	191.3	156.4	192.9	202.1	301.1	175.8
85 years and over	*	*	*	269.9	259.1	271.5	322.8	362.2
Asian or Pacific Islander female[3]								
All ages, age adjusted[2]	5.8	11.0	12.1	12.7	11.3	11.8	12.1	11.7
All ages, crude	2.6	5.2	6.3	6.9	6.2	6.5	7.0	6.8
35–44 years	*	*	*	*	*	*	*	*
45–54 years	*	*	3.6	*	*	*	*	*
55–64 years	*	15.2	9.6	8.9	6.4	6.7	7.7	6.2
65–74 years	*	26.5	29.2	31.5	28.0	29.3	39.9	29.2
75–84 years	*	80.6	113.2	115.4	91.6	96.0	94.1	88.9
85 years and over	*	232.5	227.8	261.0	273.0	286.0	268.0	299.5
Hispanic or Latino female[3,4]								
All ages, age adjusted[2]	- - -	13.4	16.9	16.6	15.6	16.3	17.7	16.3
All ages, crude	- - -	6.3	7.7	7.4	7.0	7.3	8.0	7.2
35–44 years	- - -	*	1.4	1.1	1.8	1.9	1.8	1.3
45–54 years	- - -	4.9	4.6	4.4	3.2	3.4	4.2	3.3
55–64 years	- - -	14.4	12.9	12.0	12.0	12.6	12.0	10.8
65–74 years	- - -	36.6	43.1	40.3	40.6	42.5	47.5	38.0
75–84 years	- - -	101.1	125.0	130.6	131.1	137.4	142.9	136.0
85 years and over	- - -	269.0	402.6	392.5	334.0	350.0	391.0	387.8
White, not Hispanic or Latino female[4]								
All ages, age adjusted[2]	- - -	28.5	34.0	35.9	37.1	38.9	40.8	40.7
All ages, crude	- - -	35.7	44.7	48.2	50.4	52.8	55.9	56.2
35–44 years	- - -	1.2	1.7	1.8	1.6	1.7	1.8	1.9
45–54 years	- - -	8.5	8.5	8.0	7.9	8.3	8.5	8.3
55–64 years	- - -	43.7	46.2	46.8	44.6	46.7	48.3	45.8
65–74 years	- - -	122.8	143.0	149.3	157.9	165.4	167.4	167.6
75–84 years	- - -	231.9	284.5	304.5	314.6	329.6	348.8	347.2
85 years and over	- - -	302.1	393.7	436.4	465.3	487.5	532.8	548.7

* Rates based on fewer than 20 deaths are considered unreliable and are not shown.

- - - Data not available.

[1]Starting with 1999 data, cause of death is coded according to ICD–10. To estimate change between 1998 and 1999, compare the 1999 rate with the comparability-modified rate for 1998. See Appendix II, Comparability ratio and tables V and VI.

[2]Age-adjusted rates are calculated using the year 2000 standard population starting with *Health, United States, 2001*. See Appendix II, Age adjustment.

[3]The race groups, white, black, Asian or Pacific Islander, and American Indian or Alaska Native, include persons of Hispanic and non-Hispanic origin. Persons of Hispanic origin may be of any race. Death rates for the American Indian or Alaska Native and Asian or Pacific Islander populations are known to be underestimated. See Appendix II, Race, for a discussion of sources of bias in death rates by race and Hispanic origin.

[4]Prior to 1997, excludes data from States lacking an Hispanic-origin item on the death certificate. See Appendix II, Hispanic origin.

NOTES: Population estimates used to compute rates for 1991–2000 differ from those used previously. Starting with *Health, United States, 2003*, rates for 1991–99 were revised using intercensal population estimates based on Census 2000. Rates for 2000 were revised based on Census 2000 counts. See Appendix I, Population Census and Population Estimates. Underlying cause of death code numbers are based on the applicable revision of the *International Classification of Diseases* (ICD) for data years shown. For the period 1980–98, causes were coded using ICD–9 codes that are most nearly comparable with the 113 cause list for ICD–10. See Appendix II, tables IV and V. Age groups were selected to minimize the presentation of unstable age-specific death rates based on small numbers of deaths and for consistency among comparison groups. Data for additional years are available (see Appendix III).

SOURCES: Centers for Disease Control and Prevention, National Center for Health Statistics, National Vital Statistics System; numerator data from annual mortality files; denominator data from national population estimates for race groups from table 1 and unpublished Hispanic population estimates for 1985–96 prepared by the Housing and Household Economic Statistics Division, U.S. Bureau of the Census; additional mortality tables are available at www.cdc.gov/nchs/datawh/statab/unpubd/mortabs.htm; Anderson RN, Arias E. The effect of revised populations on mortality statistics for the U.S., 2000. National vital statistics reports. Vol 51 no 9. Hyattsville, Maryland: National Center for Health Statistics. 2003.

This table will be updated with 2001 data on the web. Go to www.cdc.gov/nchs/hus.htm.

Table 42 (page 1 of 2). Death rates for human immunodeficiency virus (HIV) disease, according to sex, race, Hispanic origin, and age: United States, selected years 1987–2000

[Data are based on death certificates]

Sex, race, Hispanic origin, and age	1987	1990	1995	1997	1998	Comparability modified 1998[1]	1999[1]	2000
All persons	Deaths per 100,000 resident population							
All ages, age adjusted[2]	5.6	10.2	16.2	6.0	4.9	5.6	5.3	5.2
All ages, crude	5.6	10.1	16.2	6.1	4.9	5.6	5.3	5.1
Under 1 year	2.3	2.7	1.5	*	*	*	*	*
1–4 years	0.7	0.8	1.3	0.3	0.2	0.2	0.2	*
5–14 years	0.1	0.2	0.5	0.3	0.1	0.1	0.2	0.1
15–24 years	1.3	1.5	1.7	0.7	0.5	0.6	0.5	0.5
25–34 years	11.7	19.7	28.3	9.7	7.1	8.1	6.8	6.1
35–44 years	14.0	27.4	44.2	16.0	12.8	14.7	13.8	13.1
45–54 years	8.0	15.2	26.0	10.3	8.9	10.2	10.7	11.0
55–64 years	3.5	6.2	10.9	4.8	4.3	4.9	4.8	5.1
65–74 years	1.3	2.0	3.6	1.8	1.6	1.8	2.2	2.2
75–84 years	0.8	0.7	0.7	0.6	0.5	0.6	0.6	0.7
85 years and over	*	*	*	*	*	*	*	*
Male								
All ages, age adjusted[2]	10.4	18.5	27.3	9.6	7.6	8.7	8.2	7.9
All ages, crude	10.2	18.5	27.6	9.7	7.6	8.7	8.2	7.9
Under 1 year	2.2	2.4	1.7	*	*	*	*	*
1–4 years	0.7	0.8	1.2	0.3	*	*	*	*
5–14 years	0.2	0.3	0.5	0.3	0.1	0.1	0.2	0.1
15–24 years	2.2	2.2	2.0	0.8	0.5	0.6	0.5	0.5
25–34 years	20.7	34.5	45.5	14.4	10.0	11.4	9.5	8.0
35–44 years	26.3	50.2	75.5	25.4	20.0	22.9	21.0	19.8
45–54 years	15.5	29.1	46.2	17.1	14.8	16.9	17.5	17.8
55–64 years	6.8	12.0	19.7	8.3	7.2	8.2	8.3	8.7
65–74 years	2.4	3.7	6.4	3.4	2.9	3.3	3.8	3.8
75–84 years	1.2	1.1	1.3	1.0	0.9	1.0	1.0	1.3
85 years and over	*	*	*	*	*	*	*	*
Female								
All ages, age adjusted[2]	1.1	2.2	5.3	2.6	2.2	2.5	2.5	2.5
All ages, crude	1.1	2.2	5.3	2.6	2.2	2.5	2.5	2.5
Under 1 year	2.5	3.0	1.2	*	*	*	*	*
1–4 years	0.7	0.8	1.5	0.4	*	*	*	*
5–14 years	*	0.2	0.5	0.2	0.2	0.2	0.2	0.1
15–24 years	0.3	0.7	1.4	0.7	0.5	0.6	0.5	0.4
25–34 years	2.8	4.9	10.9	4.9	4.2	4.8	4.1	4.2
35–44 years	2.1	5.2	13.3	6.7	5.7	6.5	6.7	6.5
45–54 years	0.8	1.9	6.6	3.7	3.1	3.5	4.1	4.4
55–64 years	0.5	1.1	2.8	1.6	1.6	1.8	1.6	1.8
65–74 years	0.5	0.8	1.4	0.5	0.6	0.7	0.8	0.8
75–84 years	0.5	0.4	0.3	0.4	0.3	0.3	0.3	0.3
85 years and over	*	*	*	*	*	*	*	*
All ages, age adjusted[2]								
White male	8.7	15.7	20.4	5.9	4.5	5.2	4.9	4.6
Black or African American male	26.2	46.3	89.0	40.9	33.2	38.0	36.1	35.1
American Indian or Alaska Native male	*	3.3	10.5	3.3	3.5	4.0	4.2	3.5
Asian or Pacific Islander male	2.5	4.3	6.0	1.6	1.3	1.5	1.4	1.2
Hispanic or Latino male[3]	18.8	28.8	40.8	14.0	10.2	11.7	10.9	10.6
White, not Hispanic or Latino male[3]	10.7	14.1	17.9	4.8	3.7	4.2	4.0	3.8
White female	0.6	1.1	2.5	1.0	0.8	0.9	1.0	1.0
Black or African American female	4.6	10.1	24.4	13.7	12.0	13.7	13.1	13.2
American Indian or Alaska Native female	*	*	2.5	1.0	0.6	*	1.0	1.0
Asian or Pacific Islander female	*	*	0.6	0.2	0.3	*	0.2	0.2
Hispanic or Latino female[3]	2.1	3.8	8.8	3.3	2.8	3.2	3.0	2.9
White, not Hispanic or Latino female[3]	0.5	0.7	1.7	0.7	0.5	0.6	0.7	0.7

See footnotes at end of table.

Table 42 (page 2 of 2). Death rates for human immunodeficiency virus (HIV) disease, according to sex, race, Hispanic origin, and age: United States, selected years 1987–2000

[Data are based on death certificates]

Sex, race, Hispanic origin, and age	1987	1990	1995	1997	1998	Comparability modified 1998[1]	1999[1]	2000
Age 25–44 years	Deaths per 100,000 resident population							
All persons..........................	12.7	23.2	36.3	12.9	10.1	11.6	10.5	9.8
White male...............	19.2	35.0	46.1	12.9	9.6	11.0	9.7	8.8
Black or African American male	60.2	102.0	179.4	75.2	58.1	66.5	59.3	55.4
American Indian or Alaska Native male......	*	7.7	28.5	9.5	7.5	8.6	9.1	5.5
Asian or Pacific Islander male	4.1	8.1	12.1	3.3	2.4	2.7	2.4	1.9
Hispanic or Latino male[3]	36.8	59.3	73.9	23.3	16.6	19.0	16.5	14.3
White, not Hispanic or Latino male[3]	23.3	31.6	41.2	10.9	8.1	9.3	8.2	7.4
White female	1.2	2.3	5.9	2.3	1.8	2.1	2.2	2.1
Black or African American female..........	11.6	23.6	53.6	28.6	25.5	29.2	26.6	26.7
American Indian or Alaska Native female	*	*	*	*	*	*	*	*
Asian or Pacific Islander female	*	*	1.2	*	*	*	*	*
Hispanic or Latino female[3]...............	4.9	8.9	17.2	6.2	4.6	5.3	5.3	4.6
White, not Hispanic or Latino female[3]	1.0	1.5	4.2	1.7	1.3	1.5	1.6	1.6
Age 45–64 years								
All persons..........................	5.8	11.1	19.9	8.1	7.0	8.0	8.4	8.7
White male...............	9.9	18.6	26.0	7.9	6.6	7.6	7.8	8.1
Black or African American male	27.3	53.0	133.2	69.3	60.9	69.7	70.7	71.6
American Indian or Alaska Native male......	*	*	*	*	*	*	*	*
Asian or Pacific Islander male	*	6.5	9.1	2.3	2.4	2.7	2.3	2.1
Hispanic or Latino male[3]	25.8	37.9	67.1	25.1	18.3	20.9	21.2	23.3
White, not Hispanic or Latino male[3]	12.6	16.9	22.4	6.3	5.4	6.2	6.4	6.5
White female	0.5	0.9	2.4	1.1	0.9	1.0	1.2	1.3
Black or African American female..........	2.6	7.5	27.0	17.5	15.4	17.6	18.6	19.6
American Indian or Alaska Native female	*	*	*	*	*	*	*	*
Asian or Pacific Islander female	*	*	*	*	*	*	*	*
Hispanic or Latino female[3]...............	*	3.1	12.6	5.4	4.9	5.6	5.1	5.8
White, not Hispanic or Latino female[3]	0.5	0.7	1.5	0.7	0.5	0.6	0.8	0.9

* Rates based on fewer than 20 deaths are considered unreliable and are not shown.
[1]Starting with 1999 data, cause of death is coded according to ICD–10. To estimate change between 1998 and 1999, compare the 1999 rate with the comparability-modified rate for 1998. See Appendix II, Comparability ratio and tables V and VI.
[2]Age-adjusted rates are calculated using the year 2000 standard population starting with *Health, United States, 2001*. See Appendix II, Age adjustment.
[3]Prior to 1997, excludes data from States lacking an Hispanic-origin item on the death certificate. See Appendix II, Hispanic origin.

NOTES: Population estimates used to compute rates for 1991–2000 differ from those used previously. Starting with *Health, United States, 2003*, rates for 1991–99 were revised using intercensal population estimates based on Census 2000. Rates for 2000 were revised based on Census 2000 counts. See Appendix I, Population Census and Population Estimates. The race groups, white, black, Asian or Pacific Islander, and American Indian or Alaska Native, include persons of Hispanic and non-Hispanic origin. Persons of Hispanic origin may be of any race. Death rates for the American Indian or Alaska Native and Asian or Pacific Islander populations are known to be underestimated. See Appendix II, Race, for a discussion of sources of bias in death rates by race and Hispanic origin. Categories for the coding and classification of human immunodeficiency virus (HIV) disease were introduced in the United States in 1987. Underlying cause of death code numbers are based on the applicable revision of the *International Classification of Diseases* (ICD) for data years shown. See Appendix II, tables IV and V. Data for additional years are available (see Appendix III).

SOURCES: Centers for Disease Control and Prevention, National Center for Health Statistics, National Vital Statistics System; numerator data from annual mortality files; denominator data from national population estimates for race groups from table 1 and unpublished Hispanic population estimates for 1987–96 prepared by the Housing and Household Economic Statistics Division, U.S. Bureau of the Census; additional mortality tables are available at www.cdc.gov/nchs/datawh/statab/unpubd/mortabs.htm; Anderson RN, Arias E. The effect of revised populations on mortality statistics for the U.S., 2000. National vital statistics reports. Vol 51 no 9. Hyattsville, Maryland: National Center for Health Statistics. 2003.

This table will be updated with 2001 data on the web. Go to www.cdc.gov/nchs/hus.htm.

Table 43. Maternal mortality for complications of pregnancy, childbirth, and the puerperium, according to race, Hispanic origin, and age: United States, selected years 1950–2000

[Data are based on death certificates]

Race, Hispanic origin, and age	1950[1]	1960[1]	1970	1980	1990	1995	1997	1998	1999[2]	2000
	Number of deaths									
All persons	2,960	1,579	803	334	343	277	327	281	391	396
White	1,873	936	445	193	177	129	179	158	214	240
Black or African American	1,041	624	342	127	153	133	125	104	154	137
American Indian or Alaska Native	- - -	- - -	- - -	3	4	1	2	2	5	6
Asian or Pacific Islander	- - -	- - -	- - -	11	9	14	21	17	18	13
Hispanic or Latino[3]	- - -	- - -	- - -	- - -	47	43	57	42	67	81
White, not Hispanic or Latino[3]	- - -	- - -	- - -	- - -	125	84	121	116	149	160
All persons	Deaths per 100,000 live births									
All ages, age adjusted[4]	73.7	32.1	21.5	9.4	7.6	6.3	7.6	6.1	8.3	8.2
All ages, crude	83.3	37.1	21.5	9.2	8.2	7.1	8.4	7.1	9.9	9.8
Under 20 years	70.7	22.7	18.9	7.6	7.5	3.9	5.7	*	6.6	*
20–24 years	47.6	20.7	13.0	5.8	6.1	5.7	6.6	5.0	6.2	7.4
25–29 years	63.5	29.8	17.0	7.7	6.0	6.0	7.9	6.7	8.2	7.9
30–34 years	107.7	50.3	31.6	13.6	9.5	7.3	8.3	7.5	10.1	10.0
35 years and over[5]	222.0	104.3	81.9	36.3	20.7	15.9	16.1	14.5	23.0	22.7
White										
All ages, age adjusted[4]	53.1	22.4	14.4	6.7	5.1	3.6	5.2	4.2	5.5	6.2
All ages, crude	61.1	26.0	14.3	6.6	5.4	4.2	5.8	5.1	6.8	7.5
Under 20 years	44.9	14.8	13.8	5.8	*	*	*	*	*	*
20–24 years	35.7	15.3	8.4	4.2	3.9	3.5	4.2	3.1	4.0	5.6
25–29 years	45.0	20.3	11.1	5.4	4.8	4.0	5.4	4.9	5.4	5.9
30–34 years	75.9	34.3	18.7	9.3	5.0	4.0	5.4	4.9	7.0	7.1
35 years and over[5]	174.1	73.9	59.3	25.5	12.6	9.1	11.5	11.0	16.6	18.0
Black or African American										
All ages, age adjusted[4]	- - -	92.0	65.5	24.9	21.7	20.9	20.1	16.1	23.3	20.1
All ages, crude	- - -	103.6	60.9	22.4	22.4	22.1	20.8	17.1	25.4	22.0
Under 20 years	- - -	54.8	32.3	13.1	*	*	*	*	*	*
20–24 years	- - -	56.9	41.9	13.9	14.7	15.3	15.3	12.7	14.0	15.3
25–29 years	- - -	92.8	65.2	22.4	14.9	21.0	24.3	17.2	26.6	21.8
30–34 years	- - -	150.6	117.8	44.0	44.2	31.2	32.9	27.7	36.1	34.8
35 years and over[5]	- - -	299.5	207.5	100.6	79.7	61.4	40.4	37.2	69.9	62.8
Hispanic or Latino[3,6]										
All ages, age adjusted[4]	- - -	- - -	- - -	- - -	7.4	5.4	7.6	5.2	7.9	9.0
All ages, crude	- - -	- - -	- - -	- - -	7.9	6.3	8.0	5.7	8.8	9.9
White, not Hispanic or Latino[3]										
All ages, age adjusted[4]	- - -	- - -	- - -	- - -	4.4	3.3	4.4	4.0	4.9	5.5
All ages, crude	- - -	- - -	- - -	- - -	4.8	3.5	5.2	4.9	6.4	6.8

- - - Data not available.

* Rates based on fewer than 20 deaths are considered unreliable and are not shown.

[1]Includes deaths of persons who were not residents of the 50 States and the District of Columbia.

[2]Starting with 1999 data, changes have been made in the classification and coding of maternal deaths under ICD–10. The large increase in the number of maternal deaths between 1998 and 1999 is due to changes associated with ICD–10. See Appendix II, *International Classification of Diseases (ICD)*; Maternal death.

[3]Prior to 1997, excludes data from States lacking an Hispanic-origin item on the death certificate. See Appendix II, Hispanic origin.

[4]Rates are age adjusted to the 1970 distribution of live births by mother's age in the United States. See Appendix II, Age adjustment.

[5]Rates computed by relating deaths of women 35 years and over to live births to women 35–49 years. See Appendix II, Rate: Death and related rates.

[6]Age-specific maternal mortality rates are not calculated because rates based on fewer than 20 deaths are considered unreliable.

NOTES: Underlying cause of death code numbers are based on the applicable revision of the *International Classification of Diseases* (ICD) for data years shown. See Appendix II, tables IV and V. The race groups, white, black, Asian or Pacific Islander, and American Indian or Alaska Native, include persons of Hispanic and non-Hispanic origin. Persons of Hispanic origin may be of any race. For 1950 and 1960, rates were based on live births by race of child; for all other years, rates are based on live births by race of mother. See Appendix II, Race. Rates are not calculated for American Indian or Alaska Native and Asian or Pacific Islander mothers because rates based on fewer than 20 deaths are considered unreliable. Data for additional years are available (see Appendix III).

SOURCES: Centers for Disease Control and Prevention, National Center for Health Statistics, National Vital Statistics System; numerator data from annual mortality files; denominator data from annual natality files; Minino AM, Arias E, Kochanek KD, Murphy SL, Smith BL. Deaths: Final data for 2000. National vital statistics reports. Vol 50 no 15. Hyattsville, Maryland: National Center for Health Statistics. 2002.

This table will be updated with 2001 data on the web. Go to www.cdc.gov/nchs/hus.htm.

Table 44 (page 1 of 4). Death rates for motor vehicle-related injuries, according to sex, race, Hispanic origin, and age: United States, selected years 1950–2000

[Data are based on death certificates]

Sex, race, Hispanic origin, and age	1950[1]	1960[1]	1970	1980	1990	1995	1999[2]	2000
All persons				Deaths per 100,000 resident population				
All ages, age adjusted[3]	24.6	23.1	27.6	22.3	18.5	16.3	15.2	15.4
All ages, crude	23.1	21.3	26.9	23.5	18.8	16.3	15.2	15.4
Under 1 year.	8.4	8.1	9.8	7.0	4.9	4.7	4.8	4.4
1–14 years	9.8	8.6	10.5	8.2	6.0	5.3	4.3	4.3
1–4 years	11.5	10.0	11.5	9.2	6.3	5.2	4.2	4.2
5–14 years	8.8	7.9	10.2	7.9	5.9	5.3	4.3	4.3
15–24 years	34.4	38.0	47.2	44.8	34.1	28.9	26.2	26.9
15–19 years	29.6	33.9	43.6	43.0	33.1	28.1	25.9	26.0
20–24 years.	38.8	42.9	51.3	46.6	35.0	29.7	26.5	28.0
25–34 years	24.6	24.3	30.9	29.1	23.6	19.2	16.9	17.3
35–44 years	20.3	19.3	24.9	20.9	16.9	15.3	14.9	15.3
45–64 years	25.2	23.0	26.5	18.0	15.7	14.1	13.8	14.3
45–54 years.	22.2	21.4	25.5	18.6	15.6	13.8	13.6	14.2
55–64 years.	29.0	25.1	27.9	17.4	15.9	14.5	14.2	14.4
65 years and over	43.1	34.7	36.2	22.5	23.1	22.6	22.4	21.4
65–74 years.	39.1	31.4	32.8	19.2	18.6	17.5	17.8	16.5
75–84 years.	52.7	41.8	43.5	28.1	29.1	28.4	26.5	25.7
85 years and over	45.1	37.9	34.2	27.6	31.2	31.0	30.4	30.4
Male								
All ages, age adjusted[3]	38.5	35.4	41.5	33.6	26.5	22.8	21.3	21.7
All ages, crude	35.4	31.8	39.7	35.3	26.7	22.4	20.9	21.3
Under 1 year.	9.1	8.6	9.3	7.3	5.0	4.9	5.0	4.6
1–14 years	12.3	10.7	13.0	10.0	7.0	6.1	5.0	4.9
1–4 years	13.0	11.5	12.9	10.2	6.9	5.6	4.7	4.7
5–14 years	11.9	10.4	13.1	9.9	7.0	6.3	5.1	5.0
15–24 years	56.7	61.2	73.2	68.4	49.5	40.5	36.0	37.4
15–19 years.	46.3	51.7	64.1	62.6	45.5	36.1	33.1	33.9
20–24 years.	66.7	73.2	84.4	74.3	53.3	45.0	39.1	41.2
25–34 years	40.8	40.1	49.4	46.3	35.7	28.1	24.7	25.5
35–44 years	32.5	29.9	37.7	31.7	24.7	21.7	21.1	22.0
45–64 years	37.7	33.3	38.9	26.5	21.9	19.5	19.3	20.2
45–54 years.	33.6	31.6	37.2	27.6	22.0	19.3	19.4	20.4
55–64 years.	43.1	35.6	40.9	25.4	21.7	19.6	19.3	19.8
65 years and over	66.6	52.1	54.4	33.9	32.1	30.7	31.3	29.5
65–74 years.	59.1	45.8	47.3	27.3	24.2	22.2	23.3	21.7
75–84 years.	85.0	66.0	68.2	44.3	41.2	39.9	38.0	35.6
85 years and over	78.1	62.7	63.1	56.1	64.5	61.5	59.8	57.5
Female								
All ages, age adjusted[3]	11.5	11.7	14.9	11.8	11.0	10.3	9.6	9.5
All ages, crude	10.9	11.0	14.7	12.3	11.3	10.4	9.7	9.7
Under 1 year.	7.6	7.5	10.4	6.7	4.9	4.5	4.7	4.2
1–14 years	7.2	6.3	7.9	6.3	4.9	4.4	3.6	3.7
1–4 years	10.0	8.4	10.0	8.1	5.6	4.8	3.8	3.8
5–14 years	5.7	5.4	7.2	5.7	4.7	4.2	3.6	3.6
15–24 years	12.6	15.1	21.6	20.8	17.9	16.8	15.9	15.9
15–19 years.	12.9	16.0	22.7	22.8	20.0	19.7	18.3	17.5
20–24 years.	12.2	14.0	20.4	18.9	16.0	13.8	13.4	14.2
25–34 years	9.3	9.2	13.0	12.2	11.5	10.2	8.9	8.8
35–44 years	8.5	9.1	12.9	10.4	9.2	9.0	8.8	8.8
45–64 years	12.6	13.1	15.3	10.3	10.1	9.0	8.6	8.7
45–54 years.	10.9	11.6	14.5	10.2	9.6	8.4	8.0	8.2
55–64 years.	14.9	15.2	16.2	10.5	10.8	9.9	9.5	9.5
65 years and over	21.9	20.3	23.1	15.0	17.2	17.0	16.1	15.8
65–74 years.	20.6	19.0	21.6	13.0	14.1	13.7	13.3	12.3
75–84 years.	25.2	23.0	27.2	18.5	21.9	21.2	19.1	19.2
85 years and over	22.1	22.0	18.0	15.2	18.3	19.3	18.5	19.3
White male[4]								
All ages, age adjusted[3]	37.9	34.8	40.4	33.8	26.3	22.6	21.3	21.8
All ages, crude	35.1	31.5	39.1	35.9	26.7	22.4	21.1	21.6
Under 1 year.	9.1	8.8	9.1	7.0	4.8	4.3	5.0	4.2
1–14 years	12.4	10.6	12.5	9.8	6.6	5.9	4.8	4.8
15–24 years	58.3	62.7	75.2	73.8	52.5	42.4	37.8	39.6
25–34 years	39.1	38.6	47.0	46.6	35.4	27.9	24.6	25.1
35–44 years	30.9	28.4	35.2	30.7	23.7	21.1	20.9	21.8
45–64 years	36.2	31.7	36.5	25.2	20.6	18.7	18.8	19.7
65 years and over	67.1	52.1	54.2	32.7	31.4	30.1	31.2	29.4

See footnotes at end of table.

Table 44 (page 2 of 4). **Death rates for motor vehicle-related injuries, according to sex, race, Hispanic origin, and age: United States, selected years 1950–2000**

[Data are based on death certificates]

Sex, race, Hispanic origin, and age	1950[1]	1960[1]	1970	1980	1990	1995	1999[2]	2000
Black or African American male[4]				Deaths per 100,000 resident population				
All ages, age adjusted[3]	34.8	39.6	51.0	34.2	29.9	26.1	24.3	24.4
All ages, crude	37.2	33.1	44.3	31.1	28.1	24.1	22.2	22.5
Under 1 year	- - -	*	10.6	7.8	*	8.7	*	6.7
1–14 years[5]	10.4	11.2	16.3	11.4	8.9	7.5	6.3	5.5
15–24 years	42.5	46.4	58.1	34.9	36.1	33.9	30.5	30.2
25–34 years	54.4	51.0	70.4	44.9	39.5	32.2	29.7	32.6
35–44 years	46.7	43.6	59.5	41.2	33.5	28.7	26.3	27.2
45–64 years	54.6	47.8	61.7	39.5	33.3	26.2	26.5	27.1
65 years and over	52.6	48.2	53.4	42.4	36.3	36.9	33.6	32.1
American Indian or Alaska Native male[4]								
All ages, age adjusted[3]	- - -	- - -	- - -	78.9	48.3	40.7	37.5	35.8
All ages, crude	- - -	- - -	- - -	74.6	47.6	40.1	34.1	33.6
1–14 years	- - -	- - -	- - -	15.1	11.6	7.6	7.6	7.8
15–24 years	- - -	- - -	- - -	126.1	75.2	69.0	58.0	56.8
25–34 years	- - -	- - -	- - -	107.0	78.2	67.8	40.8	49.8
35–44 years	- - -	- - -	- - -	82.8	57.0	45.2	38.6	36.3
45–64 years	- - -	- - -	- - -	77.4	45.9	38.8	38.8	32.0
65 years and over	- - -	- - -	- - -	97.0	43.0	*	57.3	48.5
Asian or Pacific Islander male[4]								
All ages, age adjusted[3]	- - -	- - -	- - -	19.0	17.9	14.5	9.8	10.6
All ages, crude	- - -	- - -	- - -	17.1	15.8	12.6	8.9	9.8
1–14 years	- - -	- - -	- - -	8.2	6.3	4.5	2.4	2.5
15–24 years	- - -	- - -	- - -	27.2	25.7	18.5	14.8	17.0
25–34 years	- - -	- - -	- - -	18.8	17.0	12.4	9.2	10.4
35–44 years	- - -	- - -	- - -	13.1	12.2	9.9	7.4	6.9
45–64 years	- - -	- - -	- - -	13.7	15.1	14.3	8.5	10.1
65 years and over	- - -	- - -	- - -	37.3	33.6	32.1	20.8	21.1
Hispanic or Latino male[4,6]								
All ages, age adjusted[3]	- - -	- - -	- - -	- - -	29.5	24.4	20.4	21.3
All ages, crude	- - -	- - -	- - -	- - -	29.2	22.4	19.1	20.1
1–14 years	- - -	- - -	- - -	- - -	7.2	5.7	4.6	4.4
15–24 years	- - -	- - -	- - -	- - -	48.2	37.1	31.6	34.7
25–34 years	- - -	- - -	- - -	- - -	41.0	28.8	24.4	24.9
35–44 years	- - -	- - -	- - -	- - -	28.0	23.2	20.8	21.6
45–64 years	- - -	- - -	- - -	- - -	28.9	23.0	19.7	21.7
65 years and over	- - -	- - -	- - -	- - -	35.3	37.0	30.6	28.9
White, not Hispanic or Latino male[6]								
All ages, age adjusted[3]	- - -	- - -	- - -	- - -	25.7	22.1	21.3	21.7
All ages, crude	- - -	- - -	- - -	- - -	26.0	21.9	21.1	21.5
1–14 years	- - -	- - -	- - -	- - -	6.4	5.8	4.7	4.9
15–24 years	- - -	- - -	- - -	- - -	52.3	42.7	38.8	40.3
25–34 years	- - -	- - -	- - -	- - -	34.0	27.1	24.2	24.7
35–44 years	- - -	- - -	- - -	- - -	23.1	20.3	20.6	21.6
45–64 years	- - -	- - -	- - -	- - -	19.8	18.1	18.5	19.3
65 years and over	- - -	- - -	- - -	- - -	31.1	29.4	31.1	29.3
White female[4]								
All ages, age adjusted[3]	11.4	11.7	14.9	12.2	11.2	10.4	9.7	9.8
All ages, crude	10.9	11.2	14.8	12.8	11.6	10.7	10.0	10.0
Under 1 year	7.8	7.5	10.2	7.1	4.7	4.5	3.9	3.5
1–14 years	7.2	6.2	7.5	6.2	4.8	4.3	3.5	3.7
15–24 years	12.6	15.6	22.7	23.0	19.5	18.1	17.1	17.1
25–34 years	9.0	9.0	12.7	12.2	11.6	10.2	9.1	8.9
35–44 years	8.1	8.9	12.3	10.6	9.2	8.9	8.8	8.9
45–64 years	12.7	13.1	15.1	10.4	9.9	8.9	8.5	8.7
65 years and over	22.2	20.8	23.7	15.3	17.4	17.5	16.4	16.2

See footnotes at end of table.

[Data are based on death certificates]

Sex, race, Hispanic origin, and age	1950[1]	1960[1]	1970	1980	1990	1995	1999[2]	2000
Black or African American female[4]				Deaths per 100,000 resident population				
All ages, age adjusted[3]	9.3	10.4	14.1	8.5	9.6	9.0	9.0	8.4
All ages, crude	10.2	9.7	13.4	8.3	9.4	8.8	8.7	8.2
Under 1 year.	- - -	8.1	11.9	*	7.0	*	8.7	*
1–14 years[5]	7.2	6.9	10.2	6.3	5.3	4.9	4.4	3.9
15–24 years	11.6	9.9	13.4	8.0	9.9	10.5	11.8	11.7
25–34 years	10.8	9.8	13.3	10.6	11.1	10.3	8.6	9.4
35–44 years	11.1	11.0	16.1	8.3	9.4	9.7	9.6	8.2
45–64 years	11.8	12.7	16.7	9.2	10.7	9.3	8.9	9.0
65 years and over	14.3	13.2	15.7	9.5	13.5	11.4	12.8	10.4
American Indian or Alaska Native female[4]								
All ages, age adjusted[3]	- - -	- - -	- - -	32.0	17.5	18.2	18.9	19.5
All ages, crude	- - -	- - -	- - -	32.0	17.3	18.8	17.5	18.6
1–14 years	- - -	- - -	- - -	15.0	8.1	8.1	*	6.5
15–24 years	- - -	- - -	- - -	42.3	31.4	30.4	25.2	30.3
25–34 years	- - -	- - -	- - -	52.5	18.8	33.7	28.2	22.3
35–44 years	- - -	- - -	- - -	38.1	18.2	17.2	21.7	22.0
45–64 years	- - -	- - -	- - -	32.6	17.6	15.7	14.8	17.8
65 years and over	- - -	- - -	- - -	*	*	*	30.9	24.0
Asian or Pacific Islander female[4]								
All ages, age adjusted[3]	- - -	- - -	- - -	9.3	10.4	8.6	7.0	6.7
All ages, crude	- - -	- - -	- - -	8.2	9.0	7.7	6.3	5.9
1–14 years	- - -	- - -	- - -	7.4	3.6	3.2	2.0	2.3
15–24 years	- - -	- - -	- - -	7.4	11.4	11.5	7.8	6.0
25–34 years	- - -	- - -	- - -	7.3	7.3	4.8	4.3	4.5
35–44 years	- - -	- - -	- - -	8.6	7.5	5.9	4.5	4.9
45–64 years	- - -	- - -	- - -	8.5	11.8	10.4	9.5	6.4
65 years and over	- - -	- - -	- - -	18.6	24.3	18.9	14.8	18.5
Hispanic or Latino female[4,6]								
All ages, age adjusted[3]	- - -	- - -	- - -	- - -	9.6	8.8	8.0	7.9
All ages, crude	- - -	- - -	- - -	- - -	8.9	8.0	7.2	7.2
1–14 years	- - -	- - -	- - -	- - -	4.8	4.3	3.5	3.9
15–24 years	- - -	- - -	- - -	- - -	11.6	11.8	10.6	10.6
25–34 years	- - -	- - -	- - -	- - -	9.4	7.2	7.1	6.5
35–44 years	- - -	- - -	- - -	- - -	8.0	7.9	6.5	7.3
45–64 years	- - -	- - -	- - -	- - -	11.4	9.3	8.6	8.3
65 years and over	- - -	- - -	- - -	- - -	14.9	14.6	14.3	13.4

See footnotes at end of table.

Table 44 (page 4 of 4). Death rates for motor vehicle-related injuries, according to sex, race, Hispanic origin, and age: United States, selected years 1950–2000

[Data are based on death certificates]

Sex, race, Hispanic origin, and age	1950[1]	1960[1]	1970	1980	1990	1995	1999[2]	2000
White, not Hispanic or Latino female[6]				Deaths per 100,000 resident population				
All ages, age adjusted[3]	- - -	- - -	- - -	- - -	11.3	10.5	9.9	10.0
All ages, crude	- - -	- - -	- - -	- - -	11.7	10.9	10.3	10.3
1–14 years	- - -	- - -	- - -	- - -	4.7	4.2	3.5	3.5
15–24 years	- - -	- - -	- - -	- - -	20.4	19.0	18.3	18.4
25–34 years	- - -	- - -	- - -	- - -	11.7	10.5	9.4	9.3
35–44 years	- - -	- - -	- - -	- - -	9.3	8.9	9.0	9.0
45–64 years	- - -	- - -	- - -	- - -	9.7	8.6	8.4	8.7
65 years and over	- - -	- - -	- - -	- - -	17.5	17.5	16.5	16.3

- - - Data not available.

* Rates based on fewer than 20 deaths are considered unreliable and are not shown.

[1]Includes deaths of persons who were not residents of the 50 States and the District of Columbia.

[2]Starting with 1999 data, cause of death is coded according to ICD–10. To estimate change between 1998 and 1999, compare the 1999 rate with the comparability-modified rate for 1998. See Appendix II, Comparability ratio and tables V and VI.

[3]Age-adjusted rates are calculated using the year 2000 standard population starting with *Health, United States, 2001*. See Appendix II, Age adjustment.

[4]The race groups, white, black, Asian or Pacific Islander, and American Indian or Alaska Native, include persons of Hispanic and non-Hispanic origin. Persons of Hispanic origin may be of any race. Death rates for the American Indian or Alaska Native and Asian or Pacific Islander populations are known to be underestimated. See Appendix II, Race, for a discussion of sources of bias in death rates by race and Hispanic origin.

[5]In 1950 rate is for the age group under 15 years.

[6]Prior to 1997, excludes data from States lacking an Hispanic-origin item on the death certificate. See Appendix II, Hispanic origin.

NOTES: Population estimates used to compute rates for 1991–2000 differ from those used previously. Starting with *Health, United States, 2003*, rates for 1991–99 were revised using intercensal population estimates based on Census 2000. Rates for 2000 were revised based on Census 2000 counts. See Appendix I, Population Census and Population Estimates. Underlying cause of death code numbers are based on the applicable revision of the *International Classification of Diseases* (ICD) for data years shown. See Appendix II, tables IV and V. Age groups were selected to minimize the presentation of unstable age-specific death rates based on small numbers of deaths and for consistency among comparison groups. For additional injury-related statistics, see www.cdc.gov/ncipc/wisqars, a Web-based interactive database for injury data. Data for additional years are available (see Appendix III).

SOURCES: Centers for Disease Control and Prevention, National Center for Health Statistics, National Vital Statistics System; Grove RD, Hetzel AM. Vital statistics rates in the United States, 1940–1960. Washington: U.S. Government Printing Office. 1968; numerator data from National Vital Statistics System, annual mortality files; denominator data from national population estimates for race groups from table 1 and unpublished Hispanic population estimates for 1985–96 prepared by the Housing and Household Economic Statistics Division, U.S. Bureau of the Census; additional mortality tables are available at www.cdc.gov/nchs/datawh/statab/unpubd/mortabs.htm; Anderson RN, Arias E. The effect of revised populations on mortality statistics for the U.S., 2000. National vital statistics reports. Vol 51 no 9. Hyattsville, Maryland: National Center for Health Statistics. 2003.

This table will be updated with 2001 data on the web. Go to www.cdc.gov/nchs/hus.htm.

Table 45 (page 1 of 3). Death rates for homicide, according to sex, race, Hispanic origin, and age: United States, selected years 1950–2000

[Data are based on death certificates]

Sex, race, Hispanic origin, and age	1950[1]	1960[1]	1970	1980	1990	1995	1999[2]	2000
All persons			Deaths per 100,000 resident population					
All ages, age adjusted	5.1	5.0	8.8	10.4	9.4	8.3	6.0	5.9
All ages, crude	5.0	4.6	8.1	10.6	9.9	8.5	6.1	6.0
Under 1 year	4.4	4.8	4.3	5.9	8.4	8.2	8.7	9.2
1–14 years	0.6	0.6	1.1	1.5	1.8	1.9	1.4	1.3
1–4 years	0.6	0.7	1.9	2.5	2.5	2.9	2.5	2.3
5–14 years	0.5	0.5	0.9	1.2	1.5	1.5	1.1	0.9
15–24 years	5.8	5.6	11.3	15.4	19.7	19.6	12.9	12.6
15–19 years	3.9	3.9	7.7	10.5	16.9	17.8	10.4	9.5
20–24 years	8.5	7.7	15.6	20.2	22.2	21.5	15.6	16.0
25–44 years	8.9	8.5	14.9	17.5	14.7	11.9	8.7	8.7
25–34 years	9.3	9.2	16.2	19.3	17.4	14.4	10.5	10.4
35–44 years	8.4	7.8	13.5	14.9	11.6	9.4	7.1	7.1
45–64 years	5.0	5.3	8.7	9.0	6.3	5.4	4.0	4.0
45–54 years	5.9	6.1	10.0	11.0	7.5	6.0	4.6	4.7
55–64 years	3.9	4.1	7.1	7.0	5.0	4.4	3.0	3.0
65 years and over	3.0	2.7	4.6	5.5	4.0	3.1	2.5	2.4
65–74 years	3.2	2.8	4.9	5.7	3.8	3.2	2.6	2.4
75–84 years	2.5	2.3	4.0	5.2	4.3	3.0	2.5	2.4
85 years and over	2.3	2.4	4.2	5.3	4.6	3.2	2.4	2.4
Male								
All ages, age adjusted[3]	7.9	7.5	14.3	16.6	14.8	12.8	9.1	9.0
All ages, crude	7.7	6.8	13.1	17.1	15.9	13.4	9.3	9.3
Under 1 year	4.5	4.7	4.5	6.3	8.8	9.0	9.6	10.4
1–14 years	0.6	0.6	1.2	1.6	2.0	2.2	1.5	1.5
1–4 years	0.5	0.7	1.9	2.7	2.7	3.1	2.5	2.5
5–14 years	0.6	0.5	1.0	1.2	1.7	1.9	1.2	1.1
15–24 years	8.6	8.4	18.2	24.0	32.5	32.8	21.1	20.9
15–19 years	5.5	5.7	12.1	15.9	27.8	29.1	16.9	15.5
20–24 years	13.5	11.8	25.6	32.2	36.9	36.5	25.7	26.7
25–44 years	13.8	12.8	24.4	28.9	23.5	18.2	13.3	13.3
25–34 years	14.4	13.9	26.8	31.9	27.7	22.5	16.5	16.7
35–44 years	13.2	11.7	21.7	24.5	18.6	14.0	10.3	10.3
45–64 years	8.1	8.1	14.8	15.2	10.2	8.3	6.0	6.0
45–54 years	9.5	9.4	16.8	18.4	11.9	9.2	6.8	6.9
55–64 years	6.3	6.4	12.1	11.8	8.0	7.0	4.7	4.6
65 years and over	4.8	4.3	7.7	8.8	5.8	4.2	3.5	3.3
65–74 years	5.2	4.6	8.5	9.2	5.8	4.5	3.7	3.4
75–84 years	3.9	3.7	5.9	8.1	5.7	3.7	3.4	3.2
85 years and over	2.5	3.6	7.4	7.5	6.7	4.1	3.4	3.3
Female								
All ages, age adjusted[3]	2.4	2.6	3.7	4.4	4.0	3.7	2.9	2.8
All ages, crude	2.4	2.4	3.4	4.5	4.2	3.8	2.9	2.8
Under 1 year	4.2	4.9	4.1	5.6	8.0	7.4	7.8	7.9
1–14 years	0.6	0.5	1.0	1.4	1.6	1.5	1.3	1.1
1–4 years	0.7	0.7	1.9	2.2	2.3	2.6	2.4	2.1
5–14 years	0.5	0.4	0.7	1.1	1.2	1.0	0.9	0.7
15–24 years	3.0	2.8	4.6	6.6	6.2	5.9	4.3	3.9
15–19 years	2.4	1.9	3.2	4.9	5.4	5.8	3.5	3.1
20–24 years	3.7	3.8	6.2	8.2	7.0	6.0	5.1	4.7
25–44 years	4.2	4.3	5.8	6.4	6.0	5.6	4.2	4.0
25–34 years	4.5	4.6	6.0	6.9	7.1	6.3	4.4	4.1
35–44 years	3.8	4.0	5.7	5.7	4.8	4.9	4.0	4.0
45–64 years	1.9	2.5	3.1	3.4	2.8	2.6	2.0	2.1
45–54 years	2.3	2.9	3.7	4.1	3.2	2.9	2.4	2.5
55–64 years	1.4	2.0	2.5	2.8	2.3	2.1	1.5	1.6
65 years and over	1.4	1.3	2.3	3.3	2.8	2.4	1.8	1.8
65–74 years	1.3	1.3	2.2	3.0	2.2	2.1	1.7	1.6
75–84 years	1.4	1.3	2.7	3.5	3.4	2.6	1.9	2.0
85 years and over	2.1	1.6	2.5	4.3	3.8	2.9	2.0	2.0
White male[4]								
All ages, age adjusted[3]	3.8	3.9	7.2	10.4	8.3	7.3	5.4	5.2
All ages, crude	3.6	3.6	6.6	10.7	8.8	7.5	5.5	5.2
Under 1 year	4.3	3.8	2.9	4.3	6.4	7.1	7.9	8.2
1–14 years	0.4	0.5	0.7	1.2	1.3	1.5	1.1	1.2
15–24 years	3.2	5.0	7.6	15.1	15.2	15.9	10.3	9.9
25–44 years	5.4	5.5	11.6	17.2	13.0	10.4	7.7	7.4
25–34 years	4.9	5.7	12.5	18.5	14.7	12.1	8.8	8.4
35–44 years	6.1	5.2	10.8	15.2	11.1	8.7	6.7	6.5
45–64 years	4.8	4.6	8.3	9.8	6.9	5.5	4.3	4.1
65 years and over	3.8	3.1	5.4	6.7	4.1	2.9	2.8	2.5

See footnotes at end of table.

Table 45 (page 2 of 3). Death rates for homicide, according to sex, race, Hispanic origin, and age: United States, selected years 1950–2000

[Data are based on death certificates]

Sex, race, Hispanic origin, and age	1950[1]	1960[1]	1970	1980	1990	1995	1999[2]	2000
Black or African American male[4]			Deaths per 100,000 resident population					
All ages, age adjusted[3]	47.0	42.3	78.2	69.4	63.1	51.1	34.2	35.4
All ages, crude	44.7	35.0	66.0	65.7	68.5	54.5	36.1	37.2
Under 1 year	- - -	10.3	14.3	18.6	21.4	20.3	19.5	23.3
1–14 years[5]	1.8	1.5	4.4	4.1	5.8	5.8	3.5	3.1
15–24 years	53.8	43.2	98.3	82.6	137.1	129.4	84.7	85.3
25–44 years	92.8	80.5	140.2	130.0	105.4	75.8	53.0	55.8
25–34 years	104.3	86.4	154.5	142.9	123.7	95.1	69.2	73.9
35–44 years	80.0	74.4	124.0	109.3	81.2	54.9	37.2	38.5
45–64 years	46.0	44.6	82.3	70.6	41.4	33.4	20.4	21.9
65 years and over	16.5	17.3	33.3	30.9	25.7	20.3	11.9	12.8
American Indian or Alaska Native male[4]								
All ages, age adjusted[3]	- - -	- - -	- - -	23.3	16.7	14.4	13.5	10.7
All ages, crude	- - -	- - -	- - -	23.1	16.6	15.7	12.7	10.7
15–24 years	- - -	- - -	- - -	35.4	25.1	28.0	17.5	17.0
25–44 years	- - -	- - -	- - -	39.2	25.7	24.6	18.3	17.0
45–64 years	- - -	- - -	- - -	22.1	14.8	12.0	14.1	*
Asian or Pacific Islander male[4]								
All ages, age adjusted[3]	- - -	- - -	- - -	9.1	7.3	7.2	3.9	4.3
All ages, crude	- - -	- - -	- - -	8.3	7.9	7.5	4.2	4.4
15–24 years	- - -	- - -	- - -	9.3	14.9	17.2	7.8	7.8
25–44 years	- - -	- - -	- - -	11.3	9.6	7.4	4.7	4.6
45–64 years	- - -	- - -	- - -	10.4	7.0	7.7	4.3	6.1
Hispanic or Latino male[4,6]								
All ages, age adjusted[3]	- - -	- - -	- - -	- - -	27.4	20.4	12.2	11.8
All ages, crude	- - -	- - -	- - -	- - -	31.0	23.5	13.8	13.4
Under 1 year	- - -	- - -	- - -	- - -	8.7	5.9	6.7	6.6
1–14 years	- - -	- - -	- - -	- - -	3.1	3.2	1.8	1.7
15–24 years	- - -	- - -	- - -	- - -	55.4	54.7	29.1	28.5
25–44 years	- - -	- - -	- - -	- - -	46.4	28.8	17.7	17.2
25–34 years	- - -	- - -	- - -	- - -	50.9	33.0	20.6	19.9
35–44 years	- - -	- - -	- - -	- - -	39.3	22.8	13.9	13.5
45–64 years	- - -	- - -	- - -	- - -	20.5	14.7	9.2	9.1
65 years and over	- - -	- - -	- - -	- - -	9.4	5.8	5.2	4.4
White, not Hispanic or Latino male[6]								
All ages, age adjusted[3]	- - -	- - -	- - -	- - -	5.6	4.8	3.8	3.6
All ages, crude	- - -	- - -	- - -	- - -	5.8	4.9	3.9	3.6
Under 1 year	- - -	- - -	- - -	- - -	5.4	6.8	8.0	8.3
1–14 years	- - -	- - -	- - -	- - -	0.9	1.1	1.0	1.0
15–24 years	- - -	- - -	- - -	- - -	7.5	7.2	5.1	4.7
25–44 years	- - -	- - -	- - -	- - -	8.7	7.2	5.6	5.2
25–34 years	- - -	- - -	- - -	- - -	9.3	7.7	5.7	5.2
35–44 years	- - -	- - -	- - -	- - -	8.0	6.7	5.4	5.2
45–64 years	- - -	- - -	- - -	- - -	5.7	4.6	3.8	3.6
65 years and over	- - -	- - -	- - -	- - -	3.7	2.6	2.7	2.3
White female[4]								
All ages, age adjusted[3]	1.4	1.5	2.3	3.2	2.7	2.7	2.1	2.1
All ages, crude	1.4	1.4	2.1	3.2	2.8	2.7	2.1	2.1
Under 1 year	3.9	3.5	2.9	4.3	5.1	5.1	5.4	5.0
1–14 years	0.4	0.4	0.7	1.1	1.0	1.1	1.0	0.8
15–24 years	1.3	1.5	2.7	4.7	4.0	4.0	3.0	2.7
25–44 years	2.0	2.1	3.3	4.2	3.8	3.7	2.9	2.9
45–64 years	1.5	1.7	2.1	2.6	2.3	2.2	1.6	1.8
65 years and over	1.2	1.2	1.9	2.9	2.2	2.0	1.6	1.6
Black or African American female[4]								
All ages, age adjusted[3]	11.1	11.4	14.7	13.2	12.5	10.4	7.3	7.1
All ages, crude	11.5	10.4	13.2	13.5	13.4	10.9	7.6	7.2
Under 1 year	- - -	13.8	10.7	12.8	22.8	20.1	19.5	22.2
1–14 years[5]	1.8	1.2	3.1	3.3	4.7	3.4	2.9	2.7
15–24 years	16.5	11.9	17.7	18.4	18.9	16.4	11.2	10.7
25–44 years	22.5	22.7	25.3	22.6	21.0	17.1	11.6	11.0
45–64 years	6.8	10.3	13.4	10.8	6.5	5.9	4.7	4.5
65 years and over	3.6	3.0	7.4	8.0	9.4	6.8	3.4	3.5

See footnotes at end of table.

Table 45 (page 3 of 3). Death rates for homicide, according to sex, race, Hispanic origin, and age: United States, selected years 1950–2000

[Data are based on death certificates]

Sex, race, Hispanic origin, and age	1950[1]	1960[1]	1970	1980	1990	1995	1999[2]	2000
American Indian or Alaska Native female[4]				Deaths per 100,000 resident population				
All ages, age adjusted[3]	- - -	- - -	- - -	8.1	4.6	5.3	5.1	3.0
All ages, crude	- - -	- - -	- - -	7.7	4.8	5.1	5.2	2.9
15–24 years	- - -	- - -	- - -	*	*	*	*	*
25–44 years	- - -	- - -	- - -	13.7	6.9	8.3	8.4	5.9
45–64 years	- - -	- - -	- - -	*	*	*	*	*
Asian or Pacific Islander female[4]								
All ages, age adjusted[3]	- - -	- - -	- - -	3.1	2.8	2.4	2.2	1.7
All ages, crude	- - -	- - -	- - -	3.1	2.8	2.6	2.2	1.7
15–24 years	- - -	- - -	- - -	*	*	3.4	2.5	*
25–44 years	- - -	- - -	- - -	4.6	3.8	3.6	2.6	2.2
45–64 years	- - -	- - -	- - -	*	*	2.2	2.1	2.0
Hispanic or Latino female[4,6]								
All ages, age adjusted[3]	- - -	- - -	- - -	- - -	4.3	4.0	2.6	2.8
All ages, crude	- - -	- - -	- - -	- - -	4.7	4.2	2.8	2.8
Under 1 year	- - -	- - -	- - -	- - -	*	*	7.3	7.4
1–14 years	- - -	- - -	- - -	- - -	1.9	1.8	1.2	1.0
15–24 years	- - -	- - -	- - -	- - -	8.1	6.4	4.4	3.7
25–44 years	- - -	- - -	- - -	- - -	6.1	5.6	3.4	3.7
45–64 years	- - -	- - -	- - -	- - -	3.3	3.4	2.5	2.9
65 years and over	- - -	- - -	- - -	- - -	*	2.4	*	2.4
White, not Hispanic or Latino female[6]								
All ages, age adjusted[3]	- - -	- - -	- - -	- - -	2.5	2.3	2.0	1.9
All ages, crude	- - -	- - -	- - -	- - -	2.5	2.3	2.0	1.9
Under 1 year	- - -	- - -	- - -	- - -	4.4	4.4	4.4	4.1
1–14 years	- - -	- - -	- - -	- - -	0.8	0.9	0.9	0.8
15–24 years	- - -	- - -	- - -	- - -	3.3	3.4	2.6	2.3
25–44 years	- - -	- - -	- - -	- - -	3.5	3.3	2.8	2.7
45–64 years	- - -	- - -	- - -	- - -	2.2	1.9	1.5	1.6
65 years and over	- - -	- - -	- - -	- - -	2.2	1.9	1.7	1.6

- - - Data not available.

* Rates based on fewer than 20 deaths are considered unreliable and are not shown.

[1] Includes deaths of persons who were not residents of the 50 States and the District of Columbia.

[2] Starting with 1999 data, cause of death is coded according to ICD–10. To estimate change between 1998 and 1999, compare the 1999 rate with the comparability-modified rate for 1998. See Appendix II, Comparability ratio and tables V and VI.

[3] Age-adjusted rates are calculated using the year 2000 standard population starting with *Health, United States, 2001*. See Appendix II, Age adjustment.

[4] The race groups, white, black, Asian or Pacific Islander, and American Indian or Alaska Native, include persons of Hispanic and non-Hispanic origin. Persons of Hispanic origin may be of any race. Death rates for the American Indian or Alaska Native and Asian or Pacific Islander populations are known to be underestimated. See Appendix II, Race, for a discussion of sources of bias in death rates by race and Hispanic origin.

[5] In 1950 rate is for the age group under 15 years.

[6] Prior to 1997, excludes data from States lacking an Hispanic-origin item on the death certificate. See Appendix II, Hispanic origin.

NOTES: Population estimates used to compute rates for 1991–2000 differ from those used previously. Starting with *Health, United States, 2003*, rates for 1991–99 were revised using intercensal population estimates based on Census 2000. Rates for 2000 were revised based on Census 2000 counts. See Appendix I, Population Census and Population Estimates. Underlying cause of death code numbers are based on the applicable revision of the *International Classification of Diseases* (ICD) for data years shown. For the period 1980–98, causes were coded using ICD–9 codes that are most nearly comparable with the 113 cause list for ICD–10. See Appendix II, tables IV and V. Age groups were selected to minimize the presentation of unstable age-specific death rates based on small numbers of deaths and for consistency among comparison groups. For additional injury-related statistics, see www.cdc.gov/ncipc/wisqars, a Web-based interactive database for injury data. Data for additional years are available (see Appendix III).

SOURCES: Centers for Disease Control and Prevention, National Center for Health Statistics, National Vital Statistics System; Grove RD, Hetzel AM. Vital statistics rates in the United States, 1940–1960. Washington: U.S. Government Printing Office. 1968; numerator data from National Vital Statistics System, annual mortality files; denominator data from national population estimates for race groups from table 1 and unpublished Hispanic population estimates for 1985–96 prepared by the Housing and Household Economic Statistics Division, U.S. Bureau of the Census; additional mortality tables are available at www.cdc.gov/nchs/datawh/statab/unpubd/mortabs.htm; Anderson RN, Arias E. The effect of revised populations on mortality statistics for the U.S., 2000. National vital statistics reports. Vol 51 no 9. Hyattsville, Maryland: National Center for Health Statistics. 2003.

This table will be updated with 2001 data on the web. Go to www.cdc.gov/nchs/hus.htm.

[Data are based on death certificates]

Sex, race, Hispanic origin, and age	1950[1]	1960[1]	1970	1980	1990	1995	1999[2]	2000
All persons	Deaths per 100,000 resident population							
All ages, age adjusted[3]	13.2	12.5	13.1	12.2	12.5	11.8	10.5	10.4
All ages, crude	11.4	10.6	11.6	11.9	12.4	11.7	10.5	10.4
Under 1 year.	. . .	. . .	. . .	. . .	. . .	. . .	. . .	. . .
1–4 years	. . .	. . .	. . .	. . .	. . .	. . .	. . .	. . .
5–14 years	0.2	0.3	0.3	0.4	0.8	0.9	0.6	0.7
15–24 years	4.5	5.2	8.8	12.3	13.2	13.0	10.1	10.2
15–19 years.	2.7	3.6	5.9	8.5	11.1	10.3	8.0	8.0
20–24 years.	6.2	7.1	12.2	16.1	15.1	15.8	12.3	12.5
25–44 years	11.6	12.2	15.4	15.6	15.2	15.1	13.6	13.4
25–34 years.	9.1	10.0	14.1	16.0	15.2	15.0	12.7	12.0
35–44 years.	14.3	14.2	16.9	15.4	15.3	15.1	14.3	14.5
45–64 years	23.5	22.0	20.6	15.9	15.3	13.9	13.2	13.5
45–54 years.	20.9	20.7	20.0	15.9	14.8	14.4	13.9	14.4
55–64 years.	26.8	23.7	21.4	15.9	16.0	13.2	12.2	12.1
65 years and over	30.0	24.5	20.8	17.6	20.5	17.9	15.8	15.2
65–74 years.	29.6	23.0	20.8	16.9	17.9	15.7	13.4	12.5
75–84 years.	31.1	27.9	21.2	19.1	24.9	20.6	18.1	17.6
85 years and over	28.8	26.0	19.0	19.2	22.2	21.3	19.3	19.6
Male								
All ages, age adjusted[3]	21.2	20.0	19.8	19.9	21.5	20.3	17.8	17.7
All ages, crude	17.8	16.5	16.8	18.6	20.4	19.5	17.1	17.1
Under 1 year.	. . .	. . .	. . .	. . .	. . .	. . .	. . .	. . .
1–4 years	. . .	. . .	. . .	. . .	. . .	. . .	. . .	. . .
5–14 years	0.3	0.4	0.5	0.6	1.1	1.3	0.9	1.2
15–24 years	6.5	8.2	13.5	20.2	22.0	22.0	16.8	17.1
15–19 years.	3.5	5.6	8.8	13.8	18.1	17.1	13.0	13.0
20–24 years.	9.3	11.5	19.3	26.8	25.7	27.0	20.8	21.4
25–44 years	17.2	17.9	20.9	24.0	24.4	24.4	21.6	21.3
25–34 years.	13.4	14.7	19.8	25.0	24.8	24.8	20.7	19.6
35–44 years.	21.3	21.0	22.1	22.5	23.9	24.0	22.4	22.8
45–64 years	37.1	34.4	30.0	23.7	24.3	22.2	20.8	21.3
45–54 years.	32.0	31.6	27.9	22.9	23.2	22.5	21.5	22.4
55–64 years.	43.6	38.1	32.7	24.5	25.7	21.8	19.8	19.4
65 years and over	52.8	44.0	38.4	35.0	41.6	36.2	32.2	31.1
65–74 years.	50.5	39.6	36.0	30.4	32.2	28.5	24.7	22.7
75–84 years.	58.3	52.5	42.8	42.3	56.1	44.9	38.8	38.6
85 years and over	58.3	57.4	42.4	50.6	65.9	62.7	57.1	57.5
Female								
All ages, age adjusted[3]	5.6	5.6	7.4	5.7	4.8	4.3	4.0	4.0
All ages, crude	5.1	4.9	6.6	5.5	4.8	4.3	4.0	4.0
Under 1 year.	. . .	. . .	. . .	. . .	. . .	. . .	. . .	. . .
1–4 years	. . .	. . .	. . .	. . .	. . .	. . .	. . .	. . .
5–14 years	0.1	0.1	0.2	0.2	0.4	0.4	0.3	0.3
15–24 years	2.6	2.2	4.2	4.3	3.9	3.6	3.0	3.0
15–19 years.	1.8	1.6	2.9	3.0	3.7	3.1	2.7	2.7
20–24 years.	3.3	2.9	5.7	5.5	4.1	4.2	3.4	3.2
25–44 years	6.2	6.6	10.2	7.7	6.2	5.8	5.5	5.4
25–34 years.	4.9	5.5	8.6	7.1	5.6	5.1	4.6	4.3
35–44 years.	7.5	7.7	11.9	8.5	6.8	6.4	6.4	6.4
45–64 years	9.9	10.2	12.0	8.9	7.1	6.1	6.0	6.2
45–54 years.	9.9	10.2	12.6	9.4	6.9	6.6	6.6	6.7
55–64 years.	9.9	10.2	11.4	8.4	7.3	5.3	5.2	5.4
65 years and over	9.4	8.4	8.1	6.1	6.4	5.4	4.3	4.0
65–74 years.	10.1	8.4	9.0	6.5	6.7	5.4	4.1	4.0
75–84 years.	8.1	8.9	7.0	5.5	6.3	5.4	4.7	4.0
85 years and over	8.2	6.0	5.9	5.5	5.4	5.4	4.1	4.2
White male[4]								
All ages, age adjusted[3]	22.3	21.1	20.8	20.9	22.8	21.6	19.0	19.1
All ages, crude	19.0	17.6	18.0	19.9	22.0	21.1	18.7	18.8
15–24 years	6.6	8.6	13.9	21.4	23.2	23.1	17.5	17.9
25–44 years	17.9	18.5	21.5	24.6	25.4	25.8	23.2	22.9
45–64 years	39.3	36.5	31.9	25.0	26.0	23.9	22.6	23.2
65 years and over	55.8	46.7	41.1	37.2	44.2	38.5	34.4	33.3
65–74 years.	53.2	42.0	38.7	32.5	34.2	30.1	26.4	24.3
75–84 years.	61.9	55.7	45.5	45.5	60.2	47.7	41.2	41.1
85 years and over	61.9	61.3	45.8	52.8	70.3	67.9	61.5	61.6

See footnotes at end of table.

Table 46 (page 2 of 3). Death rates for suicide, according to sex, race, Hispanic origin, and age: United States, selected years 1950–2000

[Data are based on death certificates]

Sex, race, Hispanic origin, and age	1950[1]	1960[1]	1970	1980	1990	1995	1999[2]	2000
Black or African American male[4]				Deaths per 100,000 resident population				
All ages, age adjusted[3]	7.5	8.4	10.0	11.4	12.8	12.4	10.3	10.0
All ages, crude	6.3	6.4	8.0	10.3	12.0	11.7	9.6	9.4
15–24 years	4.9	4.1	10.5	12.3	15.1	17.8	14.3	14.2
25–44 years	9.8	12.6	16.1	19.2	19.6	18.3	15.0	14.3
45–64 years	12.7	13.0	12.4	11.8	13.1	11.5	9.7	9.9
65 years and over	9.0	9.9	8.7	11.4	14.9	14.6	12.6	11.5
65–74 years	10.0	11.3	8.7	11.1	14.7	13.8	11.8	11.1
75–84 years[5]	*	*	*	10.5	14.4	16.7	13.8	12.1
85 years and over	- - -	*	*	*	*	*	*	*
American Indian or Alaska Native male[4]								
All ages, age adjusted[3]	- - -	- - -	- - -	19.3	20.1	17.4	16.5	16.0
All ages, crude	- - -	- - -	- - -	20.9	20.9	18.0	16.5	15.9
15–24 years	- - -	- - -	- - -	45.3	49.1	30.8	30.8	26.2
25–44 years	- - -	- - -	- - -	31.2	27.8	29.1	25.1	24.5
45–64 years	- - -	- - -	- - -	*	*	13.6	13.2	15.4
65 years and over	- - -	- - -	- - -	*	*	*	*	*
Asian or Pacific Islander male[4]								
All ages, age adjusted[3]	- - -	- - -	- - -	10.7	9.6	9.6	9.0	8.6
All ages, crude	- - -	- - -	- - -	8.8	8.7	9.0	8.5	7.9
15–24 years	- - -	- - -	- - -	10.8	13.5	14.4	9.1	9.1
25–44 years	- - -	- - -	- - -	11.0	10.6	10.8	10.8	9.9
45–64 years	- - -	- - -	- - -	13.0	9.7	8.7	11.6	9.7
65 years and over	- - -	- - -	- - -	18.6	16.8	18.9	13.4	15.4
Hispanic or Latino male[4,6]								
All ages, age adjusted[3]	- - -	- - -	- - -	- - -	13.7	12.7	10.3	10.3
All ages, crude	- - -	- - -	- - -	- - -	11.4	10.9	8.2	8.4
15–24 years	- - -	- - -	- - -	- - -	14.7	16.0	9.9	10.9
25–44 years	- - -	- - -	- - -	- - -	16.2	14.5	11.3	11.2
45–64 years	- - -	- - -	- - -	- - -	16.1	14.2	11.8	12.0
65 years and over	- - -	- - -	- - -	- - -	23.4	21.0	19.5	19.5
White, not Hispanic or Latino male[6]								
All ages, age adjusted[3]	- - -	- - -	- - -	- - -	23.5	22.3	20.2	20.2
All ages, crude	- - -	- - -	- - -	- - -	23.1	22.2	20.3	20.4
15–24 years	- - -	- - -	- - -	- - -	24.4	24.0	19.2	19.5
25–44 years	- - -	- - -	- - -	- - -	26.4	27.1	25.2	25.1
45–64 years	- - -	- - -	- - -	- - -	26.8	24.5	23.4	24.0
65 years and over	- - -	- - -	- - -	- - -	45.4	39.0	35.0	33.9
White female[4]								
All ages, age adjusted[3]	6.0	5.9	7.9	6.1	5.2	4.7	4.4	4.3
All ages, crude	5.5	5.3	7.1	5.9	5.3	4.8	4.5	4.4
15–24 years	2.7	2.3	4.2	4.6	4.2	3.8	3.2	3.1
25–44 years	6.6	7.0	11.0	8.1	6.6	6.3	6.2	6.0
45–64 years	10.6	10.9	13.0	9.6	7.7	6.7	6.7	6.9
65 years and over	9.9	8.8	8.5	6.4	6.8	5.7	4.6	4.3
Black or African American female[4]								
All ages, age adjusted[3]	1.8	2.0	2.9	2.4	2.4	2.0	1.6	1.8
All ages, crude	1.5	1.6	2.6	2.2	2.3	2.0	1.6	1.7
15–24 years	1.8	*	3.8	2.3	2.3	2.2	1.9	2.2
25–44 years	2.3	3.0	4.8	4.3	3.8	3.3	2.5	2.6
45–64 years	2.7	3.1	2.9	2.5	2.9	2.0	1.8	2.1
65 years and over	*	*	2.6	*	1.9	2.1	1.5	1.3

See footnotes at end of table.

Table 46 (page 3 of 3). Death rates for suicide, according to sex, race, Hispanic origin, and age: United States, selected years 1950–2000

[Data are based on death certificates]

Sex, race, Hispanic origin, and age	1950[1]	1960[1]	1970	1980	1990	1995	1999[2]	2000
American Indian or Alaska Native female[4]				Deaths per 100,000 resident population				
All ages, age adjusted[3]	- - -	- - -	- - -	4.7	3.6	3.9	4.0	3.8
All ages, crude	- - -	- - -	- - -	4.7	3.7	3.8	4.1	4.0
15–24 years	- - -	- - -	- - -	*	*	*	*	*
25–44 years	- - -	- - -	- - -	10.7	*	6.4	6.8	7.2
45–64 years	- - -	- - -	- - -	*	*	*	*	*
65 years and over	- - -	- - -	- - -	*	*	*	*	*
Asian or Pacific Islander female[4]								
All ages, age adjusted[3]	- - -	- - -	- - -	5.5	4.1	4.1	3.4	2.8
All ages, crude	- - -	- - -	- - -	4.7	3.4	3.7	3.3	2.7
15–24 years	- - -	- - -	- - -	*	3.9	4.8	4.0	2.7
25–44 years	- - -	- - -	- - -	5.4	3.8	3.6	3.8	3.3
45–64 years	- - -	- - -	- - -	7.9	5.0	4.7	3.8	3.2
65 years and over	- - -	- - -	- - -	*	8.5	8.6	6.4	5.2
Hispanic or Latino female[4],[6]								
All ages, age adjusted[3]	- - -	- - -	- - -	- - -	2.3	2.0	1.9	1.7
All ages, crude	- - -	- - -	- - -	- - -	2.2	1.8	1.6	1.5
15–24 years	- - -	- - -	- - -	- - -	3.1	2.4	1.8	2.0
25–44 years	- - -	- - -	- - -	- - -	3.1	2.5	2.3	2.1
45–64 years	- - -	- - -	- - -	- - -	2.5	2.8	2.5	2.5
65 years and over	- - -	- - -	- - -	- - -	*	*	2.4	*
White, not Hispanic or Latino female[6]								
All ages, age adjusted[3]	- - -	- - -	- - -	- - -	5.4	4.9	4.7	4.7
All ages, crude	- - -	- - -	- - -	- - -	5.6	5.1	4.9	4.9
15–24 years	- - -	- - -	- - -	- - -	4.3	4.0	3.4	3.3
25–44 years	- - -	- - -	- - -	- - -	7.0	6.6	6.8	6.7
45–64 years	- - -	- - -	- - -	- - -	8.0	6.9	7.0	7.3
65 years and over	- - -	- - -	- - -	- - -	7.0	5.8	4.7	4.4

. . . Category not applicable.

* Rates based on fewer than 20 deaths are considered unreliable and are not shown.

- - - Data not available.

[1]Includes deaths of persons who were not residents of the 50 States and the District of Columbia.

[2]Starting with 1999 data, cause of death is coded according to ICD–10. To estimate change between 1998 and 1999, compare the 1999 rate with the comparability-modified rate for 1998. See Appendix II, Comparability ratio and tables V and VI.

[3]Age-adjusted rates are calculated using the year 2000 standard population starting with *Health, United States, 2001.* See Appendix II, Age adjustment.

[4]The race groups, white, black, Asian or Pacific Islander, and American Indian or Alaska Native, include persons of Hispanic and non-Hispanic origin. Persons of Hispanic origin may be of any race. Death rates for the American Indian or Alaska Native and Asian or Pacific Islander populations are known to be underestimated. See Appendix II, Race, for a discussion of sources of bias in death rates by race and Hispanic origin.

[5]In 1950 rate is for the age group 75 years and over.

[6]Prior to 1997, excludes data from States lacking an Hispanic-origin item on the death certificate. See Appendix II, Hispanic origin.

NOTES: Population estimates used to compute rates for 1991–2000 differ from those used previously. Starting with *Health, United States, 2003,* rates for 1991–99 were revised using intercensal population estimates based on Census 2000. Rates for 2000 were revised based on Census 2000 counts. See Appendix I, Population Census and Population Estimates. Underlying cause of death code numbers are based on the applicable revision of the *International Classification of Diseases* (ICD) for data years shown. For the period 1980–98, causes were coded using ICD–9 codes that are most nearly comparable with the 113 cause list for ICD–10. See Appendix II, tables IV and V. Age groups were selected to minimize the presentation of unstable age-specific death rates based on small numbers of deaths and for consistency among comparison groups. For additional injury-related statistics, see www.cdc.gov/ncipc/wisqars, a Web-based interactive database for injury data. Data for additional years are available (see Appendix III).

SOURCES: Centers for Disease Control and Prevention, National Center for Health Statistics, National Vital Statistics System; Grove RD, Hetzel AM. Vital statistics rates in the United States, 1940–1960. Washington: U.S. Government Printing Office. 1968; numerator data from National Vital Statistics System, annual mortality files; denominator data from national population estimates for race groups from table 1 and unpublished Hispanic population estimates for 1985–96 prepared by the Housing and Household Economic Statistics Division, U.S. Bureau of the Census; additional mortality tables are available at www.cdc.gov/nchs/datawh/statab/unpubd/mortabs.htm; Anderson RN, Arias E. The effect of revised populations on mortality statistics for the U.S., 2000. National vital statistics reports. Vol 51 no 9. Hyattsville, Maryland: National Center for Health Statistics. 2003.

This table will be updated with 2001 data on the web. Go to www.cdc.gov/nchs/hus.htm.

Table 47 (page 1 of 3). Death rates for firearm-related injuries, according to sex, race, Hispanic origin, and age: United States, selected years 1970–2000

[Data are based on death certificates]

Sex, race, Hispanic origin, and age	1970	1980	1990	1995	1999[1]	2000
All persons			Deaths per 100,000 resident population			
All ages, age adjusted[2]	14.3	14.8	14.6	13.4	10.3	10.2
All ages, crude	13.1	14.9	14.9	13.5	10.3	10.2
Under 1 year	*	*	*	*	*	*
1–14 years	1.6	1.4	1.5	1.6	0.9	0.7
1–4 years	1.0	0.7	0.6	0.6	0.4	0.3
5–14 years	1.7	1.6	1.9	1.9	1.0	0.9
15–24 years	15.5	20.6	25.8	26.7	17.6	16.8
15–19 years	11.4	14.7	23.3	24.1	14.4	12.9
20–24 years	20.3	26.4	28.1	29.2	21.0	20.9
25–44 years	20.9	22.5	19.3	16.9	13.1	13.1
25–34 years	22.2	24.3	21.8	19.6	14.9	14.5
35–44 years	19.6	20.0	16.3	14.3	11.6	11.9
45–64 years	17.6	15.2	13.6	11.7	10.0	10.0
45–54 years	18.1	16.4	13.9	12.0	10.2	10.5
55–64 years	17.0	13.9	13.3	11.3	9.7	9.4
65 years and over	13.8	13.5	16.0	14.1	12.5	12.2
65–74 years	14.5	13.8	14.4	12.8	11.0	10.6
75–84 years	13.4	13.4	19.4	16.3	14.2	13.9
85 years and over	10.2	11.6	14.7	14.4	13.5	14.2
Male						
All ages, age adjusted[2]	24.8	25.9	26.1	23.8	18.4	18.1
All ages, crude	22.2	25.7	26.2	23.6	18.1	17.8
Under 1 year	*	*	*	*	*	*
1–14 years	2.3	2.0	2.2	2.3	1.2	1.1
1–4 years	1.2	0.9	0.7	0.8	0.5	0.4
5–14 years	2.7	2.5	2.9	2.9	1.5	1.4
15–24 years	26.4	34.8	44.7	46.5	30.6	29.4
15–19 years	19.2	24.5	40.1	41.6	24.8	22.4
20–24 years	35.1	45.2	49.1	51.5	36.8	37.0
25–44 years	34.1	38.1	32.6	28.4	22.0	22.0
25–34 years	36.5	41.4	37.0	33.2	25.5	24.9
35–44 years	31.6	33.2	27.4	23.6	18.9	19.4
45–64 years	31.0	25.9	23.4	20.0	17.1	17.1
45–54 years	30.7	27.3	23.2	20.1	17.0	17.6
55–64 years	31.3	24.5	23.7	19.8	17.1	16.3
65 years and over	29.7	29.7	35.3	30.7	27.2	26.4
65–74 years	29.5	27.8	28.2	25.1	21.5	20.3
75–84 years	31.0	33.0	46.9	37.8	32.8	32.2
85 years and over	26.2	34.9	49.3	47.1	43.3	44.7
Female						
All ages, age adjusted[2]	4.8	4.7	4.2	3.8	2.9	2.8
All ages, crude	4.4	4.7	4.3	3.8	2.9	2.8
Under 1 year	*	*	*	*	*	*
1–14 years	0.8	0.7	0.8	0.8	0.5	0.3
1–4 years	0.9	0.5	0.5	0.5	0.4	*
5–14 years	0.8	0.7	1.0	0.9	0.5	0.4
15–24 years	4.8	6.1	6.0	5.9	3.9	3.5
15–19 years	3.5	4.6	5.7	5.6	3.4	2.9
20–24 years	6.4	7.7	6.3	6.1	4.4	4.2
25–44 years	8.3	7.4	6.1	5.5	4.3	4.2
25–34 years	8.4	7.5	6.7	5.8	4.1	4.0
35–44 years	8.2	7.2	5.4	5.2	4.4	4.4
45–64 years	5.4	5.4	4.5	3.9	3.3	3.4
45–54 years	6.4	6.2	4.9	4.2	3.6	3.6
55–64 years	4.2	4.6	4.0	3.5	2.9	3.0
65 years and over	2.4	2.5	3.1	2.8	2.2	2.2
65–74 years	2.8	3.1	3.6	3.0	2.4	2.5
75–84 years	1.7	1.7	2.9	2.8	2.1	2.0
85 years and over	*	1.3	1.3	1.8	1.5	1.7
White male[3]						
All ages, age adjusted[2]	19.7	22.1	22.0	20.1	16.2	15.9
All ages, crude	17.6	21.8	21.8	19.9	15.9	15.6
1–14 years	1.8	1.9	1.9	1.9	1.0	1.0
15–24 years	16.9	28.4	29.5	30.8	20.5	19.6
25–44 years	24.2	29.5	25.7	23.2	18.3	18.0
25–34 years	24.3	31.1	27.8	25.2	19.2	18.1
35–44 years	24.1	27.1	23.3	21.2	17.6	17.9
45–64 years	27.4	23.3	22.8	19.5	17.3	17.4
65 years and over	29.9	30.1	36.8	32.2	28.9	28.2

See footnotes at end of table.

[Data are based on death certificates]

Sex, race, Hispanic origin, and age	1970	1980	1990	1995	1999[1]	2000
Black or African American male[3]			Deaths per 100,000 resident population			
All ages, age adjusted[2]	70.8	60.1	56.3	49.2	34.1	34.2
All ages, crude	60.8	57.7	61.9	52.9	36.0	36.1
1–14 years	5.3	3.0	4.4	4.4	2.0	1.8
15–24 years	97.3	77.9	138.0	138.7	91.4	89.3
25–44 years	126.2	114.1	90.3	70.2	51.5	54.1
25–34 years	145.6	128.4	108.6	92.3	71.3	74.8
35–44 years	104.2	92.3	66.1	46.3	32.2	34.3
45–64 years	71.1	55.6	34.5	28.3	19.0	18.4
65 years and over	30.6	29.7	23.9	21.8	15.2	13.8
American Indian or Alaska Native male[3]						
All ages, age adjusted[2]	- - -	24.0	19.4	19.4	16.1	13.1
All ages, crude	- - -	27.5	20.5	20.9	16.2	13.2
15–24 years	- - -	55.3	49.1	40.9	33.5	26.9
25–44 years	- - -	43.9	25.4	31.2	21.5	16.6
45–64 years	- - -	*	*	14.2	12.0	12.2
65 years and over	- - -	*	*	*	*	*
Asian or Pacific Islander male[3]						
All ages, age adjusted[2]	- - -	7.8	8.8	9.2	5.9	6.0
All ages, crude	- - -	8.2	9.4	10.0	6.3	6.2
15–24 years	- - -	10.8	21.0	24.3	10.9	9.3
25–44 years	- - -	12.8	10.9	10.6	8.3	8.1
45–64 years	- - -	10.4	8.1	8.2	6.4	7.4
65 years and over	- - -	*	*	*	*	*
Hispanic or Latino male[3,4]						
All ages, age adjusted[2]	- - -	- - -	27.6	23.8	14.2	13.6
All ages, crude	- - -	- - -	29.9	26.2	14.6	14.2
1–14 years	- - -	- - -	2.6	2.8	1.1	1.0
15–24 years	- - -	- - -	55.5	61.7	31.6	30.8
25–44 years	- - -	- - -	42.7	31.4	17.9	17.3
25–34 years	- - -	- - -	47.3	36.4	20.6	20.3
35–44 years	- - -	- - -	35.4	24.2	14.3	13.2
45–64 years	- - -	- - -	21.4	17.2	11.2	12.0
65 years and over	- - -	- - -	19.1	16.5	14.4	12.2
White, not Hispanic or Latino male[4]						
All ages, age adjusted[2]	- - -	- - -	20.6	18.6	15.8	15.5
All ages, crude	- - -	- - -	20.4	18.5	15.9	15.7
1–14 years	- - -	- - -	1.6	1.6	1.0	1.0
15–24 years	- - -	- - -	24.1	23.5	17.2	16.2
25–44 years	- - -	- - -	23.3	21.4	18.2	17.9
25–34 years	- - -	- - -	24.7	22.5	18.6	17.2
35–44 years	- - -	- - -	21.6	20.4	17.8	18.4
45–64 years	- - -	- - -	22.7	19.5	17.8	17.8
65 years and over	- - -	- - -	37.4	32.5	29.5	29.0
White female[3]						
All ages, age adjusted[2]	4.0	4.2	3.8	3.5	2.7	2.7
All ages, crude	3.7	4.1	3.8	3.5	2.8	2.7
15–24 years	3.4	5.1	4.8	0.7	0.4	0.3
25–44 years	6.9	6.2	5.3	4.5	3.0	2.8
45–64 years	5.0	5.1	4.5	4.0	3.4	3.5
65 years and over	2.2	2.5	3.1	2.8	2.3	2.4

See footnotes at end of table.

Table 47 (page 3 of 3). Death rates for firearm-related injuries, according to sex, race, Hispanic origin, and age: United States, selected years 1970–2000

[Data are based on death certificates]

Sex, race, Hispanic origin, and age	1970	1980	1990	1995	1999[1]	2000
Black or African American female[3]			Deaths per 100,000 resident population			
All ages, age adjusted[2]	11.1	8.7	7.3	6.2	4.3	3.9
All ages, crude	10.0	8.8	7.8	6.5	4.4	4.0
15–24 years	15.2	12.3	13.3	13.2	0.9	0.5
25–44 years	19.4	16.1	12.4	9.8	9.0	7.6
45–64 years	10.2	8.2	4.8	4.1	6.7	6.5
65 years and over	4.3	3.1	3.1	2.6	3.0	3.1
American Indian or Alaska Native female[3]						
All ages, age adjusted[2]	- - -	5.8	3.3	3.8	2.6	2.9
All ages, crude	- - -	5.8	3.4	4.1	2.8	2.9
15–24 years	- - -	*	*	*	*	*
25–44 years	- - -	10.2	*	7.0	*	5.5
45–64 years	- - -	*	*	*	*	*
65 years and over	- - -	*	*	*	*	*
Asian or Pacific Islander female[3]						
All ages, age adjusted[2]	- - -	2.0	1.9	2.0	1.6	1.1
All ages, crude	- - -	2.1	2.1	2.1	1.7	1.2
15–24 years	- - -	*	*	3.9	*	*
25–44 years	- - -	3.2	2.7	2.7	2.2	1.5
45–64 years	- - -	*	*	*	2.1	*
65 years and over	- - -	*	*	*	*	*
Hispanic or Latino female[3,4]						
All ages, age adjusted[2]	- - -	- - -	3.3	3.1	2.0	1.8
All ages, crude	- - -	- - -	3.6	3.3	2.0	1.8
15–24 years	- - -	- - -	6.9	6.1	3.8	2.9
25–44 years	- - -	- - -	5.1	4.7	2.5	2.5
45–64 years	- - -	- - -	2.4	2.4	2.4	2.2
65 years and over	- - -	- - -	*	*	*	*
White, not Hispanic or Latino female[4]						
All ages, age adjusted[2]	- - -	- - -	3.7	3.4	2.8	2.8
All ages, crude	- - -	- - -	3.7	3.5	2.9	2.9
15–24 years	- - -	- - - -	4.3	4.1	2.8	2.7
25–44 years	- - -	- - -	5.1	4.8	4.2	4.2
45–64 years	- - -	- - -	4.6	4.1	3.5	3.6
65 years and over	- - -	- - -	3.2	2.8	2.4	2.4

* Rates based on fewer than 20 deaths are considered unreliable and are not shown.

- - - Data not available.

[1]Starting with 1999 data, cause of death is coded according to ICD–10. To estimate change between 1998 and 1999, compare the 1999 rate with the comparability-modified rate for 1998. See Appendix II, Comparability ratio and tables V and VI.

[2]Age-adjusted rates are calculated using the year 2000 standard population starting with *Health, United States, 2001*. See Appendix II, Age adjustment.

[3]The race groups, white, black, Asian or Pacific Islander, and American Indian or Alaska Native, include persons of Hispanic and non-Hispanic origin. Persons of Hispanic origin may be of any race. Death rates for the American Indian or Alaska Native and Asian or Pacific Islander populations are known to be underestimated. See Appendix II, Race, for a discussion of sources of bias in death rates by race and Hispanic origin.

[4]Prior to 1997, excludes data from States lacking an Hispanic-origin item on the death certificate. See Appendix II, Hispanic origin.

NOTES: Population estimates used to compute rates for 1991–2000 differ from those used previously. Starting with *Health, United States, 2003*, rates for 1991–99 were revised using intercensal population estimates based on Census 2000. Rates for 2000 were revised based on Census 2000 counts. See Appendix I, Population Census and Population Estimates. Underlying cause of death code numbers are based on the applicable revision of the *International Classification of Diseases* (ICD) for data years shown. See Appendix II, tables IV and V. Age groups were selected to minimize the presentation of unstable age-specific death rates based on small numbers of deaths and for consistency among comparison groups. For additional injury-related statistics, see www.cdc.gov/ncipc/wisqars, a Web-based interactive database for injury data. Data for additional years are available (see Appendix III).

SOURCES: Centers for Disease Control and Prevention, National Center for Health Statistics, National Vital Statistics System; numerator data from annual mortality files; denominator data from national population estimates for race groups from table 1 and unpublished Hispanic population estimates for 1985–96 prepared by the Housing and Household Economic Statistics Division, U.S. Bureau of the Census; additional mortality tables are available at www.cdc.gov/nchs/datawh/statab/unpubd/mortabs.htm; Anderson RN, Arias E. The effect of revised populations on mortality statistics for the U.S., 2000. National vital statistics reports. Vol 51 no 9. Hyattsville, Maryland: National Center for Health Statistics. 2003.

This table will be updated with 2001 data on the web. Go to www.cdc.gov/nchs/hus.htm.

Table 48. Deaths from selected occupational diseases for persons 15 years of age and over: United States, selected years 1980–2000

[Data are based on death certificates]

Cause of death[1]	1980	1985	1990	1995	1997	1998	1999[2]	2000[2]
Underlying and nonunderlying cause of death				Number of deaths				
Angiosarcoma of liver[3]	- - -	- - -	- - -	- - -	- - -	- - -	4	16
Malignant mesothelioma[4]	699	715	874	897	984	1,064	2,485	2,531
Pneumoconiosis[5]	4,151	3,783	3,644	3,151	2,928	2,790	2,739	2,859
Coal workers' pneumoconiosis	2,576	2,615	1,990	1,413	1,297	1,103	1,002	949
Asbestosis	339	534	948	1,169	1,171	1,221	1,259	1,486
Silicosis	448	334	308	242	198	178	185	151
Other (including unspecified)	814	321	413	343	275	311	310	290
Underlying cause of death								
Angiosarcoma of liver[3]	- - -	- - -	- - -	- - -	- - -	- - -	3	15
Malignant mesothelioma[4]	531	573	725	780	865	935	2,343	2,384
Pneumoconiosis	1,581	1,355	1,335	1,117	1,087	1,099	1,081	1,142
Coal workers' pneumoconiosis	982	958	734	533	486	421	409	389
Asbestosis	101	139	302 `	355	405	458	449	558
Silicosis	207	143	150	114	98	93	102	71
Other (including unspecified)	291	115	149	115	98	127	121	124

- - - Data not available.

[1]Cause-of-death titles for selected occupational diseases and corresponding code numbers according to the Ninth and Tenth Revisions, *International Classification of Diseases*. See Appendix II, table IV.

Cause of death	ICD–9 code	ICD–10 code
Angiosarcoma of liver	- - -	C22.3
Malignant mesothelioma	158.8,158.9,163	C45
Pneumoconiosis	500–505	J60-J66
Coal workers' pneumoconiosis	500	J60
Asbestosis	501	J61
Silicosis	502	J62
Other (including unspecified)	503–505	J63–J66

[2]Starting with 1999 data, cause of death is coded according to ICD–10. See Appendix II, *International Classification of Diseases* (ICD). Discontinuities exist between 1998 and 1999 due to ICD–10 coding and classification changes. Caution should be exercised in interpreting trends for these causes, especially for those causes with major ICD–10 changes (e.g., malignant mesothelioma).
[3]Prior to 1999 there was no discrete code for this condition.
[4]Prior to 1999 the combined ICD–9 categories of malignant neoplasm of peritoneum and malignant neoplasm of pleura served as a crude surrogate for malignant mesothelioma under ICD–10.
[5]For underlying and nonunderlying cause of death, counts of deaths for pneumoconiosis subgroups may sum to slightly more than total pneumoconiosis deaths due to the reporting of more than one type of pneumoconiosis on some death certificates. The total underlying and nonunderlying pneumoconiosis death count is tracked by Healthy People 2010.

NOTES: Selection of occupational diseases is based on definitions in Mullan RJ, Murthy LI. Occupational sentinel health events: An updated list for physician recognition and public health surveillance. *Am J Ind Med* 19:775–799, 1991. For more detailed information about pneumoconiosis deaths, see *Work-Related Lung Disease Surveillance Report 1999*, DHHS (NIOSH) Publication Number 2000–105 at www.cdc.gov/niosh/w99cont.html.

SOURCE: Centers for Disease Control and Prevention, National Center for Health Statistics, National Vital Statistics System; annual mortality files for underlying and multiple cause of death.

This table will be updated with 2001 data on the web. Go to www.cdc.gov/nchs/hus.htm.

Table 49 (page 1 of 2). Occupational injury deaths and rates by industry, sex, age, race, and Hispanic origin: United States, 1992–2001

[Data are compiled from various Federal, State, and local administrative sources]

Characteristic	1992[1]	1994	1995	1996	1997	1998	1999	2000	2001[2,3]
	Deaths per 100,000 employed workers[4]								
Total work force	5.2	5.3	4.9	4.8	4.7	4.5	4.5	4.3	4.3
Total, including fatalities from Sept 11, 2001	...	...	...	...	...	...	...	...	6.4
Industry[5]									
Private sector	5.5	5.7	5.1	5.1	5.0	4.8	4.8	4.6	4.5
Agriculture, forestry, and fishing	24.0	23.9	22.2	22.4	23.5	23.4	23.8	20.9	22.8
Mining	27.1	26.9	25.0	27.0	25.0	23.8	21.7	30.0	30.0
Construction	14.1	14.8	14.7	14.0	14.1	14.5	14.0	12.9	13.3
Manufacturing	3.8	3.9	3.5	3.5	3.6	3.4	3.6	3.3	3.2
Transportation and public utilities	13.4	13.4	12.6	13.4	13.2	11.8	12.7	11.8	11.2
Wholesale trade	5.3	5.8	5.1	5.4	4.9	4.5	4.6	4.3	4.3
Retail trade	3.8	3.8	3.3	3.2	3.1	2.6	2.3	2.7	2.4
Finance, insurance, and real estate	1.6	1.4	1.6	1.5	1.2	1.1	1.2	0.9	1.0
Services	2.5	2.6	2.2	2.2	2.0	2.0	1.9	2.0	1.9
Government[6]	3.7	3.4	3.9	3.1	3.2	3.0	2.8	2.8	3.1
Sex									
Male	- - -	9.0	8.3	8.2	8.1	7.7	7.7	7.4	7.4
Female	- - -	0.9	0.9	0.9	0.8	0.8	0.7	0.7	0.7
Age									
16–17 years	- - -	1.7	1.6	1.6	1.5	1.2	1.6	1.6	1.3
18–19 years	- - -	3.0	3.3	3.2	2.8	3.1	2.7	2.7	2.8
20–24 years	- - -	4.1	3.8	3.5	3.9	3.3	3.4	3.3	3.2
25–34 years	- - -	4.8	4.3	4.2	4.1	3.9	3.8	3.8	3.8
35–44 years	- - -	4.8	4.6	4.5	4.2	4.2	4.1	4.0	4.0
45–54 years	- - -	5.6	5.2	4.9	4.9	4.6	4.6	4.4	4.5
55–64 years	- - -	7.7	7.2	7.3	7.1	6.5	6.1	6.1	5.5
65 years and over	- - -	14.3	14.0	13.7	13.8	14.5	14.6	12.0	12.7
Race and Hispanic origin[7]									
White	- - -	5.1	4.7	4.7	4.6	4.5	4.4	- - -	- - -
Black or African American	- - -	5.4	5.1	4.6	4.8	4.0	4.1	- - -	- - -
Hispanic or Latino	- - -	5.7	5.5	5.4	5.1	5.2	5.2	5.6	6.0
Not Hispanic or Latino	- - -	5.3	4.9	4.8	4.7	4.5	4.4	4.2	5.2
White	- - -	- - -	- - -	- - -	- - -	- - -	- - -	4.2	4.2
Black or African American	- - -	- - -	- - -	- - -	- - -	- - -	- - -	3.9	3.8
	Number of deaths[8]								
Total work force	6,217	6,632	6,275	6,202	6,238	6,055	6,054	5,920	5,900
Total, including fatalities from Sept 11, 2001	...	...	...	...	...	...	...	...	8,786
Industry[5]									
Private sector	5,497	5,959	5,495	5,597	5,616	5,457	5,488	5,347	5,270
Agriculture, forestry, and fishing	808	852	800	806	833	840	814	720	740
Mining	181	180	156	153	158	147	122	156	170
Construction	919	1,028	1,055	1,047	1,107	1,174	1,191	1,155	1,225
Manufacturing	765	789	709	725	744	698	722	668	599
Transportation and public utilities	895	949	901	970	1,008	911	1,008	957	911
Wholesale trade	253	271	256	270	241	229	238	230	220
Retail trade	734	808	687	681	670	570	513	594	537
Finance, insurance, and real estate	122	113	125	116	97	92	107	79	86
Services	757	853	749	776	727	763	736	769	767
Not classified	63	116	57	53	31	33	37	19	15
Government[6]	720	673	780	605	622	598	566	573	630

See footnotes at end of table.

Table 49 (page 2 of 2). Occupational injury deaths and rates by industry, sex, age, race, and Hispanic origin: United States, 1992–2001

[Data are compiled from various Federal, State, and local administrative sources]

Characteristic	1992[1]	1994	1995	1996	1997	1998	1999	2000	2001[2,3]
Sex				Number of deaths[8]					
Male	5,774	6,104	5,736	5,688	5,761	5,569	5,612	5,471	5,429
Female	443	528	539	514	477	486	442	449	471
Age									
Under 16 years	27	25	26	27	21	33	26	29	20
16–17 years	41	42	42	43	41	32	46	44	33
18–19 years	107	114	130	125	113	137	122	127	122
20–24 years	544	545	486	444	503	421	451	446	440
25–34 years	1,556	1,567	1,409	1,362	1,325	1,238	1,175	1,163	1,140
35–44 years	1,538	1,619	1,571	1,586	1,524	1,525	1,510	1,473	1,474
45–54 years	1,167	1,310	1,256	1,242	1,302	1,279	1,333	1,313	1,363
55–64 years	767	866	827	855	875	836	816	831	773
65 years and over	467	525	515	504	520	541	565	488	529
Unspecified	3	19	13	14	14	13	10	6	6
Race and Hispanic origin									
White	5,173	5,460	5,120	5,111	5,108	5,041	4,990	- - -	- - -
Black or African American	624	707	697	631	677	594	626	- - -	- - -
Hispanic or Latino	533	624	619	638	658	707	730	815	891
Not Hispanic or Latino	5,684	6,008	5,656	5,564	5,580	5,348	5,323	5,100	5,009
White	4,712	4,954	4,599	4,586	4,576	4,478	4,410	4,244	4,168
Black or African American	618	695	684	615	661	583	616	575	563
American Indian or Alaska Native	36	39	27	35	34	28	54	33	48
Asian[9]	192	211	188	188	218	164	180	171	172
Native Hawaiian or Pacific Islander	- - -	- - -	- - -	- - -	- - -	- - -	- - -	14	9
Multiple races	- - -	- - -	- - -	- - -	- - -	- - -	- - -	- - -	6
Other races or not reported	126	109	158	140	91	95	64	68	43

. . . Data not applicable.

- - - Data not available.

[1]1992 and 1993 employment data by demographic characteristics are not available from the Current Population Survey (CPS) for calculation of rates.

[2]Fatalities due to the September 11 terrorist attacks are included only in the total line, as labeled, and not in the subcategories by industry and demographic characteristics.

[3]Preliminary data.

[4]Numerator excludes deaths to workers under the age of 16 years. Employment data in denominators are average annual estimates of employed civilians 16 years of age and over from the Current Population Survey (CPS) plus resident armed forces figures from the Bureau of the Census (1992–98) and Department of Defense (1999–2001).

[5]Classified according to the *Standard Industrial Classification Manual*, 1987 (see Appendix II, table VIII).

[6]Includes fatalities to workers employed by governmental organizations regardless of industry.

[7]Employment data for American Indian or Alaska Native workers and Asian or Pacific Islander workers are not available for the calculation of rates; Employment data for non-Hispanic white and non-Hispanic black workers were not available before the year 2000.

[8]Includes fatalities to all workers, regardless of age.

[9]In 1999 and earlier years, category also includes Native Hawaiian or Pacific Islander.

NOTES: Fatalities and rates are based on revised data and may differ from originally published data from the Census of Fatal Occupational Injuries (CFOI). See Appendix I, CFOI. CFOI began collecting fatality data in 1992. For data for prior years, see CDC. Fatal Occupational Injuries—United States, 1980–1997. MMWR 2001; 50(16):317–320, which reports trend data from the National Traumatic Occupational Fatalities (NTOF) surveillance system. NTOF was established at the National Institute of Occupational Safety and Health (NIOSH) to monitor occupational injury deaths through death certificates. In 1999 and earlier years the race groups white and black included persons of Hispanic and non-Hispanic origin. Some numbers for 2000 in this table were revised and differ from the previous edition of *Health, United States*. Data for additional years are available (see Appendix III).

SOURCE: Department of Labor, Bureau of Labor Statistics, Census of Fatal Occupational Injuries. Revised annual data.

Table 50. Occupational injuries with lost workdays in the private sector, according to industry: United States, selected years 1980–2001

[Data are based on employer records from a sample of business establishments]

Industry	1980	1985	1990	1995	1997	1998	1999	2000	2001
	Injuries with lost workdays per 100 full-time equivalents[1]								
Total private sector[2]	3.9	3.6	3.9	3.4	3.1	2.9	2.8	2.8	2.6
Agriculture, fishing, and forestry[2]	5.6	5.6	5.7	4.2	4.0	3.8	3.3	3.5	3.6
Mining	6.4	4.7	4.9	3.8	3.7	2.7	2.5	3.0	2.3
Construction	6.5	6.8	6.6	4.8	4.4	4.0	4.1	4.0	3.9
Manufacturing	5.2	4.4	5.3	4.6	4.2	4.2	4.0	4.0	3.6
Transportation, communication, and public utilities	5.4	4.9	5.4	5.0	4.7	4.2	4.3	4.1	4.2
Wholesale trade	3.8	3.5	3.6	3.5	3.1	3.2	3.2	3.0	2.5
Retail trade	2.9	3.1	3.4	2.9	2.8	2.6	2.5	2.4	2.4
Finance, insurance, and real estate	0.8	0.9	1.1	0.9	0.8	0.6	0.7	0.7	0.7
Services	2.3	2.5	2.7	2.7	2.4	2.3	2.1	2.2	2.1
	Number of injuries with lost workdays in thousands								
Total private sector[2]	2,491.0	2,484.7	2,987.3	2,767.6	2,682.6	2,612.0	2,575.9	2,587.0	2,409.4
Agriculture, fishing, and forestry[2]	39.3	45.2	57.2	51.7	53.8	53.8	47.5	52.4	53.5
Mining	66.2	43.9	35.6	22.8	22.6	16.9	14.2	17.0	13.9
Construction	242.6	272.8	296.3	217.9	227.4	217.0	240.2	246.1	237.6
Manufacturing	1,009.5	825.1	975.0	838.1	785.4	782.6	744.6	727.7	614.5
Transportation, communication, and public utilities	263.0	243.5	293.3	289.2	281.3	261.3	274.3	274.6	276.4
Wholesale trade	191.1	188.4	211.5	214.7	200.7	211.1	210.6	201.7	177.1
Retail trade	330.2	399.9	483.9	459.6	456.9	434.7	420.7	420.6	411.0
Finance, insurance, and real estate	38.1	45.5	63.7	52.2	47.6	39.6	45.8	45.9	45.0
Services	311.1	420.6	570.8	621.4	606.9	594.9	578.0	601.1	580.5

[1]Incidence rate calculated as (N/EH) x 200,000, where N = total number of injuries with lost workdays in a calendar year, EH = total hours worked by all full-time and part-time employees in a calendar year, and 200,000 = base for 100 full-time equivalent employees working 40 hours per week, 50 weeks per year.
[2]Excludes farms with fewer than 11 employees.

NOTES: Industry is coded based on various editions of the *Standard Industrial Classification Manual* as follows: data for 1980–87 are based on the 1972 edition, 1977 supplement; and data for 1988–2001 are based on the 1987 edition (see Appendix II, Industry). Data for additional years are available (see Appendix III).

SOURCE: U.S. Department of Labor, Bureau of Labor Statistics, Survey of Occupational Injuries and Illnesses: Workplace injuries and illnesses, 1980–2001 editions. Summary News Release. 1982–2002. Internet address: www.bls.gov/iif/home.htm.

Table 51 (page 1 of 2). Healthy People 2010 Leading Health Indicators: United States, selected years 1990–2002 and 2010 target

[Data are based on interviews and examinations of samples of the civilian noninstitutionalized population or special population subgroups; information from death certificates and birth certificates; and air quality measurements]

Leading Health Indicators, measures, and Healthy People 2010 objective numbers	1990	1995	1998	1999	2000	2001	2002	2010 Target
Physical activity								
1a. Adolescents in grades 9–12: percent who engaged in 20 minutes or more of vigorous activity 3 or more days per week (obj 22–07)	- - -	64	- - -	65	- - -	65	- - -	85
1b. Adults age 18 years and over: age-adjusted percent who engaged in moderate activity (at least 30 minutes, 5 days per week) or vigorous activity (at least 20 minutes, 3 days per week) (obj 22–02)[1] . . .	- - -	- - -	30	30	32	32	33	50
Overweight and obesity[2]								
2a. Overweight or obese children and adolescents, age 6–19 years: percent who are at or above the sex- and age-specific 95th percentile of Body Mass Index (BMI) based on CDC Growth Charts: United States (obj 19–03c)	11	- - -	- - -	- - -	15	- - -	- - -	5
2b. Obese adults age 20 years and over: age-adjusted percent with BMI of 30 Kg/m^2 or more (obj 19–02)	23	- - -	- - -	- - -	31	- - -	- - -	15
Tobacco use								
3a. Adolescents in grades 9–12: percent who smoked cigarettes one or more days in the past 30 days (obj 27–02b)	- - -	35	- - -	35	28	28	- - -	16
3b. Adults age 18 years and over: age-adjusted percent who smoked more than 100 cigarettes in their lifetime and now report smoking on some days or every day (obj 27–01a)[1]	25	25	24	23	23	23	22	12
Substance abuse[3]								
4a. Adolescents age 12–17 years: percent who reported no use of alcohol or illicit drugs in the past 30 days (obj 26–10a)	- - -	- - -	- - -	80	80	- - -	- - -	89
4b. Adults age 18 years and over: percent who reported illicit drug use in the past 30 days (obj 26–10c)	- - -	- - -	- - -	5.8	5.9	- - -	- - -	2.0
4c. Adults age 18 years and over: percent who reported binge drinking in the past 30 days (obj 26–11c).	- - -	- - -	- - -	21	22	- - -	- - -	6
Responsible sexual behavior								
5a. Adolescents in grades 9–12: percent who are not sexually active or sexually active and used condoms (obj 25–11)	- - -	83	- - -	85	- - -	86	- - -	95
5a1. Never had intercourse.	- - -	47	- - -	50	- - -	54	- - -	. . .
5a2. Used a condom at last intercourse.	- - -	21	- - -	21	- - -	19	- - -	. . .
5a3. No sexual intercourse in past 3 months . .	- - -	15	- - -	14	- - -	12	- - -	. . .
5b. Sexually active unmarried women age 18–44 years: percent who reported condom use by partners (obj 13–06a)	- - -	23	- - -	- - -	- - -	- - -	- - -	50
5c. New cases of gonorrhea per 100,000 population (obj 25–02) (supplemental measure)	277	149	132	132	129	129	- - -	19
Mental health								
6a. Adults age 18 years and over: percent with recognized depression who received treatment (obj 18–09b)[4]	- - -	23	- - -	- - -	- - -	- - -	- - -	50
6b. Age-adjusted suicide rate per 100,000 standard population (obj 18–01) (supplemental measure) . . .	12.5	12.0	11.3	10.7	10.6	- - -	- - -	5.0
Injury and violence								
7a. Age-adjusted death rate for motor vehicle traffic-related injuries per 100,000 standard population (obj 15–15a)[5].	18.0	16.1	15.6	15.0	15.2	- - -	- - -	9.2
7b. Age-adjusted homicide rate per 100,000 standard population (obj 15–32).	9.4	8.4	6.5	6.2	6.1	- - -	- - -	3.0

See footnotes at end of table.

Table 51 (page 2 of 2). Healthy People 2010 Leading Health Indicators: United States, selected years 1990–2002 and 2010 target

[Data are based on interviews and examinations of samples of the civilian noninstitutionalized population or special population subgroups; information from death certificates and birth certificates; and air quality measurements]

Leading Health Indicators, measures, and Healthy People 2010 objective numbers	1990	1995	1998	1999	2000	2001	2002	2010 Target
Environmental quality								
8a. Percent of population exposed to ozone above EPA standard (obj 08–01a)	- - -	- - -	43	43	43	41	- - -	0
8b. Persons age 4 years and over: age-adjusted percent of nonsmokers exposed to environmental tobacco smoke (obj 27–10)[2]	65	- - -	- - -	- - -	- - -	- - -	- - -	45
8c. Persons under age 18 years: hospital admissions for asthma per 10,000 population (obj 01–09a) (supplemental measure)	- - -	- - -	- - -	25.5	- - -	21.4	- - -	17.3
Immunization								
9a. Children age 19–35 months: percent who received all DTaP, polio, MMR, Hib, and HepB vaccines (obj 14–24a)	- - -	- - -	73	73	73	74	- - -	80
9b. Adults age 65 years and over: age-adjusted percent who received influenza vaccine in the past 12 months (obj 14–29a)[1]	- - -	59	64	66	65	63	66	90
9c. Adults age 65 years and over: age-adjusted percent who ever received pneumococcal vaccine (obj 14–29b)[1]	- - -	35	46	50	53	54	55	90
Access to health care								
10a. Persons under age 65 years: age-adjusted percent with health insurance (obj 01–01)[1,6]	- - -	84	83	84	83	84	84	100
10b. Persons of all ages: age-adjusted percent with a specific source of ongoing primary care (obj 01–04a)[1]	- - -	87	87	86	87	88	88	96
10c. Pregnant women: percent who received prenatal care in the first trimester (obj 16–06a)	76	81	83	83	83	83	- - -	90

- - - Data not available.

. . . Data not applicable.

[1]Data for 1997 and later years are not strictly comparable with data for earlier years due to the 1997 questionnaire redesign. See Appendix I, NHIS. Data for 2002 are provisional.

[2]NHANES data for 1990 are for the period 1988–94. NHANES data for 2000 are for the period 1999–2000, and are based on a smaller sample size and therefore are subject to greater sampling error than the estimate for 1988–94.

[3]In a major redesign of the survey in 1999, the sample size, mode of administration, and survey content changed. Data are not shown for 1998 and earlier years because only limited comparisons can be made between data from the redesigned surveys (1999 onward) and data obtained from surveys prior to 1999. See Appendix I, NHSDA.

[4]Baseline year 1997 and baseline value 23 percent are shown in 1995.

[5]Motor vehicle traffic-related injuries (ICD–9-E810–E819 prior to 1999; and for 1999 and later years ICD–10-V02–V04(.1,.9), V09.2, V12–V14(.3–.9), V19(.4–.6), V20–V28(.3–.9), V29(.4–.9), V30–V39(.4–.9), V40–V49(.4–.9), V50–V59(.4–.9), V60–V69(.4–.9), V70–V79(.4–.9), V80(.3–.5), V81.1, V82.1, V83–V86(.0–.3), V87(.0–.8), V89.2) are a subset of data in tables 29 and 44 for motor vehicle-related injuries. (For ICD–10 codes, parenthetical digits apply to each preceding alphanumeric in the range.)

[6]See Appendix II, Health insurance coverage, for a discussion of changes in measurement of this variable.

NOTES: Additional information on specific measures is presented in the following tables: measure 3b (table 59); measure 5c (table 52); measure 6b (table 46); measure 7b (table 45); measure 10a (table 130); measure 10c (table 6). Additional information related to other measures is presented in the following tables: measure 2a (table 69); measure 2b (table 68); measures 4a and 4c (table 62); measure 5b (table 17); measure 7a (table 44); measure 9a (tables 71 and 72); measure 10b (tables 74 and 76). Current data for the Leading Health Indicators can be obtained from the Healthy People 2010 DATA2010 Web site: wonder.cdc.gov/data2010. Data for additional years are available (see Appendix III).

SOURCES: Youth Risk Behavior Surveillance System (YRBSS), CDC, NCCDPHP: measures 1a, 3a, and 5a; National Youth Tobacco Survey (NYTS), CDC, OSH: measure 3a (2000); National Health Interview Survey (NHIS), CDC, NCHS: measures 1b, 3b, 9b, 9c, 10a, and 10b; National Health and Nutrition Examination Survey (NHANES), CDC, NCHS: measures 2a, 2b, and 8b; National Household Survey on Drug Abuse (NHSDA), SAMHSA: measures 4a, 4b, 4c, and 6a; National Survey of Family Growth (NSFG), CDC, NCHS: measure 5b; Sexually Transmitted Diseases (STD) Surveillance System, CDC, NCHSTP: measure 5c; National Vital Statistics System (NVSS), CDC, NCHS: measures 6b, 7a, 7b, 10c; Aerometric Information Retrieval System (AIRS), EPA, OAR: measure 8a; Healthcare Cost and Utilization Project (HCUP), AHRQ: measure 8c; National Immunization Survey (NIS), CDC, NIP and NCHS: measure 9a.

Some measures will be updated on the web. Go to www.cdc.gov/nchs/hus.htm.

Table 52. Selected notifiable disease rates, according to disease: United States, selected years 1950–2001

[Data are based on reporting by State health departments]

Disease	1950	1960	1970	1980	1990	1995	1998	1999	2000	2001
	Cases per 100,000 population									
Diphtheria	3.83	0.51	0.21	0.00	0.00	–	0.00	0.00	0.00	0.00
Haemophilus influenzae, invasive	- - -	- - -	- - -	- - -	- - -	0.45	0.44	0.48	0.51	0.57
Hepatitis A	- - -	- - -	27.87	12.84	12.64	12.13	8.59	6.25	4.91	3.77
Hepatitis B	- - -	- - -	4.08	8.39	8.48	4.19	3.80	2.82	2.95	2.79
Lyme disease	- - -	- - -	- - -	- - -	- - -	4.49	6.39	5.99	6.53	6.05
Meningococcal disease	- - -	- - -	1.23	1.25	0.99	1.25	1.01	0.92	0.83	0.83
Mumps	- - -	- - -	55.55	3.86	2.17	0.35	0.25	0.14	0.13	0.10
Pertussis (whooping cough)	79.82	8.23	2.08	0.76	1.84	1.97	2.74	2.67	2.88	2.69
Poliomyelitis, total	22.02	1.77	0.02	0.00	0.00	0.00	0.01	0.00	–	–
Paralytic[1]	- - -	1.40	0.02	0.00	0.00	0.00	0.01	0.00	–	–
Rocky Mountain spotted fever	- - -	- - -	0.19	0.52	0.26	0.23	0.14	0.21	0.18	0.25
Rubella (German measles)	- - -	- - -	27.75	1.72	0.45	0.05	0.13	0.10	0.06	0.01
Rubeola (measles)	211.01	245.42	23.23	5.96	11.17	0.12	0.04	0.04	0.03	0.04
Salmonellosis, excluding typhoid fever	- - -	3.85	10.84	14.88	19.54	17.66	16.17	14.89	14.51	14.39
Shigellosis	15.45	6.94	6.79	8.41	10.89	12.32	8.74	6.43	8.41	7.19
Tuberculosis[2]	- - -	30.83	18.28	12.25	10.33	8.70	6.79	6.43	6.01	5.68
Sexually transmitted diseases:[3]										
Syphilis[4]	146.02	68.78	45.26	30.51	54.52	26.40	14.19	12.97	11.23	11.45
Primary and secondary	16.73	9.06	10.89	12.06	20.34	6.30	2.59	2.43	2.12	2.17
Early latent	39.71	10.11	8.08	9.00	22.27	10.15	4.70	4.23	3.36	3.09
Late and late latent[5]	70.22	45.91	24.94	9.30	10.35	9.25	6.56	6.11	5.54	6.03
Congenital[6]	8.97	2.48	0.97	0.12	1.55	0.71	0.31	0.21	0.20	0.16
Chlamydia[7]	- - -	- - -	- - -	- - -	160.83	190.42	236.67	252.99	252.10	278.32
Gonorrhea[8]	192.50	145.40	297.22	445.10	277.45	149.44	131.89	132.32	129.04	128.53
Chancroid	3.34	0.94	0.70	0.30	1.69	0.23	0.07	0.05	0.03	0.01
	Number of cases									
Diphtheria	5,796	918	435	3	4	–	1	1	1	2
Haemophilus influenzae, invasive	- - -	- - -	- - -	- - -	- - -	1,180	1,194	1,309	1,398	1,597
Hepatitis A	- - -	- - -	56,797	29,087	31,441	31,582	23,229	17,047	13,397	10,609
Hepatitis B	- - -	- - -	8,310	19,015	21,102	10,805	10,258	7,694	8,036	7,843
Lyme disease	- - -	- - -	- - -	- - -	- - -	11,700	16,801	16,273	17,730	17,029
Meningococcal disease	- - -	- - -	2,505	2,840	2,451	3,243	2,725	2,501	2,256	2,333
Mumps	- - -	- - -	104,953	8,576	5,292	906	666	387	338	266
Pertussis (whooping cough)	120,718	14,809	4,249	1,730	4,570	5,137	7,405	7,288	7,867	7,580
Poliomyelitis, total	33,300	3,190	33	9	6	7	3	2	–	–
Paralytic[1]	- - -	2,525	31	9	6	7	3	2	–	–
Rocky Mountain spotted fever	- - -	- - -	380	1,163	651	590	365	579	495	695
Rubella (German measles)	- - -	- - -	56,552	3,904	1,125	128	364	267	176	23
Rubeola (measles)	319,124	441,703	47,351	13,506	27,786	309	100	100	86	116
Salmonellosis, excluding typhoid fever	- - -	6,929	22,096	33,715	48,603	45,970	43,694	40,596	39,574	40,495
Shigellosis	23,367	12,487	13,845	19,041	27,077	32,080	23,626	17,521	22,922	20,221
Tuberculosis[2]	- - -	55,494	37,137	27,749	25,701	22,860	18,361	17,531	16,377	15,989
Sexually transmitted diseases:[3]										
Syphilis[4]	217,558	122,538	91,382	68,832	135,590	69,356	38,286	35,379	31,592	32,221
Primary and secondary	23,939	16,145	21,982	27,204	50,578	16,543	7,007	6,617	5,979	6,103
Early latent	59,256	18,017	16,311	20,297	55,397	26,657	12,696	11,534	9,465	8,701
Late and late latent[5]	113,569	81,798	50,348	20,979	25,750	24,296	17,743	16,653	15,594	16,976
Congenital[6]	13,377	4,416	1,953	277	3,865	1,860	840	575	554	441
Chlamydia[7]	- - -	- - -	- - -	- - -	323,663	478,577	614,250	662,647	709,452	783,242
Gonorrhea[8]	286,746	258,933	600,072	1,004,029	690,042	392,651	356,492	360,813	363,136	361,705
Chancroid	4,977	1,680	1,416	788	4,212	607	189	142	78	38

0.00 Rate greater than zero but less than 0.005.   – Quantity zero.   - - - Data not available.

[1]Data beginning in 1986 may be updated due to retrospective case evaluations or late reports.

[2]Case reporting for tuberculosis began in 1953. Data prior to 1975 are not comparable with subsequent years' data because of changes in reporting criteria effective in 1975.

[3]Newly reported civilian cases prior to 1991; includes military cases beginning in 1991. Adjustments to the number of cases from State health departments were made for hardcopy forms and for electronic data submissions through May 3, 2002. For 1950, data for Alaska and Hawaii were not included.

[4]Includes stage of syphilis not stated.

[5]Includes cases of unknown duration.

[6]Data reported for 1989 and later years reflect change in case definition introduced in 1988. Through 1994, all cases of congenitally acquired syphilis; as of 1995, congenital syphilis less than 1 year of age. See STD Surveillance Report for congenital syphilis rates per 100,000 live births. In 2001 the rate was 11.1 congenital syphilis cases per 100,000 live births.

[7]Chlamydia was non-notifiable in 1994 and earlier years. In 1994–99 cases for New York based exclusively on those reported by New York City. Starting in 2000, includes cases for New York State.   [8]Data for 1994 do not include cases from Georgia.

NOTES: The total resident population was used to calculate all rates except sexually transmitted diseases, which used the civilian resident population. For sexually transmitted diseases, 2000 population estimates were used to calculate 2001 rates. Population data from those States where diseases were not notifiable or not available were excluded from rate calculation. See Appendix I for information on underreporting of notifiable diseases. Some numbers for sexually transmitted diseases (1988–2000) and poliomyelitis (1996–99) have been revised and differ from the previous edition of *Health, United States*. Data for additional years are available (see Appendix III).

SOURCES: Centers for Disease Control and Prevention. Summary of notifiable diseases, United States, 2001. Morbidity and mortality weekly report; 50(53). Atlanta, Georgia: Public Health Service. 2003; National Center for HIV, STD, and TB Prevention, Division of STD Prevention. Sexually transmitted disease surveillance, 2001. Atlanta, Georgia: U.S. Department of Health and Human Services, Centers for Disease Control and Prevention, 2002.

Table 53. Acquired immunodeficiency syndrome (AIDS) cases, according to age at diagnosis, sex, detailed race, and Hispanic origin: United States, selected years 1985–2002

[Data are based on reporting by State health departments]

Age at diagnosis, sex, race, and Hispanic origin	All years[1] Percent distribution[2]	All years[1]	1985	1990	1995	1999	2000	2001	2002	2002 Cases per 100,000 population[3]
					Number, by year of report					
All races	. . .	831,112	8,159	41,448	70,412	44,580	40,282	41,450	42,745	15.0
Male										
All males, 13 years and over	100.0	676,609	7,504	36,179	56,689	34,013	30,135	30,663	31,644	28.0
Not Hispanic or Latino:										
White	47.7	322,920	4,746	20,825	26,028	12,691	11,314	11,054	11,221	13.9
Black or African American	35.4	239,650	1,710	10,239	20,833	14,830	13,082	13,764	14,310	111.9
American Indian or Alaska Native .	0.3	2,203	7	81	197	135	136	149	155	17.3
Asian or Pacific Islander	0.8	5,666	49	264	489	295	291	348	381	8.2
Hispanic or Latino[4]	15.6	105,628	992	4,743	9,111	6,043	5,275	5,318	5,543	39.3
13–19 years	0.4	2,632	27	107	223	131	145	184	199	1.4
20–29 years	15.4	104,174	1,501	6,921	8,387	3,972	3,327	3,291	3,433	17.5
30–39 years	44.7	302,420	3,588	16,668	25,684	14,410	12,543	12,082	12,101	56.2
40–49 years	27.8	188,299	1,634	8,828	16,151	10,836	9,648	10,261	10,658	49.5
50–59 years	8.7	58,745	597	2,645	4,692	3,479	3,387	3,633	3,959	24.9
60 years and over	3.0	20,339	157	1,010	1,552	1,185	1,085	1,212	1,294	6.5
Female										
All females, 13 years and over	100.0	145,696	524	4,544	12,978	10,312	9,958	10,617	10,951	9.2
Not Hispanic or Latino:										
White	22.0	32,000	143	1,228	3,042	1,896	1,859	1,993	1,930	2.3
Black or African American	61.2	89,130	280	2,557	7,586	6,711	6,489	6,963	7,339	50.0
American Indian or Alaska Native .	0.3	509	2	9	38	40	70	42	42	4.5
Asian or Pacific Islander	0.6	832	1	20	73	61	74	67	68	1.4
Hispanic or Latino[4]	15.9	23,145	98	726	2,236	1,599	1,462	1,543	1,561	11.8
13–19 years	1.4	1,995	5	67	157	166	170	171	203	1.5
20–29 years	20.6	29,996	178	1,117	2,676	1,886	1,750	1,717	1,819	9.6
30–39 years	43.6	63,504	232	2,087	5,934	4,234	3,973	4,145	3,991	18.7
40–49 years	24.1	35,168	45	780	3,059	2,789	2,857	3,147	3,377	15.3
50–59 years	7.0	10,243	26	274	818	916	867	999	1,150	6.9
60 years and over	3.3	4,790	38	219	334	321	341	438	411	1.5
Children										
All children, under 13 years	100.0	8,807	131	725	745	255	189	170	150	0.3
Not Hispanic or Latino:										
White	18.2	1,601	26	157	117	30	32	30	23	0.1
Black or African American	61.6	5,422	87	390	483	171	122	111	99	1.2
American Indian or Alaska Native .	0.4	31	–	5	2	2	1	–	–	–
Asian or Pacific Islander	0.7	58	–	4	5	2	3	3	4	0.2
Hispanic or Latino[4]	19.1	1,685	18	169	135	49	30	26	24	0.2
Under 1 year	36.9	3,249	54	298	258	87	61	47	46	1.1
1–12 years	63.1	5,558	77	427	487	168	128	123	104	0.2

. . . Category not applicable.

– Quantity zero.

[1]Includes cases reported to the Centers for Disease Control and Prevention prior to 1985 and through December 31, 2002.

[2]Percents may not sum to 100 percent due to rounding.

[3]Computed using estimates of July 1, 2001, U.S. resident population by age, sex, race, and Hispanic origin, prepared for NCHS under a collaboration arrangement with the U.S. Census Bureau.

[4]Persons of Hispanic origin may be of any race.

NOTES: The AIDS case reporting definitions were expanded in 1985, 1987, and 1993. See Appendix II, AIDS. Excludes data for U.S. dependencies and possessions and independent nations in free association with the United States. Data for all years have been updated through December 31, 2002, to include temporally delayed case reports and may differ from previous editions of Health, United States.

SOURCE: Centers for Disease Control and Prevention, National Center for HIV, STD, and TB Prevention, Division of HIV/AIDS Prevention—Surveillance and Epidemiology, AIDS Surveillance, 2003 special data run.

Table 54 (page 1 of 3). **Age-adjusted cancer incidence rates for selected cancer sites, according to sex, race, and Hispanic origin: Selected geographic areas, 1990–99**

[Data are based on the Surveillance, Epidemiology, and End Results (SEER) Program's 12 population-based cancer registries]

Site, sex, race, and Hispanic origin	1990	1993	1994	1995	1996	1997	1998	1999	1990–1999 EAPC[1]
All sites									
	Number of new cases per 100,000 population[2]								
All persons	477.1	486.6	474.0	468.3	469.1	473.3	471.1	463.0	⌃–0.6
White	484.4	490.2	478.3	473.1	473.2	477.2	475.9	466.7	⌃–0.7
Black or African American	514.7	553.6	535.2	525.7	520.1	523.1	509.9	502.7	–0.7
American Indian or Alaska Native	234.2	257.8	242.4	249.6	235.2	255.7	232.8	239.8	–0.2
Asian or Pacific Islander	335.9	352.7	348.7	343.7	341.8	355.4	347.6	346.4	0.2
Hispanic or Latino	340.4	341.1	339.0	334.7	326.9	317.7	322.7	312.7	⌃–1.2
White, not Hispanic or Latino	492.3	497.7	489.0	485.3	487.5	491.4	486.7	481.1	⌃–0.6
Male	584.1	607.4	574.1	556.4	553.7	554.1	545.8	538.8	⌃–1.7
White	590.4	603.6	572.0	553.4	551.6	549.4	542.9	534.2	⌃–1.9
Black or African American	687.2	775.6	722.6	705.4	679.3	684.4	659.3	647.3	⌃–1.6
American Indian or Alaska Native	282.3	333.6	283.3	294.2	247.5	293.6	234.6	272.8	–1.3
Asian or Pacific Islander	387.4	426.1	416.7	404.4	397.4	412.5	394.3	400.4	–0.3
Hispanic or Latino	401.4	423.2	412.4	402.7	388.6	373.4	372.0	359.7	⌃–1.9
White, not Hispanic or Latino	599.0	606.0	580.0	562.9	562.5	559.8	548.9	544.4	⌃–1.8
Female	413.9	407.6	408.6	410.8	413.9	420.3	422.6	412.7	0.2
White	424.0	417.7	418.8	422.5	423.6	431.6	434.1	423.2	0.2
Black or African American	405.7	404.8	408.5	400.7	410.0	409.9	405.7	400.6	0.0
American Indian or Alaska Native	201.4	204.1	214.0	223.1	230.1	232.5	235.0	220.4	1.0
Asian or Pacific Islander	295.9	297.0	299.1	300.8	303.6	317.0	317.9	311.8	⌃0.9
Hispanic or Latino	307.5	289.7	294.6	292.7	289.2	283.1	292.2	284.5	⌃–0.7
White, not Hispanic or Latino	430.8	428.6	430.8	436.3	439.9	448.4	448.0	440.3	⌃0.4
Lung and bronchus									
Male	95.4	89.5	86.7	86.2	83.3	81.4	81.2	76.3	⌃–2.4
White	94.7	88.0	86.1	84.3	81.6	79.4	79.8	74.4	⌃–2.5
Black or African American	134.6	130.3	119.9	133.1	124.5	120.7	116.3	109.8	⌃–2.4
Asian or Pacific Islander	64.4	65.1	61.4	61.9	63.0	64.4	63.3	62.7	–0.4
Hispanic or Latino	58.2	48.4	46.2	47.7	43.3	41.5	42.7	35.9	⌃–4.1
White, not Hispanic or Latino	95.3	88.3	87.4	85.3	83.8	80.8	81.5	76.6	⌃–2.2
Female	47.4	48.8	48.9	49.1	49.9	49.8	50.0	48.2	0.3
White	48.7	50.8	50.5	51.4	51.9	52.2	51.9	49.9	0.4
Black or African American	53.2	52.8	55.5	50.0	54.0	50.1	55.7	55.7	0.2
Asian or Pacific Islander	28.2	26.5	29.1	27.9	27.8	29.9	28.7	28.6	0.5
Hispanic or Latino	24.6	26.4	21.1	22.6	23.0	22.8	22.2	20.6	⌃–1.8
White, not Hispanic or Latino	49.9	52.1	52.6	54.0	54.5	54.9	54.1	52.8	⌃0.8
Colon and rectum									
Male	72.5	66.2	64.9	62.3	63.7	65.4	64.4	61.8	⌃–1.5
White	73.1	65.9	64.9	61.7	63.8	64.8	63.9	61.4	⌃–1.7
Black or African American	73.1	74.8	70.8	70.8	64.9	71.1	71.8	67.8	⌃–1.2
Asian or Pacific Islander	61.3	58.2	59.1	59.2	58.4	61.9	59.4	55.9	–0.3
Hispanic or Latino	45.3	41.9	43.9	41.6	45.7	45.3	44.7	41.8	–0.7
White, not Hispanic or Latino	74.4	66.5	66.0	62.6	64.6	64.9	64.9	63.4	⌃–1.6
Female	50.3	47.5	46.4	45.6	45.7	46.7	47.9	45.6	⌃–0.8
White	49.9	47.1	45.7	45.2	45.2	46.3	47.3	44.6	⌃–0.9
Black or African American	61.1	55.6	56.8	54.6	53.7	57.4	55.8	56.1	–0.6
Asian or Pacific Islander	38.1	40.6	39.0	38.7	39.8	35.8	41.3	40.2	–0.2
Hispanic or Latino	32.3	29.1	31.3	30.3	29.4	28.4	29.5	29.4	⌃–1.1
White, not Hispanic or Latino	50.9	48.6	47.1	46.0	46.7	48.1	49.1	46.2	⌃–0.7
Prostate									
Male	166.5	205.0	175.1	163.3	162.8	167.4	163.2	170.0	–2.7
White	167.7	198.0	168.0	157.1	157.1	161.1	155.7	162.3	⌃–3.3
Black or African American	217.7	325.2	288.7	261.5	254.6	256.7	258.0	255.7	–1.1
American Indian or Alaska Native	73.1	85.8	52.2	57.4	65.9	64.5	46.9	48.3	⌃–4.7
Asian or Pacific Islander	89.0	123.1	113.2	105.1	96.1	100.5	96.1	107.1	–1.2
Hispanic or Latino	113.8	145.7	136.8	125.8	119.3	121.0	120.5	116.9	–1.6
White, not Hispanic or Latino	169.4	194.5	167.9	158.4	158.8	162.4	153.6	162.7	⌃–3.4
Breast									
Female	129.2	127.0	128.3	130.2	131.6	135.0	137.6	135.8	⌃0.7
White	134.3	131.9	133.7	135.3	136.1	140.0	142.6	140.8	⌃0.7
Black or African American	116.5	117.0	120.5	121.8	121.7	122.3	121.2	120.9	⌃0.5
American Indian or Alaska Native	36.6	59.0	52.7	60.0	72.5	53.3	59.2	54.4	2.3
Asian or Pacific Islander	86.5	84.6	81.3	88.4	91.9	101.8	103.5	102.0	⌃2.8
Hispanic or Latino	84.3	75.7	82.2	84.1	84.9	79.7	85.0	83.6	0.0
White, not Hispanic or Latino	138.6	138.2	141.0	142.3	144.5	148.4	150.7	150.5	⌃1.0

See footnotes at end of table.

[Data are based on the Surveillance, Epidemiology, and End Results (SEER) Program's 12 population-based cancer registries]

Site, sex, race, and Hispanic origin	1990	1993	1994	1995	1996	1997	1998	1999	1990–1999 EAPC[1]
Cervix uteri	Number of new cases per 100,000 population[2]								
Female	11.9	10.7	10.6	9.9	10.7	9.8	9.8	9.1	^–2.3
White	11.3	10.1	9.9	9.1	9.9	9.1	9.2	8.8	^–2.3
Black or African American	16.2	14.1	13.5	14.3	13.5	13.0	12.3	12.3	^–2.7
Asian or Pacific Islander	12.0	12.1	14.5	11.3	13.2	11.3	11.4	8.6	–1.8
Hispanic or Latino	21.1	19.5	19.5	17.5	17.7	15.3	15.1	16.1	^–3.7
White, not Hispanic or Latino	9.5	8.5	8.2	7.7	8.3	7.8	7.9	7.3	^–2.2
Corpus uteri									
Female	24.7	23.9	24.3	24.8	24.4	25.2	24.8	24.3	0.1
White	26.5	25.3	25.7	26.3	25.7	26.7	26.2	25.6	0.0
Black or African American	17.1	17.7	18.0	17.7	19.0	17.9	18.1	17.3	0.9
Asian or Pacific Islander	13.2	14.7	16.0	18.1	16.9	18.3	17.5	18.0	^3.0
Hispanic or Latino	16.2	15.1	15.3	15.9	15.1	16.3	16.6	15.3	–0.1
White, not Hispanic or Latino	27.1	26.5	27.2	27.5	27.0	27.7	27.3	26.6	0.1
Ovary									
Female	17.9	17.8	16.9	17.3	16.8	16.8	16.7	16.7	^–0.9
White	18.9	18.7	17.8	18.3	18.0	17.8	17.6	17.6	^–0.9
Black or African American	12.9	13.3	13.8	12.5	10.9	11.8	12.5	11.8	–0.5
Asian or Pacific Islander	12.7	13.4	11.9	12.5	11.9	13.6	12.4	13.1	0.6
Hispanic or Latino	14.3	14.2	13.4	13.2	13.6	12.7	14.1	12.4	–1.2
White, not Hispanic or Latino	19.6	19.1	18.4	18.8	18.5	18.3	17.8	18.5	^–0.9
Oral cavity and pharynx									
Male	19.2	18.1	17.7	16.9	17.3	16.7	16.2	14.9	^–2.3
White	18.7	17.8	17.2	16.8	16.8	16.4	15.8	14.6	^–2.4
Black or African American	26.1	23.8	23.8	22.1	23.0	19.5	21.0	18.7	^–2.7
Asian or Pacific Islander	15.1	12.9	14.3	12.2	14.7	15.2	13.7	11.4	–0.9
Hispanic or Latino	10.9	10.3	11.0	12.4	10.4	9.6	9.2	9.1	^–2.4
White, not Hispanic or Latino	19.3	18.7	17.8	16.7	17.3	17.2	16.4	15.6	^–2.2
Female	7.3	7.2	6.7	6.9	6.9	6.9	6.5	6.1	^–1.4
White	7.4	7.3	6.7	7.0	6.8	6.7	6.6	5.9	^–1.7
Black or African American	6.3	7.3	7.1	6.7	7.3	7.0	6.5	5.8	–0.5
Asian or Pacific Islander	6.0	5.9	5.6	5.3	5.7	6.6	4.5	6.4	–0.8
Hispanic or Latino	3.6	4.6	4.5	3.5	3.5	3.4	3.2	3.9	–1.0
White, not Hispanic or Latino	7.7	7.6	7.0	7.2	7.3	7.2	7.1	6.1	^–1.7
Stomach									
Male	14.7	14.3	14.2	13.5	13.7	13.2	12.6	12.5	^–1.9
White	12.9	12.3	12.3	11.9	11.8	11.1	10.8	10.8	^–2.1
Black or African American	22.0	20.3	22.5	17.6	21.4	20.8	18.8	15.1	^–3.0
Asian or Pacific Islander	27.0	28.3	24.9	24.5	24.5	25.4	22.0	23.3	·–2.2
Hispanic or Latino	19.6	19.5	20.8	17.6	15.4	16.8	16.5	16.6	^–2.4
White, not Hispanic or Latino	12.0	11.2	11.2	10.8	11.1	10.0	9.6	9.5	^–2.6
Female	6.7	6.4	6.2	6.2	6.1	6.1	6.3	6.3	^–1.0
White	5.7	5.4	5.0	5.1	5.0	4.9	5.1	5.2	^–1.6
Black or African American	9.9	8.9	10.1	9.9	9.3	10.9	10.9	10.0	0.4
Asian or Pacific Islander	15.5	15.3	15.0	13.1	13.8	12.3	12.7	12.5	^–2.7
Hispanic or Latino	10.8	10.1	8.2	10.2	9.1	9.1	9.6	8.1	^–2.5
White, not Hispanic or Latino	5.0	4.8	4.4	4.4	4.3	4.0	4.2	4.6	^–2.2
Pancreas									
Male	13.1	12.5	12.9	12.6	12.4	12.7	12.5	11.8	^–0.6
White	12.7	12.1	12.3	12.3	12.1	12.3	12.4	11.6	^–0.6
Black or African American	19.6	18.2	18.5	18.3	18.3	17.2	15.9	16.4	^–1.6
Asian or Pacific Islander	11.2	12.3	14.3	10.6	10.9	12.7	10.7	9.1	–1.0
Hispanic or Latino	10.9	9.9	9.4	11.1	10.1	10.6	8.4	7.9	–2.1
White, not Hispanic or Latino	12.4	11.9	12.5	12.1	12.1	12.3	12.7	12.1	–0.1
Female	10.0	9.8	9.9	9.9	10.0	10.0	9.8	9.1	^–0.7
White	9.8	9.5	9.7	9.6	9.6	9.5	9.5	8.8	^–0.8
Black or African American	12.9	15.7	15.1	15.7	14.9	16.9	13.7	12.5	–0.8
Asian or Pacific Islander	10.0	8.0	6.8	8.0	7.9	8.3	8.5	8.6	–0.2
Hispanic or Latino	9.7	9.2	8.9	8.0	8.1	8.5	8.2	8.1	^–2.1
White, not Hispanic or Latino	9.6	9.4	9.4	9.6	9.7	9.2	9.6	8.6	–0.8

See footnotes at end of table.

Table 54 (page 3 of 3). **Age-adjusted cancer incidence rates for selected cancer sites, according to sex, race, and Hispanic origin: Selected geographic areas, 1990–99**

[Data are based on the Surveillance, Epidemiology, and End Results (SEER) Program's 12 population-based cancer registries]

Site, sex, race, and Hispanic origin	1990	1993	1994	1995	1996	1997	1998	1999	1990–1999 EAPC[1]
Urinary bladder	Number of new cases per 100,000 population[2]								
Male	37.2	36.5	35.7	34.8	35.0	35.1	35.7	34.9	^–0.7
White	40.6	39.6	39.2	38.1	38.3	38.5	39.2	38.0	^–0.7
Black or African American	19.8	23.2	18.8	18.7	18.5	19.7	19.1	20.3	–0.5
Asian or Pacific Islander	15.7	16.9	16.3	16.9	16.3	15.9	16.9	17.6	1.5
Hispanic or Latino	21.7	18.3	19.5	16.7	16.1	15.4	15.7	15.3	^–3.2
White, not Hispanic or Latino	41.7	40.9	40.0	39.5	40.2	40.3	40.5	39.7	^–0.6
Female	9.5	9.4	9.0	9.3	8.9	9.2	8.9	9.1	^–0.5
White	9.9	10.1	9.8	10.0	9.7	9.8	9.6	9.6	^–0.4
Black or African American	8.6	7.9	7.1	7.4	7.2	8.1	6.5	8.5	–0.8
Asian or Pacific Islander	5.4	3.9	3.9	4.5	3.9	5.3	4.9	4.2	0.0
Hispanic or Latino	5.3	5.0	4.9	4.7	4.7	4.4	3.8	3.7	^–3.8
White, not Hispanic or Latino	10.1	10.4	9.9	10.4	10.0	10.5	10.1	10.1	0.0
Non-Hodgkin's lymphoma									
Male	22.7	23.3	24.6	24.9	24.4	23.6	22.4	23.0	0.0
White	23.7	24.5	25.6	25.9	25.4	24.2	23.3	23.7	–0.2
Black or African American	17.8	17.3	20.1	21.1	18.6	22.2	16.4	17.5	0.3
Asian or Pacific Islander	16.5	15.7	18.3	16.9	17.1	16.8	15.9	18.9	1.0
Hispanic or Latino	16.9	16.9	17.8	20.5	20.3	15.9	17.3	15.0	–1.2
White, not Hispanic or Latino	24.6	25.4	26.5	26.8	26.2	24.8	24.2	24.8	–0.2
Female	14.5	14.5	15.2	15.0	15.0	15.7	15.9	15.4	^1.0
White	15.4	15.2	16.1	15.6	15.6	16.3	16.5	16.2	^0.8
Black or African American	10.4	10.0	8.7	9.9	11.2	12.0	12.4	10.4	2.0
Asian or Pacific Islander	9.2	11.0	12.4	11.9	9.7	11.5	11.4	11.4	2.1
Hispanic or Latino	13.1	12.2	13.0	11.4	12.3	12.6	11.7	11.8	–0.2
White, not Hispanic or Latino	15.3	15.4	16.2	16.0	15.8	16.7	16.9	16.5	^1.0
Leukemia									
Male	16.9	16.3	16.0	17.0	15.9	16.1	15.7	14.5	^–1.3
White	17.7	17.1	17.0	18.2	16.5	17.0	16.4	15.0	^–1.4
Black or African American	15.3	13.7	11.4	12.5	12.8	12.9	12.1	11.8	^–1.9
Asian or Pacific Islander	8.6	9.7	10.3	10.1	11.1	9.4	10.1	10.6	0.9
Hispanic or Latino	11.3	10.8	9.7	14.2	11.4	11.0	10.5	9.6	–1.2
White, not Hispanic or Latino	17.6	17.3	17.4	18.6	16.5	17.1	16.6	15.1	^–1.3
Female	9.7	9.8	9.6	9.8	9.6	9.4	9.3	8.3	^–1.3
White	10.1	10.1	10.0	10.3	10.0	9.9	9.8	8.5	^–1.2
Black or African American	8.3	9.4	7.6	7.9	7.9	7.6	7.6	7.2	^–2.3
Asian or Pacific Islander	5.9	7.5	7.1	6.3	6.8	5.7	6.7	6.3	0.1
Hispanic or Latino	8.2	6.9	7.8	7.8	6.7	7.6	7.5	6.4	–1.5
White, not Hispanic or Latino	10.0	10.1	9.7	10.2	10.0	9.9	9.4	8.4	^–1.3

^ Estimated annual percent change (EAPC) is significantly different from 0 ($p < 0.05$).
[1]EAPC has been calculated by fitting a linear regression model to the natural logarithm of the yearly rates from 1990–99.
[2]Age adjusted by 5-year age groups to the year 2000 U.S. standard population. See Appendix II, Age adjustment.

NOTES: Estimates are based on 12 SEER areas November 2001 submission and differ from published estimates based on 9 SEER areas or other submission dates. Estimates for Hispanic population exclude data from Alaska, Detroit, and Hawaii. See Appendix I, SEER. Numbers have been revised and differ from previous editions of *Health, United States*. The race groups, white, black, Asian or Pacific Islander, and American Indian or Alaska Native, include persons of Hispanic and non-Hispanic origin. Conversely, persons of Hispanic origin may be of any race. Estimates for American Indian or Alaska Native are not shown for some sites because of the small number of annual cases.

SOURCE: National Institutes of Health, National Cancer Institute, Surveillance, Epidemiology, and End Results (SEER) Program at www.seer.cancer.gov.

This table will be updated with 2000 data on the web. Go to www.cdc.gov/nchs/hus.htm.

Table 55. Five-year relative cancer survival rates for selected cancer sites, according to race and sex: Selected geographic areas, 1974–79, 1980–82, 1983–85, 1986–88, 1989–91, and 1992–98

[Data are based on the Surveillance, Epidemiology, and End Results Program's 9 population-based cancer registries]

Sex and site	White						Black or African American					
	1974–79	1980–82	1983–85	1986–88	1989–91	1992–98	1974–79	1980–82	1983–85	1986–88	1989–91	1992–98
Both sexes	Percent of patients											
All sites	50.9	52.1	53.9	56.7	60.3	63.8	39.2	39.7	39.8	42.6	46.2	52.6
Oral cavity and pharynx.	54.9	55.6	55.3	55.2	55.4	58.8	36.5	31.0	35.2	34.7	32.6	34.9
Esophagus.	5.5	7.3	9.3	10.7	11.8	14.7	3.3	5.4	6.2	7.2	8.9	8.3
Stomach	15.2	16.5	16.2	19.1	18.4	20.9	15.7	19.4	18.9	19.3	24.8	20.0
Colon	51.9	55.7	58.4	61.6	63.1	62.7	47.3	49.3	49.3	52.9	53.9	52.8
Rectum	49.8	53.1	55.9	59.1	60.5	62.4	40.4	37.9	43.9	51.1	54.3	52.7
Pancreas	2.4	2.8	2.9	3.1	4.1	4.3	3.2	4.5	5.0	6.2	3.8	3.9
Lung and bronchus	13.1	13.5	13.8	13.5	14.3	15.0	11.3	12.1	11.3	11.9	10.7	12.3
Urinary bladder.	74.9	78.9	78.2	80.7	82.1	82.3	51.5	58.3	59.6	62.3	61.9	64.5
Non-Hodgkin's lymphoma . . .	48.2	51.9	54.4	52.9	51.9	56.1	50.3	50.2	45.1	50.2	43.7	46.1
Leukemia.	36.6	39.5	42.0	44.2	45.8	47.3	30.8	32.9	33.6	38.0	34.1	38.4
Male												
All sites	43.4	46.7	48.5	51.8	57.7	63.5	32.1	34.3	34.5	37.7	43.3	54.0
Oral cavity and pharynx.	54.4	54.6	54.4	52.2	52.1	57.8	31.2	26.5	29.9	29.3	27.9	29.5
Esophagus.	5.2	6.5	7.8	11.2	11.8	14.7	2.3	4.6	5.0	7.0	8.0	9.0
Stomach	13.8	15.6	14.6	16.2	15.1	19.5	15.3	18.5	18.5	15.3	22.3	19.2
Colon	51.0	56.0	58.9	62.5	63.7	63.0	45.4	46.7	48.3	52.6	53.8	53.2
Rectum	48.9	51.7	55.2	58.8	60.2	61.6	36.7	36.1	43.1	46.2	56.0	51.6
Pancreas	2.6	2.5	2.7	2.9	3.8	4.3	2.4	3.2	4.4	6.4	3.3	4.2
Lung and bronchus	11.6	12.2	12.1	12.0	12.7	13.3	10.0	10.9	10.3	11.9	9.5	10.8
Prostate gland	70.3	74.5	76.3	82.7	91.8	97.8	60.8	64.7	63.9	69.3	80.6	92.6
Urinary bladder.	75.9	79.9	79.5	82.3	84.4	84.4	58.9	62.8	64.8	67.4	65.5	69.4
Non-Hodgkin's lymphoma . . .	47.2	50.9	53.4	50.1	47.7	52.7	44.7	47.2	43.6	46.6	38.7	41.4
Leukemia.	35.6	39.6	41.6	45.5	46.4	48.4	30.7	30.1	32.5	36.7	29.2	37.9
Female												
All sites	57.4	57.1	58.8	61.5	62.9	64.2	46.9	46.0	45.4	47.9	49.3	51.0
Colon	52.6	55.4	58.0	60.7	62.5	62.4	48.7	51.3	50.1	53.1	53.9	52.5
Rectum	50.7	54.7	56.7	59.5	60.8	63.5	43.8	40.2	44.7	56.0	52.6	53.8
Pancreas	2.3	3.0	3.2	3.4	4.4	4.4	4.1	5.8	5.5	6.0	4.3	3.7
Lung and bronchus	16.7	16.2	17.0	15.8	16.6	17.0	15.5	15.5	14.1	11.7	13.0	14.7
Melanoma of skin	85.8	88.3	89.4	91.3	91.5	91.8	69.9	*	70.1	*	94.0	61.9
Breast	75.4	77.1	79.2	83.9	86.1	87.6	63.1	65.7	63.4	69.2	71.1	72.5
Cervix uteri	69.7	68.2	70.6	71.7	72.3	72.1	63.0	61.3	60.4	55.5	62.6	59.9
Corpus uteri	87.7	82.8	84.5	84.4	85.6	86.0	59.4	55.1	54.2	57.1	57.5	60.5
Ovary	37.2	38.7	40.2	41.9	49.6	52.5	40.5	39.1	41.6	38.6	41.6	52.5
Non-Hodgkin's lymphoma . . .	49.3	52.9	55.5	56.2	57.1	60.2	57.5	53.7	46.9	54.8	50.8	53.8

* Data for population groups with fewer than 25 cases are not shown.

NOTES: Rates are based on followup of patients through 1999. The rate is the ratio of the observed survival rate for the patient group to the expected survival rate for persons in the general population similar to the patient group with respect to age, sex, race, and calendar year of observation. It estimates the chance of surviving the effects of cancer. The race groups white and black include persons of Hispanic and non-Hispanic origin. Numbers have been revised and differ from previous editions of Health, United States.

SOURCE: National Institutes of Health, National Cancer Institute, Surveillance, Epidemiology, and End Results (SEER) Program at www.seer.cancer.gov.

Table 56 (page 1 of 3). Limitation of activity caused by chronic conditions, according to selected characteristics: United States, selected years 1997–2001

[Data are based on household interviews of a sample of the civilian noninstitutionalized population]

Characteristic	1997	1999	2000	2001
All ages	Percent of persons with any activity limitation[1]			
Total[2,3]	13.3	12.2	11.7	12.1
Age				
Under 18 years	6.6	6.0	6.0	6.7
Under 5 years	3.5	3.1	3.2	3.3
5–17 years	7.8	7.0	7.0	8.0
18–44 years	7.0	6.3	5.8	6.1
18–24 years	5.1	4.4	3.6	4.6
25–44 years	7.6	6.9	6.5	6.6
45–54 years	14.2	13.1	12.4	13.1
55–64 years	22.2	21.1	19.7	20.7
65 years and over	38.7	35.6	34.7	34.5
65–74 years	30.0	27.5	26.1	26.0
75 years and over	50.2	45.6	45.1	44.7
Sex[3]				
Male	13.1	12.1	11.7	12.2
Female	13.4	12.2	11.5	11.9
Race[3,4]				
White only	13.1	12.0	11.5	11.8
Black or African American only	17.1	15.3	14.3	15.6
American Indian and Alaska Native only	23.1	18.8	20.1	18.9
Asian only	7.5	6.8	6.6	6.7
Native Hawaiian and Other Pacific Islander only	- - -	*	*	*
2 or more races	- - -	20.3	19.8	19.8
Black or African American; White	- - -	14.9	*20.3	14.9
American Indian and Alaska Native; White	- - -	26.0	25.3	22.0
Hispanic origin and race[3,4]				
Hispanic or Latino	12.8	10.4	10.3	10.6
Mexican	12.5	9.6	10.4	10.3
Not Hispanic or Latino	13.5	12.4	11.9	12.4
White only	13.2	12.2	11.7	12.1
Black or African American only	17.0	15.2	14.3	15.5
Poverty status[3,5]				
Poor	26.8	24.6	23.2	24.1
Near poor	19.0	19.1	17.5	18.8
Nonpoor	10.5	10.0	9.5	9.9
Hispanic origin and race and poverty status[3,4,5]				
Hispanic or Latino:				
Poor	19.7	16.4	16.9	17.2
Near poor	13.1	11.4	11.4	11.2
Nonpoor	9.8	7.9	7.4	7.9
Not Hispanic or Latino:				
White only:				
Poor	29.5	27.6	25.6	26.4
Near poor	20.7	21.5	19.7	20.8
Nonpoor	10.7	10.2	9.8	10.2
Black or African American only:				
Poor	29.4	28.0	24.7	27.0
Near poor	20.0	19.1	18.3	22.1
Nonpoor	10.7	10.1	9.7	10.3
Geographic region[3]				
Northeast	13.0	11.3	10.6	11.1
Midwest	13.1	12.9	12.3	13.4
South	13.9	12.6	11.7	12.3
West	13.0	11.7	12.1	11.5
Location of residence[3]				
Within MSA[6]	12.7	11.4	10.9	11.3
Outside MSA[6]	15.5	15.1	14.6	15.3

See footnotes at end of table.

Table 56 (page 2 of 3). Limitation of activity caused by chronic conditions, according to selected characteristics: United States, selected years 1997–2001

[Data are based on household interviews of a sample of the civilian noninstitutionalized population]

Characteristic	1997	1999	2000	2001	1997	1999	2000	2001
65 years of age and over	Percent with ADL limitation[7]				Percent with IADL limitation[7]			
All adults 65 years of age and over[2,8]	6.7	6.3	6.3	6.4	13.7	12.4	12.7	12.6
Age								
65–74 years	3.4	3.1	3.3	3.4	6.9	6.2	6.6	6.7
75 years and over	10.4	9.9	9.5	9.6	21.2	19.1	19.3	18.9
Sex[8]								
Male.	5.2	4.9	5.1	6.1	9.1	8.4	9.2	9.6
Female.	7.7	7.2	7.0	6.6	16.9	15.1	15.1	14.6
Race[4,8]								
White only.	6.3	5.8	5.8	5.7	13.1	11.6	12.1	11.8
Black or African American only	11.7	12.0	10.2	11.7	21.3	20.9	19.2	18.7
American Indian and Alaska Native only	*	*	*	*	*	*25.2	*	*
Asian only.	*	*	*7.4	*9.1	*9.1	*9.1	*10.1	15.8
Native Hawaiian and Other Pacific Islander only	- - -	*	*	*	- - -	*	*	*
2 or more races.	- - -	*	*	*	- - -	*	*	*16.1
Hispanic origin and race[4,8]								
Hispanic or Latino	10.8	8.6	8.6	11.2	16.3	14.1	13.4	17.0
Mexican.	11.4	8.9	9.4	10.6	18.8	15.6	16.3	17.0
Not Hispanic or Latino	6.5	6.2	6.1	6.1	13.6	12.3	12.6	12.3
White only	6.1	5.7	5.7	5.5	13.0	11.5	12.1	11.6
Black or African American only.	11.7	12.0	10.1	11.8	21.2	21.0	19.1	18.7
Poverty status[5,8]								
Poor.	13.0	10.1	9.6	12.7	26.9	22.3	20.2	24.8
Near poor	7.5	6.7	7.1	7.4	16.3	15.1	15.3	15.0
Nonpoor	5.3	5.5	5.2	5.0	10.1	9.7	9.4	9.7
Hispanic origin and race and poverty status[4,5,8]								
Hispanic or Latino:								
Poor	15.5	*8.4	12.3	14.1	25.8	17.9	17.6	23.5
Near poor	11.3	*8.6	*7.6	10.5	16.5	14.1	14.1	14.6
Nonpoor	*	*8.1	*6.5	*8.4	*9.7	*10.4	*7.9	*11.7
Not Hispanic or Latino:								
White only:								
Poor	12.7	8.8	8.9	11.2	27.2	21.2	20.0	25.2
Near poor.	6.7	5.7	6.4	6.1	15.8	14.3	14.8	14.0
Nonpoor.	5.0	5.3	4.8	4.4	10.0	9.2	9.2	9.0
Black or African American only:								
Poor	12.9	13.9	9.9	18.2	27.4	27.9	21.8	29.1
Near poor.	12.0	15.2	11.2	13.4	21.4	23.5	20.5	19.3
Nonpoor.	*10.6	*8.9	*11.9	*12.0	*13.0	18.4	15.5	18.3

See footnotes at end of table.

Table 56 (page 3 of 3). Limitation of activity caused by chronic conditions, according to selected characteristics: United States, selected years 1997–2001

[Data are based on household interviews of a sample of the civilian noninstitutionalized population]

Characteristic	1997	1999	2000	2001	1997	1999	2000	2001
Geographic region[8]	Percent with ADL limitation[7]				Percent with IADL limitation[7]			
Northeast	6.1	5.8	5.7	6.6	12.2	11.2	11.5	11.3
Midwest	5.8	5.4	5.6	4.9	13.1	12.3	13.2	12.5
South	8.2	7.1	7.4	7.5	15.8	13.2	13.1	13.3
West	5.9	6.7	5.7	6.0	12.4	12.3	12.6	12.6
Location of residence[8]								
Within MSA[6]	6.6	6.3	6.4	6.1	13.5	12.1	12.6	12.2
Outside MSA[6]	7.2	6.4	6.0	7.3	14.4	13.4	13.2	13.7

* Estimates are considered unreliable. Data preceded by an asterisk have a relative standard error (RSE) of 20–30 percent. Data not shown have a RSE of greater than 30 percent.

- - - Data not available.

[1]Limitation of activity is assessed by asking respondents a series of questions about limitations in their ability to perform activities usual for their age group because of a physical, mental, or emotional problem. See Appendix II, Limitation of activity; Activities of daily living; Condition; Instrumental activities of daily living.

[2]Includes all other races not shown separately and unknown poverty status.

[3]Estimates for all persons are age adjusted to the year 2000 standard population using six age groups: Under 18 years, 18–44 years, 45–54 years, 55–64 years, 65–74 years, and 75 years and over. See Appendix II, Age adjustment.

[4]The race groups, white, black, American Indian and Alaska Native (AI/AN), Asian, Native Hawaiian and Other Pacific Islander, and 2 or more races, include persons of Hispanic and non-Hispanic origin. Persons of Hispanic origin may be of any race. Starting with data year 1999 race-specific estimates are tabulated according to 1997 Standards for Federal data on Race and Ethnicity and are not strictly comparable with estimates for earlier years. The five single race categories plus multiple race categories shown in the table conform to 1997 Standards. The 1999 race-specific estimates are for persons who reported only one racial group; the category "2 or more races" includes persons who reported more than one racial group. Prior to data year 1999, data were tabulated according to 1977 Standards with four racial groups and the category "Asian only" included Native Hawaiian and Other Pacific Islander. Estimates for single race categories prior to 1999 included persons who reported one race or, if they reported more than one race, identified one race as best representing their race. The effect of the 1997 Standard on the 1999 estimates can be seen by comparing 1999 data tabulated according to the two Standards: Age-adjusted estimates based on the 1977 Standard of the percent of persons with activity limitation are: identical for white and black persons; 1.1 percentage points higher for AI/AN persons; and 0.5 percentage points higher for Asian and Pacific Islander persons; for persons 65 years of age and older with ADL limitation: identical for white persons; and 0.1 percentage points lower for black persons; for persons 65 years of age and older with IADL limitation: identical for white persons; 0.2 percentage points lower for black persons; 3.0 percentage points lower for AI/AN persons; and 0.2 percentage points lower for Asian and Pacific Islander persons than estimates based on the 1997 Standards. See Appendix II, Race.

[5]Poor persons are defined as below the poverty threshold. Near poor persons have incomes of 100 percent to less than 200 percent of the poverty threshold. Nonpoor persons have incomes of 200 percent or greater than the poverty threshold. Poverty status was unknown for 20 percent of persons in the sample in 1997, 25 percent in 1998, 28 percent in 1999, 27 percent in 2000, and 28 percent in 2001. See Appendix II, Family income; Poverty level.

[6]MSA is metropolitan statistical area.

[7]These estimates are for elderly noninstitutionalized persons. ADL is activities of daily living and IADL is instrumental activities of daily living. Respondents were asked about needing the help of another person with personal care (ADL) and routine needs such as chores and shopping (IADL) because of a physical, mental, or emotional problem. See Appendix II, Activities of daily living; Condition; Instrumental activities of daily living.

[8]Estimates are age adjusted to the year 2000 standard population using two age groups: 65–74 years and 75 years and over. See Appendix II, Age adjustment.

NOTE: Standard errors for selected years are available in the spreadsheet version of this table. See www.cdc.gov/nchs/hus.htm.

SOURCE: Centers for Disease Control and Prevention, National Center for Health Statistics, National Health Interview Survey, family core questionnaire.

Table 57 (page 1 of 2). Respondent-assessed health status according to selected characteristics: United States, selected years 1991–2001

[Data are based on household interviews of a sample of the civilian noninstitutionalized population]

Characteristic	1991	1995	1997[1]	1998[1]	1999[1]	2000[1]	2001[1]
	Percent of persons with fair or poor health[2]						
Total[3,4]	10.4	10.6	9.2	9.1	8.9	9.0	9.2
Age							
Under 18 years	2.6	2.6	2.1	1.8	1.6	1.7	1.8
Under 6 years	2.7	2.7	1.9	1.5	1.4	1.5	1.6
6–17 years	2.6	2.5	2.1	1.9	1.8	1.8	1.9
18–44 years	6.1	6.6	5.3	5.3	5.1	5.1	5.4
18–24 years	4.8	4.5	3.4	3.2	3.4	3.2	3.3
25–44 years	6.4	7.2	5.9	5.9	5.6	5.7	6.0
45–54 years	13.4	13.4	11.7	11.6	11.5	11.9	11.7
55–64 years	20.7	21.4	18.2	18.0	18.5	17.9	19.2
65 years and over	29.0	28.3	26.7	26.7	26.1	27.0	26.6
65–74 years	26.0	25.6	23.1	23.9	22.7	22.6	23.0
75 years and over	33.6	32.2	31.5	30.4	30.2	32.2	30.8
Sex[3]							
Male	10.0	10.1	8.8	8.8	8.6	8.8	9.0
Female	10.8	11.1	9.7	9.4	9.2	9.3	9.5
Race[3,5]							
White only	9.6	9.7	8.3	8.2	8.0	8.2	8.2
Black or African American only	16.8	17.2	15.8	15.7	14.6	14.6	15.4
American Indian and Alaska Native only	18.3	18.7	17.3	17.6	14.7	17.2	14.5
Asian only	7.8	9.3	7.8	7.1	8.6	7.4	8.1
Native Hawaiian and Other Pacific Islander only	- - -	- - -	- - -	- - -	*	*	*
2 or more races	- - -	- - -	- - -	- - -	12.9	16.4	13.8
Black or African American; White	- - -	- - -	- - -	- - -	*20.5	14.6	*10.1
American Indian and Alaska Native; White	- - -	- - -	- - -	- - -	14.5	18.8	15.0
Hispanic origin and race[3,5]							
Hispanic or Latino	15.6	15.1	13.0	13.1	11.9	12.9	12.7
Mexican	17.0	16.7	13.1	13.5	12.3	12.9	12.5
Not Hispanic or Latino	#	#	8.9	8.8	8.6	8.7	8.9
White only	9.1	9.1	8.0	7.8	7.7	7.9	7.9
Black or African American only	16.8	17.3	15.8	15.8	14.6	14.6	15.5
Poverty status[3,6]							
Poor	22.8	23.7	21.4	22.2	21.7	20.9	21.0
Near poor	14.7	15.5	14.6	15.6	14.9	15.3	15.5
Nonpoor	6.8	6.7	6.1	5.7	6.1	6.3	6.2
Hispanic origin and race and poverty status[3,5,6]							
Hispanic or Latino:							
Poor	23.6	22.7	19.8	21.7	18.9	19.1	18.8
Near poor	18.0	16.9	14.0	15.3	14.2	16.5	15.2
Nonpoor	9.3	8.7	8.8	7.9	8.2	8.4	9.2
Not Hispanic or Latino:							
White only:							
Poor	21.9	22.8	20.6	21.3	20.5	20.1	19.4
Near poor	14.0	14.8	14.1	15.3	14.5	14.7	14.6
Nonpoor	6.4	6.2	5.7	5.3	5.7	5.8	5.8
Black or African American only:							
Poor	25.8	27.7	25.6	26.3	27.2	25.3	26.5
Near poor	17.0	19.3	19.5	19.3	18.2	19.4	20.9
Nonpoor	10.9	9.9	9.6	9.0	8.6	9.6	9.3

See footnotes at end of table.

Table 57 (page 2 of 2). Respondent-assessed health status according to selected characteristics: United States, selected years 1991–2001

[Data are based on household interviews of a sample of the civilian noninstitutionalized population]

Characteristic	1991	1995	1997[1]	1998[1]	1999[1]	2000[1]	2001[1]
Geographic region[3]	Percent of persons with fair or poor health[2]						
Northeast	8.3	9.1	8.0	7.9	7.5	7.6	7.4
Midwest	9.1	9.7	8.1	8.0	8.0	8.0	8.8
South	13.1	12.3	10.8	10.9	10.5	10.7	10.8
West	9.7	10.1	8.8	8.4	8.7	8.8	8.6
Location of residence[3]							
Within MSA[7]	9.9	10.1	8.7	8.5	8.3	8.5	8.7
Outside MSA[7]	11.9	12.6	11.1	11.4	11.1	11.1	11.0

* Estimates are considered unreliable. Data preceded by an asterisk have a relative standard error (RSE) of 20–30 percent. Data not shown have a RSE of greater than 30 percent.

- - - Data not available.

\#Estimates calculated upon request.

[1]Data starting in 1997 are not strictly comparable with data for earlier years due to the 1997 questionnaire redesign. See Appendix I, National Health Interview Survey.

[2]See Appendix II, Health status, respondent-assessed.

[3]Estimates are age adjusted to the year 2000 standard population using six age groups: Under 18 years, 18–44 years, 45–54 years, 55–64 years, 65–74 years, and 75 years and over. See Appendix II, Age adjustment.

[4]Includes all other races not shown separately and unknown poverty status.

[5]The race groups, white, black, American Indian and Alaska Native (AI/AN), Asian, Native Hawaiian and Other Pacific Islander, and 2 or more races, include persons of Hispanic and non-Hispanic origin. Persons of Hispanic origin may be of any race. Starting with data year 1999 race-specific estimates are tabulated according to 1997 Standards for Federal data on Race and Ethnicity and are not strictly comparable with estimates for earlier years. The five single race categories plus multiple race categories shown in the table conform to 1997 Standards. The 1999 race-specific estimates are for persons who reported only one racial group; the category "2 or more races" includes persons who reported more than one racial group. Prior to data year 1999, data were tabulated according to 1977 Standards with four racial groups and the category "Asian only" included Native Hawaiian and Other Pacific Islander. Estimates for single race categories prior to 1999 included persons who reported one race or, if they reported more than one race, identified one race as best representing their race. The effect of the 1997 Standard on the 1999 estimates can be seen by comparing 1999 data tabulated according to the two Standards: Age-adjusted estimates based on the 1977 Standards of the percent of persons in fair or poor health are: identical for the white and black groups; 0.1 percentage points lower for the Asian and Pacific Islander group; and 0.8 percentage points higher for the AI/AN group than estimates based on the 1997 Standards. See Appendix II, Race.

[6]Poor persons are defined as below the poverty threshold. Near poor persons have incomes of 100 percent to less than 200 percent of the poverty threshold. Nonpoor persons have incomes of 200 percent or greater than the poverty threshold. Missing family income data were imputed for 16–18 percent of persons in 1991 and 1995. Poverty status was unknown for 20 percent of persons in the sample in 1997, 25 percent in 1998, 28 percent in 1999, 27 percent in 2000, and 29 percent in 2001. See Appendix II, Family Income; Poverty level.

[7]MSA is metropolitan statistical area.

NOTE: Standard errors for selected years are available in the spreadsheet version of this table. See www.cdc.gov/nchs/hus.htm.

SOURCE: Centers for Disease Control and Prevention, National Center for Health Statistics, National Health Interview Survey, family core questionnaire.

Table 58 (page 1 of 2). Suicidal ideation, suicide attempts, and injurious suicide attempts among students in grades 9–12, by sex, grade level, race, and Hispanic origin: United States, selected years 1991–2001

[Data are based on a national sample of high school students, grades 9–12]

Sex, grade level, race, and Hispanic origin	1991	1993	1995	1997	1999	2001
	Percent of students who seriously considered suicide[1]					
Total	29.0	24.1	24.1	20.5	19.3	19.0
Male						
Total	20.8	18.8	18.3	15.1	13.7	14.2
9th grade	17.6	17.7	18.2	16.1	11.9	14.7
10th grade	19.5	18.0	16.7	14.5	13.7	13.8
11th grade	25.3	20.6	21.7	16.6	13.7	14.1
12th grade	20.7	18.3	16.3	13.5	15.6	13.7
Not Hispanic or Latino:						
White	21.7	19.1	19.1	14.4	12.5	14.9
Black or African American	13.3	15.4	16.7	10.6	11.7	9.2
Hispanic or Latino	18.0	17.9	15.7	17.1	13.6	12.2
Female						
Total	37.2	29.6	30.4	27.1	24.9	23.6
9th grade	40.3	30.9	34.4	28.9	24.4	26.2
10th grade	39.7	31.6	32.8	30.0	30.1	24.1
11th grade	38.4	28.9	31.1	26.2	23.0	23.6
12th grade	30.7	27.3	23.9	23.6	21.2	18.9
Not Hispanic or Latino:						
White	38.6	29.7	31.6	26.1	23.2	24.2
Black or African American	29.4	24.5	22.2	22.0	18.8	17.2
Hispanic or Latino	34.6	34.1	34.1	30.3	26.1	26.5
	Percent of students who attempted suicide[1]					
Total	7.3	8.6	8.7	7.7	8.3	8.8
Male						
Total	3.9	5.0	5.6	4.5	5.7	6.2
9th grade	4.5	5.8	6.8	6.3	6.1	8.2
10th grade	3.3	5.9	5.4	3.8	6.2	6.7
11th grade	4.1	3.4	5.8	4.4	4.8	4.9
12th grade	3.8	4.5	4.7	3.7	5.4	4.4
Not Hispanic or Latino:						
White	3.3	4.4	5.2	3.2	4.5	5.3
Black or African American	3.3	5.4	7.0	5.6	7.1	7.5
Hispanic or Latino	3.7	7.4	5.8	7.2	6.6	8.0
Female						
Total	10.7	12.5	11.9	11.6	10.9	11.2
9th grade	13.8	14.4	14.9	15.1	14.0	13.2
10th grade	12.2	13.1	15.1	14.3	14.8	12.2
11th grade	8.7	13.6	11.4	11.3	7.5	11.5
12th grade	7.8	9.1	6.6	6.2	5.8	6.5
Not Hispanic or Latino:						
White	10.4	11.3	10.4	10.3	9.0	10.3
Black or African American	9.4	11.2	10.8	9.0	7.5	9.8
Hispanic or Latino	11.6	19.7	21.0	14.9	18.9	15.9

See footnotes at end of table.

Table 58 (page 2 of 2). Suicidal ideation, suicide attempts, and injurious suicide attempts among students in grades 9–12, by sex, grade level, race, and Hispanic origin: United States, selected years 1991–2001

[Data are based on a national sample of high school students, grades 9–12]

Sex, grade level, race, and Hispanic origin	1991	1993	1995	1997	1999	2001
	Percent of students with an injurious suicide attempt[1,2]					
Total	1.7	2.7	2.8	2.6	2.6	2.6
Male						
Total	1.0	1.6	2.2	2.0	2.1	2.1
9th grade	1.0	2.1	2.3	3.2	2.6	2.6
10th grade	0.5	1.3	2.4	1.4	1.8	2.5
11th grade	1.5	1.1	2.0	2.6	2.1	1.6
12th grade	0.9	1.5	2.2	1.0	1.7	1.5
Not Hispanic or Latino:						
White	1.0	1.4	2.1	1.5	1.6	1.7
Black or African American.........	0.4	2.0	2.8	1.8	3.4	3.6
Hispanic or Latino	0.5	2.0	2.9	2.1	1.4	2.5
Female						
Total	2.5	3.8	3.4	3.3	3.1	3.1
9th grade	2.8	3.5	6.3	5.0	3.8	3.8
10th grade	2.6	5.1	3.8	3.7	4.0	3.6
11th grade	2.1	3.9	2.9	2.8	2.8	2.8
12th grade	2.4	2.9	1.3	2.0	1.3	1.7
Not Hispanic or Latino:						
White	2.3	3.6	2.9	2.6	2.3	2.9
Black or African American.........	2.9	4.0	3.6	3.0	2.4	3.1
Hispanic or Latino	2.7	5.5	6.6	3.8	4.6	4.2

[1]Response is for the 12 months preceding the survey.
[2]A suicide attempt that required medical attention.

NOTES: Only youth attending school participated in the survey. Persons of Hispanic origin may be of any race.

SOURCE: Centers for Disease Control and Prevention, National Center for Chronic Disease Prevention and Health Promotion, National Youth Risk Behavior Survey (YRBS).

Table 59 (page 1 of 2). Current cigarette smoking by persons 18 years of age and over according to sex, race, and age: United States, selected years 1965–2001

[Data are based on household interviews of a sample of the civilian noninstitutionalized population]

Sex, race, and age	1965	1974	1979	1983	1985	1990	1995	1997[1]	1998[1]	1999[1]	2000[1]	2001[1]
18 years and over, age adjusted[2]	\multicolumn{12}{c}{Percent of persons who are current cigarette smokers[3]}
All persons	41.9	37.0	33.3	31.9	29.9	25.3	24.6	24.6	24.0	23.3	23.1	22.7
Male	51.2	42.8	37.0	34.8	32.2	28.0	26.5	27.1	25.9	25.2	25.2	24.7
Female	33.7	32.2	30.1	29.4	27.9	22.9	22.7	22.2	22.1	21.6	21.1	20.8
White male[4]	50.4	41.7	36.4	34.2	31.3	27.6	26.2	26.8	26.0	25.0	25.5	24.9
Black or African American male[4]	58.8	53.6	43.9	41.7	40.2	32.8	29.4	32.4	29.0	28.4	25.7	27.6
White female[4]	33.9	32.0	30.3	29.6	27.9	23.5	23.4	22.8	23.0	22.5	22.0	22.1
Black or African American female[4]	31.8	35.6	30.5	31.3	30.9	20.8	23.5	22.5	21.1	20.5	20.7	17.9
18 years and over, crude												
All persons	42.4	37.1	33.5	32.1	30.1	25.5	24.7	24.7	24.1	23.5	23.3	22.8
Male	51.9	43.1	37.5	35.1	32.6	28.4	27.0	27.6	26.4	25.7	25.7	25.2
Female	33.9	32.1	29.9	29.5	27.9	22.8	22.6	22.1	22.0	21.5	21.0	20.7
White male[4]	51.1	41.9	36.8	34.5	31.7	28.0	26.6	27.2	26.3	25.3	25.8	25.1
Black or African American male[4]	60.4	54.3	44.1	40.6	39.9	32.5	28.5	32.2	29.0	28.6	26.1	27.6
White female[4]	34.0	31.7	30.1	29.4	27.7	23.4	23.1	22.5	22.6	22.1	21.6	21.7
Black or African American female[4]	33.7	36.4	31.1	32.2	31.0	21.2	23.5	22.5	21.1	20.6	20.8	18.0
All males												
18–24 years	54.1	42.1	35.0	32.9	28.0	26.6	27.8	31.7	31.3	29.5	28.5	30.4
25–34 years	60.7	50.5	43.9	38.8	38.2	31.6	29.5	30.3	28.5	29.1	29.0	27.2
35–44 years	58.2	51.0	41.8	41.0	37.6	34.5	31.5	32.1	30.2	30.0	30.2	27.4
45–64 years	51.9	42.6	39.3	35.9	33.4	29.3	27.1	27.6	27.7	25.8	26.4	26.4
65 years and over	28.5	24.8	20.9	22.0	19.6	14.6	14.9	12.8	10.4	10.5	10.2	11.5
White male[4]												
18–24 years	53.0	40.8	34.3	32.5	28.4	27.4	28.4	34.0	34.1	30.5	30.9	32.5
25–34 years	60.1	49.5	43.6	38.6	37.3	31.6	29.9	30.4	29.2	30.8	29.9	29.0
35–44 years	57.3	50.1	41.3	40.8	36.6	33.5	31.2	32.1	29.6	29.5	30.6	27.8
45–64 years	51.3	41.2	38.3	35.0	32.1	28.7	26.3	26.5	27.0	24.5	25.8	25.1
65 years and over	27.7	24.3	20.5	20.6	18.9	13.7	14.1	11.5	10.0	10.0	9.8	10.7
Black or African American male[4]												
18–24 years	62.8	54.9	40.2	34.2	27.2	21.3	*14.6	23.5	19.7	23.6	20.8	21.6
25–34 years	68.4	58.5	47.5	39.9	45.6	33.8	25.1	31.6	25.2	22.7	23.3	23.8
35–44 years	67.3	61.5	48.6	45.5	45.0	42.0	36.3	33.9	36.1	34.8	30.8	29.9
45–64 years	57.9	57.8	50.0	44.8	46.1	36.7	33.9	39.4	37.3	35.7	32.2	34.3
65 years and over	36.4	29.7	26.2	38.9	27.7	21.5	28.5	26.0	16.3	17.3	14.2	21.1

See footnotes at end of table.

Table 59 (page 2 of 2). Current cigarette smoking by persons 18 years of age and over according to sex, race, and age: United States, selected years 1965–2001

[Data are based on household interviews of a sample of the civilian noninstitutionalized population]

Sex, race, and age	1965	1974	1979	1983	1985	1990	1995	1997[1]	1998[1]	1999[1]	2000[1]	2001[1]
All females	Percent of persons who are current cigarette smokers[3]											
18–24 years	38.1	34.1	33.8	35.5	30.4	22.5	21.8	25.7	24.5	26.3	25.1	23.4
25–34 years	43.7	38.8	33.7	32.6	32.0	28.2	26.4	24.8	24.6	23.5	22.5	23.0
35–44 years	43.7	39.8	37.0	33.8	31.5	24.8	27.1	27.2	26.4	26.5	26.2	25.7
45–64 years	32.0	33.4	30.7	31.0	29.9	24.8	24.0	21.5	22.5	21.0	21.6	21.4
65 years and over	9.6	12.0	13.2	13.1	13.5	11.5	11.5	11.5	11.2	10.7	9.3	9.2
White female[4]												
18–24 years	38.4	34.0	34.5	36.5	31.8	25.4	24.9	29.4	28.1	29.6	28.7	27.2
25–34 years	43.4	38.6	34.1	32.2	32.0	28.5	27.3	26.1	26.9	25.5	25.1	25.5
35–44 years	43.9	39.3	37.2	34.8	31.0	25.0	27.0	27.5	26.6	26.9	26.6	27.0
45–64 years	32.7	33.0	30.6	30.6	29.7	25.4	24.3	20.9	22.5	21.2	21.4	21.6
65 years and over	9.8	12.3	13.8	13.2	13.3	11.5	11.7	11.7	11.2	10.5	9.1	9.4
Black or African American female[4]												
18–24 years	37.1	35.6	31.8	32.0	23.7	10.0	*8.8	11.5	*8.1	14.8	14.2	10.0
25–34 years	47.8	42.2	35.2	38.0	36.2	29.1	26.7	22.5	21.5	18.2	15.5	16.8
35–44 years	42.8	46.4	37.7	32.7	40.2	25.5	31.9	30.1	30.0	28.8	30.2	24.0
45–64 years	25.7	38.9	34.2	36.3	33.4	22.6	27.5	28.4	25.4	22.3	25.6	22.6
65 years and over	7.1	*8.9	*8.5	*13.1	14.5	11.1	13.3	10.7	11.5	13.5	10.2	9.3

* Estimates are considered unreliable. Data preceded by an asterisk have a relative standard error of 20–30 percent.

[1]Data starting in 1997 are not strictly comparable with data for earlier years due to the 1997 questionnaire redesign. See Appendix I, National Health Interview Survey. Cigarette smoking data were not collected in 1996.

[2]Estimates are age adjusted to the year 2000 standard population using five age groups: 18–24 years, 25–34 years, 35–44 years, 45–64 years, 65 years and over. See Appendix II, Age adjustment.

[3]Beginning in 1993 current cigarette smokers reported ever smoking 100 cigarettes in their lifetime and smoking now on every day or some days. See Appendix II, Cigarette smoking.

[4]The race groups, white and black, include persons of Hispanic and non-Hispanic origin. Starting with data year 1999 race-specific estimates are tabulated according to 1997 Standards for Federal data on Race and Ethnicity and are not strictly comparable with estimates for earlier years. The single race categories shown in the table conform to 1997 Standards. The 1999 race-specific estimates are for persons who reported only one racial group. Prior to data year 1999, data were tabulated according to 1977 Standards. Estimates for single race categories prior to 1999 included persons who reported one race or, if they reported more than one race, identified one race as best representing their race. The effect of the 1997 Standard on the 1999 estimates can be seen by comparing 1999 data tabulated according to the two Standards: Age-adjusted estimates based on the 1977 Standards of the percent of current smokers are: identical for white males and females; 0.1 percentage points higher for black males; and 0.2 percentage points higher for black females than estimates based on the 1997 Standards. See Appendix II, Race. For additional data on cigarette smoking by racial groups, see table 61 of Health, United States, 2003.

NOTES: Data for additional years are available (see Appendix III). Standard errors for selected years are available in the spreadsheet version of this table. See www.cdc.gov/nchs/hus.htm. For more data on cigarette smoking see the National Health Interview Survey home page: www.cdc.gov/nchs/nhis.htm.

SOURCES: Centers for Disease Control and Prevention, National Center for Health Statistics, National Health Interview Survey. Data are from the core questionnaire (1965) and the following questionnaire supplements: hypertension (1974), smoking (1979), alcohol and health practices (1983), health promotion and disease prevention (1985, 1990–91), cancer control and cancer epidemiology (1992), and year 2000 objectives (1993–95). Starting in 1997 data are from the family core and sample adult questionnaires.

Table 60. Age-adjusted prevalence of current cigarette smoking by persons 25 years of age and over, according to sex, race, and education: United States, selected years 1974–2001

[Data are based on household interviews of a sample of the civilian noninstitutionalized population]

Sex, race, and education	1974	1979	1983	1985	1990	1995	1997[1]	1998[1]	1999[1]	2000[1]	2001[1]
25 years and over, age adjusted[2]	\multicolumn{11}{c}{Percent of persons who are current cigarette smokers[3]}										
All persons[4]	36.9	33.1	31.6	30.0	25.4	24.5	24.0	23.4	22.7	22.6	22.1
No high school diploma or GED	43.7	40.7	40.7	40.8	36.7	35.6	33.5	34.4	32.2	31.9	30.9
High school diploma or GED.	36.2	33.6	33.5	32.0	29.1	29.1	29.9	28.9	28.0	29.2	28.2
Some college, no bachelor's degree	35.9	33.2	30.3	29.5	23.4	22.6	23.7	23.5	23.3	21.7	22.3
Bachelor's degree or higher	27.2	22.6	20.5	18.5	13.9	13.6	11.4	10.9	11.1	10.9	10.8
All males[4]	42.9	37.3	35.1	32.8	28.2	26.4	26.4	25.1	24.5	24.8	23.9
No high school diploma or GED	52.3	47.6	47.1	45.7	42.0	39.7	39.1	37.5	36.2	36.4	34.7
High school diploma or GED.	42.4	38.9	37.4	35.5	33.1	32.7	32.2	32.0	30.4	32.1	30.3
Some college, no bachelor's degree	41.8	36.5	33.3	32.9	25.9	23.7	25.5	25.4	24.8	23.3	24.4
Bachelor's degree or higher	28.3	22.7	21.7	19.6	14.5	13.8	12.5	11.0	11.8	11.6	11.2
White males[4,5]	41.9	36.7	34.4	31.7	27.6	25.9	25.8	24.8	24.2	24.7	23.8
No high school diploma or GED	51.5	47.6	47.7	45.0	41.8	38.7	38.5	37.4	36.3	38.6	35.4
High school diploma or GED.	42.0	38.5	37.0	34.8	32.9	32.9	31.8	32.2	30.5	32.5	30.5
Some college, no bachelor's degree	41.6	36.4	32.9	32.2	25.4	23.3	25.6	25.2	24.7	23.6	24.6
Bachelor's degree or higher	27.8	22.5	21.0	19.1	14.4	13.4	12.0	10.9	11.8	11.3	11.2
Black or African American males[4,5]	53.4	44.4	42.8	42.1	34.5	31.6	33.8	30.4	29.1	26.5	28.4
No high school diploma or GED	58.1	49.7	46.0	50.5	41.6	41.9	44.6	42.9	43.8	38.3	37.9
High school diploma or GED.	*50.7	48.6	47.7	41.8	37.4	36.6	39.0	32.8	32.5	29.1	33.4
Some college, no bachelor's degree	*45.3	39.2	44.9	41.8	28.1	26.4	27.0	28.4	23.4	20.0	24.2
Bachelor's degree or higher	*41.4	*36.8	*31.7	*32.0	*20.8	*17.3	14.5	*15.3	11.3	14.7	11.3
All females[4]	32.0	29.5	28.5	27.5	22.9	22.9	21.7	21.7	20.9	20.6	20.4
No high school diploma or GED	36.6	34.8	35.2	36.5	31.8	31.7	28.2	31.3	28.2	27.3	27.2
High school diploma or GED.	32.2	29.8	30.7·	29.5	26.1	26.4	27.9	26.2	25.9	26.7	26.5
Some college, no bachelor's degree	30.1	30.0	27.3	26.3	21.0	21.6	22.0	21.8	21.9	20.4	20.5
Bachelor's degree or higher	25.9	22.5	18.9	17.1	13.3	13.3	10.3	10.7	10.4	10.1	10.5
White females[4,5]	31.7	29.7	28.6	27.3	23.3	23.1	21.9	22.3	21.4	21.1	21.4
No high school diploma or GED	36.8	35.8	35.6	36.7	33.4	32.4	29.7	33.0	29.5	28.6	29.6
High school diploma or GED.	31.9	29.9	30.8	29.4	26.5	26.8	28.3	27.1	27.2	27.9	28.4
Some college, no bachelor's degree	30.4	30.7	27.8	26.7	21.2	22.2	22.1	22.2	22.3	21.1	21.3
Bachelor's degree or higher	25.5	21.9	18.7	16.5	13.4	13.5	10.5	11.5	10.5	10.2	10.9
Black or African American females[4,5]	35.6	30.3	31.2	32.0	22.4	25.7	24.1	23.0	21.4	21.6	19.1
No high school diploma or GED	36.1	31.6	36.5	39.4	26.3	32.3	27.1	32.8	30.1	31.2	26.3
High school diploma or GED.	40.9	32.6	34.6	32.1	24.1	27.8	29.1	24.3	22.4	25.4	21.3
Some college, no bachelor's degree	32.3	*28.9	*27.1	23.9	22.7	20.8	24.3	21.7	22.3	20.4	17.4
Bachelor's degree or higher	*36.3	*43.3	*36.8	26.6	17.0	17.3	12.5	9.0	13.4	10.8	11.6

* Estimates are considered unreliable. Data preceded by an asterisk have a relative standard error of 20–30 percent.

[1]Data starting in 1997 are not strictly comparable with data for earlier years due to the 1997 questionnaire redesign. See Appendix I, National Health Interview Survey. Cigarette smoking data were not collected in 1996.

[2]Estimates are age adjusted to the year 2000 standard population using four age groups: 25–34 years, 35–44 years, 45–64 years, 65 years and over. See Appendix II, Age adjustment. For age groups where percent smoking was 0 or 100, the age-adjustment procedure was modified to substitute the percent smoking from the next lower education group.

[3]Beginning in 1993 current cigarette smokers reported ever smoking 100 cigarettes in their lifetime and smoking now on every day or some days. See Appendix II, Cigarette smoking.

[4]Includes unknown education. Education categories shown are for 1997 and subsequent years. GED stands for General Educational Development high school equivalency diploma. In 1974–95 the following categories based on number of years of school completed were used: less than 12 years, 12 years, 13–15 years, 16 years or more. See Appendix II, Education.

[5]The race groups, white and black, include persons of Hispanic and non-Hispanic origin. Starting with data year 1999 race-specific estimates are tabulated according to 1997 Standards for Federal data on Race and Ethnicity and are not strictly comparable with estimates for earlier years. The single race categories shown in the table conform to 1997 Standards. The 1999 race-specific estimates are for persons who reported only one racial group. Prior to data year 1999, data were tabulated according to 1977 Standards. Estimates for single race categories prior to 1999 included persons who reported one race or, if they reported more than one race, identified one race as best representing their race. The effect of the 1997 Standard on the 1999 estimates can be seen by comparing 1999 data tabulated according to the two Standards: Age-adjusted estimates based on the 1977 Standards of the percent of current smokers are: identical for white males; 0.2 percentage points higher for black males and females; and 0.1 percentage points higher for white females than estimates based on the 1997 Standards. See Appendix II, Race. For additional data on cigarette smoking by racial groups, see table 61 of *Health, United States, 2003*.

NOTES: Data for additional years are available (see Appendix III). Standard errors for selected years are available in the spreadsheet version of this table. See www.cdc.gov/nchs/hus.htm. For more data on cigarette smoking see the National Health Interview Survey home page: www.cdc.gov/nchs/nhis.htm.

SOURCES: Centers for Disease Control and Prevention, National Center for Health Statistics, National Health Interview Survey. Data are from the following questionnaire supplements: hypertension (1974), smoking (1979), alcohol and health practices (1983), health promotion and disease prevention (1985, 1990–91), cancer control and cancer epidemiology (1992), and year 2000 objectives (1993–95). Starting in 1997 data are from the family core and sample adult questionnaires.

Table 61 (page 1 of 2). Current cigarette smoking by adults according to sex, race, Hispanic origin, age, and education: United States, average annual 1990–92, 1995–98, and 1999–2001

[Data are based on household interviews of a sample of the civilian noninstitutionalized population]

Characteristic	Male			Female		
	1990–92	1995–98[1]	1999–2001[1]	1990–92	1995–98[1]	1999–2001[1]
18 years of age and over, age adjusted[2]	Percent of persons who are current cigarette smokers[3]					
All persons[4]	27.9	26.5	25.1	23.7	22.1	21.2
Race[5]						
White only	27.4	26.4	25.2	24.3	22.9	22.2
Black or African American only	33.9	30.7	27.2	23.1	21.8	19.7
American Indian and Alaska Native only	34.2	40.5	30.4	36.7	28.9	34.7
Asian only	24.8	18.1	20.3	6.3	11.0	6.7
Native Hawaiian and Other Pacific Islander only	- - -	- - -	*	- - -	- - -	*
2 or more races	- - -	- - -	34.5	- - -	- - -	30.8
American Indian and Alaska Native; White . .	- - -	- - -	38.7	- - -	- - -	39.0
Hispanic origin and race[5]						
Hispanic or Latino	25.7	24.4	22.3	15.8	13.7	12.1
Mexican	26.2	24.5	22.0	14.8	12.0	10.6
Not Hispanic or Latino	28.1	26.9	25.5	24.4	23.1	22.3
White only	27.7	26.9	25.6	25.2	24.1	23.5
Black or African American only	33.9	30.7	27.3	23.2	21.9	19.7
18 years of age and over, crude						
All persons[4]	28.4	27.0	25.5	23.6	22.0	21.0
Race[5]						
White only	27.8	26.8	25.4	24.1	22.6	21.8
Black or African American only	33.2	30.6	27.4	23.3	21.8	19.8
American Indian and Alaska Native only	35.5	39.2	32.0	37.3	31.2	36.9
Asian only	24.9	20.0	21.3	6.3	11.2	6.9
Native Hawaiian and Other Pacific Islander only	- - -	- - -	*	- - -	- - -	*
2 or more races	- - -	- - -	35.9	- - -	- - -	31.6
American Indian and Alaska Native; White . .	- - -	- - -	41.0	- - -	- - -	40.3
Hispanic origin and race[5]						
Hispanic or Latino	26.5	25.5	23.2	16.6	13.8	12.5
Mexican	27.1	25.2	22.8	15.0	11.6	10.9
Not Hispanic or Latino	28.5	27.2	25.8	24.2	22.9	22.0
White only	28.0	27.0	25.6	24.8	23.5	22.8
Black or African American only	33.3	30.6	27.5	23.3	21.9	19.8
18–24 years:						
Hispanic or Latino	19.3	26.5	22.8	12.8	12.0	12.9
Not Hispanic or Latino:						
White only	28.9	35.5	32.7	28.7	31.6	30.8
Black or African American only	17.7	21.3	21.9	10.8	9.8	13.0
25–34 years:						
Hispanic or Latino	29.9	25.9	23.4	19.2	12.6	12.5
Not Hispanic or Latino:						
White only	32.7	30.5	30.8	30.9	28.5	27.4
Black or African American only	34.6	28.5	23.3	29.2	22.0	16.9
35–44 years:						
Hispanic or Latino	32.1	26.2	25.4	19.9	17.6	14.1
Not Hispanic or Latino:						
White only	32.3	31.5	29.6	27.3	28.1	28.3
Black or African American only	44.1	34.7	32.0	31.3	30.3	27.5
45–64 years:						
Hispanic or Latino	26.6	26.8	24.7	17.1	14.7	13.5
Not Hispanic or Latino:						
White only	28.4	26.8	25.2	26.1	22.3	22.1
Black or African American only	38.0	38.8	34.0	26.1	26.9	23.6
65 years and over:						
Hispanic or Latino	16.1	14.7	12.5	6.6	9.4	5.9
Not Hispanic or Latino:						
White only	14.2	10.6	10.0	12.3	11.6	9.9
Black or African American only	25.2	20.9	17.6	10.7	11.2	11.0

See footnotes at end of table.

Table 61 (page 2 of 2). Current cigarette smoking by adults according to sex, race, Hispanic origin, age, and education: United States, average annual 1990–92, 1995–98, and 1999–2001

[Data are based on household interviews of a sample of the civilian noninstitutionalized population]

	Male			Female		
Characteristic	1990–92	1995–98[1]	1999–2001[1]	1990–92	1995–98[1]	1999–2001[1]
Education, Hispanic origin, and race[5,6]	Percent of persons who are current cigarette smokers[3]					
25 years of age and over, age adjusted[7]						
No high school diploma or GED:						
Hispanic or Latino..............	30.2	27.6	24.2	15.8	13.3	12.1
Not Hispanic or Latino:						
White only.................	46.1	43.9	43.5	40.4	40.7	39.3
Black or African American only	45.4	44.6	40.0	31.3	30.0	29.4
High school diploma or GED:						
Hispanic or Latino..............	29.6	26.7	24.2	18.4	16.4	12.5
Not Hispanic or Latino:						
White only.................	32.9	32.8	31.9	28.4	28.8	29.2
Black or African American only	38.2	35.7	31.5	25.4	26.6	23.0
Some college or more:						
Hispanic or Latino..............	20.4	16.6	17.2	14.3	13.5	11.1
Not Hispanic or Latino:						
White only.................	19.3	18.3	17.6	18.1	17.2	16.7
Black or African American only	25.6	23.3	19.2	22.8	18.9	17.0

* Estimates are considered unreliable. Data preceded by an asterisk have a relative standard error (RSE) of 20–30 percent. Data not shown have a RSE of greater than 30 percent.

- - - Data not available.

[1]Data starting in 1997 are not strictly comparable with data for earlier years due to the 1997 questionnaire redesign. See Appendix I, National Health Interview Survey. Cigarette smoking data were not collected in 1996.

[2]Estimates are age adjusted to the year 2000 standard population using five age groups: 18–24 years, 25–34 years, 35–44 years, 45–64 years, and 65 years and over. See Appendix II, Age adjustment. For age groups where percent smoking is 0 or 100, the age adjustment procedure was modified to substitute the percent smoking from the previous 3-year period.

[3]Beginning in 1993 current cigarette smokers reported ever smoking 100 cigarettes in their lifetime and smoking now on every day or some days. See Appendix II, Cigarette smoking.

[4]Includes all other races not shown separately.

[5]The race groups, white, black, American Indian and Alaska Native (AI/AN), Asian, Native Hawaiian and Other Pacific Islander, and 2 or more races, include persons of Hispanic and non-Hispanic origin. Persons of Hispanic origin may be of any race. Starting with data years 1999–2001 race-specific estimates are tabulated according to 1997 Standards for Federal data on Race and Ethnicity and are not strictly comparable with estimates for earlier years. The five single race categories plus multiple race categories shown in the table conform to 1997 Standards. The 1999–2001 race-specific estimates are for persons who reported only one racial group; the category "2 or more races" includes persons who reported more than one racial group. Prior to data years 1999–2001, data were tabulated according to 1977 Standards with four racial groups and the category "Asian only" included Native Hawaiian and Other Pacific Islander. Estimates for single race categories prior to 1999–2001 included persons who reported one race or, if they reported more than one race, identified one race as best representing their race. The effect of the 1997 Standard on the 1999–2001 estimates can be seen by comparing 1999–2001 data tabulated according to the two Standards: Age-adjusted estimates based on the 1977 Standards of the percent of current smokers for adults 18 years of age and over are: identical for white males; 0.2 percentage points higher for black males; 1.1 percentage points higher for AI/AN males; 0.9 percentage points higher for Asian and Pacific Islander males; identical for white females; 0.1 percentage points higher for black females; 1.0 percentage points higher for AI/AN females; and 1.6 percentage points higher for Asian and Pacific Islander females than estimates based on the 1997 Standards. See Appendix II, Race.

[6]Education categories shown are for 1997 and subsequent years. GED stands for General Educational Development high school equivalency diploma. In years prior to 1997 the following categories based on number of years of school completed were used: less than 12 years, 12 years, 13 years or more. See Appendix II, Education.

[7]Estimates are age adjusted to the year 2000 standard using four age groups: 25–34 years, 35–44 years, 45–64 years, and 65 years and over. See Appendix II, Age adjustment.

NOTES: Data for additional years are available (see Appendix III). Standard errors for selected years are available in the spreadsheet version of this table. See www.cdc.gov/nchs/hus.htm. For more data on cigarette smoking see the National Health Interview Survey home page: www.cdc.gov/nchs/nhis.htm.

SOURCES: Centers for Disease Control and Prevention, National Center for Health Statistics, National Health Interview Survey. Data are from the following questionnaire supplements: health promotion and disease prevention (1990–91), cancer control and cancer epidemiology (1992), and year 2000 objectives (1993–95). Starting in 1997 data are from the family core and sample adult questionnaires.

Table 62 (page 1 of 2). Use of selected substances in the past month by persons 12 years of age and over, according to age, sex, race, and Hispanic origin: United States, selected years 1999–2001

[Data are based on household interviews of a sample of the civilian noninstitutionalized population 12 years of age and over]

Age, sex, race, and Hispanic origin	Any illicit drug[1]			Marijuana			Nonmedical use of any psychotherapeutic drug[2]		
	1999	2000	2001	1999	2000	2001	1999	2000	2001
	Percent of population								
12 years and over....................	6.3	6.3	7.1	4.7	4.8	5.4	1.8	1.7	2.1
Age									
12–13 years...............	3.9	3.0	3.8	1.5	1.1	1.5	1.8	1.6	1.8
14–15 years...............	9.8	9.8	10.9	6.9	6.9	7.6	3.4	3.0	3.5
16–17 years...:..........	15.4	16.4	17.8	13.2	13.7	14.9	3.4	4.3	4.4
18–25 years...............	16.4	15.9	18.8	14.2	13.6	16.0	3.7	3.6	4.8
26–34 years...............	6.8	7.8	8.8	5.4	5.9	6.8	1.5	2.1	2.4
35 years and over...........	3.4	3.3	3.5	2.2	2.3	2.4	1.3	1.0	1.3
Sex									
Male.............	8.1	7.7	8.7	6.5	6.2	7.0	1.9	1.8	2.2
Female.............	4.6	5.0	5.5	3.1	3.5	3.8	1.7	1.7	2.0
Age and sex									
12–17 years...............	9.8	9.7	10.8	7.2	7.2	8.0	2.9	3.0	3.2
Male.............	10.1	9.8	11.4	7.8	7.7	8.9	2.6	2.7	2.7
Female.............	9.4	9.5	10.2	6.7	6.6	7.1	3.1	3.3	3.8
Hispanic origin and race[3]									
Not Hispanic or Latino:									
White only...............	6.2	6.4	7.2	4.7	4.9	5.6	1.9	1.8	2.3
Black or African American only..........	7.5	6.4	7.4	5.9	5.2	5.6	1.4	1.2	1.6
American Indian and Alaska Native only ...	10.4	12.6	9.9	6.9	10.1	8.0	3.5	3.9	2.3
Native Hawaiian and Other Pacific Islander only...............	*	6.2	7.5	*	2.5	7.1	0.3	3.5	1.1
Asian only...............	3.2	2.7	2.8	2.3	1.4	1.7	0.9	1.1	0.8
2 or more races...............	10.3	14.8	12.6	8.5	12.5	9.6	2.7	2.3	5.3
Hispanic or Latino, any race.............	6.1	5.3	6.4	4.2	3.6	4.2	1.7	1.7	1.9

	Alcohol use			Binge alcohol use[4]			Heavy alcohol use[5]		
	1999	2000	2001	1999	2000	2001	1999	2000	2001
Age	Percent of population								
12 years and over....................	46.4	46.6	48.3	20.2	20.6	20.5	5.7	5.6	5.7
12–13 years...............	4.4	4.6	4.4	1.8	2.0	1.9	0.2	0.2	0.2
14–15 years...............	15.4	15.7	16.6	9.0	9.3	9.2	1.6	1.8	1.7
16–17 years...............	29.6	29.1	30.8	19.3	20.3	20.8	5.4	6.0	5.7
18–25 years...............	57.2	56.8	58.8	37.9	37.8	38.7	13.3	12.8	13.6
26–34 years...............	57.4	58.3	59.9	29.3	30.3	30.1	7.5	7.6	7.8
35 years and over...........	46.6	46.8	48.7	16.0	16.4	16.2	4.2	4.1	4.2
Sex									
Male.............	53.2	53.6	54.8	28.1	28.3	28.2	9.2	8.7	9.2
Female.............	40.2	40.2	42.3	12.9	13.5	13.4	2.4	2.7	2.6
Age and sex									
12–17 years...............	16.5	16.4	17.3	10.1	10.4	10.6	2.4	2.6	2.5
Male.............	16.7	16.2	17.2	11.3	11.2	11.2	3.0	3.2	3.1
Female.............	16.3	16.5	17.3	8.9	9.6	9.9	1.8	2.0	1.9
Hispanic origin and race[3]									
Not Hispanic or Latino:									
White only...............	50.3	50.7	52.7	21.1	21.2	21.5	6.2	6.2	6.4
Black or African American only..........	34.3	33.7	35.1	16.3	17.7	16.8	3.6	4.0	4.1
American Indian and Alaska Native only ...	33.9	35.1	35.0	20.0	26.2	21.8	5.8	7.2	7.1
Native Hawaiian and Other Pacific Islander only...............	*	*	*	*	*	17.0	*	*	4.0
Asian only...............	30.7	28.0	31.9	10.8	11.6	10.1	2.5	1.4	1.5
2 or more races...............	41.4	41.6	43.2	20.2	17.5	19.4	7.7	5.2	6.7
Hispanic or Latino, any race.............	38.6	39.8	39.5	21.7	22.7	21.3	5.4	4.4	4.4

See footnotes at end of table.

Table 62 (page 2 of 2). Use of selected substances in the past month by persons 12 years of age and over, according to age, sex, race, and Hispanic origin: United States, selected years 1999–2001

[Data are based on household interviews of a sample of the civilian noninstitutionalized population 12 years of age and over]

Age, sex, race, and Hispanic origin	Any tobacco[6]			Cigarettes			Cigars		
	1999	2000	2001	1999	2000	2001	1999	2000	2001
	Percent of population								
12 years and over....................	30.2	29.3	29.5	25.8	24.9	24.9	5.5	4.8	5.4
Age									
12–13 years.......................	4.8	4.0	3.9	4.1	3.4	3.2	1.1	0.8	1.0
14–15 years.......................	16.4	14.2	13.4	14.3	12.1	11.4	5.1	4.3	3.7
16–17 years.......................	30.3	28.9	28.1	26.1	25.2	24.4	9.7	8.6	8.1
18–25 years.......................	44.6	42.9	43.9	39.7	38.3	39.1	11.5	10.4	10.4
26–34 years.......................	38.2	35.6	36.2	31.5	29.7	30.5	7.0	5.7	5.9
35 years and over..................	27.4	27.3	27.3	23.3	22.9	22.7	3.9	3.4	4.4
Sex									
Male	36.6	35.2	35.6	28.3	26.9	27.1	9.5	8.4	9.4
Female	24.3	23.9	23.8	23.4	23.1	23.0	1.7	1.5	1.6
Age and sex									
12–17 years.......................	17.3	15.6	15.1	14.9	13.4	13.0	5.4	4.5	4.3
Male.............................	18.7	16.3	15.8	14.8	12.8	12.4	7.7	6.4	5.8
Female...........................	15.8	14.8	14.4	15.0	14.1	13.6	2.9	2.5	2.6
Hispanic origin and race[3]									
Not Hispanic or Latino:									
White only......................	31.9	31.0	31.3	27.0	25.9	26.1	5.8	5.0	5.6
Black or African American only	26.6	26.7	27.7	22.5	23.3	23.9	5.9	5.1	5.8
American Indian and Alaska Native only ...	43.1	55.0	44.9	36.0	42.3	38.0	6.3	10.7	8.6
Native Hawaiian and Other Pacific Islander only	*	*	28.5	*	*	27.7	4.4	3.1	2.8
Asian only......................	18.7	17.9	13.6	16.7	16.5	12.9	1.9	1.6	1.4
2 or more races.................	34.0	38.9	34.1	29.8	32.3	31.1	5.3	5.1	5.3
Hispanic or Latino, any race	24.7	22.2	22.9	22.6	20.7	20.9	4.3	3.5	4.2

* Estimates are considered unreliable; relative standard error greater than 17.5 percent of the log transformation of the proportion or minimum effective sample size less than 68 or minimum nominal sample size less than 100 or prevalence close to 0 or 100 percent. See Appendix I, National Household Survey on Drug Abuse.
[1]Any illicit drug includes marijuana/hashish, cocaine (including crack), heroin, hallucinogens (including LSD and PCP), inhalants, or any prescription-type psychotherapeutic drug used nonmedically.
[2]Psychotherapeutic drugs include prescription-type pain relievers, tranquilizers, stimulants, or sedatives; does not include over-the-counter drugs.
[3]Persons of Hispanic origin may be of any race. Race and Hispanic origin were collected using the 1997 Standards for Federal data on Race and Ethnicity. Single race categories shown include persons who reported only one racial group. The category 2 or more races includes persons who reported more than one racial group. See Appendix II, Race.
[4]Binge alcohol use is defined as drinking five or more drinks on the same occasion on at least 1 day in the past 30 days. By "occasion" is meant at the same time or within a couple hours of each other.
[5]Heavy alcohol use is defined as drinking five or more drinks on the same occasion on each of 5 or more days in the past 30 days; all heavy alcohol users are also "binge" alcohol users.
[6]Any tobacco product includes cigarettes, smokeless tobacco (i.e., chewing tobacco or snuff), cigars, or pipe tobacco.

NOTES: Because of methodological differences among the National Household Survey on Drug Abuse (NHSDA), Monitoring the Future Study (MTF), and Youth Risk Behavior Survey (YRBS), rates of substance use measured by these surveys are not directly comparable. See Appendix I, NHSDA, MTF, and YRBS.

SOURCES: Substance Abuse and Mental Health Services Administration, Office of Applied Studies, National Household Survey on Drug Abuse, www.drugabusestatistics.samhsa.gov/.

Table 63 (page 1 of 3). Use of selected substances by high school seniors, eighth-, and tenth-graders, according to sex and race: United States, selected years 1980–2002

[Data are based on a survey of high school seniors and eighth-graders in the coterminous United States]

Substance, sex, race, and grade in school	1980	1990	1991	1995	1998	1999	2000	2001	2002
Cigarettes				Percent using substance in the past month					
All seniors	30.5	29.4	28.3	33.5	35.1	34.6	31.4	29.5	26.7
Male	26.8	29.1	29.0	34.5	36.3	35.4	32.8	29.7	27.4
Female.	33.4	29.2	27.5	32.0	33.3	33.5	29.7	28.7	25.5
White	31.0	32.5	31.8	37.3	41.0	39.1	36.6	34.1	30.9
Black or African American	25.2	12.0	9.4	15.0	14.9	14.9	13.6	12.9	11.3
All tenth-graders.	- - -	- - -	20.8	27.9	27.6	25.7	23.9	21.3	17.7
Male	- - -	- - -	20.8	27.7	26.2	25.2	23.8	20.9	16.7
Female.	- - -	- - -	20.7	27.9	29.1	25.8	23.6	21.5	18.6
White	- - -	- - -	23.9	31.2	32.4	29.1	27.3	24.0	20.8
Black or African American	- - -	- - -	6.4	12.2	13.8	11.0	11.3	10.9	9.1
All eighth-graders.	- - -	- - -	14.3	19.1	19.1	17.5	14.6	12.2	10.7
Male	- - -	- - -	15.5	18.8	18.0	16.7	14.3	12.2	11.0
Female.	- - -	- - -	13.1	19.0	19.8	17.7	14.7	12.0	10.4
White	- - -	- - -	15.0	21.7	21.1	19.0	16.4	12.8	11.1
Black or African American	- - -	- - -	5.3	8.2	10.8	10.7	8.4	8.0	7.3
Marijuana									
All seniors	33.7	14.0	13.8	21.2	22.8	23.1	21.6	22.4	21.5
Male	37.8	16.1	16.1	24.6	26.5	26.3	24.7	25.6	25.3
Female.	29.1	11.5	11.2	17.2	18.8	19.7	18.3	19.1	17.4
White	34.2	15.6	15.0	21.5	24.2	23.4	22.0	23.9	22.8
Black or African American	26.5	5.2	6.5	17.8	18.3	20.4	17.5	16.5	16.4
All tenth-graders.	- - -	- - -	8.7	17.2	18.7	19.4	19.7	19.8	17.8
Male	- - -	- - -	10.1	19.2	20.3	21.8	23.3	22.7	19.3
Female.	- - -	- - -	7.3	15.0	17.2	17.0	16.2	16.8	16.4
White	- - -	- - -	9.4	17.7	19.5	20.2	20.1	20.4	19.1
Black or African American	- - -	- - -	3.8	15.1	14.5	14.7	17.0	16.5	14.4
All eighth-graders.	- - -	- - -	3.2	9.1	9.7	9.7	9.1	9.2	8.3
Male	- - -	- - -	3.8	9.8	10.3	10.5	10.2	11.0	9.5
Female.	- - -	- - -	2.6	8.2	8.8	8.8	7.8	7.3	7.1
White	- - -	- - -	3.0	9.0	8.9	8.5	8.3	8.6	7.9
Black or African American	- - -	- - -	2.1	7.0	9.4	10.0	8.5	7.7	7.1
Cocaine									
All seniors	5.2	1.9	1.4	1.8	2.4	2.6	2.1	2.1	2.3
Male	6.0	2.3	1.7	2.2	3.0	3.3	2.7	2.5	2.7
Female.	4.3	1.3	0.9	1.3	1.7	1.8	1.6	1.6	1.8
White	5.4	1.8	1.3	1.7	2.7	2.8	2.2	2.3	2.8
Black or African American	2.0	0.5	0.8	0.4	0.4	0.5	1.0	0.6	0.2
All tenth-graders.	- - -	- - -	0.7	1.7	2.1	1.9	1.8	1.3	1.6
Male	- - -	- - -	0.7	1.8	2.4	2.2	2.1	1.5	1.8
Female.	- - -	- - -	0.6	1.5	1.8	1.6	1.4	1.2	1.4
White	- - -	- - -	0.6	1.7	2.0	1.9	1.7	1.2	1.7
Black or African American	- - -	- - -	0.2	0.4	0.8	0.3	0.4	0.3	0.4
All eighth-graders.	- - -	- - -	0.5	1.2	1.4	1.3	1.2	1.2	1.1
Male	- - -	- - -	0.7	1.1	1.5	1.4	1.3	1.1	1.1
Female.	- - -	- - -	0.4	1.2	1.2	1.2	1.1	1.2	1.1
White	- - -	- - -	0.4	1.0	1.0	1.1	1.1	1.1	1.0
Black or African American	- - -	- - -	0.4	0.4	0.6	0.3	0.5	0.4	0.5

See footnotes at end of table.

[Data are based on a survey of high school seniors and eighth-graders in the coterminous United States]

Substance, sex, race, and grade in school	1980	1990	1991	1995	1998	1999	2000	2001	2002
Inhalants				Percent using substance in the past month					
All seniors	1.4	2.7	2.4	3.2	2.3	2.0	2.2	1.7	1.5
Male	1.8	3.5	3.3	3.9	2.9	2.5	2.9	2.3	2.2
Female	1.0	2.0	1.6	2.5	1.7	1.5	1.7	1.1	0.8
White	1.4	3.0	2.4	3.7	2.6	2.1	2.1	1.8	1.3
Black or African American	1.0	1.5	1.5	1.1	1.0	0.4	2.1	1.3	1.2
All tenth-graders	- - -	- - -	2.7	3.5	2.9	2.6	2.6	2.5	2.4
Male	- - -	- - -	2.9	3.8	3.2	2.9	3.0	2.5	2.3
Female	- - -	- - -	2.6	3.2	2.6	2.2	2.2	2.4	2.4
White	- - -	- - -	2.9	3.9	3.3	2.9	2.8	2.5	2.6
Black or African American	- - -	- - -	2.0	1.2	1.1	0.8	1.5	0.9	1.5
All eighth-graders	- - -	- - -	4.4	6.1	4.8	5.0	4.5	4.0	3.8
Male	- - -	- - -	4.1	5.6	4.8	4.6	4.1	3.6	3.5
Female	- - -	- - -	4.7	6.6	4.7	5.3	4.8	4.3	3.9
White	- - -	- - -	4.5	7.0	5.3	5.6	4.5	4.1	3.9
Black or African American	- - -	- - -	2.3	2.3	2.2	2.3	2.3	2.6	2.7
MDMA (Ecstasy)									
All seniors	- - -	- - -	- - -	- - -	1.5	2.5	3.6	2.8	2.4
Male	- - -	- - -	- - -	- - -	2.3	2.6	4.1	3.7	2.6
Female	- - -	- - -	- - -	- - -	0.8	2.5	3.1	2.0	2.1
White	- - -	- - -	- - -	- - -	1.8	2.7	3.9	2.8	2.5
Black or African American	- - -	- - -	- - -	- - -	0.2	0.0	1.9	0.9	0.5
All tenth-graders	- - -	- - -	- - -	- - -	1.3	1.8	2.6	2.6	1.8
Male	- - -	- - -	- - -	- - -	1.4	1.7	2.5	3.5	1.6
Female	- - -	- - -	- - -	- - -	1.1	1.9	2.5	1.6	1.8
White	- - -	- - -	- - -	- - -	1.3	2.1	2.5	2.6	2.3
Black or African American	- - -	- - -	- - -	- - -	0.7	0.3	1.8	1.0	0.5
All eighth-graders	- - -	- - -	- - -	- - -	0.9	0.8	1.4	1.8	1.4
Male	- - -	- - -	- - -	- - -	1.0	0.9	1.6	1.9	1.5
Female	- - -	- - -	- - -	- - -	0.7	0.7	1.2	1.8	1.3
White	- - -	- - -	- - -	- - -	0.9	0.9	1.4	2.0	1.0
Black or African American	- - -	- - -	- - -	- - -	0.4	0.4	0.8	1.1	0.6
Alcohol[1]									
All seniors	72.0	57.1	54.0	51.3	52.0	51.0	50.0	49.8	48.6
Male	77.4	61.3	58.4	55.7	57.6	55.3	54.0	54.7	52.3
Female	66.8	52.3	49.0	47.0	46.9	46.8	46.1	45.1	45.1
White	75.8	62.2	57.7	54.8	57.6	54.9	55.3	55.3	52.7
Black or African American	47.7	32.9	34.4	37.4	33.6	30.8	29.3	29.6	30.7
All tenth-graders	- - -	- - -	42.8	38.8	38.8	40.0	41.0	39.0	35.4
Male	- - -	- - -	45.5	39.7	40.0	42.3	43.3	41.1	35.3
Female	- - -	- - -	40.3	37.8	37.7	38.1	38.6	36.8	35.7
White	- - -	- - -	45.7	41.3	42.5	43.4	44.3	41.0	39.0
Black or African American	- - -	- - -	30.2	24.9	24.2	24.6	24.7	26.0	23.2
All eighth-graders	- - -	- - -	25.1	24.6	23.0	24.0	22.4	21.5	19.6
Male	- - -	- - -	26.3	25.0	24.0	24.8	22.5	22.3	19.1
Female	- - -	- - -	23.8	24.0	21.9	23.3	22.0	20.6	20.0
White	- - -	- - -	26.0	25.4	24.0	25.6	23.9	22.5	20.4
Black or African American	- - -	- - -	17.8	17.3	15.4	16.8	15.1	14.9	14.7

See footnotes at end of table.

Table 63 (page 3 of 3). Use of selected substances by high school seniors, eighth-, and tenth-graders, according to sex and race: United States, selected years 1980–2002

[Data are based on a survey of high school seniors and eighth-graders in the coterminous United States]

Substance, sex, race, and grade in school	1980	1990	1991	1995	1998	1999	2000	2001	2002
Binge drinking[2]				Percent in last 2 weeks					
All seniors	41.2	32.2	29.8	29.8	31.5	30.8	30.0	29.7	28.6
Male	52.1	39.1	37.8	36.9	39.2	38.1	36.7	36.0	34.2
Female.	30.5	24.4	21.2	23.0	24.0	23.6	23.5	23.7	23.0
White.	44.6	36.2	32.9	32.9	36.6	34.8	34.4	34.5	32.9
Black or African American	17.0	11.6	11.8	15.5	12.7	11.9	11.0	12.6	10.4
All tenth-graders.	- - -	- - -	22.9	24.0	24.4	25.6	26.2	24.9	22.4
Male	- - -	- - -	26.4	26.4	26.7	29.7	29.8	28.6	23.8
Female.	- - -	- - -	19.5	21.5	22.2	21.8	22.5	21.4	21.0
White.	- - -	- - -	24.4	25.7	26.8	27.7	28.5	26.4	24.6
Black or African American	- - -	- - -	14.4	12.3	12.5	12.9	12.9	12.3	12.4
All eighth-graders	- - -	- - -	12.9	14.5	13.7	15.2	14.1	13.2	12.4
Male	- - -	- - -	14.3	15.1	14.4	16.4	14.4	13.7	12.5
Female.	- - -	- - -	11.4	13.9	12.7	13.9	13.6	12.4	12.1
White.	- - -	- - -	12.6	14.5	13.5	15.2	14.6	13.1	12.3
Black or African American	- - -	- - -	9.9	10.0	9.1	10.8	9.3	8.8	9.9

- - - Data not available.

0.0 Quantity more than zero but less than 0.05.

[1]In 1993 the alcohol question was changed to indicate that a "drink" meant "more than a few sips." 1993 data, available electronically, are based on a half sample.

[2]Five or more alcoholic drinks in a row at least once in the prior 2-week period.

NOTES: Because of methodological differences among the National Household Survey on Drug Abuse (NHSDA), Monitoring the Future Study (MTF), and Youth Risk Behavior Survey (YRBS), rates of substance use measured by these surveys are not directly comparable. See Appendix I, NHSDA, MTF, and YRBS. Data for additional years are available (see Appendix III).

SOURCE: National Institutes of Health, National Institute on Drug Abuse (NIDA), Monitoring the Future Study, Annual surveys.

Table 64 (page 1 of 2). Cocaine-related emergency department episodes, according to age, sex, race, and Hispanic origin: United States, selected years 1990–2001

[Data are weighted national estimates based on a sample of emergency departments]

Age, sex, race, and Hispanic origin	1990	1991	1995	1996	1997	1998	1999	2000	2001
All races, both sexes[1]					Number of episodes				
All ages[2]	80,355	101,189	135,711	152,420	161,083	172,011	168,751	174,881	193,034
6–17 years	1,877	2,210	2,051	2,595	3,642	4,362	3,299	4,402	3,514
18–25 years	19,614	21,766	21,110	22,060	25,218	24,507	25,264	25,753	28,666
26–34 years	35,639	46,137	54,881	58,729	57,143	59,008	54,058	51,007	53,693
35 years and over	23,054	30,582	57,341	68,717	74,600	83,730	85,869	93,357	106,810
Male									
Not Hispanic or Latino:									
White:									
All ages[2]	15,512	19,385	25,634	28,644	32,778	32,767	35,378	36,508	43,387
6–17 years	527	486	493	604	898	1,302	666	897	935
18–25 years	3,810	5,284	5,459	4,967	6,644	6,069	7,367	7,294	9,726
26–34 years	6,724	8,777	10,426	11,405	11,697	11,302	11,421	11,143	12,282
35 years and over	4,432	4,747	9,226	11,645	13,464	14,075	15,893	17,148	20,424
Black or African American:									
All ages[2]	27,745	36,597	48,872	51,685	54,257	55,562	49,944	49,612	53,282
6–17 years	241	244	304	348	388	236	404	305	91
18–25 years	5,104	5,743	4,735	3,886	4,725	4,153	4,066	3,836	3,756
26–34 years	12,160	16,232	18,756	18,558	18,052	17,578	13,433	11,608	11,924
35 years and over	10,202	14,110	25,016	28,741	30,850	33,511	31,978	33,758	37,437
Hispanic or Latino[3]:									
All ages[2]	4,821	6,571	7,886	12,575	11,540	14,844	15,111	16,774	18,293
6–17 years	144	201	181	431	402	725	899	612	485
18–25 years	1,774	1,831	1,892	3,725	3,467	3,871	4,027	4,268	4,108
26–34 years	1,758	2,723	2,901	4,342	3,575	4,694	4,582	5,510	6,080
35 years and over	1,125	1,801	2,907	4,054	4,077	5,536	5,540	6,375	7,615
Female									
Not Hispanic or Latino:									
White:									
All ages[2]	8,331	9,541	13,566	15,593	17,593	19,687	20,884	22,419	27,365
6–17 years	486	529	495	542	1,021	1,125	837	1,208	838
18–25 years	2,663	2,765	2,962	3,344	3,742	4,368	4,348	4,259	5,675
26–34 years	3,636	4,427	5,976	6,540	6,771	6,621	8,022	7,471	8,936
35 years and over	1,539	1,808	4,126	5,155	6,043	7,504	7,667	9,414	11,801
Black or African American:									
All ages[2]	14,833	19,149	24,138	25,713	27,298	28,361	27,625	25,480	26,257
6–17 years	177	210	153	89	100	80	125	99	175
18–25 years	3,820	3,892	3,307	2,803	3,407	2,245	2,012	1,947	1,824
26–34 years	7,418	9,481	10,831	11,082	11,004	11,312	9,994	7,962	6,927
35 years and over	3,369	5,512	9,822	11,712	12,752	14,687	15,473	15,453	17,305
Hispanic or Latino[3]:									
All ages[2]	1,719	2,356	3,515	5,042	5,063	6,238	5,224	6,598	6,491
6–17 years	64	183	128	250	675	625	146	901	550
18–25 years	634	616	901	1,296	1,287	1,505	1,167	1,699	1,112
26–34 years	663	1,044	1,280	2,116	1,698	2,278	2,091	1,967	2,409
35 years and over	357	513	1,203	1,378	1,402	1,821	1,811	2,029	2,419

See notes at end of table.

Table 64 (page 2 of 2). **Cocaine-related emergency department episodes, according to age, sex, race, and Hispanic origin: United States, selected years 1990–2001**

[Data are weighted national estimates based on a sample of emergency departments]

Age and sex	1990	1991	1995	1996	1997	1998	1999	2000	2001
Both sexes				Episodes per 100,000 population[4]					
6 years and over, age adjusted[5]	- - -	41.0	56.2	63.0	66.4	70.7	69.2	70.8	77.6
6 years and over, crude[6].	- - -	45.2	58.3	64.8	67.7	71.5	69.4	70.7	76.1
6–11 years	- - -	*	*	*	*	*	*	*	*
12–17 years	- - -	10.6	9.3	11.5	16.0	18.8	14.0	18.8	14.5
18–25 years	- - -	76.9	76.2	80.1	91.8	88.2	89.5	88.9	85.5
26–34 years	- - -	120.5	153.7	166.7	164.5	173.1	161.9	154.6	176.4
35 years and over	- - -	26.5	46.0	54.0	57.4	63.2	63.7	67.7	76.2
Male									
6 years and over, age adjusted[5]	- - -	56.2	77.5	87.1	91.2	96.4	93.4	95.7	104.5
6 years and over, crude[2].	- - -	61.6	79.9	88.7	92.2	96.7	93.0	94.8	101.8
6–11 years	- - -	*	*	*	*	*	*	*	*
12–17 years	- - -	9.5	10.5	12.9	15.3	20.7	17.4	16.7	14.3
18–25 years	- - -	102.7	98.1	101.9	116.1	115.2	120.5	118.5	112.8
26–34 years	- - -	152.8	196.2	212.7	211.3	219.7	195.5	193.8	220.8
35 years and over	- - -	40.7	69.2	81.2	85.6	92.2	92.0	97.1	108.0
Female									
6 years and over, age adjusted[5]	- - -	26.5	35.5	40.0	42.6	46.1	46.0	46.3	51.4
6 years and over, crude[2].	- - -	29.1	37.0	41.3	43.5	46.7	46.4	46.4	50.4
6–11 years	- - -	*	*	*	*	*	*	*	*
12–17 years	- - -	11.0	7.8	10.0	16.6	16.7	10.2	20.9	14.5
18–25 years	- - -	53.0	54.1	57.5	66.4	61.7	57.7	58.2	55.6
26–34 years	- - -	86.1	108.6	118.9	117.0	125.0	127.3	112.9	130.0
35 years and over	- - -	13.6	24.8	29.2	31.3	36.6	37.9	40.1	46.6

- - - Data not available.

* Estimates with a relative standard error of 50 percent or higher are considered unreliable and are not shown.

[1]Includes other races and unknown race, Hispanic origin, and/or sex.

[2]Includes unknown age.

[3]Persons of Hispanic origin may be of any race.

[4]Rates are based on the average civilian, noninstitutionalized population for each year estimated by SAMHSA based on a procedure using three Census Bureau data files: The Civilian Noninstitutional Population of the U.S. by Age, Race, and Sex (CNP tables); 1990 Census Counts by Age, Sex, and Race (ASR file); and County-Level Population Estimates (CPOP file).

[5]Age adjusted to the year 2000 standard population using five age groups. See Appendix II, Age adjustment.

[6]Includes unknown sex and age.

SOURCE: Substance Abuse and Mental Health Services Administration (SAMHSA), Office of Applied Studies, Drug Abuse Warning Network, www.drugabusestatistics.samhsa.gov/.

Table 65 (page 1 of 3). Alcohol consumption by persons 18 years of age and over, according to selected characteristics: United States, selected years 1997–2001

[Data are based on household interviews of a sample of the civilian noninstitutionalized population]

Characteristic	Both sexes			Male			Female		
	1997	2000	2001	1997	2000	2001	1997	2000	2001
Drinking status[1]	Percent distribution								
18 years and over, age adjusted[2]									
All	100.0	100.0	100.0	100.0	100.0	100.0	100.0	100.0	100.0
Lifetime abstainer	21.2	24.1	22.6	14.0	17.5	15.2	27.6	29.9	29.2
Former drinker	15.7	14.4	14.9	16.2	14.9	16.0	15.3	14.2	14.0
Infrequent	9.0	8.2	8.5	7.7	7.0	7.7	10.1	9.2	9.1
Regular	6.7	6.3	6.4	8.5	7.8	8.3	5.2	5.0	4.8
Current drinker	63.1	61.5	62.5	69.8	67.7	68.8	57.0	55.8	56.8
Infrequent	15.0	14.7	12.8	11.7	11.1	9.2	18.1	18.2	16.2
Regular	48.1	46.7	48.7	58.1	56.6	58.4	38.9	37.7	39.7
18 years and over, crude									
All	100.0	100.0	100.0	100.0	100.0	100.0	100.0	100.0	100.0
Lifetime abstainer	21.1	24.0	22.5	14.0	17.5	15.2	27.7	30.1	29.3
Former drinker	15.5	14.3	14.8	15.6	14.3	15.5	15.4	14.3	14.1
Infrequent	8.9	8.1	8.4	7.5	6.8	7.5	10.1	9.3	9.2
Regular	6.6	6.2	6.4	8.1	7.5	8.0	5.2	5.0	4.9
Current drinker	63.4	61.7	62.7	70.5	68.2	69.3	57.0	55.6	56.6
Infrequent	15.0	14.7	12.9	11.7	11.1	9.3	18.1	18.1	16.2
Regular	48.4	46.9	48.8	58.8	57.2	58.9	38.8	37.5	39.5
Age	Percent current drinkers among all persons								
All persons:									
18–44 years.	69.4	67.4	69.0	74.8	73.0	75.0	64.2	61.9	63.2
18–24 years	62.2	59.4	63.6	66.7	64.0	69.6	57.7	54.9	57.7
25–44 years	71.6	69.9	70.8	77.2	76.0	76.8	66.1	64.1	65.0
45–64 years.	63.3	62.0	62.5	70.8	68.1	67.8	56.2	56.3	57.5
45–54 years	67.1	65.1	65.6	73.8	70.3	70.1	60.7	60.1	61.2
55–64 years	57.3	57.2	57.6	65.8	64.6	64.2	49.4	50.6	51.6
65 years and over	43.4	42.1	42.0	52.7	50.0	50.9	36.6	36.2	35.5
65–74 years	48.6	46.9	45.8	56.7	52.6	55.2	42.0	42.2	38.2
75 years and over	36.6	36.3	37.6	46.7	46.6	45.1	30.2	29.7	32.6
Race[2,3]									
White only.	66.0	64.6	65.8	71.8	69.7	71.0	60.7	59.9	61.0
Black or African American only	47.8	46.8	46.6	56.9	56.2	56.9	40.9	39.4	38.6
American Indian and Alaska Native only	53.9	54.2	51.5	66.1	62.6	62.8	45.2	46.9	38.6
Asian only.	45.8	43.0	44.7	60.1	55.9	59.7	31.6	29.3	30.1
Native Hawaiian and Other Pacific Islander only	- - -	*	*	- - -	*	*	- - -	*	*
2 or more races.	- - -	61.6	68.5	- - -	70.5	69.9	- - -	52.7	67.1
Hispanic origin and race[2,3]									
Hispanic or Latino	53.4	52.1	49.8	64.6	63.7	61.2	42.1	41.2	39.0
Mexican.	53.0	50.6	49.8	66.9	64.4	63.0	38.9	36.8	36.7
Not Hispanic or Latino	64.1	52.1	49.8	70.2	63.7	61.2	58.7	41.2	39.0
White only	67.5	66.0	67.7	72.7	70.4	72.0	62.9	61.9	63.7
Black or African American only.	47.8	46.8	46.5	57.1	56.4	57.0	40.7	39.3	38.4
Geographic region[2]									
Northeast	68.7	68.0	68.4	74.4	73.2	73.8	63.8	63.7	63.7
Midwest	66.8	65.6	67.1	73.0	70.7	71.7	61.1	61.1	63.0
South	56.2	54.3	55.5	63.9	62.1	63.2	49.2	47.1	48.5
West	64.9	62.8	64.0	71.5	68.4	70.5	58.9	57.2	57.6
Location of residence[2]									
Within MSA[4]	64.7	63.0	64.1	71.0	69.0	70.4	59.1	57.5	58.3
Outside MSA[4]	57.4	56.0	56.9	65.7	62.6	62.8	49.5	50.3	51.6

See footnotes at end of table.

Table 65 (page 2 of 3). Alcohol consumption by persons 18 years of age and over, according to selected characteristics: United States, selected years 1997–2001

[Data are based on household interviews of a sample of the civilian noninstitutionalized population]

Characteristic	Both sexes			Male			Female		
	1997	2000	2001	1997	2000	2001	1997	2000	2001
Level of alcohol consumption in past year for current drinkers[5]	Percent distribution of current drinkers								
18 years and over, age adjusted[2]									
All drinking levels.	100.0	100.0	100.0	100.0	100.0	100.0	100.0	100.0	100.0
Light.	69.6	70.6	68.8	59.5	60.4	59.1	81.0	82.0	79.6
Moderate	22.5	22.2	23.4	31.8	32.0	32.6	12.0	11.5	13.0
Heavier.	7.9	7.1	7.9	8.7	7.7	8.3	7.0	6.5	7.3
18 years and over, crude									
All drinking levels.	100.0	100.0	100.0	100.0	100.0	100.0	100.0	100.0	100.0
Light.	69.8	70.8	69.0	59.6	60.5	59.2	81.4	82.3	79.9
Moderate	22.3	22.1	23.2	31.7	31.8	32.4	11.7	11.3	12.9
Heavier.	7.9	7.1	7.8	8.8	7.7	8.4	6.9	6.4	7.2
Number of days in the past year with 5 or more drinks	Percent distribution of current drinkers								
18 years and over, crude									
All current drinkers.	100.0	100.0	100.0	100.0	100.0	100.0	100.0	100.0	100.0
No days.	65.9	68.2	67.6	54.7	56.9	57.2	78.6	80.6	79.0
At least 1 day	34.1	31.8	32.4	45.3	43.1	42.8	21.4	19.4	21.0
1–11 days	18.5	17.4	17.1	22.0	21.2	19.9	14.6	13.3	14.0
12 or more days.	15.6	14.4	15.3	23.4	21.9	22.8	6.8	6.1	7.0
Hispanic origin, race, and age[3]	Percent of persons with 5 or more drinks on at least one day among current drinkers								
All persons:									
18 years and over, age adjusted[2].	32.4	30.3	30.6	43.3	41.2	40.5	20.2	18.5	19.9
18 years and over, crude.	34.1	31.8	32.4	45.3	43.1	42.7	21.4	19.4	20.9
18–44 years.	42.4	40.4	41.4	54.6	52.3	52.2	28.7	27.0	29.2
18–24 years.	51.6	52.2	51.8	61.5	60.8	60.1	40.2	42.4	41.7
25–44 years.	40.0	37.1	38.3	52.8	49.9	49.7	25.7	22.8	25.7
45–64 years.	25.3	23.5	23.8	36.1	35.0	34.7	12.9	10.8	11.9
45–54 years.	28.5	25.5	26.4	40.1	37.9	38.0	15.3	12.0	14.0
55–64 years.	19.6	19.9	18.9	28.9	29.9	28.7	8.3	8.7	8.0
65 years and over	11.2	9.1	8.2	17.8	14.8	13.1	4.4	3.4	3.1
65–74 years.	13.9	11.3	10.2	21.6	18.3	15.5	5.5	4.2	4.0
75 years and over.	6.7	5.8	5.3	11.0	9.5	9.1	*2.5	*	*
Race[2,3]									
White only.	33.3	31.0	31.8	44.4	41.8	42.0	20.9	19.2	20.7
Black or African American only.	23.6	23.9	20.6	31.7	34.1	27.5	14.9	12.7	12.5
American Indian and Alaska Native only	54.5	45.0	34.6	70.5	47.0	35.9	38.4	34.7	*27.9
Asian only.	25.5	20.3	23.2	30.7	25.4	28.9	16.6	10.8	*12.9
Native Hawaiian and Other Pacific Islander only.	- - -	*	*	- - -	*	*	- - -	*	*
2 or more races.	- - -	44.0	41.6	- - -	53.1	59.9	- - -	31.5	24.3
Hispanic origin and race[2,3]									
Hispanic or Latino	36.8	31.9	32.2	46.3	43.0	41.9	22.3	16.0	17.9
Mexican.	39.0	37.5	35.6	50.1	49.0	45.9	20.3	17.9	17.7
Not Hispanic or Latino	31.9	31.9	32.2	42.7	43.0	41.9	20.0	16.0	17.9
White only.	33.2	31.2	32.0	44.5	42.1	42.2	21.0	19.7	21.3
Black or African American only.	23.4	23.8	20.5	31.7	33.8	27.4	14.4	12.7	12.5

See footnotes at end of table.

Table 65 (page 3 of 3). Alcohol consumption by persons 18 years of age and over, according to selected characteristics: United States, selected years 1997–2001

[Data are based on household interviews of a sample of the civilian noninstitutionalized population]

Characteristic	Both sexes			Male			Female		
	1997	2000	2001	1997	2000	2001	1997	2000	2001
Geographic region	Percent of persons with 5 or more drinks on at least one day among current drinks								
Northeast	31.3	28.9	30.0	43.1	39.7	41.4	18.9	18.1	18.8
Midwest	33.8	33.3	33.6	44.7	44.7	44.4	21.6	21.5	22.4
South	30.9	27.4	27.9	40.5	37.1	36.1	19.2	15.6	18.0
West	33.4	32.0	31.7	44.6	43.1	41.4	20.8	18.8	20.1
Location of residence[2]									
Within MSA[4]	31.6	30.0	30.1	42.4	40.4	39.9	19.8	18.5	19.1
Outside MSA[4]	34.8	31.3	32.8	45.7	43.1	42.2	21.2	18.5	22.5

* Estimates are considered unreliable. Data preceded by an asterisk have a relative standard error (RSE) of 20–30 percent. Data not shown have a RSE of greater than 30 percent.

- - - Data not available.

[1]Drinking status categories are based on self-reported responses to questions about alcohol consumption. Lifetime abstainers had fewer than 12 drinks in their lifetime. Former drinkers had at least 12 drinks in their lifetime and none in the past year. Former infrequent drinkers are former drinkers who had fewer than 12 drinks in any one year. Former regular drinkers are former drinkers who had at least 12 drinks in any one year. Current drinkers had 12 drinks in their lifetime and at least one drink in the past year. Current infrequent drinkers are current drinkers who had fewer than 12 drinks in the past year. Current regular drinkers are current drinkers who had at least 12 drinks in the past year. See Appendix II, Alcohol consumption.

[2]Estimates are age adjusted to the year 2000 standard population using four age groups: 18–24 years, 25–44 years, 45–64 years, and 65 years and over. See Appendix II, Age adjustment.

[3]The race groups, white, black, American Indian and Alaska Native (AI/AN), Asian, Native Hawaiian and Other Pacific Islander, and 2 or more races, include persons of Hispanic and non-Hispanic origin. Persons of Hispanic origin may be of any race. Starting with data year 1999 race-specific estimates are tabulated according to 1997 Standards for Federal data on Race and Ethnicity and are not strictly comparable with estimates for earlier years. The five single race categories plus multiple race categories shown in the table conform to 1997 Standards. The 1999 race-specific estimates are for persons who reported only one racial group; the category "2 or more races" includes persons who reported more than one racial group. Prior to data year 1999, data were tabulated according to 1977 Standards with four racial groups and the category "Asian only" included Native Hawaiian and Other Pacific Islander. Estimates for single race categories prior to 1999 included persons who reported one race or, if they reported more than one race, identified one race as best representing their race. The effect of the 1997 Standard on the 1999 estimates can be seen by comparing 1999 data tabulated according to the two Standards: Age-adjusted estimates based on the 1977 Standards of the percent of persons who are current drinkers are: identical for the white men; 0.3 percentage points higher for black men; 1.6 percentage points higher for AI/AN men; 0.2 percentage points lower for Asian and Pacific Islander men; identical for white women; 0.2 percentage points higher for black women; 1.8 percentage points lower for AI/AN women; and 2.4 percentage points higher for Asian and Pacific Islander women than estimates based on the 1997 Standards. See Appendix II, Race.

[4]MSA is metropolitan statistical area.

[5]Level of alcohol consumption categories are based on self-reported responses to questions about average alcohol consumption and defined as follows: light drinkers: 3 drinks or fewer per week; moderate drinkers: more than 3 drinks and up to 14 drinks per week for men and more than 3 drinks and up to 7 drinks per week for women; heavier drinkers: more than 14 drinks per week for men and more than 7 drinks per week for women. (Most drinking guidelines consider more than 7 drinks per week to be a heavier level of consumption for women. U.S. Department of Agriculture: Dietary Guidelines for Americans, 2000, 5th edition.)

NOTES: Data for additional years are available (see Appendix III). Standard errors for selected years are available in the spreadsheet version of this table. See www.cdc.gov/nchs/hus.htm. For more data on alcohol consumption see the National Health Interview Survey home page: www.cdc.gov/nchs/nhis.htm.

SOURCE: Centers for Disease Control and Prevention, National Center for Health Statistics, National Health Interview Survey, family core and sample adult questionnaires.

Table 66. Hypertension among persons 20 years of age and over, according to sex, age, race, and Hispanic origin: United States, 1960–62, 1971–74, 1976–80, 1988–94, and 1999–2000

[Data are based on physical examinations of a sample of the civilian noninstitutionalized population]

Sex, age, race, and Hispanic origin[1]	1960–62	1971–74	1976–80[2]	1988–94[3]	1999–2000[3]
20–74 years, age adjusted[4]		Percent of population (standard error)			
Both sexes[5,6]	38.1	39.8	40.4	23.9 (0.6)	28.7 (1.6)
Male	41.3	43.9	45.2	26.4 (0.9)	29.8 (1.9)
Female[5]	35.0	35.8	35.8	21.4 (0.7)	27.5 (1.7)
Not Hispanic or Latino:					
White only, male	- - -	- - -	45.0	25.6 (1.0)	28.8 (2.0)
White only, female[5]	- - -	- - -	33.7	19.7 (0.8)	24.5 (1.9)
Black or African American only, male	- - -	- - -	50.7	36.5 (1.0)	37.8 (2.9)
Black or African American only, female[5]	- - -	- - -	51.1	36.4 (0.9)	40.9 (2.4)
Mexican male	- - -	- - -	25.6	25.9 (1.2)	30.6 (2.6)
Mexican female[5]	- - -	- - -	22.5	22.3 (1.0)	25.0 (1.8)
20 years and over, age adjusted[4]					
Both sexes[5,6]	- - -	- - -	- - -	27.8 (0.6)	32.8 (1.5)
Male	- - -	- - -	- - -	29.4 (0.9)	33.1 (1.7)
Female[5]	- - -	- - -	- - -	25.9 (0.6)	32.1 (1.6)
Not Hispanic or Latino:					
White only, male	- - -	- - -	- - -	28.6 (1.0)	32.2 (1.9)
White only, female[5]	- - -	- - -	- - -	24.4 (0.7)	29.5 (1.8)
Black or African American only, male	- - -	- - -	- - -	39.7 (1.1)	41.6 (2.7)
Black or African American only, female[5]	- - -	- - -	- - -	39.9 (0.9)	44.7 (2.2)
Mexican male	- - -	- - -	- - -	29.5 (1.2)	34.5 (2.6)
Mexican female[5]	- - -	- - -	- - -	26.4 (0.9)	29.9 (1.7)
20 years and over, crude					
Both sexes[5,6]	- - -	- - -	- - -	26.3 (0.8)	32.2 (1.5)
Male	- - -	- - -	- - -	26.6 (1.0)	31.2 (1.7)
Female[5]	- - -	- - -	- - -	26.0 (0.9)	33.1 (1.8)
Not Hispanic or Latino:					
White only, male	- - -	- - -	- - -	27.1 (1.2)	32.3 (1.8)
White only, female[5]	- - -	- - -	- - -	26.1 (1.1)	32.6 (2.2)
Black or African American only, male	- - -	- - -	- - -	33.1 (1.2)	35.1 (3.0)
Black or African American only, female[5]	- - -	- - -	- - -	33.8 (1.2)	40.6 (3.1)
Mexican male	- - -	- - -	- - -	18.8 (1.3)	24.0 (2.9)
Mexican female[5]	- - -	- - -	- - -	17.1 (0.8)	21.1 (2.2)
Male					
20–34 years	22.8	24.8	28.9	8.6 (1.0)	*11.8 (2.6)
35–44 years	37.7	39.1	40.5	20.8 (1.7)	19.2 (2.8)
45–54 years	47.6	55.0	53.6	34.0 (2.2)	36.9 (3.3)
55–64 years	60.3	62.5	61.8	42.9 (2.6)	50.7 (4.3)
65–74 years	68.8	67.2	67.1	57.3 (2.5)	68.3 (4.9)
75 years and over	- - -	- - -	- - -	64.2 (2.2)	70.7 (3.2)
Female[5]					
20–34 years	9.3	11.2	11.1	3.3 (0.6)	*3.1 (0.9)
35–44 years	24.0	28.2	28.8	12.6 (1.1)	18.6 (2.9)
45–54 years	43.4	43.6	47.1	25.1 (2.1)	33.4 (3.4)
55–64 years	66.4	62.5	61.1	44.1 (2.5)	57.9 (3.2)
65–74 years	81.5	78.3	71.8	60.6 (1.6)	73.4 (3.5)
75 years and over	- - -	- - -	- - -	76.5 (1.7)	84.9 (3.2)

* Estimates are considered unreliable. Data preceded by an asterisk have a relative standard error of 20–30 percent.   - - - Data not available.

[1]Persons of Mexican origin may be of any race. Starting with data year 1999 race-specific estimates are tabulated according to 1997 Standards for Federal data on Race and Ethnicity and are not strictly comparable with estimates for earlier years. The two non-Hispanic race categories shown in the table conform to 1997 Standards. The 1999–2000 race-specific estimates are for persons who reported only one racial group. Prior to data year 1999, data were tabulated according to 1977 Standards. Estimates for single race categories prior to 1999 included persons who reported one race or, if they reported more than one race, identified one race as best representing their race. The effect of the 1997 Standard on the 1999–2000 estimates can be seen by comparing 1999–2000 data tabulated according to the two Standards: Estimates based on the 1977 Standards of the percent of the population 20–74 years, age adjusted, with hypertension are: 0.1 percentage points higher for white males; 0.2 percentage points higher for white females; 0.2 percentage points higher for black males; and 0.1 percentage points higher for black females than estimates based on the 1997 Standards. See Appendix II, Race.

[2]Data for Mexicans are for 1982–84. See Appendix I, National Health and Nutrition Examination Survey (NHANES).

[3]Standard errors of estimates for 1988–94 and 1999–2000 are shown. 1999–2000 estimates are based on a smaller sample size than estimates for earlier time periods and therefore are subject to greater sampling error.

[4]Age adjusted to the 2000 standard population using five age groups except for 1999–2000 estimates, which are age adjusted using three age groups (20–39, 40–59, and 60–74 or 60 years and over) due to a smaller sample size; however, use of three rather than five groups had virtually no effect on age-adjusted estimates. See Appendix II, Age adjustment.

[5]Excludes pregnant women.   [6]Includes persons of all races and Hispanic origins, not just those shown separately.

NOTES: A person with hypertension is defined by either having elevated blood pressure (systolic pressure of at least 140 mmHg or diastolic pressure of at least 90 mmHg) or taking antihypertensive medication. Percents are based on a single measurement of blood pressure to provide comparable data across the five time periods. Some data for 1988–94 have been revised and differ from the previous edition of Health, United States. Estimates for persons 20 years and over are used for setting and tracking Healthy People 2010 objectives.

SOURCES: Centers for Disease Control and Prevention, National Center for Health Statistics, National Health and Nutrition Examination Survey, Hispanic Health and Nutrition Examination Survey (1982–84), and National Health Examination Survey (1960–62).

Table 67 (page 1 of 2). Serum cholesterol levels among persons 20 years of age and over, according to sex, age, race, and Hispanic origin: United States, 1960–62, 1971–74, 1976–80, 1988–94, and 1999–2000

[Data are based on physical examinations of a sample of the civilian noninstitutionalized population]

Sex, age, race, and Hispanic origin[1]	1960–62	1971–74	1976–80[2]	1988–94[3]	1999–2000[3]
20–74 years, age adjusted[4]	Percent of population with high serum cholesterol (standard error)				
Both sexes[5]	33.3	28.6	27.8	19.7 (0.6)	18.0 (0.9)
Male	30.6	27.9	26.4	18.8 (0.8)	17.7 (1.1)
Female	35.6	29.1	28.8	20.5 (0.8)	18.2 (1.3)
Not Hispanic or Latino:					
White only, male	- - -	- - -	26.4	18.7 (0.9)	18.3 (1.4)
White only, female	- - -	- - -	29.6	20.7 (1.0)	19.3 (1.7)
Black or African American only, male	- - -	- - -	25.5	16.4 (1.0)	10.7 (2.1)
Black or African American only, female	- - -	- - -	26.3	19.9 (0.8)	16.5 (2.5)
Mexican male	- - -	- - -	20.3	18.7 (1.5)	17.8 (1.9)
Mexican female	- - -	- - -	20.5	17.7 (1.2)	13.1 (1.3)
20 years and over, age adjusted[4]					
Both sexes[5]	- - -	- - -	- - -	20.8 (0.6)	18.3 (0.8)
Male	- - -	- - -	- - -	19.0 (0.7)	17.2 (1.1)
Female	- - -	- - -	- - -	22.0 (0.8)	19.1 (1.2)
Not Hispanic or Latino:					
White only, male	- - -	- - -	- - -	18.8 (0.8)	17.8 (1.3)
White only, female	- - -	- - -	- - -	22.2 (1.0)	19.9 (1.6)
Black or African American only, male	- - -	- - -	- - -	16.9 (0.9)	10.6 (1.9)
Black or African American only, female	- - -	- - -	- - -	21.4 (0.9)	17.7 (2.4)
Mexican male	- - -	- - -	- - -	18.5 (1.6)	17.8 (1.9)
Mexican female	- - -	- - -	- - -	18.7 (1.3)	13.9 (1.3)
20 years and over, crude					
Both sexes[5]	- - -	- - -	- - -	19.6 (0.6)	17.8 (0.9)
Male	- - -	- - -	- - -	17.7 (0.7)	16.7 (1.1)
Female	- - -	- - -	- - -	21.3 (0.9)	18.7 (1.2)
Not Hispanic or Latino:					
White only, male	- - -	- - -	- - -	18.0 (0.8)	17.7 (1.4)
White only, female	- - -	- - -	- - -	22.5 (1.1)	20.2 (1.6)
Black or African American only, male	- - -	- - -	- - -	14.7 (1.0)	*10.1 (2.1)
Black or African American only, female	- - -	- - -	- - -	18.2 (0.9)	15.9 (2.2)
Mexican male	- - -	- - -	- - -	15.4 (1.3)	14.8 (2.0)
Mexican female	- - -	- - -	- - -	14.3 (1.1)	11.3 (1.4)
Male					
20–34 years	15.1	12.4	11.9	8.2 (0.9)	11.0 (1.5)
35–44 years	33.9	31.8	27.9	19.4 (1.6)	21.1 (3.3)
45–54 years	39.2	37.5	36.9	26.6 (2.3)	22.9 (3.4)
55–64 years	41.6	36.2	36.8	28.0 (2.1)	16.5 (2.4)
65–74 years	38.0	34.7	31.7	21.9 (2.2)	19.2 (2.8)
75 years and over	- - -	- - -	- - -	20.4 (1.8)	*10.1 (2.1)
Female					
20–34 years	12.4	10.9	9.8	7.3 (1.0)	9.3 (1.4)
35–44 years	23.1	19.3	20.7	12.3 (1.3)	12.8 (2.5)
45–54 years	46.9	38.7	40.5	26.7 (2.1)	23.7 (4.2)
55–64 years	70.1	53.1	52.9	40.9 (1.9)	26.2 (3.1)
65–74 years	68.5	57.7	51.6	41.3 (2.4)	37.4 (4.0)
75 years and over	- - -	- - -	- - -	38.2 (2.2)	27.6 (2.5)

See footnotes at end of table.

Table 67 (page 2 of 2). Serum cholesterol levels among persons 20 years of age and over, according to sex, age, race, and Hispanic origin: United States, 1960–62, 1971–74, 1976–80, 1988–94, and 1999–2000

[Data are based on physical examinations of a sample of the civilian noninstitutionalized population]

Sex, age, race, and Hispanic origin[1]	1960–62	1971–74	1976–80[2]	1988–94[3]	1999–2000[3]
20–74 years, age adjusted[4]		Mean serum cholesterol level, mg/dL (standard error)			
Both sexes[5]	222	216	215	205 (0.8)	204 (1.0)
Male	220	216	213	204 (0.9)	204 (1.2)
Female	224	217	216	205 (0.8)	203 (1.4)
Not Hispanic or Latino:					
White only, male	- - -	- - -	213	204 (1.0)	204 (1.6)
White only, female	- - -	- - -	216	206 (1.1)	206 (1.7)
Black or African American only, male	- - -	- - -	211	201 (1.3)	192 (2.5)
Black or African American only, female	- - -	- - -	216	204 (0.6)	200 (2.8)
Mexican male	- - -	- - -	209	206 (1.6)	207 (1.7)
Mexican female	- - -	- - -	209	204 (1.3)	198 (2.0)
20 years and over, age adjusted[4]					
Both sexes[5]	- - -	- - -	- - -	206 (0.7)	204 (0.9)
Male	- - -	- - -	- - -	204 (0.9)	203 (1.1)
Female	- - -	- - -	- - -	207 (0.8)	205 (1.3)
Not Hispanic or Latino:					
White only, male	- - -	- - -	- - -	205 (1.0)	204 (1.5)
White only, female	- - -	- - -	- - -	208 (1.1)	207 (1.6)
Black or African American only, male	- - -	- - -	- - -	202 (1.3)	192 (2.3)
Black or African American only, female	- - -	- - -	- - -	207 (0.7)	201 (2.7)
Mexican male	- - -	- - -	- - -	206 (1.5)	207 (1.7)
Mexican female	- - -	- - -	- - -	206 (1.3)	199 (1.9)
20 years and over, crude					
Both sexes[5]	- - -	- - -	- - -	204 (0.8)	203 (1.0)
Male	- - -	- - -	- - -	202 (0.9)	202 (1.1)
Female	- - -	- - -	- - -	206 (0.9)	204 (1.5)
Not Hispanic or Latino:					
White only, male	- - -	- - -	- - -	203 (1.0)	203 (1.5)
White only, female	- - -	- - -	- - -	208 (1.3)	207 (1.6)
Black or African American only, male	- - -	- - -	- - -	198 (1.3)	190 (2.5)
Black or African American only, female	- - -	- - -	- - -	201 (0.7)	198 (2.8)
Mexican male	- - -	- - -	- - -	199 (1.6)	203 (1.8)
Mexican female	- - -	- - -	- - -	198 (1.5)	195 (2.0)
Male					
20–34 years	198	194	192	186 (1.2)	189 (2.0)
35–44 years	227	221	217	206 (1.6)	205 (2.8)
45–54 years	231	229	227	216 (1.8)	215 (2.9)
55–64 years	233	229	229	216 (2.2)	210 (2.5)
65–74 years	230	226	221	212 (1.9)	210 (2.6)
75 years and over	- - -	- - -	- - -	205 (1.9)	194 (2.4)
Female					
20–34 years	194	191	189	184 (1.3)	186 (2.2)
35–44 years	214	207	207	195 (1.4)	197 (2.1)
45–54 years	237	232	232	217 (2.3)	213 (3.1)
55–64 years	262	245	249	235 (1.6)	223 (2.8)
65–74 years	266	250	246	233 (1.9)	229 (3.2)
75 years and over	- - -	- - -	- - -	229 (2.0)	219 (2.5)

* Estimates are considered unreliable. Data preceded by an asterisk have a relative standard error of 20–30 percent.   - - - Data not available.

[1]Persons of Mexican origin may be of any race. Starting with data year 1999 race-specific estimates are tabulated according to 1997 Standards for Federal data on Race and Ethnicity and are not strictly comparable with estimates for earlier years. The two non-Hispanic race categories shown in the table conform to 1997 Standards. The 1999–2000 race-specific estimates are for persons who reported only one racial group. Prior to data year 1999, data were tabulated according to 1977 Standards. Estimates for single race categories prior to 1999 included persons who reported one race or, if they reported more than one race, identified one race as best representing their race. The effect of the 1997 Standard on the 1999–2000 estimates can be seen by comparing 1999–2000 data tabulated according to the two Standards: Estimates based on the 1977 Standards of the percent of the population 20–74 years, age adjusted, with high serum cholesterol are: 0.1 percentage points lower for white males; 0.1 percentage points higher for white females; 0.1 percentage points lower for black males; and unchanged for black females than estimates based on the 1997 Standards. See Appendix II, Race.
[2]Data for Mexicans are for 1982–84. See Appendix I, National Health and Nutrition Examination Survey (NHANES).
[3]Standard errors of estimates for 1988–94 and 1999–2000 are shown. 1999–2000 estimates are based on a smaller sample size than estimates for earlier time periods and therefore are subject to greater sampling error.
[4]Age adjusted to the 2000 standard population using five age groups except for 1999–2000 estimates, which are age adjusted using three age groups (20–39, 40–59, and 60–74 or 60 years and over) due to a smaller sample size; however, use of three rather than five groups had virtually no effect on age-adjusted estimates. See Appendix II, Age adjustment.   [5]Includes persons of all races and Hispanic origins, not just those shown separately.

NOTES: High serum cholesterol is defined as greater than or equal to 240 mg/dL (6.20 mmol/L). Risk levels have been defined by the Second report of the National Cholesterol Education Program Expert Panel on Detection, Evaluation and Treatment of High Blood Cholesterol in Adults. National Heart, Lung, and Blood Institute, National Institutes of Health. September 1993. (Summarized in *JAMA* 269(23):3015–23. June 16, 1993.)

SOURCES: Centers for Disease Control and Prevention, National Center for Health Statistics, National Health and Nutrition Examination Survey, Hispanic Health and Nutrition Examination Survey (1982–84), and National Health Examination Survey (1960–62).

Table 68 (page 1 of 4). Overweight, obesity, and healthy weight among persons 20 years of age and over, according to sex, age, race, and Hispanic origin: United States, 1960–62, 1971–74, 1976–80, 1988–94, and 1999–2000

[Data are based on measured height and weight of a sample of the civilian noninstitutionalized population]

Sex, age, race, and Hispanic origin[1]	Overweight[2]				
	1960–62	1971–74	1976–80[3]	1988–94[4]	1999–2000[4]
20–74 years, age adjusted[5]	Percent of population (standard error)				
Both sexes[6,7]	44.8	47.7	47.4	56.0 (0.9)	64.5 (1.5)
Male	49.5	54.7	52.9	61.0 (1.0)	67.0 (1.5)
Female[6]	40.2	41.1	42.0	51.2 (1.1)	62.0 (2.0)
Not Hispanic or Latino:					
White only, male	- - -	- - -	53.8	61.6 (1.2)	67.3 (2.0)
White only, female[6]	- - -	- - -	38.7	47.2 (1.4)	57.2 (2.7)
Black or African American only, male	- - -	- - -	51.3	58.2 (1.2)	60.3 (2.3)
Black or African American only, female[6]	- - -	- - -	62.6	68.5 (1.4)	77.7 (1.9)
Mexican male	- - -	- - -	61.6	69.4 (1.1)	74.4 (2.8)
Mexican female[6]	- - -	- - -	61.7	69.6 (1.7)	71.8 (2.5)
20 years and over, age adjusted[5]					
Both sexes[6,7]	- - -	- - -	- - -	56.0 (0.8)	64.5 (1.4)
Male	- - -	- - -	- - -	60.9 (1.0)	67.2 (1.4)
Female[6]	- - -	- - -	- - -	51.4 (1.0)	61.9 (1.9)
Not Hispanic or Latino:					
White only, male	- - -	- - -	- - -	61.6 (1.2)	67.4 (1.8)
White only, female[6]	- - -	- - -	- - -	47.5 (1.3)	57.3 (2.5)
Black or African American only, male	- - -	- - -	- - -	57.8 (1.2)	60.7 (1.9)
Black or African American only, female[6]	- - -	- - -	- - -	68.2 (1.3)	77.3 (2.0)
Mexican male	- - -	- - -	- - -	68.9 (1.1)	74.7 (2.6)
Mexican female[6]	- - -	- - -	- - -	68.9 (1.6)	71.9 (2.4)
20 years and over, crude					
Both sexes[6,7]	- - -	- - -	- - -	54.9 (0.8)	64.1 (1.4)
Male	- - -	- - -	- - -	59.4 (1.0)	66.5 (1.4)
Female[6]	- - -	- - -	- - -	50.7 (1.0)	61.8 (1.9)
Not Hispanic or Latino:					
White only, male	- - -	- - -	- - -	60.6 (1.2)	67.3 (1.8)
White only, female[6]	- - -	- - -	- - -	47.4 (1.2)	57.8 (2.6)
Black or African American only, male	- - -	- - -	- - -	56.7 (1.2)	58.9 (2.3)
Black or African American only, female[6]	- - -	- - -	- - -	66.0 (1.4)	76.5 (2.2)
Mexican male	- - -	- - -	- - -	63.9 (1.5)	72.0 (3.7)
Mexican female[6]	- - -	- - -	- - -	65.9 (1.4)	69.4 (3.1)
Male					
20–34 years	42.7	42.8	41.2	47.5 (1.4)	58.0 (2.5)
35–44 years	53.5	63.2	57.2	65.5 (1.7)	67.6 (2.7)
45–54 years	53.9	59.7	60.2	66.1 (2.1)	71.3 (3.5)
55–64 years	52.2	58.5	60.2	70.5 (2.1)	72.5 (3.5)
65–74 years	47.8	54.6	54.2	68.5 (2.1)	77.2 (3.6)
75 years and over	- - -	- - -	- - -	56.5 (2.0)	66.4 (3.5)
Female[6]					
20–34 years	21.2	25.8	27.9	37.0 (1.4)	51.5 (2.8)
35–44 years	37.2	40.5	40.7	49.6 (2.4)	63.6 (4.1)
45–54 years	49.3	49.0	48.7	60.3 (2.5)	64.7 (3.7)
55–64 years	59.9	54.5	53.7	66.3 (1.6)	73.1 (3.7)
65–74 years	60.9	55.9	59.5	60.3 (1.8)	70.1 (4.0)
75 years and over	- - -	- - -	- - -	52.3 (1.5)	59.6 (3.7)

See footnotes at end of table.

[Data are based on measured height and weight of a sample of the civilian noninstitutionalized population]

Sex, age, race, and Hispanic origin[1]	Obesity[8]				
	1960–62	1971–74	1976–80[3]	1988–94[4]	1999–2000[4]
20–74 years, age adjusted[5]	Percent of population (standard error)				
Both sexes[6,7]	13.3	14.6	15.1	23.3 (0.7)	30.9 (1.6)
Male	10.7	12.2	12.8	20.6 (0.7)	27.7 (1.7)
Female[6]	15.7	16.8	17.1	26.0 (1.0)	34.0 (2.0)
Not Hispanic or Latino:					
White only, male	- - -	- - -	12.4	20.7 (0.9)	27.4 (1.9)
White only, female[6]	- - -	- - -	15.4	23.3 (1.2)	30.4 (2.3)
Black or African American only, male	- - -	- - -	16.5	21.3 (1.0)	28.9 (2.4)
Black or African American only, female[6]	- - -	- - -	31.0	39.1 (1.4)	50.4 (2.8)
Mexican male	- - -	- - -	15.7	24.4 (1.1)	29.4 (2.5)
Mexican female[6]	- - -	- - -	26.6	36.1 (1.4)	40.1 (3.8)
20 years and over, age adjusted[5]					
Both sexes[6,7]	- - -	- - -	- - -	22.9 (0.7)	30.5 (1.4)
Male	- - -	- - -	- - -	20.2 (0.7)	27.5 (1.6)
Female[6]	- - -	- - -	- - -	25.5 (0.9)	33.4 (1.8)
Not Hispanic or Latino:					
White only, male	- - -	- - -	- - -	20.3 (0.8)	27.3 (1.8)
White only, female[6]	- - -	- - -	- - -	22.9 (1.1)	30.1 (2.1)
Black or African American only, male	- - -	- - -	- - -	20.9 (1.0)	28.1 (2.3)
Black or African American only, female[6]	- - -	- - -	- - -	38.3 (1.4)	49.7 (2.8)
Mexican male	- - -	- - -	- - -	23.8 (1.0)	28.9 (2.3)
Mexican female[6]	- - -	- - -	- - -	35.2 (1.4)	39.7 (3.6)
20 years and over, crude					
Both sexes[6,7]	- - -	- - -	- - -	22.3 (0.6)	30.3 (1.4)
Male	- - -	- - -	- - -	19.5 (0.7)	27.1 (1.6)
Female[6]	- - -	- - -	- - -	25.0 (0.9)	33.3 (1.8)
Not Hispanic or Latino:					
White only, male	- - -	- - -	- - -	19.9 (0.8)	27.2 (1.8)
White only, female[6]	- - -	- - -	- - -	22.7 (1.1)	30.3 (2.1)
Black or African American only, male	- - -	- - -	- - -	20.7 (1.0)	28.1 (2.6)
Black or African American only, female[6]	- - -	- - -	- - -	36.7 (1.4)	49.4 (2.8)
Mexican male	- - -	- - -	- - -	20.6 (1.2)	29.3 (2.8)
Mexican female[6]	- - -	- - -	- - -	33.3 (1.3)	37.9 (4.1)
Male					
20–34 years	9.2	9.7	8.9	14.1 (1.0)	24.1 (1.9)
35–44 years	12.1	13.5	13.5	21.5 (1.2)	25.2 (3.0)
45–54 years	12.5	13.7	16.7	23.2 (1.7)	30.1 (4.4)
55–64 years	9.2	14.1	14.1	27.2 (2.2)	32.9 (4.1)
65–74 years	10.4	10.9	13.2	24.1 (1.8)	33.4 (3.9)
75 years and over	- - -	- - -	- - -	13.2 (2.1)	20.4 (2.8)
Female[6]					
20–34 years	7.2	9.7	11.0	18.5 (1.1)	25.8 (2.6)
35–44 years	14.7	17.7	17.8	25.5 (2.1)	33.9 (3.0)
45–54 years	20.3	18.9	19.6	32.4 (1.9)	38.1 (4.1)
55–64 years	24.4	24.1	22.9	33.7 (1.8)	43.1 (4.2)
65–74 years	23.2	22.0	21.5	26.9 (1.5)	38.8 (3.8)
75 years and over	- - -	- - -	- - -	19.2 (1.3)	25.1 (4.0)

See footnotes at end of table.

[Data are based on measured height and weight of a sample of the civilian noninstitutionalized population]

Sex, age, race, and Hispanic origin[1]	Healthy weight[9]				
	1960–62	1971–74	1976–80[3]	1988–94[4]	1999–2000[4]
20–74 years, age adjusted[5]	Percent of population (standard error)				
Both sexes[6,7]	51.2	48.8	49.6	41.7 (0.9)	33.6 (1.4)
Male	48.3	43.0	45.4	37.9 (1.0)	31.8 (1.5)
Female[6]	54.1	54.3	53.7	45.3 (1.1)	35.3 (2.0)
Not Hispanic or Latino:					
White only, male	- - -	- - -	45.3	37.4 (1.2)	31.3 (2.0)
White only, female[6]	- - -	- - -	56.7	49.2 (1.4)	39.1 (2.6)
Black or African American only, male	- - -	- - -	46.6	40.0 (1.2)	38.1 (2.2)
Black or African American only, female[6]	- - -	- - -	35.0	28.9 (1.2)	22.0 (1.9)
Mexican male	- - -	- - -	37.1	29.8 (1.1)	25.0 (2.7)
Mexican female[6]	- - -	- - -	36.4	29.0 (1.7)	26.9 (2.6)
20 years and over, age adjusted[5]					
Both sexes[6,7]	- - -	- - -	- - -	41.6 (0.8)	33.5 (1.3)
Male	- - -	- - -	- - -	37.9 (1.0)	31.7 (1.4)
Female[6]	- - -	- - -	- - -	45.0 (1.0)	35.3 (1.9)
Not Hispanic or Latino:					
White only, male	- - -	- - -	- - -	37.3 (1.1)	31.3 (1.8)
White only, female[6]	- - -	- - -	- - -	48.7 (1.3)	39.0 (2.5)
Black or African American only, male	- - -	- - -	- - -	40.1 (1.2)	37.4 (1.9)
Black or African American only, female[6]	- - -	- - -	- - -	29.2 (1.2)	22.3 (2.0)
Mexican male	- - -	- - -	- - -	30.2 (1.0)	24.8 (2.5)
Mexican female[6]	- - -	- - -	- - -	29.7 (1.6)	26.6 (2.4)
20 years and over, crude					
Both sexes[6,7]	- - -	- - -	- - -	42.6 (0.8)	33.9 (1.3)
Male	- - -	- - -	- - -	39.4 (1.0)	32.3 (1.4)
Female[6]	- - -	- - -	- - -	45.7 (1.0)	35.4 (1.9)
Not Hispanic or Latino:					
White only, male	- - -	- - -	- - -	38.2 (1.2)	31.4 (1.8)
White only, female[6]	- - -	- - -	- - -	48.8 (1.2)	38.6 (2.5)
Black or African American only, male	- - -	- - -	- - -	41.5 (1.2)	39.3 (2.2)
Black or African American only, female[6]	- - -	- - -	- - -	31.2 (1.3)	23.1 (2.1)
Mexican male	- - -	- - -	- - -	35.2 (1.5)	27.4 (3.5)
Mexican female[6]	- - -	- - -	- - -	32.4 (1.5)	29.1 (3.1)
Male					
20–34 years	55.3	54.7	57.1	51.1 (1.5)	39.8 (2.5)
35–44 years	45.2	35.2	41.3	33.4 (1.7)	31.4 (2.7)
45–54 years	44.8	38.5	38.7	33.6 (2.0)	28.7 (3.5)
55–64 years	44.9	38.3	38.7	28.6 (2.1)	26.5 (3.2)
65–74 years	46.2	42.1	42.3	30.1 (2.2)	21.5 (3.3)
75 years and over	- - -	- - -	- - -	40.9 (1.9)	32.7 (3.4)
Female[6]					
20–34 years	67.6	65.8	65.0	57.9 (1.3)	43.9 (2.5)
35–44 years	58.4	56.7	55.6	47.1 (2.5)	33.6 (4.0)
45–54 years	47.6	49.3	48.7	37.2 (2.3)	33.3 (3.8)
55–64 years	38.1	41.1	43.5	31.5 (1.5)	26.9 (3.7)
65–74 years	36.4	40.6	37.8	37.0 (2.0)	27.7 (3.9)
75 years and over	- - -	- - -	- - -	43.0 (1.6)	37.4 (3.7)

See footnotes at end of table.

Table 68 (page 4 of 4). Overweight, obesity, and healthy weight among persons 20 years of age and over, according to sex, age, race, and Hispanic origin: United States, 1960–62, 1971–74, 1976–80, 1988–94, and 1999–2000

[Data are based on measured height and weight of a sample of the civilian noninstitutionalized population]

- - - Data not available.

[1]Persons of Mexican origin may be of any race. Starting with data year 1999 race-specific estimates are tabulated according to 1997 Standards for Federal data on Race and Ethnicity and are not strictly comparable with estimates for earlier years. The two non-Hispanic race categories shown in the table conform to 1997 Standards. The 1999–2000 race-specific estimates are for persons who reported only one racial group. Prior to data year 1999, data were tabulated according to 1977 Standards. Estimates for single race categories prior to 1999 included persons who reported one race or, if they reported more than one race, identified one race as best representing their race. The effect of the 1997 Standard on the 1999–2000 estimates can be seen by comparing 1999–2000 data tabulated according to the two Standards: Estimates based on the 1977 Standards of the percent of the population 20–74 years, age adjusted, who were overweight are: 0.2 percentage points higher for white males; 0.3 percentage points higher for white females; 0.2 percentage points lower for black males; and 0.3 percentage points higher for black females than estimates based on the 1997 Standards. See Appendix II, Race.

[2]Body mass index (BMI) greater than or equal to 25.

[3]Data for Mexicans are for 1982–84. See Appendix I, National Health and Nutrition Examination Survey (NHANES).

[4]Standard errors of estimates for 1988–94 and 1999–2000 are shown. 1999–2000 estimates are based on a smaller sample size than estimates for earlier time periods and therefore are subject to greater sampling error.

[5]Age adjusted to the 2000 standard population using five age groups except for 1999–2000 estimates, which are age adjusted using three age groups (20–39, 40–59, and 60–74 or 60 years and over) due to a smaller sample size; however, use of three rather than five groups had virtually no effect on age-adjusted estimates. See Appendix II, Age adjustment.

[6]Excludes pregnant women.

[7]Includes persons of all races and Hispanic origins, not just those shown separately.

[8]Body mass index (BMI) greater than or equal to 30.

[9]BMI of 18.5 to less than 25 kilograms/meter^2 (see Appendix II, Body mass index).

NOTES: Percents do not sum to 100 because the percent of persons with BMI less than 18.5 is not shown and the percent of persons with obesity is a subset of the percent with overweight. Height was measured without shoes; two pounds were deducted from data for 1960–62 to allow for weight of clothing. Some data for 1988–94 have been revised and differ from the previous edition of *Health, United States*.

SOURCES: Centers for Disease Control and Prevention, National Center for Health Statistics, National Health and Nutrition Examination Survey, Hispanic Health and Nutrition Examination Survey (1982–84), and National Health Examination Survey (1960–62).

Table 69. Overweight children and adolescents 6–19 years of age, according to sex, age, race, and Hispanic origin: United States, selected years 1963–65 through 1999–2000

[Data are based on physical examinations of a sample of the civilian noninstitutionalized population]

Age, sex, race, and Hispanic origin[1]	1963–65 1966–70[2]	1971–74	1976–80[3]	1988–94[4]	1999–2000[4]
6–11 years of age	Percent of population (standard error)				
Both sexes[5]	4.2	4.0	6.5	11.3 (1.0)	15.3 (1.7)
Boys	4.0	4.3	6.6	11.6 (1.3)	16.0 (2.3)
Not Hispanic or Latino:					
White only	- - -	- - -	6.1	10.7 (2.0)	*11.9 (3.0)
Black or African American only	- - -	- - -	6.8	12.3 (1.4)	17.6 (2.8)
Mexican	- - -	- - -	13.3	17.5 (2.4)	27.3 (3.1)
Girls[6]	4.5	3.6	6.4	11.0 (1.4)	14.5 (2.4)
Not Hispanic or Latino:					
White only	- - -	- - -	5.2	*9.8 (2.0)	*12.0 (3.6)
Black or African American only	- - -	- - -	11.2	17.0 (1.6)	22.1 (3.3)
Mexican	- - -	- - -	9.8	15.3 (2.5)	19.6 (3.1)
12–19 years of age					
Both sexes[5]	4.6	6.1	5.0	10.5 (0.9)	15.5 (1.2)
Boys	4.5	6.1	4.8	11.3 (1.3)	15.5 (1.6)
Not Hispanic or Latino:					
White only	- - -	- - -	3.8	11.6 (1.9)	13.0 (2.5)
Black or African American only	- - -	- - -	6.1	10.7 (1.4)	20.5 (2.6)
Mexican	- - -	- - -	7.7	14.1 (1.8)	27.5 (3.0)
Girls[6]	4.7	6.2	5.3	9.7 (1.1)	15.5 (1.6)
Not Hispanic or Latino:					
White only	- - -	- - -	4.6	8.9 (1.7)	12.2 (2.1)
Black or African American only	- - -	- - -	10.7	16.3 (2.1)	25.7 (2.6)
Mexican	- - -	- - -	8.8	*13.4 (3.1)	19.4 (2.8)

* Estimates are considered unreliable. Data preceded by an asterisk have a relative standard error of 20–30 percent.

- - - Data not available.

[1]Persons of Mexican origin may be of any race. Starting with data year 1999 race-specific estimates are tabulated according to 1997 Standards for Federal data on Race and Ethnicity and are not strictly comparable with estimates for earlier years. The two non-Hispanic race categories shown in the table conform to 1997 Standards. The 1999–2000 race-specific estimates are for persons who reported only one racial group. Prior to data year 1999, data were tabulated according to 1977 Standards. Estimates for single race categories prior to 1999 included persons who reported one race or, if they reported more than one race, identified one race as best representing their race. The effect of the 1997 Standard on the 1999–2000 estimates can be seen by comparing 1999–2000 data tabulated according to the two Standards: Estimates based on the 1977 Standards of the percent of the children 6–11 years who were overweight are: 0.1 percentage points higher for white males; 0.5 percentage points lower for black males; 0.4 percentage points lower for white females; and 0.1 percentage points higher for black females than estimates based on the 1997 Standards. Estimates based on the 1977 Standards of the percent of adolescents 12–19 years of age who were overweight are: 0.2 percentage points lower for white males; 0.2 percentage points higher for black males; 0.2 percentage points higher for white females; and 0.9 percentage points higher for black females than estimates based on the 1997 Standards. See Appendix II, Race.

[2]Data for 1963–65 are for children 6–11 years of age; data for 1966–70 are for adolescents 12–17 years of age, not 12–19 years.

[3]Data for Mexicans are for 1982–84. See Appendix I, National Health and Nutrition Examination Survey (NHANES).

[4]Standard errors of estimates for 1988–94 and 1999–2000 are shown. 1999–2000 estimates are based on a smaller sample size than estimates for earlier time periods and therefore are subject to greater sampling error.

[5]Includes persons of all races and Hispanic origins, not just those shown separately.

[6]Excludes pregnant women starting with 1971–74. Pregnancy status not available for 1963–65 and 1966–70.

NOTES: Overweight is defined as body mass index (BMI) at or above the sex- and age-specific 95th percentile BMI cutoff points from the 2000 CDC Growth Charts: United States. Advance data from vital and health statistics; no 314. Hyattsville, Maryland: National Center for Health Statistics. 2000. Age is at time of examination at mobile examination center. Crude rates, not age-adjusted rates, are shown. Some data for 1976–80, 1988–94, and 1999–2000 have been revised and differ from the previous edition of *Health, United States*.

SOURCES: Centers for Disease Control and Prevention, National Center for Health Statistics, National Health and Nutrition Examination Survey, Hispanic Health and Nutrition Examination Survey (1982–84), and National Health Examination Survey (1963–65 and 1966–70).

Table 70 (page 1 of 3). Health care visits to doctor's offices, emergency departments, and home visits within the past 12 months, according to selected characteristics: United States, selected years 1997–2001

[Data are based on household interviews of a sample of the civilian noninstitutionalized population]

	Number of health care visits[1]											
	None			1–3 visits			4–9 visits			10 or more visits		
Characteristic	1997	1999	2001	1997	1999	2001	1997	1999	2001	1997	1999	2001
	Percent distribution											
All persons[2,3]	16.5	17.5	16.5	46.2	45.8	45.8	23.6	23.3	24.4	13.7	13.4	13.3
Age												
Under 18 years	11.8	12.4	11.6	54.1	54.4	54.6	25.2	25.0	26.1	8.9	8.2	7.6
Under 6 years	5.0	5.9	5.5	44.9	45.9	45.8	37.0	36.8	37.9	13.0	11.3	10.8
6–17 years	15.3	15.5	14.6	58.7	58.5	58.9	19.3	19.4	20.5	6.8	6.7	6.1
18–44 years	21.7	24.2	23.3	46.7	45.8	46.1	19.0	17.8	18.9	12.6	12.3	11.8
18–24 years	22.0	24.8	25.4	46.8	46.1	44.7	20.0	17.8	19.5	11.2	11.4	10.5
25–44 years	21.6	24.0	22.6	46.7	45.7	46.5	18.7	17.8	18.7	13.0	12.6	12.2
45–64 years	16.9	16.9	15.6	42.9	42.4	42.9	24.7	25.0	25.7	15.5	15.7	15.9
45–54 years	17.9	18.4	17.1	43.9	43.2	44.9	23.4	22.8	23.6	14.8	15.7	14.4
55–64 years	15.3	14.7	13.3	41.3	41.1	39.6	26.7	28.4	28.9	16.7	15.8	18.2
65 years and over	8.9	7.9	7.1	34.7	34.3	32.3	32.5	34.1	35.6	23.8	23.7	25.0
65–74 years	9.8	8.6	8.1	36.9	36.9	35.8	31.6	33.2	33.5	21.6	21.3	22.6
75 years and over	7.7	7.2	5.8	31.8	31.1	28.2	33.8	35.1	38.1	26.6	26.6	27.9
Sex[3]												
Male	21.3	23.1	21.3	47.1	45.5	46.5	20.6	20.6	21.6	11.0	10.8	10.7
Female	11.8	12.0	11.9	45.4	46.1	45.1	26.5	25.9	27.1	16.3	15.9	15.9
Race[3,4]												
White only	16.0	16.9	15.9	46.1	45.7	45.7	23.9	23.8	24.8	14.0	13.6	13.5
Black or African American only	16.8	18.4	16.4	46.1	46.2	46.4	23.2	21.9	24.0	13.9	13.5	13.2
American Indian and Alaska Native only	17.1	20.6	*21.4	38.0	34.3	36.4	24.2	27.8	25.4	20.7	17.2	16.9
Asian only	22.8	23.1	20.8	49.1	47.3	48.3	19.7	19.4	22.3	8.3	10.2	8.6
Native Hawaiian and Other Pacific Islander only	- - -	*	*	- - -	*	*	- - -	*	*	- - -	*	*
2 or more races	- - -	15.2	18.0	- - -	40.8	41.2	- - -	22.2	23.5	- - -	21.8	17.3
Hispanic origin and race[3,4]												
Hispanic or Latino	24.9	26.2	27.0	42.3	44.3	40.2	20.3	19.2	20.7	12.5	10.3	12.0
Mexican	28.9	30.2	31.4	40.8	43.0	39.2	18.5	18.2	19.6	11.8	8.7	9.8
Not Hispanic or Latino	15.4	16.2	15.0	46.7	46.0	46.5	24.0	23.9	25.0	13.9	13.9	13.5
White only	14.7	15.5	14.3	46.6	46.0	46.4	24.4	24.5	25.4	14.3	14.1	13.9
Black or African American only	16.9	18.4	16.4	46.1	46.2	46.4	23.1	21.9	24.0	13.8	13.5	13.1
Respondent-assessed health status[3]												
Fair or poor	7.8	9.8	9.0	23.3	25.9	22.1	29.0	24.3	27.7	39.9	40.1	41.3
Good to excellent	17.2	18.1	17.3	48.4	47.7	48.0	23.3	23.2	24.3	11.1	11.0	10.5
Poverty status[3,5]												
Poor	20.3	21.5	21.7	37.1	39.2	37.2	22.7	21.3	23.4	19.9	18.0	17.7
Near poor	19.9	22.2	20.4	42.8	41.6	41.4	21.8	21.5	22.9	15.5	14.7	15.3
Nonpoor	14.0	14.9	14.0	48.0	47.0	47.4	25.0	25.0	25.8	13.0	13.1	12.8

See footnotes at end of table.

Table 70 (page 2 of 3). Health care visits to doctor's offices, emergency departments, and home visits within the past 12 months, according to selected characteristics: United States, selected years 1997–2001

[Data are based on household interviews of a sample of the civilian noninstitutionalized population]

	Number of health care visits[1]											
	None			1–3 visits			4–9 visits			10 or more visits		
Characteristic	1997	1999	2001	1997	1999	2001	1997	1999	2001	1997	1999	2001
Hispanic origin and race and poverty status[3,4,5]						Percent distribution						
Hispanic or Latino:												
Poor	30.6	31.2	34.3	33.8	38.2	32.7	20.0	18.7	18.1	15.6	11.8	14.9
Near poor	29.1	30.2	28.9	39.0	42.1	39.3	20.9	17.5	20.2	11.0	10.1	11.6
Nonpoor	18.7	21.0	19.9	48.6	46.8	44.6	20.3	21.9	24.7	12.3	10.2	10.8
Not Hispanic or Latino:												
White only:												
Poor	16.3	17.2	16.2	37.7	38.9	38.7	24.0	23.3	26.4	22.1	20.7	18.8
Near poor	17.1	19.8	17.1	43.7	40.8	41.3	22.3	23.3	24.1	17.0	16.1	17.6
Nonpoor	13.2	14.0	13.1	47.6	46.9	47.5	25.7	25.5	26.1	13.4	13.6	13.3
Black or African American only:												
Poor	17.8	18.0	17.3	37.4	39.9	38.1	23.3	23.1	24.0	21.5	19.0	20.5
Near poor	18.9	19.9	18.1	43.0	44.0	44.9	23.4	20.5	23.4	14.7	15.6	13.6
Nonpoor	15.6	16.3	14.6	50.5	48.2	47.4	23.3	23.7	26.6	10.6	11.8	11.4
Health insurance status[6,7]												
Under 65 years of age:												
Insured	14.3	15.4	14.1	49.0	48.6	49.1	23.6	23.2	24.2	13.1	12.7	12.6
Private	14.7	15.9	14.4	50.6	49.9	50.6	23.1	22.9	24.0	11.6	11.3	11.0
Medicaid	9.8	10.7	10.4	35.5	35.6	35.4	26.5	26.0	26.3	28.2	27.6	27.8
Uninsured	33.7	37.3	37.5	42.8	41.6	41.4	15.3	13.2	14.6	8.2	7.9	6.5
65 years of age and over:												
Medicare HMO	8.9	5.7	5.0	35.8	34.2	30.0	33.1	34.6	41.1	22.3	25.5	23.9
Private	7.3	6.7	5.5	35.9	34.9	34.6	34.0	34.9	35.2	22.7	23.5	24.8
Medicaid	9.3	*7.3	6.1	19.2	21.4	18.7	27.9	34.8	31.6	43.7	36.5	43.5
Medicare fee-for-service only	15.5	14.0	14.1	34.0	35.8	30.5	28.1	31.0	34.2	22.4	19.2	21.2
Poverty status and health insurance status[5,6,7]												
Under 65 years of age:												
Poor:												
Insured	13.7	14.6	14.0	38.8	41.4	41.1	24.5	23.2	24.9	22.9	20.7	20.0
Uninsured	36.7	39.8	43.2	38.8	39.3	34.6	14.9	12.6	15.3	9.5	8.3	6.9
Near poor:												
Insured	15.6	17.0	15.8	45.5	44.9	44.7	22.3	22.6	22.7	16.6	15.5	16.8
Uninsured	34.5	38.0	35.3	41.8	40.2	40.9	15.6	13.4	16.6	8.1	8.4	7.2
Nonpoor:												
Insured	13.4	14.7	13.6	50.3	49.1	49.8	24.2	24.2	25.0	12.1	12.0	11.6
Uninsured	29.1	32.9	31.9	45.4	43.7	46.0	17.0	14.6	15.5	8.4	8.8	6.6
Geographic region[3]												
Northeast	13.2	12.8	11.8	45.9	46.4	47.2	26.0	25.6	26.6	14.9	15.2	14.3
Midwest	15.9	16.2	14.9	47.7	46.7	47.2	22.8	23.8	24.0	13.6	13.3	13.9
South	17.2	18.9	17.7	46.1	45.5	45.2	23.3	22.5	24.4	13.5	13.2	12.8
West	19.1	20.9	20.5	44.8	44.8	44.1	22.8	21.9	22.8	13.3	12.4	12.7

See footnotes at end of table.

Table 70 (page 3 of 3). Health care visits to doctor's offices, emergency departments, and home visits within the past 12 months, according to selected characteristics: United States, selected years 1997–2001

[Data are based on household interviews of a sample of the civilian noninstitutionalized population]

	Number of health care visits[1]											
	None			1–3 visits			4–9 visits			10 or more visits		
Characteristic	1997	1999	2001	1997	1999	2001	1997	1999	2001	1997	1999	2001
Location of residence[3]	Percent distribution											
Within MSA[8]	16.2	17.4	16.4	46.4	45.9	45.7	23.7	23.4	24.6	13.7	13.2	13.2
Outside MSA[8]	17.3	17.7	16.7	45.4	45.1	46.1	23.3	22.9	23.6	13.9	14.4	13.6

* Estimates are considered unreliable. Data not shown have a relative standard error (RSE) of greater than 30 percent. Data preceded by an asterisk have a RSE of 20–30 percent.

- - - Data not available.

[1]This table presents a summary measure of ambulatory and home health care visits during a 12-month period. See Appendix II, Health care contact; Emergency department visit; Home visit.

[2]Includes all other races not shown separately, unknown poverty status, and unknown health insurance status.

[3]Estimates are age adjusted to the year 2000 standard population using six age groups: Under 18 years, 18–44 years, 45–54 years, 55–64 years, 65–74 years, and 75 years and over. See Appendix II, Age adjustment.

[4]The race groups, white, black, American Indian and Alaska Native (AI/AN), Asian, Native Hawaiian and Other Pacific Islander, and 2 or more races, include persons of Hispanic and non-Hispanic origin. Persons of Hispanic origin may be of any race. Starting with data year 1999 race-specific estimates are tabulated according to 1997 Standards for Federal data on Race and Ethnicity and are not strictly comparable with estimates for earlier years. The five single race categories plus multiple race categories shown in the table conform to 1997 Standards. The 1999 race-specific estimates are for persons who reported only one racial group; the category "2 or more races" includes persons who reported more than one racial group. Prior to data year 1999, data were tabulated according to 1977 Standards with four racial groups and the category "Asian only" included Native Hawaiian and Other Pacific Islander. Estimates for single race categories prior to 1999 included persons who reported one race or, if they reported more than one race, identified one race as best representing their race. The effect of the 1997 Standard on the 1999 estimates can be seen by comparing 1999 data tabulated according to the two Standards: Age-adjusted estimates based on the 1977 Standard of the percent of persons with a specified number of health care contacts are: (no visits) identical for white and black persons; 0.1 percentage points higher for AI/AN persons; 0.4 percentage points lower for Asian and Pacific Islander persons; (1–3 visits) identical for white persons; 0.1 percentage points lower for black persons; 1.3 percentage points higher for AI/AN persons; 0.1 percentage points lower for Asian and Pacific Islander persons; (4–9 visits) identical for white persons; 0.2 percentage points higher for black persons; 2.2 percentage points lower for AI/AN persons; 0.4 percentage points higher for Asian and Pacific Islander persons; (10 or more visits) identical for white and black persons; 0.9 percentage points higher for AI/AN persons; and 0.1 percentage points higher for Asian and Pacific Islander persons than estimates based on the 1997 Standards. See Appendix II, Race.

[5]Poor persons are defined as below the poverty threshold. Near poor persons have incomes of 100 percent to less than 200 percent of poverty threshold. Nonpoor persons have incomes of 200 percent or greater than the poverty threshold. Poverty status was unknown for 20 percent of persons in the sample in 1997, 25 percent in 1998, 28 percent in 1999, 27 percent in 2000, and 28 percent in 2001. See Appendix II, Family income; Poverty level.

[6]Estimates for persons under 65 years of age are age adjusted to the year 2000 standard using four age groups: Under 18 years, 18–44 years, 45–54 years, and 55–64 years of age. Estimates for persons 65 years of age and over are age adjusted to the year 2000 standard using two age groups: 65–74 years and 75 years and over. See Appendix II, Age adjustment.

[7]Health insurance categories are mutually exclusive. Persons who reported both Medicaid and private coverage are classified as having private coverage. Persons 65 years of age and over who reported Medicare HMO (health maintenance organization) and some other type of health insurance coverage are classified as having Medicare HMO. Starting in 1997 Medicaid includes state-sponsored health plans and State Children's Health Insurance Program (SCHIP). The category "insured" also includes military, other State, and Medicare coverage. See Appendix II, Health insurance coverage.

[8]MSA is metropolitan statistical area.

NOTES: Some numbers in this table for health insurance estimates were revised and differ from previous editions of *Health, United States*. In 1997 the National Health Interview Survey questionnaire was redesigned. See Appendix I, National Health Interview Survey. Data for additional years are available (see Appendix III). Standard errors for selected years are available in the spreadsheet version of this table. See www.cdc.gov/nchs/hus.htm.

SOURCE: Centers for Disease Control and Prevention, National Center for Health Statistics, National Health Interview Survey, family core and sample adult questionnaires.

Table 71 (page 1 of 2). Vaccinations of children 19–35 months of age for selected diseases, according to race, Hispanic origin, poverty status, and residence in metropolitan statistical area (MSA): United States, 1995–2001

[Data are based on telephone interviews of a sample of the civilian noninstitutionalized population supplemented by a survey of immunization providers for interview participants]

| | | Race and Hispanic origin | | | | | Poverty status | | Location of residence | | |
| | | | Not Hispanic or Latino | | | | | | Inside MSA[1] | | |
Vaccination and year	All	White	Black or African American	American Indian or Alaska Native	Asian or Pacific Islander	Hispanic or Latino[2]	Below poverty	At or above poverty	Central city	Remaining areas	Outside MSA[1]
					Percent of children 19–35 months of age						
Combined series (4:3:1:3):[3]											
1995	74	76	70	69	76	68	67	77	72	75	75
1996	76	79	74	82	78	71	69	79	74	78	77
1997	76	79	73	73	71	73	71	79	74	78	77
1998	79	82	73	78	79	75	74	82	77	81	81
1999	78	81	74	75	77	75	73	81	77	79	80
2000	76	79	71	69	75	73	71	78	73	78	79
2001	77	79	71	76	77	77	72	79	75	78	79
DTP/DT/DTaP (4 doses or more):[4]											
1995	78	80	74	71	84	75	71	81	77	79	78
1996	81	83	79	85	85	77	74	84	79	83	81
1997	82	84	77	80	80	78	76	84	80	83	81
1998	84	87	77	83	89	81	80	86	82	85	85
1999	83	86	79	80	87	80	79	85	82	84	83
2000	82	84	76	75	85	79	76	84	80	83	83
2001	82	84	76	77	84	83	77	84	81	83	82
Polio (3 doses or more):											
1995	88	89	84	86	90	87	85	89	87	88	89
1996	91	92	90	90	90	89	88	92	89	92	92
1997	91	92	89	90	89	90	89	92	90	91	92
1998	91	92	88	85	93	89	90	92	89	91	93
1999	90	90	87	88	90	89	87	91	89	90	90
2000	90	91	87	90	93	88	87	90	88	90	91
2001	89	90	85	88	90	91	87	90	88	90	91
Measles, Mumps, Rubella:											
1995	90	91	87	88	95	88	86	91	90	90	89
1996	91	91	90	89	93	88	87	92	90	91	91
1997	90	91	89	92	90	88	86	92	90	91	91
1998	92	93	89	91	92	91	90	93	92	92	93
1999	92	92	90	92	93	90	90	92	91	92	90
2000	91	92	88	87	90	90	89	91	90	91	91
2001	91	92	89	94	90	92	89	92	91	92	91
Hib (3 doses or more):[5]											
1995	91	93	88	93	90	89	88	93	91	92	92
1996	91	93	89	91	92	89	87	93	90	93	92
1997	93	94	91	86	89	90	90	94	91	93	94
1998	93	95	90	90	92	92	91	95	92	94	94
1999	94	95	92	91	90	92	91	95	92	95	93
2000	93	95	93	90	92	91	90	95	92	94	95
2001	93	94	90	91	92	93	90	94	91	94	93
Hepatitis B (3 doses or more):											
1995	68	68	66	52	80	70	65	69	69	71	59
1996	82	82	82	79	85	81	78	83	81	83	81
1997	84	85	82	83	88	81	81	85	82	85	85
1998	87	88	84	82	89	86	85	88	85	88	87
1999	88	89	87	*	88	87	87	89	87	89	88
2000	90	91	89	91	91	88	87	91	89	90	92
2001	89	90	85	86	90	90	87	90	88	90	89
Varicella:[6]											
1997	26	28	21	20	36	22	17	29	26	29	17
1998	43	42	42	28	53	47	41	44	45	45	34
1999	58	56	58	*	64	61	55	58	59	61	47
2000	68	66	67	62	77	70	64	69	69	70	60
2001	76	75	75	69	82	80	74	77	78	78	68

See footnotes at end of table.

Table 71 (page 2 of 2). Vaccinations of children 19–35 months of age for selected diseases, according to race, Hispanic origin, poverty status, and residence in metropolitan statistical area (MSA): United States, 1995–2001

[Data are based on telephone interviews of a sample of the civilian noninstitutionalized population supplemented by a survey of immunization providers for interview participants]

| | Not Hispanic or Latino | | | | Hispanic or Latino[2] | |
| | White | | Black or African American | | | |
Vaccination and year	Below poverty	At or above poverty	Below poverty	At or above poverty	Below poverty	At or above poverty
	Percent of children 19–35 months of age					
Combined series (4:3:1:3):[3]						
1995	69	78	70	73	63	72
1996	68	80	69	79	68	73
1997	72	79	71	77	70	77
1998	77	83	72	74	73	79
1999	76	82	72	77	73	78
2000	73	80	69	72	70	74
2001	71	80	69	74	73	79

* Estimates are considered unreliable. Percents not shown if the unweighted sample size for the numerator was less than 30 or relative standard error greater than 0.5 or confidence interval half width greater than 10.

[1]Metropolitan statistical area.

[2]Persons of Hispanic origin may be of any race.

[3]The 4:3:1:3 combined series consists of 4 or more doses of diphtheria and tetanus toxoids and pertussis vaccine (DTP), diphtheria and tetanus toxoids (DT), or diphtheria and tetanus toxoids and acellular pertussis vaccine (DTaP), 3 or more doses of oral poliovirus vaccine, 1 or more doses of a measles-containing vaccine (MCV), and 3 or more doses of *Haemophilus influenzae* type b vaccine (Hib).

[4]Diphtheria and tetanus toxoids and pertussis vaccine, diphtheria and tetanus toxoids, and diphtheria and tetanus toxoids and acellular pertussis vaccine.

[5]*Haemophilus influenzae* type b vaccine (Hib).

[6]Recommended in 1996. Data collection for varicella began in July 1996.

NOTES: Final estimates from the National Immunization Survey include an adjustment for children with missing immunization provider data. Poverty status is based on family income and family size using Bureau of the Census poverty thresholds. Children missing information about poverty status were omitted from analysis by poverty level. In 2001, 13.7 percent of all children, 19.6 percent of Hispanic, 11.2 percent of non-Hispanic white, and 14.8 percent of non-Hispanic black children were missing information about poverty status and were omitted. See Appendix I, National Immunization Survey. Some data for previous years have been revised and differ from previous editions of *Health, United States*.

SOURCE: Centers for Disease Control and Prevention, National Center for Health Statistics and National Immunization Program, National Immunization Survey. Data are available on the CDC Web site at www.cdc.gov/nip/coverage/ and www.cdc.gov/nis/.

Table 72 (page 1 of 2). Vaccination coverage among children 19–35 months of age according to geographic division, State, and selected urban areas: United States, 1995–2001

[Data are based on telephone interviews of a sample of the civilian noninstitutionalized population supplemented by a survey of immunization providers for interview participants]

Geographic division and State	1995	1996	1997	1998	1999	2000	2001
	Percent of children 19–35 months of age with 4:3:1:3 series[1]						
United States	74	76	76	79	78	76	77
New England:							
Maine	88	86	87	86	83	83	82
New Hampshire	89	83	85	82	85	83	84
Vermont	87	87	87	86	91	83	88
Massachusetts	81	87	88	87	85	85	81
Rhode Island	83	84	82	86	87	82	84
Connecticut	86	88	86	90	86	85	84
Middle Atlantic:							
New York	74	80	75	85	81	75	81
New Jersey	70	75	76	82	81	76	76
Pennsylvania	77	79	79	83	86	78	82
East North Central:							
Ohio	71	78	72	78	78	72	75
Indiana	74	70	72	78	74	76	74
Illinois	78	75	74	78	77	75	76
Michigan	68	75	75	78	74	75	74
Wisconsin	74	77	81	78	85	80	83
West North Central:							
Minnesota	75	84	78	82	85	86	79
Iowa	83	81	77	82	83	83	79
Missouri	75	75	79	85	75	78	78
North Dakota	79	80	80	79	80	81	83
South Dakota	79	81	77	74	82	78	79
Nebraska	71	78	74	76	82	79	80
Kansas	70	72	84	82	79	76	76
South Atlantic:							
Delaware	68	81	80	79	78	75	79
Maryland	77	79	81	77	79	78	78
District of Columbia	69	76	71	71	78	71	74
Virginia	69	76	72	80	80	74	78
West Virginia	71	71	81	82	81	76	81
North Carolina	80	78	80	83	82	87	85
South Carolina	78	85	81	88	81	80	81
Georgia	77	81	78	80	82	81	80
Florida	74	79	74	79	80	74	77
East South Central:							
Kentucky	81	76	78	82	88	81	79
Tennessee	74	79	79	82	78	81	84
Alabama	73	74	87	82	78	81	83
Mississippi	79	81	80	84	82	81	84
West South Central:							
Arkansas	73	70	80	73	77	72	74
Louisiana	77	79	77	78	77	75	69
Oklahoma	74	72	70	75	73	71	76
Texas	71	71	74	74	72	69	74
Mountain:							
Montana	71	75	75	82	83	77	82
Idaho	66	65	71	76	69	74	74
Wyoming	71	77	75	80	83	79	81
Colorado	75	80	74	76	76	74	75
New Mexico	74	78	73	71	73	68	71
Arizona	69	70	71	76	72	72	73
Utah	65	65	69	76	80	77	74
Nevada	67	67	70	76	73	74	72
Pacific:							
Washington	76	78	79	81	75	77	76
Oregon	71	70	72	76	72	79	73
California	70	74	74	76	75	75	75
Alaska	74	72	75	81	80	77	74
Hawaii	75	80	77	79	82	75	73

See footnotes at end of table.

Table 72 (page 2 of 2). Vaccination coverage among children 19–35 months of age according to geographic division, State, and selected urban areas: United States, 1995–2001

[Data are based on telephone interviews of a sample of the civilian noninstitutionalized population supplemented by a survey of immunization providers for interview participants]

Geographic division and urban areas	1995	1996	1997	1998	1999	2000	2001
	Percent of children 19–35 months of age with 4:3:1:3 series[1]						
New England:							
Boston, Massachusetts	85	85	86	89	84	79	85
Middle Atlantic:							
New York City, New York.	72	78	72	81	78	68	76
Newark, New Jersey.	67	64	68	64	67	63	64
Philadelphia, Pennsylvania	67	74	81	80	81	74	74
East North Central:							
Cuyahoga County (Cleveland), Ohio.	72	79	70	75	74	73	73
Franklin County (Columbus), Ohio	75	80	73	78	78	77	78
Marion County (Indianapolis), Indiana.	77	72	80	78	79	69	72
Chicago, Illinois	70	72	66	64	71	65	69
Detroit, Michigan	54	60	60	70	66	59	63
Milwaukee County (Milwaukee), Wisconsin	69	70	72	73	74	69	70
South Atlantic:							
Baltimore, Maryland	*	80	84	81	72	70	72
District of Columbia	67	76	71	71	78	71	74
Fulton/DeKalb Counties (Atlanta), Georgia	*	76	74	71	83	80	75
Dade County (Miami), Florida	78	79	75	75	84	78	78
Duval County (Jacksonville), Florida.	69	76	69	79	78	79	76
East South Central:							
Davidson County (Nashville), Tennessee	72	80	76	80	73	73	82
Shelby County (Memphis), Tennessee	69	70	70	71	75	77	74
Jefferson County (Birmingham), Alabama	86	76	83	85	85	79	87
West South Central:							
Orleans Parish (New Orleans), Louisiana	78	72	69	79	72	70	68
Bexar County (San Antonio), Texas	76	74	79	79	70	68	73
Dallas County (Dallas), Texas	70	68	75	71	72	67	67
El Paso County (El Paso), Texas	72	61	63	78	73	70	69
Houston, Texas	64	62	62	61	63	65	69
Mountain:							
Maricopa County (Phoenix), Arizona.	67	72	70	77	71	71	72
Pacific:							
King County (Seattle), Washington.	84	82	81	86	77	75	72
Los Angeles County (Los Angeles), California . .	68	75	72	76	76	77	73
San Diego County (San Diego), California	72	74	76	77	75	76	80
Santa Clara County (Santa Clara), California . .	76	80	69	84	82	76	77

* Estimates are considered unreliable. Percents not shown if the unweighted sample size for the numerator was less than 30 or relative standard error greater than 0.5 or confidence interval half width greater than 10.

[1]The 4:3:1:3 combined series consists of 4 or more doses of diphtheria and tetanus toxoids and pertussis vaccine (DTP), diphtheria and tetanus toxoids (DT), or diphtheria and tetanus toxoids and acellular pertussis vaccine (DTaP), 3 or more doses of oral poliovirus vaccine, 1 or more doses of a measles-containing vaccine (MCV), and 3 or more doses of *Haemophilus influenzae* type b vaccine (Hib).

NOTES: Urban areas were chosen because they were high risk for under-vaccination. Final estimates from the National Immunization Survey include an adjustment for children with missing immunization provider data. Some data for previous years have been revised and differ from previous editions of *Health, United States*.

SOURCE: Centers for Disease Control and Prevention, National Center for Health Statistics and National Immunization Program, National Immunization Survey. Data are available on the CDC Web site at www.cdc.gov/nip/coverage/ and www.cdc.gov/nis/.

Table 73 (page 1 of 2). No health care visits to an office or clinic within the past 12 months among children under 18 years of age, according to selected characteristics: United States, average annual 1997–98 and 2000–01

[Data are based on household interviews of a sample of the civilian noninstitutionalized population]

Characteristic	Under 18 years of age		Under 6 years of age		6–17 years of age	
	1997–98	2000–01	1997–98	2000–01	1997–98	2000–01
	Percent of children without a health care visit[1]					
All children[2]	12.8	12.7	5.7	6.6	16.3	15.8
Race[3]						
White only	12.2	12.0	5.5	6.6	15.5	14.6
Black or African American only	14.3	15.1	6.5	6.3	18.1	19.0
American Indian and Alaska Native only	13.8	22.4	*	*	*17.6	*25.0
Asian only	16.3	15.2	*5.6	*8.7	22.1	18.9
Native Hawaiian and Other Pacific Islander only	- - -	*	- - -	*	- - -	*
2 or more races	- - -	8.5	- - -	*	- - -	13.6
Hispanic origin and race[3]						
Hispanic or Latino	19.3	19.7	9.7	10.0	25.3	25.5
Not Hispanic or Latino	11.6	11.4	4.8	5.8	14.9	14.0
White only	10.7	10.3	4.3	5.5	13.7	12.6
Black or African American only	14.5	14.8	6.5	6.5	18.3	18.5
Poverty status[4]						
Poor	17.7	18.5	8.1	10.4	23.8	22.9
Near poor	16.1	17.1	7.0	8.8	20.8	21.5
Nonpoor	9.7	9.5	3.9	4.0	12.5	12.1
Hispanic origin and race and poverty status[3,4]						
Hispanic or Latino:						
Poor	23.4	23.2	11.8	11.5	31.2	30.4
Near poor	20.1	21.8	9.3	12.9	27.3	27.4
Nonpoor	12.9	13.6	7.1	*4.8	16.2	18.4
Not Hispanic or Latino:						
White only:						
Poor	13.7	16.1	*5.4	*11.0	19.3	18.9
Near poor	14.0	14.1	6.0	6.9	18.1	17.9
Nonpoor	9.1	8.6	3.4	3.8	11.6	10.7
Black or African American only:						
Poor	16.1	16.1	*7.5	*8.2	21.0	19.8
Near poor	16.6	18.1	*7.0	*7.8	21.1	23.0
Nonpoor	12.2	12.4	*4.0	*4.1	15.6	15.9
Health insurance status[5]						
Insured	10.4	10.5	4.5	5.2	13.4	13.2
Private	10.4	10.3	4.3	4.7	13.1	12.9
Medicaid	10.1	11.0	5.0	6.3	14.4	14.2
Uninsured	28.8	30.6	14.6	18.8	34.9	35.7
Poverty status and health insurance status[4]						
Poor:						
Insured	13.2	13.6	5.7	7.5	18.4	17.2
Uninsured	34.5	37.8	19.6	23.8	40.6	44.4
Near poor:						
Insured	12.5	13.7	4.4	5.9	16.9	18.0
Uninsured	27.9	31.5	16.9	22.9	32.7	35.5
Nonpoor:						
Insured	8.9	8.9	3.6	3.6	11.4	11.4
Uninsured	23.0	21.9	*8.8	*13.2	28.6	25.2

See footnotes at end of table.

Table 73 (page 2 of 2). No health care visits to an office or clinic within the past 12 months among children under 18 years of age, according to selected characteristics: United States, average annual 1997–98 and 2000–01

[Data are based on household interviews of a sample of the civilian noninstitutionalized population]

Characteristic	Under 18 years of age		Under 6 years of age		6–17 years of age	
	1997–98	2000–01	1997–98	2000–01	1997–98	2000–01
Geographic region	Percent of children without a health care visit[1]					
Northeast	7.0	6.5	3.1	4.6	8.9	7.3
Midwest	12.2	10.5	5.9	5.3	15.3	12.9
South	14.3	15.1	5.6	7.4	18.5	18.9
West	16.3	16.8	7.9	8.2	20.7	21.3
Location of residence						
Within MSA[6]	12.3	12.3	5.4	6.5	15.9	15.2
Outside MSA[6]	14.6	14.6	6.9	6.8	17.9	18.1

* Estimates are considered unreliable. Data preceded by an asterisk have a relative standard error (RSE) of 20–30 percent. Data not shown have a RSE of greater than 30 percent.

- - - Data not available.

[1]Respondents were asked how many times a doctor or other health care professional was seen in the past 12 months at a doctor's office, clinic, or some other place. Excluded are visits to emergency rooms, hospitalizations, home visits, and telephone calls. Beginning in 2000 dental visits were also excluded. See Appendix II, Health care contact.

[2]Includes all other races not shown separately, unknown poverty status, and unknown health insurance status.

[3]The race groups, white, black, American Indian and Alaska Native (AI/AN), Asian, Native Hawaiian and Other Pacific Islander, and 2 or more races, include persons of Hispanic and non-Hispanic origin. Persons of Hispanic origin may be of any race. Starting with data years 1999–2000 race-specific estimates are tabulated according to 1997 Standards for Federal data on Race and Ethnicity and are not strictly comparable with estimates for earlier years. The five single race categories plus multiple race categories shown in the table conform to 1997 Standards. The 1999–2000 race-specific estimates are for persons who reported only one racial group; the category "2 or more races" includes persons who reported more than one racial group. Prior to data years 1999–2000, data were tabulated according to 1977 Standards with four racial groups and the category "Asian only" included Native Hawaiian and Other Pacific Islander. Estimates for single race categories prior to 1999–2000 included persons who reported one race or, if they reported more than one race, identified one race as best representing their race. The effect of the 1997 Standard on the 1999–2000 estimates can be seen by comparing 1999–2000 data tabulated according to the two Standards: Estimates based on the 1977 Standard of the percent of children under 18 years of age without a recent health care visit are: 0.1 percentage points higher for white children; 0.3 percentage points lower for black children; 1.0 percentage points lower for AI/AN children; and 1.2 percentage points lower for Asian and Pacific Islander children than estimates based on the 1997 Standards. See Appendix II, Race.

[4]Poor persons are defined as below the poverty threshold. Near poor persons have incomes of 100 percent to less than 200 percent of the poverty threshold. Nonpoor persons have incomes of 200 percent or greater than the poverty threshold. Poverty status was unknown for 17 percent of children in the sample in 1997, 21 percent in 1998, 24 percent in 1999, and 23 percent in 2000 and 2001. See Appendix II, Family income; Poverty level.

[5]Health insurance categories are mutually exclusive. Persons who reported both Medicaid and private coverage are classified as having private coverage. Starting in 1997 Medicaid includes state-sponsored health plans and State Child Health Insurance Program (SCHIP). The category "insured" also includes military, other State, and Medicare coverage. See Appendix II, Health insurance coverage.

[6]MSA is metropolitan statistical area.

NOTES: Some numbers in this table for health insurance estimates were revised and differ from previous editions of *Health, United States*. Data for additional years are available (see Appendix III). In 1997 the National Health Interview Survey questionnaire was redesigned. See Appendix I, National Health Interview Survey. Standard errors for selected years are available in the spreadsheet version of this table. See www.cdc.gov/nchs/hus.htm.

SOURCE: Centers for Disease Control and Prevention, National Center for Health Statistics, National Health Interview Survey, family core and sample child questionnaires.

Table 74 (page 1 of 2). No usual source of health care among children under 18 years of age, according to selected characteristics: United States, average annual 1993–94, 1997–98, and 2000–01

[Data are based on household interviews of a sample of the civilian noninstitutionalized population]

Characteristic	Under 18 years of age			Under 6 years of age			6–17 years of age		
	1993–94	1997–98[1]	2000–01[1]	1993–94	1997–98[1]	2000–01[1]	1993–94	1997–98[1]	2000–01[1]
	Percent of children without a usual source of health care[2]								
All children[3]	7.7	6.7	6.4	5.2	4.5	4.4	9.0	7.8	7.3
Race[4]									
White only	7.0	5.8	5.6	4.7	4.1	4.2	8.3	6.7	6.3
Black or African American only	10.3	8.9	7.4	7.6	5.6	4.0	11.9	10.4	9.0
American Indian and Alaska Native only	*9.3	*10.8	*6.7	*	*	*	*8.7	*	*
Asian only	9.7	10.7	9.9	*3.4	*	*7.5	13.5	14.4	11.3
Native Hawaiian and Other Pacific Islander only	- - -	- - -	*	- - -	- - -	*	- - -	- - -	*
2 or more races	- - -	- - -	6.0	- - -	- - -	*	- - -	- - -	*8.0
Hispanic origin and race[4]									
Hispanic or Latino	14.3	13.2	14.1	9.3	7.6	9.3	17.7	16.7	17.0
Not Hispanic or Latino	6.7	5.6	4.8	4.4	3.8	3.2	7.8	6.4	5.6
White only	5.7	4.5	3.9	3.7	3.4	2.8	6.7	5.0	4.4
Black or African American only	10.2	8.8	7.4	7.7	5.4	4.0	11.6	10.4	9.0
Poverty status[5]									
Poor	13.9	12.4	12.2	9.4	8.2	8.2	16.8	15.0	14.4
Near poor	9.8	10.1	9.4	6.7	6.5	7.1	11.6	12.0	10.7
Nonpoor	3.7	3.5	3.3	1.8	2.0	2.2	4.6	4.2	3.8
Hispanic origin and race and poverty status[4,5]									
Hispanic or Latino:									
Poor	19.6	17.0	19.2	12.7	8.4	12.8	24.8	22.7	23.3
Near poor	15.3	16.0	15.6	9.9	10.2	11.4	18.9	19.9	18.1
Nonpoor	5.0	5.7	6.2	*2.7	*3.1	*4.2	6.5	7.3	7.3
Not Hispanic or Latino:									
White only:									
Poor	10.2	11.4	9.6	6.5	10.7	*	12.7	12.0	11.0
Near poor	8.7	6.6	6.5	6.3	4.5	*5.4	10.1	7.7	7.1
Nonpoor	3.4	2.8	2.6	1.6	1.6	1.7	4.2	3.3	3.0
Black or African American only:									
Poor	13.7	9.1	8.7	10.9	*5.4	*4.7	15.5	11.2	10.5
Near poor	9.1	12.5	8.3	*6.0	*7.2	*5.0	10.8	15.0	9.8
Nonpoor	4.6	6.4	4.1	*	*4.0	*	5.8	7.4	4.8
Health insurance status[6]									
Insured	5.0	3.6	3.5	3.3	2.6	2.5	5.9	4.2	4.0
Private	3.8	3.1	2.9	1.9	2.0	1.9	4.6	3.6	3.4
Medicaid	8.9	5.5	5.1	6.4	4.1	3.8	11.3	6.7	6.0
Uninsured	23.5	27.8	28.9	18.0	19.0	20.7	26.0	31.6	32.5
Poverty status and health insurance status[5]									
Poor:									
Insured	9.1	6.2	5.5	6.0	4.8	3.5	11.5	7.2	6.7
Uninsured	29.4	35.5	38.4	25.0	26.5	29.0	31.5	39.2	42.9
Near poor:									
Insured	6.0	5.1	5.3	4.0	3.4	4.3	7.2	6.1	5.9
Uninsured	22.9	27.1	27.0	18.0	18.4	20.4	25.3	30.9	30.1
Nonpoor:									
Insured	2.9	2.5	2.5	1.5	1.6	1.7	3.6	3.0	2.8
Uninsured	14.5	19.7	19.7	6.4	*10.6	*13.2	18.1	23.4	22.2

See footnotes at end of table.

Table 74 (page 2 of 2). No usual source of health care among children under 18 years of age, according to selected characteristics: United States, average annual 1993–94, 1997–98, and 2000–01

[Data are based on household interviews of a sample of the civilian noninstitutionalized population]

Characteristic	Under 18 years of age			Under 6 years of age			6–17 years of age		
	1993–94	1997–98[1]	2000–01[1]	1993–94	1997–98[1]	2000–01[1]	1993–94	1997–98[1]	2000–01[1]
Geographic region	Percent of children without a usual source of health care[2]								
Northeast	4.1	3.1	2.3	2.9	*2.5	2.0	4.8	3.5	2.5
Midwest	5.2	4.6	4.8	4.1	4.0	3.6	5.9	4.9	5.4
South	10.9	8.4	7.6	7.3	5.3	4.9	12.7	9.9	9.0
West	8.6	9.8	9.4	5.3	5.5	6.2	10.6	12.0	11.1
Location of residence									
Within MSA[7]	7.7	6.8	6.4	5.0	4.4	4.6	9.2	8.0	7.3
Outside MSA[7]	7.8	6.4	6.3	6.0	4.7	3.5	8.7	7.2	7.6

* Estimates are considered unreliable. Data preceded by an asterisk have a relative standard error of 20–30 percent. Data not shown have a relative standard error of greater than 30 percent.

- - - Data not available.

[1]Data starting in 1997 are not strictly comparable with data for earlier years due to the 1997 questionnaire redesign. See Appendix I, National Health Interview Survey.

[2]Persons who report the emergency department as the place of their usual source of care are defined as having no usual source of care. See Appendix II, Usual source of care.

[3]Includes all other races not shown separately, unknown poverty status, and unknown health insurance status.

[4]The race groups, white, black, American Indian and Alaska Native (AI/AN), Asian, Native Hawaiian and Other Pacific Islander, and 2 or more races, include persons of Hispanic and non-Hispanic origin. Persons of Hispanic origin may be of any race. Starting with data years 1999–2000 race-specific estimates are tabulated according to 1997 Standards for Federal data on Race and Ethnicity and are not strictly comparable with estimates for earlier years. The five single race categories plus multiple race categories shown in the table conform to 1997 Standards. The 1999–2000 race-specific estimates are for persons who reported only one racial group; the category "2 or more races" includes persons who reported more than one racial group. Prior to data years 1999–2000, data were tabulated according to 1977 Standards with four racial groups and the category "Asian only" included Native Hawaiian and Other Pacific Islander. Estimates for single race categories prior to 1999–2000 included persons who reported one race or, if they reported more than one race, identified one race as best representing their race. The effect of the 1997 Standard on the 1999–2000 estimates can be seen by comparing 1999–2000 data tabulated according to the two Standards: Estimates based on the 1977 Standard of the percent of children under 18 years of age with no usual source of care are: identical for white children; 0.1 percentage points lower for black children; 0.6 percentage points lower for AI/AN children; and 1.0 percentage points lower for Asian and Pacific Islander children than estimates based on the 1997 Standards. See Appendix II, Race.

[5]Poor persons are defined as below the poverty threshold. Near poor persons have incomes of 100 percent to less than 200 percent of the poverty threshold. Nonpoor persons have incomes of 200 percent or greater than the poverty threshold. Missing family income data were imputed for 14 percent of children in 1993–96. Poverty status was unknown for 17 percent of children in the sample in 1997, 21 percent in 1998, 24 percent in 1999, and 23 percent in 2000 and 2001. See Appendix II, Family income; Poverty level.

[6]Health insurance categories are mutually exclusive. Persons who reported both Medicaid and private coverage are classified as having private coverage. Medicaid includes other public assistance through 1996. Starting in 1997 Medicaid includes state-sponsored health plans and State Child Health Insurance Program (SCHIP). The category "insured" also includes military, other State, and Medicare coverage. Health insurance status was unknown for 8–9 percent of children in the sample in 1993–96, and 1 percent in 1997–2001. See Appendix II, Health insurance coverage.

[7]MSA is metropolitan statistical area.

NOTES: Some numbers in this table for health insurance estimates were revised and differ from previous editions of *Health, United States.* Data for additional years are available (see Appendix III). For more data on usual source of care, see National Health Interview Survey home page: www.cdc.gov/nchs/nhis/htm. Standard errors for selected years are available in the spreadsheet version of this table. See www.cdc.gov/nchs/hus.htm.

SOURCES: Centers for Disease Control and Prevention, National Center for Health Statistics, National Health Interview Survey, access to care and health insurance supplements (1993–96). Starting in 1997 data are from the family core and sample child questionnaires.

Table 75 (page 1 of 3). Emergency department visits within the past 12 months among children under 18 years of age, according to selected characteristics: United States, selected years 1997–2001

[Data are based on household interviews of a sample of the civilian noninstitutionalized population]

Characteristic	Under 18 years of age			Under 6 years of age			6–17 years of age		
	1997	1999	2001	1997	1999	2001	1997	1999	2001
	Percent of children with 1 or more emergency department visits[1]								
All children[2]	19.9	17.9	20.7	24.3	23.3	24.9	17.7	15.3	18.6
Race[3]									
White only	19.4	17.1	20.2	22.6	21.9	24.2	17.8	14.8	18.2
Black or African American only	24.0	22.5	22.6	33.1	32.3	29.2	19.4	18.2	19.7
American Indian and Alaska Native only	*24.1	33.3	27.0	*24.3	*29.5	*	*24.0	*36.2	*26.5
Asian only	12.6	9.4	11.4	20.8	*13.4	*8.6	8.6	*7.4	*13.0
Native Hawaiian and Other Pacific Islander only	- - -	*	*	- - -	*	*	- - -	*	*
2 or more races	- - -	23.3	31.1	- - -	28.7	33.7	- - -	*19.7	29.2
Hispanic origin and race[3]									
Hispanic or Latino	21.1	15.9	19.4	25.7	21.4	26.1	18.1	12.6	15.4
Not Hispanic or Latino	19.7	18.3	20.9	24.0	23.8	24.7	17.6	15.7	19.2
White only	19.2	17.4	20.6	22.2	22.1	24.3	17.7	15.3	18.9
Black or African American only	23.6	22.5	22.6	32.7	32.5	28.8	19.2	18.2	19.8
Poverty status[4]									
Poor	25.4	24.4	25.2	29.9	31.6	28.1	22.5	20.6	23.5
Near poor	22.6	22.2	22.1	28.8	30.4	28.5	19.4	17.8	18.6
Nonpoor	17.4	15.4	19.5	21.0	19.0	23.5	15.8	13.8	17.7
Hispanic origin and race and poverty status[3,4]									
Hispanic or Latino:									
Poor	22.0	16.4	21.7	24.8	21.0	26.3	20.1	13.0	18.7
Near poor	20.8	15.2	17.4	28.9	21.7	24.8	15.6	11.6	13.1
Nonpoor	20.3	17.2	21.0	22.7	23.0	28.4	18.9	14.3	16.8
Not Hispanic or Latino:									
White only:									
Poor	26.3	26.3	28.2	28.0	34.9	30.0	25.1	22.4	27.2
Near poor	23.0	24.5	23.0	26.5	33.0	28.7	21.2	20.1	19.8
Nonpoor	17.4	15.1	19.4	20.6	18.1	23.1	15.9	13.8	17.7
Black or African American only:									
Poor	29.8	29.8	26.2	40.9	42.5	31.9	22.8	23.4	23.3
Near poor	23.6	23.5	26.0	33.6	33.7	35.8	19.1	18.7	21.2
Nonpoor	17.8	18.8	20.2	23.8	27.1	27.0	15.5	15.6	17.3
Health insurance status[5]									
Insured	19.8	18.1	21.0	24.4	23.1	25.1	17.5	15.7	18.9
Private	17.5	15.4	18.6	20.9	18.9	22.0	15.9	13.9	17.1
Medicaid	28.2	28.8	28.5	33.0	35.2	32.4	24.1	24.2	25.9
Uninsured	20.2	16.4	17.4	23.0	25.5	22.1	18.9	12.7	15.5
Poverty status and health insurance status[4]									
Poor:									
Insured	26.6	26.9	27.6	31.4	32.8	30.3	23.2	23.4	26.0
Uninsured	20.9	15.8	15.0	20.9	25.8	*16.7	20.9	11.9	14.2
Near poor:									
Insured	22.7	23.3	22.6	29.2	31.2	28.8	19.2	18.7	19.0
Uninsured	22.2	18.3	19.3	27.3	26.6	*25.8	20.1	14.8	16.7
Nonpoor:									
Insured	17.3	15.4	19.3	20.8	18.7	23.3	15.7	13.9	17.5
Uninsured	18.8	16.1	19.8	23.7	25.8	24.3	16.7	12.0	18.3
Geographic region									
Northeast	18.5	17.1	20.1	20.7	20.3	23.7	17.4	15.5	18.6
Midwest	19.5	18.4	21.2	26.0	24.1	25.6	16.4	15.8	19.2
South	21.8	19.2	22.2	25.6	25.7	27.0	19.9	16.1	19.8
West	18.5	15.9	18.1	23.5	21.4	22.1	15.9	13.1	15.9
Location of residence									
Within MSA[6]	19.7	16.7	19.8	23.9	22.0	24.1	17.4	14.0	17.6
Outside MSA[6]	20.8	22.4	24.3	26.2	29.1	28.5	18.6	19.7	22.4

See footnotes at end of table.

Table 75 (page 2 of 3). Emergency department visits within the past 12 months among children under 18 years of age, according to selected characteristics: United States, selected years 1997–2001

[Data are based on household interviews of a sample of the civilian noninstitutionalized population]

Characteristic	Under 18 years of age			Under 6 years of age			6–17 years of age		
	1997	1999	2001	1997	1999	2001	1997	1999	2001
	Percent of children with 2 or more emergency department visits[1]								
All children[2]	7.1	5.5	6.8	9.6	8.7	9.5	5.8	4.0	5.5
Race[3]									
White only	6.6	4.7	6.4	8.4	7.3	8.9	5.7	3.4	5.2
Black or African American only	9.6	9.1	8.5	14.9	15.8	14.3	6.9	6.1	5.9
American Indian and Alaska Native only. . .	*	*	*13.5	*	*	*	*	*	*
Asian only	*5.7	*	*4.9	*12.9	*	*	*	*	*
Native Hawaiian and Other Pacific Islander only	- - -	*	*	- - -	*	*	- - -	*	*
2 or more races	- - -	10.5	8.8	- - -	*15.7	*9.3	- - -	*	*8.4
Hispanic origin and race[3]									
Hispanic or Latino	8.9	5.2	6.4	11.8	7.9	8.7	7.0	3.6	5.1
Not Hispanic or Latino	6.8	5.5	6.9	9.2	8.8	9.7	5.7	4.0	5.6
White only	6.2	4.7	6.5	7.8	7.4	9.3	5.5	3.4	5.2
Black or African American only	9.3	9.1	8.4	14.6	15.9	14.0	6.8	6.1	5.9
Poverty status[4]									
Poor	11.2	10.5	10.5	14.4	15.5	12.9	9.1	7.7	9.2
Near poor	8.6	7.6	8.5	12.7	12.4	13.1	6.4	5.0	6.0
Nonpoor	5.2	3.9	5.6	6.7	6.1	8.0	4.6	3.0	4.4
Hispanic origin and race and poverty status[3,4]									
Hispanic or Latino:									
Poor	10.6	5.7	7.8	13.9	*8.1	7.9	8.4	*	7.7
Near poor	8.1	6.0	5.7	12.2	*9.9	8.8	*5.4	*	*3.9
Nonpoor	7.4	5.5	6.0	8.2	*9.2	9.8	7.0	*3.6	*3.8
Not Hispanic or Latino:									
White only:									
Poor	11.0	10.8	12.5	12.4	18.5	*16.0	10.1	*7.3	10.7
Near poor	8.4	7.7	9.0	11.8	13.0	14.7	6.6	*5.0	5.9
Nonpoor	5.0	3.5	5.3	6.0	5.2	7.6	4.5	2.8	4.3
Black or African American only:									
Poor	12.9	14.6	11.6	19.6	22.2	17.3	*8.7	10.9	*8.7
Near poor	9.5	9.5	10.0	*14.0	*15.7	*16.5	*7.5	*	*6.8
Nonpoor	5.1	6.3	6.7	*8.1	*13.1	12.1	*4.0	*3.7	*4.3
Health insurance status[5]									
Insured	7.0	5.6	6.9	9.6	8.6	9.6	5.7	4.1	5.6
Private	5.2	3.8	5.4	6.8	5.7	7.4	4.5	3.0	4.5
Medicaid	13.1	12.6	11.7	16.2	17.1	14.6	10.4	9.4	9.8
Uninsured	7.7	4.9	5.6	9.8	9.0	8.3	6.8	*3.2	4.5
Poverty status and health insurance status[4]									
Poor:									
Insured	12.0	12.1	11.8	15.4	16.9	14.0	9.6	9.2	10.5
Uninsured	8.0	*4.8	*5.5	*8.7	*	*	*7.7	*	*4.5
Near poor:									
Insured	8.6	8.3	8.9	12.7	13.4	14.1	6.4	5.4	6.0
Uninsured	8.3	*5.1	*6.5	*12.2	*	*	6.8	*	*
Nonpoor:									
Insured	5.1	3.9	5.5	6.4	5.9	7.8	4.5	3.0	4.4
Uninsured	7.1	*4.5	*5.5	*11.8	*	*	*5.0	*	*

See footnotes at end of table.

Table 75 (page 3 of 3). Emergency department visits within the past 12 months among children under 18 years of age, according to selected characteristics: United States, selected years 1997–2001

[Data are based on household interviews of a sample of the civilian noninstitutionalized population]

Characteristic	Under 18 years of age			Under 6 years of age			6–17 years of age		
	1997	1999	2001	1997	1999	2001	1997	1999	2001
Geographic region	Percent of children with 2 or more emergency department visits[1]								
Northeast	6.2	4.9	6.1	7.6	6.5	6.8	5.4	4.0	5.8
Midwest	6.6	5.8	7.1	10.4	9.8	11.3	4.8	4.0	5.1
South	8.0	6.1	7.8	10.1	9.8	11.3	6.9	4.3	6.0
West.	7.1	4.7	5.6	10.0	7.6	7.0	5.6	3.3	4.8
Location of residence									
Within MSA[6]	7.2	5.0	6.8	9.6	8.0	9.2	5.9	3.4	5.5
Outside MSA[6]	6.8	7.4	7.1	9.7	11.3	10.8	5.6	5.8	5.5

* Estimates are considered unreliable. Data preceded by an asterisk have a relative standard error (RSE) of 20–30 percent. Data not shown have a RSE of greater than 30 percent.

- - - Data not available.

[1]See Appendix II, Emergency department visit.

[2]Includes all other races not shown separately, unknown poverty status, and unknown health insurance status.

[3]The race groups, white, black, American Indian and Alaska Native (AI/AN), Asian, Native Hawaiian and Other Pacific Islander, and 2 or more races, include persons of Hispanic and non-Hispanic origin. Persons of Hispanic origin may be of any race. Starting with data year 1999 race-specific estimates are tabulated according to 1997 Standards for Federal data on Race and Ethnicity and are not strictly comparable with estimates for earlier years. The five single race categories plus multiple race categories shown in the table conform to 1997 Standards. The 1999 race-specific estimates are for persons who reported only one racial group; the category "2 or more races" includes persons who reported more than one racial group. Prior to data year 1999, data were tabulated according to 1977 Standards with four racial groups and the category "Asian only" included Native Hawaiian and Other Pacific Islander. Estimates for single race categories prior to 1999 included persons who reported one race or, if they reported more than one race, identified one race as best representing their race. The effect of the 1997 Standard on the 1999 estimates can be seen by comparing 1999 data tabulated according to the two Standards: Estimates based on the 1977 Standard of the percent of children under 18 years of age with 1 or more emergency department visits are: 0.1 percentage points higher for white children; 0.2 percentage points higher for black children; 2.1 percentage points lower for AI/AN children; and 2.0 percentage points higher for Asian and Pacific Islander children than estimates based on the 1997 Standards. See Appendix II, Race.

[4]Poor persons are defined as below the poverty threshold. Near poor persons have incomes of 100 percent to less than 200 percent of the poverty threshold. Nonpoor persons have incomes of 200 percent or greater than the poverty threshold. Poverty status was unknown for 17 percent of children in the sample in 1997, 21 percent in 1998, 24 percent in 1999, 23 percent in 2000, and 23 percent in 2001. See Appendix II, Family income; Poverty level.

[5]Health insurance categories are mutually exclusive. Persons who reported both Medicaid and private coverage are classified as having private coverage. Starting in 1997 Medicaid includes state-sponsored health plans and State Child Health Insurance Program (SCHIP). The category "insured" also includes military, other State, and Medicare coverage. See Appendix II, Health insurance coverage.

[6]MSA is metropolitan statistical area.

NOTES: Some numbers in this table for health insurance estimates were revised and differ from previous editions of *Health, United States*. Data for additional years are available (see Appendix III). Standard errors for selected years are available in the spreadsheet version of this table. See www.cdc.gov/nchs/hus.htm.

SOURCE: Centers for Disease Control and Prevention, National Center for Health Statistics, National Health Interview Survey, family core and sample child questionnaires.

Table 76 (page 1 of 2). No usual source of health care among adults 18–64 years of age, according to selected characteristics: United States, average annual 1993–94, 1995–96, 1999–2000, and 2000–01

[Data are based on household interviews of a sample of the civilian noninstitutionalized population]

Characteristic	1993–94	1995–96	1999–2000[1]	2000–01[1]
	Percent of adults without a usual source of health care[2]			
All adults 18–64 years of age[3,4]	18.5	16.6	17.7	16.5
Age				
18–44 years	21.7	19.6	21.5	20.3
18–24 years	26.6	22.6	26.9	26.1
25–44 years	20.3	18.8	19.7	18.4
45–64 years	12.8	11.3	10.9	9.9
45–54 years	14.1	12.2	12.0	10.9
55–64 years	11.1	9.8	9.2	8.3
Sex[4]				
Male	23.3	21.0	23.8	21.8
Female	13.9	12.5	11.7	11.4
Race[4,5]				
White only	18.2	16.3	16.8	15.8
Black or African American only	19.2	17.6	18.7	16.8
American Indian and Alaska Native only	19.1	15.9	18.7	15.9
Asian only	24.0	20.7	21.4	18.5
Native Hawaiian and Other Pacific Islander only	- - -	- - -	*	*
2 or more races	- - -	- - -	20.4	21.1
American Indian and Alaska Native; White . .	- - -	- - -	26.5	24.0
Hispanic origin and race[4,5]				
Hispanic or Latino	28.8	26.2	30.4	30.8
Mexican	30.5	28.1	33.7	34.6
Not Hispanic or Latino	17.5	15.5	16.0	14.6
White only	17.0	15.0	15.2	13.9
Black or African American only	18.9	17.4	18.7	16.7
Poverty status[4,6]				
Poor	28.2	24.9	27.4	27.4
Near poor	24.6	22.3	26.5	25.3
Nonpoor	14.8	13.5	13.8	12.4
Hispanic origin and race and poverty status[4,5,6]				
Hispanic or Latino:				
Poor	38.0	32.6	39.7	43.7
Near poor	35.7	31.6	37.4	36.0
Nonpoor	18.3	18.2	20.5	19.3
Not Hispanic or Latino:				
White only:				
Poor	27.1	22.8	22.7	21.5
Near poor	22.7	20.3	23.5	22.5
Nonpoor	14.4	13.0	12.9	11.6
Black or African American only:				
Poor	23.8	21.1	22.5	20.7
Near poor	21.6	21.2	23.6	20.7
Nonpoor	14.6	13.6	14.4	12.7
Health insurance status[4,7]				
Insured	13.3	11.4	11.0	9.7
Private	13.1	11.3	11.2	9.7
Medicaid	15.2	12.5	9.5	9.6
Uninsured	41.5	40.9	47.3	46.3
Poverty status and health insurance status[4,6]				
Poor:				
Insured	16.8	13.6	12.4	11.6
Uninsured	45.7	42.1	49.8	51.7
Near poor:				
Insured	15.3	13.1	13.1	12.4
Uninsured	42.9	41.5	49.3	47.8
Nonpoor:				
Insured	12.3	10.8	10.5	9.0
Uninsured	37.0	39.4	44.2	41.4

See footnotes at end of table.

Table 76 (page 2 of 2). No usual source of health care among adults 18–64 years of age, according to selected characteristics: United States, average annual 1993–94, 1995–96, 1999–2000, and 2000–01

[Data are based on household interviews of a sample of the civilian noninstitutionalized population]

Characteristic	1993–94	1995–96	1999–2000[1]	2000–01[1]
Geographic region[4]	Percent of adults without a usual source of health care[2]			
Northeast.................................	14.5	13.3	12.9	12.1
Midwest..................................	15.8	14.5	16.8	15.2
South	21.6	18.4	19.6	17.8
West.....................................	20.5	19.5	19.8	20.0
Location of residence[4]				
Within MSA[8].............................	18.8	16.9	17.8	16.7
Outside MSA[8]	17.4	15.4	16.9	15.8

* Estimates are considered unreliable. Data not shown have a relative standard error of greater than 30 percent.

- - - Data not available.

[1]Data starting in 1997 are not strictly comparable with data for earlier years due to the 1997 questionnaire redesign. See Appendix I, National Health Interview Survey.

[2]Persons who report the emergency department as the place of their usual source of care are defined as having no usual source of care. See Appendix II, Usual source of care.

[3]Includes all other races not shown separately, unknown poverty status, and unknown health insurance status.

[4]Estimates are for persons 18–64 years of age and are age adjusted to the year 2000 standard population using three age groups: 18–44 years, 45–54 years, and 55–64 years of age. See Appendix II, Age adjustment.

[5]The race groups, white, black, American Indian and Alaska Native (AI/AN), Asian, Native Hawaiian and Other Pacific Islander, and 2 or more races, include persons of Hispanic and non-Hispanic origin. Persons of Hispanic origin may be of any race. Starting with data years 1999–2000 race-specific estimates are tabulated according to 1997 Standards for Federal data on Race and Ethnicity and are not strictly comparable with estimates for earlier years. The five single race categories plus multiple race categories shown in the table conform to 1997 Standards. The 1999–2000 race-specific estimates are for persons who reported only one racial group; the category "2 or more races" includes persons who reported more than one racial group. Prior to data years 1999–2000, data were tabulated according to 1977 Standards with four racial groups and the category "Asian only" included Native Hawaiian and Other Pacific Islander. Estimates for single race categories prior to 1999–2000 included persons who reported one race or, if they reported more than one race, identified one race as best representing their race. The effect of the 1997 Standard on the 1999–2000 estimates can be seen by comparing 1999–2000 data tabulated according to the two Standards: Estimates based on the 1977 Standard of the percent of adults under 65 years of age with no usual source of care are: identical for white and black adults; 2.0 percentage points higher for AI/AN adults; and 0.5 percentage points lower for Asian and Pacific Islander adults than estimates based on the 1997 Standards. See Appendix II, Race.

[6]Poor persons are defined as below the poverty threshold. Near poor persons have incomes of 100 percent to less than 200 percent of the poverty threshold. Nonpoor persons have incomes of 200 percent or greater than the poverty threshold. Missing family income data were imputed for 16 percent of adults in 1993–96. Poverty status was unknown for 20 percent of adults under 65 years of age in the sample in 1997–2001. See Appendix II, Family income; Poverty level.

[7]Health insurance categories are mutually exclusive. Persons who reported both Medicaid and private coverage are classified as having private coverage. Medicaid includes other public assistance through 1996. Starting in 1997 Medicaid includes state-sponsored health plans and State Child Health Insurance Program (SCHIP). The category "insured" also includes military, other State, and Medicare coverage. In 1993–96 health insurance coverage was unknown for 8–9 percent of adults in the sample. Beginning in 1997 health insurance coverage was unknown for 1 percent of adults in the sample. See Appendix II, Health insurance coverage.

[8]MSA is metropolitan statistical area.

NOTES: Some numbers in this table for health insurance estimates were revised and differ from previous editions of *Health, United States*. Data for additional years are available (see Appendix III). For more data on usual source of care see the National Health Interview Survey home page: www.cdc.gov/nchs/nhis.htm. Standard errors for selected years are available in the spreadsheet version of this table. See www.cdc.gov/nchs/hus.htm.

SOURCE: Centers for Disease Control and Prevention, National Center for Health Statistics, National Health Interview Survey, access to care and health insurance supplements (1993–96). Starting in 1997 data are from the family core and sample adult questionnaires.

Table 77 (page 1 of 2). Emergency department visits within the past 12 months among adults 18 years of age and over, according to selected characteristics: United States, selected years 1997–2001

[Data are based on household interviews of a sample of the civilian noninstitutionalized population]

Characteristic	1 or more emergency department visits				2 or more emergency department visits			
	1997	1999	2000	2001	1997	1999	2000	2001
	Percent of adults with emergency department visit[1]							
All adults 18 years of age and over[2,3]	19.6	17.2	20.2	19.7	6.7	5.2	6.9	6.4
Age								
18–44 years	20.7	17.7	20.6	19.8	6.8	5.6	7.0	6.5
18–24 years	26.3	21.7	25.9	24.0	9.1	7.3	8.9	8.7
25–44 years	19.0	16.5	18.9	18.4	6.2	5.0	6.4	5.8
45–64 years	16.2	14.6	17.6	18.0	5.6	4.3	5.6	5.6
45–54 years	15.7	14.3	17.9	17.7	5.5	4.3	5.8	5.5
55–64 years	16.9	15.1	17.0	18.5	5.7	4.3	5.3	5.9
65 years and over	22.0	19.9	23.7	22.3	8.1	5.6	8.6	7.5
65–74 years	20.3	17.3	21.6	19.7	7.1	4.7	7.4	7.1
75 years and over	24.3	23.1	26.2	25.4	9.3	6.7	10.1	8.0
Sex[3]								
Male	19.1	16.1	18.8	18.9	5.9	4.3	5.8	5.7
Female	20.2	18.2	21.6	20.5	7.5	6.0	8.0	7.2
Race[3,4]								
White only	19.0	16.6	19.4	19.1	6.2	4.7	6.4	6.1
Black or African American only	25.9	22.2	26.5	25.2	11.1	8.8	10.7	9.4
American Indian and Alaska Native only	24.8	29.2	30.5	33.9	13.1	*11.7	*12.8	15.5
Asian only	11.6	9.7	13.6	12.7	*2.9	*	*3.8	*2.6
Native Hawaiian and Other Pacific Islander only	- - -	*	*	*	- - -	*	*	*
2 or more races	- - -	24.4	32.9	25.5	- - -	11.4	11.4	8.8
American Indian and Alaska Native; White	- - -	26.0	33.9	25.4	- - -	*13.9	*9.2	*6.1
Hispanic origin and race[3,4]								
Hispanic or Latino	19.2	15.3	18.4	18.4	7.4	4.5	7.1	7.0
Mexican American	17.8	14.4	17.4	15.6	6.4	4.1	7.1	5.6
Not Hispanic or Latino	19.7	17.5	20.6	20.0	6.7	5.3	6.9	6.4
White only	19.1	16.9	19.8	19.4	6.2	4.8	6.4	6.1
Black or African American only	25.9	22.2	26.5	25.3	11.0	8.8	10.7	9.4
Poverty status[3,5]								
Poor	29.2	27.6	30.2	27.5	13.7	11.7	14.3	13.1
Near poor	24.9	21.7	25.1	26.2	10.0	8.0	10.6	10.4
Nonpoor	17.5	15.4	18.6	18.2	5.0	4.1	5.3	5.1
Hispanic origin and race and poverty status[3,4,5]								
Hispanic or Latino:								
Poor	22.9	17.1	24.4	19.9	10.2	6.6	11.3	10.1
Near poor	19.2	15.9	19.4	20.1	8.4	5.0	7.6	7.7
Nonpoor	17.9	14.5	17.1	17.6	5.5	3.8	6.1	5.3
Not Hispanic or Latino:								
White only:								
Poor	30.8	29.4	30.6	29.6	14.1	11.7	14.3	13.7
Near poor	25.5	22.2	26.8	27.9	9.8	7.6	11.5	11.0
Nonpoor	17.2	15.5	18.2	18.0	4.8	4.1	5.0	5.1
Black or African American only:								
Poor	35.5	33.5	38.0	32.1	17.9	16.8	19.0	15.7
Near poor	30.8	27.8	29.9	28.8	12.9	13.0	13.1	12.8
Nonpoor	20.7	18.4	24.1	22.3	7.8	5.7	8.4	7.0
Health insurance status[6,7]								
18–64 years of age:								
Insured	18.8	16.1	19.5	19.2	6.1	4.7	6.4	6.2
Private	16.9	14.5	17.6	17.2	4.7	3.7	5.1	4.7
Medicaid	37.6	35.4	42.3	39.7	19.7	17.4	21.0	21.7
Uninsured	20.0	18.3	19.6	18.9	7.5	7.0	7.0	6.6
65 years of age and over:								
Medicare HMO	20.2	20.1	24.4	23.6	6.7	5.7	8.5	8.8
Private	21.3	19.3	23.3	21.0	6.9	5.3	7.9	6.4
Medicaid	35.2	30.0	35.9	36.0	20.2	12.8	18.3	18.7
Medicare fee-for-service only	22.0	19.2	20.1	21.5	9.4	4.4	7.3	6.9

See footnotes at end of table.

Table 77 (page 2 of 2). Emergency department visits within the past 12 months among adults 18 years of age and over, according to selected characteristics: United States, selected years 1997–2001

[Data are based on household interviews of a sample of the civilian noninstitutionalized population]

Characteristic	1 or more emergency department visits				2 or more emergency department visits			
	1997	1999	2000	2001	1997	1999	2000	2001
Poverty status and health insurance status[5,6]	Percent of adults with emergency department visit[1]							
18–64 years of age:								
Poor:								
Insured	32.1	29.8	33.6	30.8	15.9	13.3	17.4	15.5
Uninsured	24.4	22.7	26.0	20.0	10.0	10.3	10.6	8.5
Near poor:								
Insured	26.6	23.1	27.3	28.0	10.3	8.7	11.6	11.7
Uninsured	21.3	18.6	20.1	23.6	9.1	7.5	7.7	9.0
Nonpoor:								
Insured	16.6	14.7	17.6	17.2	4.5	3.7	4.9	4.6
Uninsured	19.0	16.3	19.2	17.8	5.4	6.5	6.4	5.0
Geographic region[3]								
Northeast	19.5	16.9	20.0	19.8	6.9	5.1	6.2	6.1
Midwest	19.3	17.2	20.1	19.6	6.2	5.1	6.9	6.0
South	20.9	17.7	21.3	20.9	7.3	5.7	7.6	7.3
West	17.7	16.4	18.7	17.6	6.0	4.5	6.3	5.6
Location of residence[3]								
Within MSA[8]	19.1	16.6	19.6	19.4	6.4	4.9	6.6	6.3
Outside MSA[8]	21.5	19.5	22.5	21.3	7.8	6.4	7.8	7.0

* Estimates are considered unreliable. Data preceded by an asterisk have a relative standard error (RSE) of 20–30 percent. Data not shown have a RSE of greater than 30 percent.

- - - Data not available.

[1]See Appendix II, Emergency department visit.

[2]Includes all other races not shown separately, unknown poverty status, and unknown health insurance status.

[3]Estimates are for persons 18 years of age and over and are age adjusted to the year 2000 standard using five age groups: 18–44 years, 45–54 years, 55–64 years, 65–74 years, and 75 years and over. See Appendix II, Age adjustment.

[4]The race groups, white, black, American Indian and Alaska Native (AI/AN), Asian, Native Hawaiian and Other Pacific Islander, and 2 or more races, include persons of Hispanic and non-Hispanic origin. Persons of Hispanic origin may be of any race. Starting with data year 1999 race-specific estimates are tabulated according to 1997 Standards for Federal data on Race and Ethnicity and are not strictly comparable with estimates for earlier years. The five single race categories plus multiple race categories shown in the table conform to 1997 Standards. The 1999 race-specific estimates are for persons who reported only one racial group; the category "2 or more races" includes persons who reported more than one racial group. Prior to data years 1999, data were tabulated according to 1977 Standards with four racial groups and the category "Asian only" included Native Hawaiian and Other Pacific Islander. Estimates for single race categories prior to 1999 included persons who reported one race or, if they reported more than one race, identified one race as best representing their race. The effect of the 1997 Standard on the 1999 estimates can be seen by comparing 1999 data tabulated according to the two Standards: Age-adjusted estimates based on the 1977 Standard of the percent of adults with 1 or more emergency department visits are: 0.1 percentage points higher for white and black adults; 2.0 percentage points lower for AI/AN adults; and 0.3 percentage points higher for Asian and Pacific Islander adults than estimates based on the 1997 Standards. See Appendix II, Race.

[5]Poor persons are defined as below the poverty threshold. Near poor persons have incomes of 100 percent to less than 200 percent of the poverty threshold. Nonpoor persons have incomes of 200 percent or greater than the poverty threshold. Poverty status was unknown for 22 percent of adults in the sample in 1997, 27 percent in 1998, 29 percent in 1999 and 2000, and 30 percent in 2001. See Appendix II, Family income; Poverty level.

[6]Estimates for persons 18–64 years of age are age adjusted to the year 2000 Standard using three age groups: 18–44 years, 45–54 years, and 55–64 years of age. Estimates for persons 65 years of age and over are age adjusted to the year 2000 Standard using two age groups: 65–74 years and 75 years and over. See Appendix II, Age adjustment.

[7]Health insurance categories are mutually exclusive. Persons who reported both Medicaid and private coverage are classified as having private coverage. Persons 65 years of age and over who reported Medicare HMO (health maintenance organization) and some other type of health insurance coverage are classified as having Medicare HMO. Starting in 1997 Medicaid includes state-sponsored health plans and State Child Health Insurance Program (SCHIP). The category "insured" also includes military, other State, and Medicare coverage. See Appendix II, Health insurance coverage.

[8]MSA is metropolitan statistical area.

NOTES: Some numbers in this table for health insurance estimates were revised and differ from previous editions of *Health, United States*. Data for additional years are available (see Appendix III). Standard errors for selected years are available in the spreadsheet version of this table. See www.cdc.gov/nchs/hus.htm.

SOURCE: Centers for Disease Control and Prevention, National Center for Health Statistics, National Health Interview Survey, family core and sample adult questionnaires.

Table 78 (page 1 of 2). Dental visits in the past year according to selected characteristics: United States, selected years 1997–2001

[Data are based on household interviews of a sample of the civilian noninstitutionalized population]

Characteristic	2 years of age and over[1]			2–17 years of age			18–64 years of age			65 years of age and over[2]		
	1997	1999	2001	1997	1999	2001	1997	1999	2001	1997	1999	2001
	Percent of persons with a dental visit in the past year[3]											
Total[4]	64.9	65.2	65.6	72.7	72.6	73.3	64.1	64.6	64.6	54.8	55.0	56.3
Sex												
Male	62.6	62.5	62.6	72.3	72.3	72.7	60.4	60.4	60.2	55.4	54.7	56.1
Female	67.2	67.8	68.5	73.0	72.8	73.9	67.7	68.5	68.9	54.4	55.2	56.5
Race[5]												
White only	66.5	67.2	67.4	74.0	74.5	74.9	65.7	66.6	66.6	56.8	56.8	58.5
Black or African American only	56.5	56.2	56.9	68.8	67.6	68.0	57.0	55.8	57.2	35.4	39.7	37.5
American Indian and Alaska Native only	51.5	56.2	53.9	66.8	58.2	72.9	49.9	55.2	47.7	*	*50.6	*50.7
Asian only	61.8	63.6	64.9	69.9	69.6	74.4	60.3	63.1	64.3	53.9	53.2	53.4
Native Hawaiian and Other Pacific Islander only	- - -	*	*	- - -	*	*	- - -	*	*	- - -	*	*
2 or more races	- - -	58.6	56.3	- - -	73.0	69.3	- - -	57.8	57.1	- - -	*35.1	*34.5
Black or African American; White	- - -	63.7	52.7	- - -	68.7	57.6	- - -	58.8	55.5	- - -	*	*
American Indian and Alaska Native; White	- - -	55.8	58.7	- - -	70.3	79.2	- - -	53.5	53.6	- - -	*	*39.0
Hispanic origin and race[5]												
Hispanic or Latino	52.9	52.3	51.2	61.0	59.3	60.5	50.8	50.6	49.2	47.8	44.0	42.6
Not Hispanic or Latino	66.4	66.9	67.5	74.7	74.9	75.8	65.7	66.3	66.7	55.2	55.6	57.2
White only	68.2	68.9	69.6	76.4	77.0	77.8	67.5	68.3	68.7	57.2	57.3	59.4
Black or African American only	56.5	56.1	56.9	68.8	67.7	68.1	56.9	55.7	57.1	35.3	39.6	37.6
Poverty status[6]												
Poor	47.2	46.2	47.0	62.0	57.8	61.0	46.4	46.0	45.8	30.3	31.9	30.6
Near poor	48.9	48.5	49.7	61.6	61.6	63.2	46.4	46.1	46.9	39.6	38.9	40.0
Nonpoor	72.3	72.0	72.0	79.7	79.9	79.3	71.1	70.8	70.5	66.3	64.4	67.0
Hispanic origin and race and poverty status[5,6]												
Hispanic or Latino:												
Poor	41.9	41.5	38.7	56.8	49.6	54.2	39.0	39.7	35.1	33.0	32.1	29.8
Near poor	46.2	43.8	43.2	54.1	54.0	59.2	42.6	41.0	39.8	49.2	34.8	30.6
Nonpoor	65.1	63.8	64.4	74.8	72.0	71.1	62.5	62.0	62.8	56.5	58.9	60.8
Not Hispanic or Latino:												
White only:												
Poor	49.9	49.8	51.5	63.3	62.6	62.9	50.3	50.6	52.1	31.1	31.9	32.3
Near poor	51.0	50.2	52.9	64.8	63.2	64.4	48.2	48.0	51.0	41.2	39.6	42.1
Nonpoor	73.6	73.6	73.7	80.7	81.8	81.7	72.5	72.4	72.0	67.6	65.4	68.6
Black or African American only:												
Poor	46.7	44.9	45.1	66.7	61.0	63.2	44.5	42.1	42.9	26.2	33.5	25.2
Near poor	44.9	47.6	47.3	60.1	66.3	64.2	44.7	45.2	44.9	23.6	30.9	33.4
Nonpoor	65.4	64.2	64.1	75.5	72.7	72.4	66.2	64.7	65.4	48.9	51.5	46.1

See footnotes at end of table.

Table 78 (page 2 of 2). Dental visits in the past year according to selected characteristics: United States, selected years 1997–2001

[Data are based on household interviews of a sample of the civilian noninstitutionalized population]

Characteristic	2 years of age and over[1]			2–17 years of age			18–64 years of age			65 years of age and over[2]		
	1997	1999	2001	1997	1999	2001	1997	1999	2001	1997	1999	2001
Geographic region	Percent of persons with a dental visit in the past year[3]											
Northeast	69.6	70.9	72.2	77.5	78.5	79.6	69.6	71.5	72.2	55.5	54.3	59.6
Midwest	68.3	68.1	68.4	76.4	76.8	77.4	67.4	67.6	68.0	57.6	54.3	55.0
South	60.0	60.6	60.2	68.0	68.0	68.8	59.4	59.4	58.7	49.0	52.4	52.0
West	64.9	64.7	65.7	71.5	69.9	70.7	62.9	63.3	64.4	61.9	61.9	62.6
Location of residence												
Within MSA[7]	66.5	67.1	67.0	73.6	73.1	73.9	65.7	66.8	66.0	57.6	58.1	59.1
Outside MSA[7]	59.1	58.3	60.3	69.3	70.7	70.7	58.0	56.2	59.1	46.1	45.0	47.2

* Estimates are considered unreliable. Data preceded by an asterisk have a relative standard error (RSE) of 20–30 percent. Data not shown have a RSE greater than 30 percent.

- - - Data not available.

[1]Estimates are age adjusted to the year 2000 standard using six age groups: 2–17 years, 18–44 years, 45–54 years, 55–64 years, 65–74 years, and 75 years and over. See Appendix II, Age adjustment.

[2]Estimates for the elderly are the percent of persons 65 years of age and over with a dental visit in the past year. Data from the 1997–2001 National Health Interview Survey estimate that 28–30 percent of persons 65 years of age and over (elderly) were edentulous (having lost all their natural teeth). In 1997–2001 about 70 percent of elderly dentate persons compared with 17–20 percent of elderly edentate persons had a dental visit in the past year.

[3]Respondents were asked "About how long has it been since you last saw or talked to a dentist?" See Appendix II, Dental visit.

[4]Includes all other races not shown separately and unknown poverty status.

[5]The race groups, white, black, American Indian and Alaska Native (AI/AN), Asian, Native Hawaiian and Other Pacific Islander, and 2 or more races, include persons of Hispanic and non-Hispanic origin. Persons of Hispanic origin may be of any race. Starting with data year 1999 race-specific estimates are tabulated according to 1997 Standards for Federal data on Race and Ethnicity and are not strictly comparable with estimates for earlier years. The five single race categories plus multiple race categories shown in the table conform to 1997 Standards. The 1999 race-specific estimates are for persons who reported only one racial group; the category "2 or more races" includes persons who reported more than one racial group. Prior to data year 1999, data were tabulated according to 1977 Standards with four racial groups and the category "Asian only" included Native Hawaiian and Other Pacific Islander. Estimates for single race categories prior to 1999 included persons who reported one race or, if they reported more than one race, identified one race as best representing their race. The effect of the 1997 Standard on the 1999 estimates can be seen by comparing 1999 data tabulated according to the two Standards: Age-adjusted estimates based on the 1977 Standard of the percent of persons with a recent dental visit are: 0.1 percentage points lower for white and black persons; identical for AI/AN persons; and 0.2 percentage points lower for Asian and Pacific Islander persons than estimates based on the 1997 Standards. See Appendix II, Race.

[6]Poor persons are defined as below the poverty threshold. Near poor persons have incomes of 100 percent to less than 200 percent of the poverty threshold. Nonpoor persons have incomes of 200 percent or greater than the poverty threshold. Poverty status was unknown for 20 percent of persons in the sample in 1997, 25 percent in 1998, 28 percent in 1999, 27 percent in 2000, and 28 percent in 2001. See Appendix II, Family income; Poverty level.

[7]MSA is metropolitan statistical area.

NOTES: In 1997 the National Health Interview Survey questionnaire was redesigned. See Appendix I, National Health Interview Survey. Data for additional years are available (see Appendix III). Standard errors for selected years are available in the spreadsheet version of this table. See www.cdc.gov/nchs/hus.htm.

SOURCE: Centers for Disease Control and Prevention, National Center for Health Statistics, National Health Interview Survey, sample child and sample adult questionnaires.

Table 79. Untreated dental caries according to age, sex, race and Hispanic origin, and poverty status: United States, 1971–74, 1982–84, and 1988–94

[Data are based on dental examinations of a sample of the civilian noninstitutionalized population]

Sex, race and Hispanic origin, and poverty status	2–5 years 1971–1974	2–5 years 1982–1984	2–5 years 1988–1994	6–17 years 1971–1974	6–17 years 1982–1984	6–17 years 1988–1994	18–64 years 1971–1974	18–64 years 1982–1984	18–64 years 1988–1994	65–74 years 1971–1974	65–74 years 1982–1984	65–74 years 1988–1994
	Percent of persons with untreated dental caries											
Total[1]	24.4	- - -	18.7	55.0	- - -	23.1	48.4	- - -	28.2	29.7	- - -	25.4
Sex												
Male	26.1	- - -	19.2	54.8	- - -	22.6	48.4	- - -	31.2	30.2	- - -	29.9
Female	22.7	- - -	18.1	55.2	- - -	23.7	48.5	- - -	25.3	28.3	- - -	21.5
Race and Hispanic origin[2]												
Not Hispanic or Latino:												
White	23.7	- - -	14.4	52.3	- - -	18.9	45.2	- - -	23.6	28.1	- - -	22.7
Black or African American	28.2	- - -	25.1	70.9	- - -	33.0	68.1	- - -	47.9	41.5	- - -	46.7
Mexican	- - -	23.1	34.9	- - -	42.8	37.2	- - -	45.4	39.9	- - -	44.3	43.8
Poverty status[3]												
Poor	30.7	- - -	28.8	70.4	- - -	36.3	63.6	- - -	47.3	34.3	- - -	46.7
Near poor	29.8	- - -	24.3	60.2	- - -	29.2	56.3	- - -	42.7	35.6	- - -	39.3
Nonpoor	17.5	- - -	9.7	46.3	- - -	14.5	43.1	- - -	19.5	26.2	- - -	19.4
Race, Hispanic origin, and poverty status[2,3]												
Not Hispanic or Latino:												
White:												
Poor	31.9	- - -	25.4	68.1	- - -	32.5	58.4	- - -	42.3	33.3	- - -	39.0
Near poor and nonpoor	22.1	- - -	12.4	50.3	- - -	16.7	44.3	- - -	21.6	28.0	- - -	22.7
Black or African American:												
Poor	29.0	- - -	27.5	73.4	- - -	35.6	73.1	- - -	59.0	39.8	- - -	50.1
Near poor and nonpoor	26.5	- - -	23.0	67.4	- - -	31.2	65.8	- - -	43.4	41.1	- - -	43.6
Mexican:												
Poor	- - -	22.6	38.5	- - -	46.4	45.8	- - -	56.3	52.4	- - -	54.4	55.5
Near poor and nonpoor	- - -	22.0	30.5	- - -	39.3	27.6	- - -	41.0	31.5	- - -	30.8	35.6

- - - Data not available.

[1]Includes all other races not shown separately and unknown poverty status.

[2]In 1971–74, data are for white persons and black persons. Persons of Mexican origin may be of any race.

[3]Poverty status is based on family income and family size. Poor persons are defined as below the poverty threshold. Near poor persons have incomes of 100 percent to less than 200 percent of the poverty threshold. Nonpoor persons have incomes of 200 percent or greater than the poverty threshold. Persons with unknown poverty status are excluded (4 percent in 1971–74, 8 percent in 1982–84, and 6 percent in 1988–94). See Appendix II, Family income; Poverty level.

NOTES: Excludes edentulous persons (persons without teeth) of all ages. The majority of edentulous persons are 65 years of age and over. Estimates of edentulism among the elderly are 46 percent in 1971–74, 37 percent in 1982–84, and 33 percent in 1988–94.

SOURCES: Centers for Disease Control and Prevention, National Center for Health Statistics, National Health and Nutrition Examination Survey (NHANES) I, Hispanic Health and Nutrition Examination Survey, and NHANES III.

Table 80 (page 1 of 2). Use of mammography for women 40 years of age and over according to selected characteristics: United States, selected years 1987–2000

[Data are based on household interviews of a sample of the civilian noninstitutionalized population]

Characteristic	1987	1990	1991	1993	1994	1998	1999	2000
	Percent of women having a mammogram within the past 2 years[1]							
40 years and over, age adjusted[2,3]	29.0	51.7	54.7	59.7	61.0	67.0	70.3	70.3
40 years and over, crude[2]	28.7	51.4	54.6	59.7	60.9	66.9	70.3	70.3
Age								
40–49 years	31.9	55.1	55.6	59.9	61.3	63.4	67.2	64.2
50–64 years	31.7	56.0	60.3	65.1	66.5	73.7	76.5	78.6
65 years and over	22.8	43.4	48.1	54.2	55.0	63.8	66.8	68.0
65–74 years.	26.6	48.7	55.7	64.2	63.0	69.4	73.9	74.0
75 years and over	17.3	35.8	37.8	41.0	44.6	57.2	58.9	61.3
Race[4]								
40 years and over, crude:								
White only	29.6	52.2	55.6	60.0	60.6	67.4	70.6	71.4
Black or African American only.	24.0	46.4	48.0	59.1	64.3	66.0	71.0	67.8
American Indian and Alaska Native only	*	43.2	54.5	49.8	65.8	45.2	63.0	47.3
Asian only	*	46.0	45.9	55.1	55.8	60.2	58.3	53.3
Native Hawaiian and Other Pacific								
Islander only	- - -	- - -	- - -	- - -	- - -	- - -	*	*
2 or more races	- - -	- - -	- - -	- - -	- - -	- - -	70.2	69.2
Hispanic origin and race[4]								
40 years and over, crude:								
Hispanic or Latino	18.3	45.2	49.2	50.9	51.9	60.2	65.7	61.4
Not Hispanic or Latino	29.4	51.8	54.9	60.3	61.5	67.5	70.7	71.0
White only	30.3	52.7	56.0	60.6	61.3	68.0	71.1	72.1
Black or African American only	23.8	46.0	47.7	59.2	64.4	66.0	71.0	67.9
Age, Hispanic origin, and race[4]								
40–49 years:								
Hispanic or Latino	*15.3	45.1	44.0	52.6	47.5	55.2	61.6	54.2
Not Hispanic or Latino:								
White only	34.3	57.0	58.1	61.6	62.0	64.4	68.3	67.1
Black or African American only	27.8	48.4	48.0	55.6	67.2	65.0	69.2	60.9
50–64 years:								
Hispanic or Latino	23.0	47.5	61.7	59.2	60.1	67.2	69.7	66.4
Not Hispanic or Latino:								
White only	33.6	58.1	61.5	66.2	67.5	75.3	77.9	80.5
Black or African American only	26.4	48.4	52.4	65.5	63.6	71.2	75.0	77.7
65 years and over:								
Hispanic or Latino	*	41.1	40.9	*35.7	48.0	59.0	67.2	68.2
Not Hispanic or Latino:								
White only	24.0	43.8	49.1	54.7	54.9	64.3	66.8	68.3
Black or African American only	14.1	39.7	41.6	56.3	61.0	60.6	68.1	65.5
Age and poverty status[5]								
40 years and over, crude:								
Poor	16.4	30.8	35.2	41.1	44.2	50.5	56.9	55.2
Near poor or nonpoor	31.3	54.1	57.5	61.8	63.4	69.3	71.5	72.2
40–49 years:								
Poor	23.0	32.2	33.0	36.1	43.0	44.9	52.5	47.2
Near poor or nonpoor	33.4	57.0	58.1	62.1	63.4	65.0	68.7	65.9
50–64 years:								
Poor	15.1	29.9	37.3	47.3	46.2	53.5	61.1	62.7
Near poor or nonpoor	34.3	58.5	63.0	66.8	68.8	76.7	77.4	80.6
65 years and over:								
Poor	13.6	30.8	35.2	40.4	43.9	52.3	57.3	55.4
Near poor or nonpoor	25.5	46.2	51.1	56.4	57.7	66.2	67.8	70.0

See footnotes at end of table.

Table 80 (page 2 of 2). Use of mammography for women 40 years of age and over according to selected characteristics: United States, selected years 1987–2000

[Data are based on household interviews of a sample of the civilian noninstitutionalized population]

Characteristic	1987	1990	1991	1993	1994	1998	1999	2000
Age and education[6]	Percent of women having a mammogram within the past 2 years[1]							
40 years and over, crude:								
No high school diploma or GED	17.8	36.4	40.0	46.4	48.2	54.5	56.7	57.7
High school diploma or GED	31.3	52.7	55.8	59.0	61.0	66.7	69.2	69.6
Some college or more	37.7	62.8	65.2	69.5	69.7	72.8	77.3	76.1
40–49 years of age:								
No high school diploma or GED	15.1	38.5	40.8	43.6	50.4	47.3	48.8	46.9
High school diploma or GED	32.6	53.1	52.0	56.6	55.8	59.1	60.8	59.0
Some college or more	39.2	62.3	63.7	66.1	68.7	68.3	74.4	70.5
50–64 years of age:								
No high school diploma or GED	21.2	41.0	43.6	51.4	51.6	58.8	62.3	66.3
High school diploma or GED	33.8	56.5	60.8	62.4	67.8	73.3	77.2	76.6
Some college or more	40.5	68.0	72.7	78.5	74.7	79.8	81.2	84.1
65 years of age and over:								
No high school diploma or GED	16.5	33.0	37.7	44.2	45.6	54.7	56.6	57.5
High school diploma or GED	25.9	47.5	54.0	57.4	59.1	66.8	68.4	72.0
Some college or more	32.3	56.7	57.9	64.8	64.3	71.3	77.1	74.1

* Estimates are considered unreliable. Data preceded by an asterisk have a relative standard error (RSE) of 20–30 percent. Data not shown have a RSE greater than 30 percent.

- - - Data not available.

[1]Questions concerning use of mammography differed slightly on the National Health Interview Survey across the years for which data are shown. See Appendix II, Mammography.

[2]Includes all other races not shown separately, unknown poverty status, and unknown education.

[3]Estimates are age adjusted to the year 2000 standard using four age groups: 40–49 years, 50–64 years, 65–74 years, and 75 years and over. See Appendix II, Age adjustment.

[4]The race groups, white, black, American Indian and Alaska Native (AI/AN), Asian, Native Hawaiian and Other Pacific Islander, and 2 or more races, include persons of Hispanic and non-Hispanic origin. Persons of Hispanic origin may be of any race. Starting with data year 1999 race-specific estimates are tabulated according to 1997 Standards for Federal data on Race and Ethnicity and are not strictly comparable with estimates for earlier years. The five single race categories plus multiple race categories shown in the table conform to 1997 Standards. The 1999 race-specific estimates are for persons who reported only one racial group; the category "2 or more races" includes persons who reported more than one racial group. Prior to data year 1999, data were tabulated according to 1977 Standards with four racial groups and the category "Asian only" included Native Hawaiian and Other Pacific Islander. Estimates for single race categories prior to 1999 included persons who reported one race or, if they reported more than one race, identified one race as best representing their race. The effect of the 1997 Standard on the 1999 estimates can be seen by comparing 1999 data tabulated according to the two Standards: Estimates based on the 1977 Standard of the percent of women 40 years of age and over with a recent mammogram are: 0.1 percentage points higher for white women; 0.2 percentage points higher for black women; 3.6 percentage points lower for AI/AN women; and 1.1 percentage points higher for Asian and Pacific Islander women than estimates based on the 1997 Standards. See Appendix II, Race.

[5]Poor persons are defined as below the poverty threshold. Near poor persons have incomes of 100 percent to less than 200 percent of the poverty threshold. Nonpoor persons have incomes of 200 percent or greater than the poverty threshold. Missing family income data were imputed for 13–16 percent of adults in the sample in 1990–94. Poverty status was unknown for 25 percent of persons in the sample in 1998, 28 percent in 1999, and 27 percent in 2000. See Appendix II, Family income; Poverty level.

[6]Education categories shown are for 1998 and subsequent years. GED stands for General Educational Development high school equivalency diploma. In years prior to 1998 the following categories based on number of years of school completed were used: less than 12 years, 12 years, 13 years or more. See Appendix II, Education.

NOTES: Standard errors for selected years are available in the spreadsheet version of this table. See www.cdc.gov/nchs/hus.htm. Data starting in 1997 are not strictly comparable with data for earlier years due to the 1997 questionnaire redesign. See Appendix I, National Health Interview Survey.

SOURCE: Centers for Disease Control and Prevention, National Center for Health Statistics, National Health Interview Survey. Data are from the following supplements: cancer control (1987), health promotion and disease prevention (1990–91), and year 2000 objectives (1993–94). Starting in 1998 data are from the family core and sample adult questionnaires.

Table 81 (page 1 of 2). Use of Pap smears for women 18 years of age and over according to selected characteristics: United States, selected years 1987–2000

[Data are based on household interviews of a sample of the civilian noninstitutionalized population]

Characteristic	1987	1993	1994	1998	1999	2000
	Percent of women having a Pap smear within the past 3 years[1]					
18 years and over, age adjusted[2,3]	74.1	77.5	76.6	79.2	80.8	81.4
18 years and over, crude[2]	74.4	77.6	76.6	79.1	80.8	81.3
Age						
18–49 years	82.6	84.2	82.4	84.4	86.5	85.2
50–64 years	68.2	74.4	75.6	79.9	80.2	83.7
65 years and over	50.8	58.0	57.6	59.8	61.0	64.6
65–74 years.	57.9	64.7	64.9	67.0	70.0	71.6
75 years and over	40.4	47.8	47.3	51.2	50.8	56.8
Race[4]						
18 years and over, crude:						
White only	74.1	77.2	76.3	78.9	80.6	81.4
Black or African American only.	80.7	82.6	83.0	84.2	85.7	85.1
American Indian and Alaska Native only	85.4	78.2	73.3	74.6	92.2	76.9
Asian only	51.9	69.6	67.2	68.5	64.4	66.3
Native Hawaiian and Other Pacific Islander only	- - -	- - -	- - -	- - -	*	*
2 or more races	- - -	- - -	- - -	- - -	86.9	80.2
Hispanic origin and race[4]						
18 years and over, crude:						
Hispanic or Latino	67.6	77.2	74.3	75.2	76.3	76.9
Not Hispanic or Latino	74.9	77.6	76.9	79.6	81.3	81.8
White only	74.7	77.2	76.5	79.3	81.0	81.9
Black or African American only	80.9	82.7	83.3	84.2	86.0	85.2
Age, Hispanic origin, and race[4]						
18–49 years:						
Hispanic or Latino	74.2	81.1	80.1	77.0	77.5	78.5
Not Hispanic or Latino:						
White only	83.3	84.7	82.6	85.5	88.1	86.7
Black or African American only	89.3	87.8	89.2	88.9	90.3	88.5
50–64 years:						
Hispanic or Latino	50.7	72.3	67.6	76.6	78.4	75.9
Not Hispanic or Latino:						
White only	70.1	74.8	76.1	80.4	80.4	85.0
Black or African American only	70.9	77.9	78.5	81.6	82.9	83.9
65 years and over:						
Hispanic or Latino	41.7	57.3	44.1	59.8	63.7	66.9
Not Hispanic or Latino:						
White only	51.8	57.5	58.4	59.7	60.5	64.3
Black or African American only	44.8	61.5	60.9	61.7	64.5	67.3
Age and poverty status[5]						
18 years and over, crude:						
Below poverty	64.2	69.4	68.1	69.4	73.9	72.1
Near or nonpoor.	77.0	78.8	78.2	81.7	82.9	83.5
18–49 years:						
Below poverty.	76.6	76.1	78.0	76.8	79.8	76.5
Near or nonpoor	84.0	85.7	83.3	86.1	88.1	86.8
50–64 years:						
Below poverty.	50.5	62.2	57.9	63.6	72.1	73.0
Near or nonpoor	70.8	75.5	77.6	82.7	80.9	84.4
65 years and over:						
Below poverty.	33.2	47.2	44.3	47.1	50.7	53.7
Near or nonpoor	55.8	59.6	60.8	62.2	62.6	67.4

See footnotes at end of table.

Table 81 (page 2 of 2). Use of Pap smears for women 18 years of age and over according to selected characteristics: United States, selected years 1987–2000

[Data are based on household interviews of a sample of the civilian noninstitutionalized population]

Characteristic	1987	1993	1994	1998	1999	2000
Age and education[6]	Percent of women having a Pap smear within the past 3 years[1]					
25 years and over, crude:						
No high school diploma or GED	57.1	61.8	60.7	65.0	66.1	70.0
High school diploma or GED	76.4	78.1	75.8	77.4	79.3	79.9
Some college or more	84.0	84.3	85.1	86.9	87.8	88.1
25–49 years of age:						
No high school diploma or GED	73.8	73.3	71.8	76.9	77.6	80.1
High school diploma or GED	84.1	84.8	80.9	83.7	86.3	85.4
Some college or more	89.4	89.2	88.9	90.6	92.3	91.0
50–64 years of age:						
No high school diploma or GED	55.0	63.4	65.7	66.8	71.9	73.3
High school diploma or GED	70.9	75.2	75.7	80.2	79.2	81.4
Some college or more	78.7	80.6	81.9	84.8	83.8	88.8
65 years of age and over:						
No high school diploma or GED	44.0	50.8	48.0	52.4	51.8	56.7
High school diploma or GED	55.4	61.9	61.4	60.7	63.7	67.0
Some college or more	59.4	62.9	66.9	67.9	68.8	69.8

* Estimates are considered unreliable. Data not shown have a relative standard error greater than 30 percent.

- - - Data not available.

[1]Questions concerning use of Pap smears differed slightly on the National Health Interview Survey across the years for which data are shown. See Appendix II, Pap smear.

[2]Includes all other races not shown separately, unknown poverty status, and unknown education.

[3]Estimates are age adjusted to the year 2000 standard using four age groups: 18–49 years, 50–64 years, 65–74 years, and 75 years and over. See Appendix II, Age adjustment.

[4]The race groups, white, black, American Indian and Alaska Native (AI/AN), Asian, Native Hawaiian and Other Pacific Islander, and 2 or more races, include persons of Hispanic and non-Hispanic origin. Persons of Hispanic origin may be of any race. Starting with data year 1999 race-specific estimates are tabulated according to 1997 Standards for Federal data on Race and Ethnicity and are not strictly comparable with estimates for earlier years. The five single race categories plus multiple race categories shown in the table conform to 1997 Standards. The 1999 race-specific estimates are for persons who reported only one racial group; the category "2 or more races" includes persons who reported more than one racial group. Prior to data year 1999, data were tabulated according to 1977 Standards with four racial groups and the category "Asian only" included Native Hawaiian and Other Pacific Islander. Estimates for single race categories prior to 1999 included persons who reported one race or, if they reported more than one race, identified one race as best representing their race. The effect of the 1997 Standard on the 1999 estimates can be seen by comparing 1999 data tabulated according to the two Standards: Estimates based on the 1977 Standard of the percent of women 18 years of age and over with a recent Pap smear are: identical for white and black women; 0.4 percentage points lower for AI/AN women; and 1.5 percentage points higher for Asian and Pacific Islander women than estimates based on the 1997 Standards. See Appendix II, Race.

[5]Poor persons are defined as below the poverty threshold. Near poor persons have incomes of 100 percent to less than 200 percent of the poverty threshold. Nonpoor persons have incomes of 200 percent or greater than the poverty threshold. Missing family income data were imputed for 13–16 percent of adults in the sample in 1990–94. Poverty status was unknown for 25 percent of persons in the sample in 1998, 28 percent in 1999, and 27 percent in 2000. See Appendix II, Family income; Poverty level.

[6]Education categories shown are for 1998 and subsequent years. In years prior to 1998 the following categories based on number of years of school completed were used: less than 12 years, 12 years, 13 years or more. GED stands for General Educational Development high school equivalency diploma. See Appendix II, Education.

NOTES: Standard errors for selected years are available in the spreadsheet version of this table. See www.cdc.gov/nchs/hus.htm. Data starting in 1997 are not strictly comparable with data for earlier years due to the 1997 questionnaire redesign. See Appendix I, National Health Interview Survey.

SOURCES: Centers for Disease Control and Prevention, National Center for Health Statistics, National Health Interview Survey. Data are from the following supplements: cancer control (1987), year 2000 objectives (1993–94). Starting in 1998 data are from the family core and sample adult questionnaires.

Table 82 (page 1 of 2). Ambulatory care visits to physician offices and hospital outpatient and emergency departments by selected characteristics: United States, selected years 1995–2000

[Data are based on reporting by a sample of office-based physicians and hospital outpatient and emergency departments]

Age, sex, and race	All places[1]				Physician offices			
	1995	1998	1999	2000	1995	1998	1999	2000
	Number of visits in thousands							
Total	860,859	1,005,078	944,122	1,014,848	697,082	829,280	756,734	823,542
Under 18 years	194,644	213,486	183,072	212,165	150,351	168,520	135,627	163,459
18–44 years	285,184	328,475	300,051	315,774	219,065	260,379	227,005	243,011
45–64 years	188,320	237,700	240,688	255,894	159,531	203,296	201,911	216,783
45–54 years	104,891	132,146	130,824	142,233	88,266	112,316	108,597	119,474
55–64 years	83,429	105,555	109,864	113,661	71,264	90,979	93,315	97,309
65 years and over	192,712	225,416	220,311	231,014	168,135	197,085	192,190	200,289
65–74 years	102,605	115,526	106,066	116,505	90,544	102,306	92,642	102,447
75 years and over	90,106	109,890	114,245	114,510	77,591	94,779	99,548	97,842
	Number of visits per 100 persons							
Total, age adjusted[2]	334	377	352	374	271	312	283	304
Total, crude	329	373	347	370	266	308	279	300
Under 18 years	275	297	254	293	213	235	188	226
18–44 years	264	303	277	291	203	240	209	224
45–64 years	364	419	410	422	309	358	344	358
45–54 years	339	384	368	385	286	327	305	323
55–64 years	401	473	477	481	343	407	405	412
65 years and over	612	697	679	706	534	609	592	612
65–74 years	560	643	596	656	494	569	521	577
75 years and over	683	764	779	766	588	659	679	654
Sex and age								
Male, age adjusted[2]	290	321	309	325	232	261	246	261
Male, crude	277	310	297	314	220	251	235	251
Under 18 years	273	303	255	302	209	239	189	231
18–44 years	190	201	206	203	139	149	150	148
45–54 years	275	302	300	316	229	251	247	260
55–64 years	351	435	427	428	300	379	361	367
65–74 years	508	608	580	614	445	538	510	539
75 years and over	711	739	758	771	616	640	663	670
Female, age adjusted[2]	377	431	393	420	309	360	317	345
Female, crude	378	433	396	424	310	362	320	348
Under 18 years	277	291	252	285	217	231	187	221
18–44 years	336	401	345	377	265	328	267	298
45–54 years	400	462	432	451	339	399	361	384
55–64 years	446	506	522	529	382	433	445	453
65–74 years	603	672	610	692	534	595	530	609
75 years and over	666	780	792	763	571	671	689	645
Race and age[3]								
White, age adjusted[2]	339	376	356	380	282	316	292	315
White, crude	338	376	357	381	281	317	293	316
Under 18 years	295	292	258	306	237	235	197	243
18–44 years	267	305	284	301	211	248	222	239
45–54 years	334	380	368	386	286	328	312	330
55–64 years	397	462	474	480	345	406	410	416
65–74 years	557	639	597	641	496	572	526	568
75 years and over	689	768	781	764	598	669	687	658
Black or African American, age adjusted[2]	309	400	355	353	204	281	239	239
Black or African American, crude	281	373	322	324	178	259	211	214
Under 18 years	193	315	237	264	100	217	144	167
18–44 years	260	317	267	257	158	207	155	149
45–54 years	387	426	398	383	281	310	277	269
55–64 years	414	561	543	495	294	411	404	373
65–74 years	553	660	611	656	429	511	485	512
75 years and over	534	725	780	745	395	537	608	568

See footnotes at end of table.

[Data are based on reporting by a sample of office-based physicians and hospital outpatient and emergency departments]

Age, sex, and race	Hospital outpatient departments				Hospital emergency departments			
	1995	1998	1999	2000	1995	1998	1999	2000
	Number of visits in thousands							
Total	67,232	75,412	84,623	83,289	96,545	100,385	102,765	108,017
Under 18 years	17,636	18,551	21,758	21,076	26,657	26,415	25,688	27,630
18–44 years	24,299	26,032	29,514	26,947	41,820	42,064	43,532	45,816
45–64 years	14,811	17,980	20,891	20,772	13,978	16,425	17,886	18,339
45–54 years	8,029	9,859	11,541	11,558	8,595	9,970	10,686	11,201
55–64 years	6,782	8,120	9,350	9,214	5,383	6,455	7,200	7,138
65 years and over	10,486	12,849	12,461	14,494	14,090	15,482	15,659	16,232
65–74 years	6,004	6,869	6,969	7,515	6,057	6,350	6,455	6,543
75 years and over.	4,482	5,979	5,493	6,979	8,033	9,132	9,205	9,690
	Number of visits per 100 persons							
Total, age adjusted[2]	26	28	31	31	37	37	38	40
Total, crude	26	28	31	30	37	37	38	39
Under 18 years	25	26	30	29	38	37	36	38
18–44 years	22	24	27	25	39	39	40	42
45–64 years	29	32	36	34	27	29	31	30
45–54 years	26	29	32	31	28	29	30	30
55–64 years	33	36	41	39	26	29	31	30
65 years and over	33	40	38	44	45	48	48	50
65–74 years	33	38	39	42	33	35	36	37
75 years and over.	34	42	37	47	61	63	63	65
Sex and age								
Male, age adjusted[2]	21	23	26	26	37	36	37	38
Male, crude	21	23	25	25	36	36	37	38
Under 18 years.	25	26	29	29	40	39	37	41
18–44 years	14	16	18	17	37	37	38	38
45–54 years	20	23	25	26	26	28	29	30
55–64 years	26	28	37	32	25	28	30	30
65–74 years	29	35	35	38	34	35	35	36
75 years and over.	34	42	34	42	61	57	61	59
Female, age adjusted[2]	31	33	37	35	37	38	39	41
Female, crude	31	33	37	35	37	38	39	41
Under 18 years.	25	26	31	29	35	35	34	35
18–44 years	31	32	36	33	40	41	42	46
45–54 years	32	34	40	36	29	30	31	31
55–64 years	38	44	44	45	26	30	32	31
65–74 years	36	41	43	46	32	35	37	37
75 years and over.	34	41	39	49	61	67	64	69
Race and age[3]								
White, age adjusted[2]	23	25	28	28	34	35	35	37
White, crude	23	25	28	28	34	35	35	37
Under 18 years.	23	23	28	27	35	34	33	36
18–44 years	20	21	25	23	36	36	37	39
45–54 years	23	25	28	28	25	27	27	28
55–64 years	28	30	36	36	24	26	28	28
65–74 years	29	33	36	38	32	33	34	35
75 years and over.	31	38	34	44	60	61	61	63
Black or African American, age adjusted[2] . .	48	55	54	51	58	63	62	62
Black or African American, crude	45	52	51	48	58	62	60	62
Under 18 years.	39	43	42	40	53	55	51	57
18–44 years	38	44	45	40	64	67	68	68
45–54 years	55	63	66	61	51	54	55	53
55–64 years	73	90	83	70	47	59	57	52
65–74 years	*77	86	69	85	47	64	58	59
75 years and over.	66	85	*79	85	73	103	93	92

* Estimates are considered unreliable. Data preceded by an asterisk have a relative standard error of 20–30 percent.
[1]All places includes visits to physician offices and hospital outpatient and emergency departments.
[2]Estimates are age adjusted to the year 2000 standard population using six age groups: under 18 years, 18–44 years, 45–54 years, 55–64 years, 65–74 years, and 75 years and over. See Appendix II, Age adjustment.
[3]Beginning in 1999 the instruction for the race item on the Patient Record Form was changed so that more than one race could be recorded. In previous years only one racial category could be checked. Estimates for racial groups presented in this table are for visits where only one race was recorded. Estimates for visits where multiple races were checked were unreliable and are not presented.

NOTES: Some numbers were revised and differ from the previous edition of *Health, United States*. Rates are based on the civilian noninstitutionalized population as of July 1 adjusted for net underenumeration using the 1990 National Population Adjustment Matrix from the U.S. Bureau of the Census. Rates will be overestimated to the extent that visits by institutionalized persons are counted in the numerator (for example, hospital emergency department visits by nursing home residents) and institutionalized persons are omitted from the denominator. Data for additional years are available (see Appendix III).

SOURCES: Centers for Disease Control and Prevention, National Center for Health Statistics, National Ambulatory Medical Care Survey and National Hospital Ambulatory Medical Care Survey.

This table will be updated with 2001 data on the web. Go to www.cdc.gov/nchs/hus.htm.

Table 83 (page 1 of 2). Injury-related visits to hospital emergency departments by sex, age, and intent and mechanism of injury: United States, average annual 1995–96, 1997–98, and 1999–2000

[Data are based on reporting by a sample of hospital emergency departments]

Sex, age, and intent and mechanism of injury[1]	1995–96	1997–98	1999–2000	1995–96	1997–98	1999–2000
Both sexes	Injury-related visits in thousands			Injury-related visits per 10,000 persons		
All ages[2,3]	36,081	36,111	39,029	1,360.9	1,344.2	1,428.1
Male						
All ages[2,3]	20,030	19,838	21,286	1,530.7	1,500.0	1,585.3
Under 18 years[2]	6,238	6,057	6,364	1,720.2	1,651.9	1,722.2
Unintentional injuries[4]	5,478	5,192	5,457	1,510.5	1,416.1	1,476.7
Falls	1,402	1,241	1,303	386.5	338.4	352.6
Struck by or against objects or persons	1,011	1,468	1,378	278.9	400.5	372.8
Motor vehicle traffic	453	405	432	125.0	110.6	116.9
Cut or pierce	493	482	455	136.0	131.5	123.2
Intentional injuries	290	229	242	80.0	62.4	65.6
18–24 years[2]	2,980	2,805	3,096	2,396.9	2,222.5	2,361.6
Unintentional injuries[4]	2,423	2,169	2,416	1,948.7	1,718.8	1,842.7
Falls	299	255	307	240.8	202.1	233.9
Struck by or against objects or persons	387	456	405	311.0	361.7	308.6
Motor vehicle traffic	347	404	469	279.4	320.2	357.5
Cut or pierce	304	310	394	244.8	245.7	300.5
Intentional injuries	335	269	322	269.2	213.1	245.9
25–44 years[2]	7,245	6,788	7,251	1,767.4	1,660.4	1,796.9
Unintentional injuries[4]	5,757	5,122	5,528	1,404.3	1,252.8	1,370.0
Falls	817	779	850	199.4	190.5	210.8
Struck by or against objects or persons	619	849	781	151.0	207.8	193.6
Motor vehicle traffic	912	831	848	222.6	203.2	210.1
Cut or pierce	860	741	764	209.8	181.1	189.4
Intentional injuries	701	526	511	171.0	128.8	126.5
45–64 years[2]	2,240	2,755	2,972	883.4	1,020.4	1,030.9
Unintentional injuries[4]	1,845	2,108	2,325	727.6	781.0	806.7
Falls	445	512	582	175.6	189.5	202.0
Struck by or against objects or persons	186	202	232	73.3	74.8	80.6
Motor vehicle traffic	244	312	316	96.3	115.6	109.6
Cut or pierce	203	289	294	79.9	107.2	101.9
Intentional injuries	86	107	99	33.8	39.7	34.3
65 years and over[2]	1,327	1,434	1,603	1,000.7	1,056.6	1,158.7
Unintentional injuries[4]	1,009	1,109	1,207	760.6	817.2	872.1
Falls	505	492	579	380.9	362.3	418.1
Struck by or against objects or persons	*39	84	112	*29.4	*61.9	*80.7
Motor vehicle traffic	99	124	114	74.7	91.7	*82.5
Cut or pierce	*81	117	102	*61.1	86.4	74.0
Intentional injuries	*	19	10	*	*	*

See footnotes at end of table.

Table 83 (page 2 of 2). Injury-related visits to hospital emergency departments by sex, age, and intent and mechanism of injury: United States, average annual 1995–96, 1997–98, and 1999–2000

[Data are based on reporting by a sample of hospital emergency departments]

Sex, age, and intent and mechanism of injury[1]	1995–96	1997–98	1999–2000	1995–96	1997–98	1999–2000
Female	Injury-related visits in thousands			Injury-related visits per 10,000 persons		
All ages[2,3]	16,051	16,273	17,743	1,186.4	1,183.1	1,267.4
Under 18 years[2]	4,372	4,100	4,443	1,263.9	1,172.0	1,259.0
Unintentional injuries[4]	3,760	3,395	3,722	1,087.0	970.5	1,054.7
Falls	1,040	821	1,025	300.7	234.6	290.6
Struck by or against objects or persons	477	704	728	137.9	201.4	206.4
Motor vehicle traffic	447	403	430	129.3	115.4	122.0
Cut or pierce	253	265	232	73.0	75.9	65.7
Intentional injuries	220	178	149	63.6	50.9	42.3
18–24 years[2]	1,900	2,025	2,219	1,523.4	1,606.2	1,688.1
Unintentional injuries[4]	1,430	1,494	1,579	1,146.7	1,185.3	1,200.9
Falls	268	222	234	214.5	176.2	178.0
Struck by or against objects or persons	134	180	170	107.4	143.1	129.6
Motor vehicle traffic	373	473	469	298.8	374.9	357.1
Cut or pierce	131	121	156	105.3	96.0	118.3
Intentional injuries	239	227	219	191.7	179.9	166.8
25–44 years[2]	5,098	5,050	5,584	1,205.8	1,194.2	1,332.7
Unintentional injuries[4]	3,877	3,720	3,976	916.8	879.9	948.9
Falls	817	830	947	193.3	196.2	225.9
Struck by or against objects or persons	380	447	382	89.8	105.7	91.3
Motor vehicle traffic	872	821	788	206.2	194.3	188.0
Cut or pierce	338	378	434	79.8	89.3	103.5
Intentional injuries	422	400	425	99.8	94.7	101.5
45–64 years[2]	2,369	2,649	2,933	873.7	919.1	952.9
Unintentional injuries[4]	1,857	1,980	2,180	685.2	686.8	708.2
Falls	600	659	749	221.5	228.5	243.5
Struck by or against objects or persons	160	224	192	58.8	77.6	62.3
Motor vehicle traffic	343	331	324	126.5	114.7	105.2
Cut or pierce	127	192	175	46.9	66.6	56.8
Intentional injuries	*64	88	125	*23.5	30.4	40.5
65 years and over[2]	2,313	2,449	2,564	1,256.1	1,314.2	1,367.8
Unintentional injuries[4]	1,931	2,009	2,013	1,049.0	1,078.0	1,073.8
Falls	1,230	1,239	1,219	667.9	664.7	650.4
Struck by or against objects or persons	82	146	103	44.8	78.2	54.8
Motor vehicle traffic	169	163	132	91.6	87.5	70.6
Cut or pierce	*42	68	72	*22.7	*36.7	*38.3
Intentional injuries	*	31	20	*	*	*

* Estimates are considered unreliable. Data preceded by an asterisk have a relative standard error (RSE) of 20–30 percent. Data not shown have a RSE of greater than 30 percent.

[1]Intent and mechanism of injury are based on the first-listed external cause of injury code (E code). Intentional injuries include suicide attempts and assaults. See Appendix II, First-listed external cause of injury and Appendix II, table VII for listing of E codes.

[2]Includes all injury-related visits not shown separately in table including those with undetermined intent (less than 1 percent in 1999–2000), insufficient or no information to code cause of injury (about 13 percent in 1999–2000), and resulting from adverse effects of medical treatment (about 3 percent in 1999–2000).

[3]Rates are age adjusted to the year 2000 standard population using six age groups: under 18 years, 18–24 years, 25–44 years, 45–64 years, 65–74 years, and 75 years and over. See Appendix II, Age adjustment.

[4]Includes unintentional injury-related visits with mechanism of injury not shown in table.

NOTES: An emergency department visit was considered injury related if the checkbox for injury was indicated, the physician's diagnosis was injury related (ICD–9–CM 800–999), an external cause of injury code was present (ICD–9–CM E800-E999), or the patient's reason for the visit was injury related. Rates are based on the civilian noninstitutionalized population as of July 1 adjusted for net underenumeration using the 1990 National Population Adjustment Matrix from the Bureau of the Census. Data for additional years are available (see Appendix III).

SOURCE: Centers for Disease Control and Prevention, National Center for Health Statistics, National Hospital Ambulatory Medical Care Survey.

This table will be updated with 2000–01 data on the web. Go to www.cdc.gov/nchs/hus.htm.

Table 84 (page 1 of 2). Ambulatory care visits to primary care and specialist physicians, according to selected characteristics and type of physician: United States, 1980, 1990, and 2000

[Data are based on reporting by a sample of office-based physicians]

| Age, sex, and race | Type of primary care physician[1] | | | | | | | | | | | |
| | All primary care | | | General and family practice | | | Internal medicine | | | Pediatrics | | |
	1980	1990	2000	1980	1990	2000	1980	1990	2000	1980	1990	2000
	Percent of all physician office visits											
Total	56.6	54.9	51.1	33.5	29.9	24.1	12.1	13.8	15.3	10.9	11.2	11.7
Under 18 years.	76.6	78.3	78.6	26.1	26.5	19.9	2.0	2.9	*	48.5	48.9	57.3
18–44 years.	43.6	44.3	41.7	34.3	31.9	28.2	8.6	11.8	12.7	0.7	0.7	*0.9
45–64 years.	56.0	50.9	46.7	36.3	32.1	26.4	19.5	18.6	20.1	*	*	*
45–54 years	54.6	49.4	46.7	37.4	32.0	27.8	17.1	17.1	18.7	*	*	*
55–64 years	57.3	52.4	46.7	35.4	32.1	24.7	21.8	20.0	21.7	*	*	*
65 years and over.	60.3	51.5	45.0	37.5	28.1	20.2	22.7	23.3	24.5	*	*	*
65–74 years	59.5	51.2	44.6	37.4	28.1	19.7	22.1	23.0	24.5	*	*	*
75 years and over	61.3	51.8	45.4	37.6	28.0	20.8	23.5	23.7	24.5	*	*	*
Sex and age												
Male:												
Under 18 years	77.1	77.9	77.4	25.6	24.1	18.3	2.0	3.0	*	49.4	50.7	58.0
18–44 years	50.5	51.7	50.4	38.0	35.9	34.2	11.5	15.0	14.4	*	*	*1.7
45–64 years	55.0	50.5	48.9	34.4	31.0	28.7	20.5	19.2	19.8	*	*	*
65 years and over	57.9	51.1	43.1	35.6	27.7	19.3	22.3	23.3	23.8	*	*	*
Female:												
Under 18 years	76.0	78.8	79.9	26.6	29.1	21.7	2.0	2.8	*	47.4	46.9	56.5
18–44 years	40.4	41.0	37.6	32.5	30.0	25.3	7.3	10.3	11.9	*	*	*
45–64 years	56.7	51.1	45.2	37.7	32.8	24.9	18.9	18.2	20.2	*	*	*
65 years and over	61.8	51.7	46.3	38.7	28.3	20.9	22.9	23.3	25.0	*	*	*
Race and age[2]												
White:												
Under 18 years	76.5	78.2	77.3	26.4	27.1	21.2	2.0	2.3	*	48.2	48.8	54.7
18–44 years	43.8	43.2	41.0	34.5	31.9	29.2	8.6	10.6	11.0	*	*	*0.8
45–64 years	55.4	49.4	44.6	36.0	31.5	27.3	19.2	17.6	17.1	*	*	*
65 years and over	60.0	50.7	43.6	36.6	27.5	20.3	23.3	23.1	23.0	*	*	*
Black or African American:												
Under 18 years	77.1	82.1	86.4	23.7	20.2	*	*	*	*	51.2	52.1	75.0
18–44 years	41.4	50.4	44.3	31.7	31.9	22.0	9.0	18.1	20.9	*	*	*
45–64 years	61.3	58.2	59.4	38.6	31.2	23.3	22.6	26.9	35.9	*	*	*
65 years and over	63.3	57.8	52.1	49.0	28.9	*18.5	14.2	28.7	33.4	*	*	*

See footnotes at end of table.

Table 84 (page 2 of 2). Ambulatory care visits to primary care and specialist physicians, according to selected characteristics and type of physician: United States, 1980, 1990, and 2000

[Data are based on reporting by a sample of office-based physicians]

Age, sex, and race	Type of specialist physician[1]								
	All specialists			Obstetrics and gynecology			All other specialists		
	1980	1990	2000	1980	1990	2000	1980	1990	2000
	Percent of all physician office visits								
Total	43.4	45.1	48.9	9.6	9.0	7.9	33.8	36.1	40.9
Under 18 years.	23.4	21.7	21.4	1.3	1.2	*1.1	22.2	20.5	20.3
18–44 years.	56.4	55.7	58.3	21.7	21.5	20.7	34.7	34.1	37.5
45–64 years.	44.0	49.1	53.3	4.2	4.8	4.6	39.8	44.3	48.8
45–54 years	45.4	50.6	53.3	5.6	6.5	5.6	39.8	44.2	47.7
55–64 years	42.7	47.6	53.3	2.9	3.2	3.3	39.8	44.4	50.1
65 years and over.	39.7	48.5	55.0	1.4	1.2	1.5	38.4	47.3	53.5
65–74 years	40.5	48.8	55.4	1.7	1.6	2.1	38.8	47.2	53.4
75 years and over	38.7	48.2	54.6	1.0	*0.7	*1.0	37.7	47.5	53.6
Sex and age									
Male:									
Under 18 years	22.9	22.1	22.6	. . .	. . .	*	22.7	21.9	22.3
18–44 years	49.5	48.3	49.6	. . .	. . .	*	49.2	48.2	48.5
45–64 years	45.0	49.5	51.1	. . .	. . .	*	44.4	49.4	50.6
65 years and over	42.1	48.9	56.9	. . .	. . .	*	41.8	48.8	56.9
Female:									
Under 18 years	24.0	21.2	20.1	2.5	2.3	2.1	21.5	18.9	18.0
18–44 years	59.6	59.0	62.4	31.7	31.4	30.2	27.9	27.6	32.2
45–64 years	43.3	48.9	54.8	6.7	7.9	7.3	36.6	40.9	47.5
65 years and over	38.2	48.3	53.7	2.1	1.9	2.6	36.1	46.4	51.1
Race and age[2]									
White:									
Under 18 years	23.5	21.8	22.7	1.1	1.0	*1.2	22.4	20.8	21.5
18–44 years	56.2	56.8	59.0	21.0	21.8	20.8	35.2	35.0	38.2
45–64 years	44.6	50.6	55.4	4.1	4.9	4.8	40.4	45.7	50.6
65 years and over	40.0	49.3	56.4	1.4	1.3	1.5	38.6	48.1	54.9
Black or African American:									
Under 18 years	22.9	17.9	*13.6	2.8	*3.4	*	20.1	14.5	*12.7
18–44 years	58.6	49.6	55.7	27.1	18.6	20.7	31.5	31.0	35.0
45–64 years	38.7	41.8	40.6	4.8	4.0	*2.4	33.9	37.9	38.3
65 years and over	36.7	42.2	47.9	*	*	*	35.4	41.3	47.0

* Estimates are considered unreliable. Data preceded by an asterisk have a relative standard error (RSE) of 20–30 percent. Data not shown have a RSE of greater than 30 percent.

. . . Category not applicable.

[1]Type of physician is based on physician's self-designated primary area of practice. Primary care physicians are defined as practitioners in the fields of general and family practice, general internal medicine, and general pediatrics. Primary care physicians in general and family practice exclude specialists such as sports medicine and geriatrics. Primary care internal medicine physicians exclude internal medicine specialists such as allergists, cardiologists, endocrinologists, etc. Primary care pediatricians exclude pediatric specialists such as adolescent medicine specialists, neonatologists, pediatric allergists, pediatric cardiologists, etc. Specialist physicians include obstetricians and gynecologists in addition to other specialists not included in general and family practice, internal medicine, pediatrics, and all other specialists. See Appendix II, Physician specialty.

[2]Beginning in 1999 the instruction for the race item on the Patient Record Form was changed so that more than one race could be recorded. In previous years only one racial category could be checked. Estimates for racial groups presented in this table are for visits where only one race was recorded. Estimates for visits where multiple races were checked were unreliable and are not presented.

NOTES: This table presents data on ambulatory care visits to physician offices and excludes ambulatory care visits to other sites such as hospital outpatient and emergency departments. In 1980 the survey excluded Alaska and Hawaii. Data for all other years include all 50 States. Excludes visits with type of physician unknown. Data for additional years are available (see Appendix III).

SOURCE: Centers for Disease Control and Prevention, National Center for Health Statistics, National Ambulatory Medical Care Survey.

This table will be updated with 2001 data on the web. Go to www.cdc.gov/nchs/hus.htm.

Table 85. Substance abuse clients in specialty treatment units according to substance abused, geographic division, and State: United States, 1998–2002

[Data are based on a 1-day census of treatment providers]

Geographic division and State	All clients			Clients with both alcoholism and drug abuse			Alcoholism only clients			Drug abuse only clients		
	1998	2000	2002	1998	2000	2002	1998	2000	2002	1998	2000	2002
	Clients per 100,000 population											
United States	461.9	434.9	488.0	228.6	211.5	235.4	109.8	98.0	103.1	123.5	125.4	149.4
New England	703.7	617.6	648.9	365.5	289.0	291.6	160.8	118.5	126.3	177.4	210.1	231.0
Maine	809.2	462.0	613.0	406.2	241.7	309.3	290.2	152.8	165.9	112.7	67.5	137.9
New Hampshire	338.4	324.1	303.1	174.6	180.7	141.3	132.5	95.8	118.2	31.3	47.6	43.6
Vermont	507.0	536.3	456.2	278.2	275.0	261.3	166.4	198.6	124.0	62.4	62.7	70.9
Massachusetts	824.4	671.4	682.9	461.2	331.1	328.2	171.8	126.4	129.4	191.4	213.8	225.4
Rhode Island	768.0	704.2	689.2	355.4	257.6	212.2	155.0	107.8	143.1	257.5	338.8	334.0
Connecticut	585.5	674.5	754.0	258.4	280.0	303.2	101.0	86.2	104.9	226.1	308.3	345.9
Middle Atlantic	554.3	556.7	650.0	259.7	272.9	319.9	86.7	79.1	82.8	207.9	204.7	247.3
New York	773.0	779.0	925.5	330.2	376.7	456.7	114.2	102.6	115.8	328.6	299.7	353.1
New Jersey	367.1	349.2	461.5	178.6	150.3	189.0	56.3	48.2	47.8	132.2	150.7	224.7
Pennsylvania	357.0	369.5	374.3	209.7	202.4	207.8	66.4	65.3	58.1	80.9	101.8	108.4
East North Central	473.8	421.0	475.8	224.5	194.1	219.9	141.1	121.4	127.5	108.3	105.5	128.4
Ohio	452.5	409.9	408.2	253.9	226.6	233.0	119.7	105.2	96.0	79.0	78.2	79.2
Indiana	339.7	313.9	548.9	148.8	159.3	277.0	116.4	90.4	148.8	74.5	64.2	123.1
Illinois	466.5	419.8	453.4	230.2	179.0	184.4	113.3	104.3	104.9	122.9	136.4	164.1
Michigan	614.6	541.6	547.4	249.3	217.5	224.8	198.8	171.5	154.9	166.5	152.7	167.7
Wisconsin	431.8	351.6	456.9	189.0	157.4	195.9	172.3	139.2	171.6	70.5	55.0	89.3
West North Central	355.0	322.2	344.9	199.9	179.9	199.3	97.3	79.3	79.4	57.8	63.0	66.3
Minnesota	264.0	205.9	229.6	140.4	100.2	128.7	67.1	54.7	54.3	56.5	51.0	46.6
Iowa	300.9	229.0	334.6	150.5	117.1	189.7	107.9	76.1	88.4	42.4	35.8	56.5
Missouri	387.0	378.9	404.4	249.2	216.9	237.3	73.7	73.1	75.6	64.1	88.9	91.5
North Dakota	549.3	251.6	330.9	258.7	120.4	176.3	224.0	114.4	116.0	66.6	16.8	38.6
South Dakota	445.9	290.6	407.8	201.9	148.4	216.1	211.2	115.9	149.3	32.8	26.4	42.4
Nebraska	396.2	323.1	374.2	220.2	162.5	238.5	122.4	96.6	76.5	53.6	64.0	59.3
Kansas	411.6	544.7	408.9	231.0	351.7	235.0	109.1	111.1	95.3	71.6	81.9	78.6
South Atlantic	382.0	406.1	427.0	191.7	199.9	196.4	94.2	99.1	88.6	96.0	107.1	142.0
Delaware	603.5	589.8	623.2	306.3	371.3	473.3	127.5	122.5	60.5	169.6	96.0	89.4
Maryland	557.6	696.6	808.1	256.0	293.3	327.5	117.2	133.0	153.2	184.3	270.3	327.4
District of Columbia	1,447.8	1,395.4	1,309.5	879.7	616.3	569.2	199.6	195.8	135.3	368.5	583.2	605.0
Virginia	364.5	388.1	391.3	184.9	205.9	185.6	102.3	103.1	98.4	77.3	79.2	107.2
West Virginia	295.8	317.4	304.6	103.5	123.2	157.8	142.0	143.2	89.0	50.3	51.0	57.9
North Carolina	402.0	471.8	407.1	214.6	237.6	203.1	115.5	140.6	96.6	71.9	93.6	107.4
South Carolina	306.6	414.1	339.0	116.3	191.5	162.6	112.6	138.0	102.5	77.6	84.6	73.9
Georgia	252.0	199.3	276.9	115.5	100.5	135.6	65.4	47.5	67.6	71.1	51.3	73.6
Florida	365.1	352.3	398.4	199.1	185.0	171.3	70.2	71.8	65.2	95.8	95.4	162.0
East South Central	327.8	307.8	301.5	151.8	136.7	141.1	89.1	79.9	70.0	86.9	91.1	90.4
Kentucky	442.4	534.6	541.6	199.1	236.8	247.5	161.4	178.1	162.1	81.9	119.6	132.1
Tennessee	280.0	195.5	201.2	110.9	77.8	94.0	71.4	42.4	33.2	97.7	75.3	74.1
Alabama	244.8	233.0	254.1	117.1	81.7	110.4	47.4	37.7	43.2	80.3	113.6	100.5
Mississippi	391.3	328.7	237.6	221.7	199.0	134.3	86.7	80.0	58.1	83.0	49.7	45.2
West South Central	329.3	268.8	244.3	186.1	150.0	129.9	63.8	42.2	37.6	79.5	76.6	76.8
Arkansas	326.1	141.2	175.5	190.6	73.7	95.6	66.6	22.2	28.7	68.9	45.4	51.3
Louisiana	472.6	311.2	327.6	268.8	157.8	160.6	88.0	42.3	55.2	115.8	111.1	111.8
Oklahoma	315.2	260.9	309.6	125.4	143.2	179.6	96.7	70.6	65.7	93.2	47.0	64.3
Texas	299.7	278.0	224.2	177.3	159.9	119.5	52.1	39.9	30.3	70.3	78.2	74.4
Mountain	584.8	596.8	630.2	278.1	261.2	291.0	175.1	194.5	178.2	131.7	141.2	161.0
Montana	321.9	244.1	318.0	172.8	108.2	190.7	107.8	96.8	83.6	41.3	39.1	43.7
Idaho	278.4	257.2	359.7	178.6	169.5	223.0	58.4	55.9	82.5	41.3	31.9	54.3
Wyoming	406.2	523.9	450.6	193.0	317.7	253.7	160.2	154.5	138.8	53.0	51.7	58.1
Colorado	722.4	843.4	909.4	326.7	333.5	406.5	267.3	351.1	350.4	128.4	158.7	152.5
New Mexico	714.0	669.7	678.7	296.6	281.7	308.6	275.3	215.3	183.7	142.1	172.7	186.4
Arizona	532.6	661.0	668.3	236.5	277.4	276.1	137.9	201.8	148.2	158.2	181.9	244.0
Utah	704.7	409.6	490.4	351.7	206.4	286.9	145.4	79.4	88.2	207.5	123.8	115.4
Nevada	548.4	464.5	428.3	322.2	229.3	170.8	116.7	90.1	95.5	109.5	145.1	162.0
Pacific	525.1	466.4	628.1	256.8	229.8	309.6	120.1	98.2	145.0	148.2	138.4	173.5
Washington	674.8	676.4	745.9	398.4	391.7	429.4	182.7	169.1	189.2	93.7	115.6	127.3
Oregon	653.4	759.7	815.9	347.8	431.4	461.9	138.5	149.4	160.6	167.0	178.9	193.4
California	491.4	401.7	597.3	223.7	180.7	275.3	106.2	79.0	136.6	161.5	142.0	185.4
Alaska	583.0	536.1	564.1	287.8	250.2	317.7	252.2	228.7	198.9	43.0	57.2	47.5
Hawaii	299.6	254.3	346.6	169.1	128.1	169.1	64.6	38.3	72.1	66.0	87.9	105.4

NOTES: Estimates for 1998 and 2000 were revised from previous editions of Health, United States. Rates for the 1990s are based on postcensal estimates of the resident population 12 years of age and over as of July 1. Client data are as of October 1. Treatment rates at the State level can vary from year to year for a variety of reasons, including failure of large facilities to respond to the survey in some years, and normal variation in the number of people in treatment on a given day.

SOURCES: Substance Abuse and Mental Health Services Administration, Office of Applied Studies, Uniform Facility Data Set (UFDS), 1997–98; National Survey of Substance Abuse Treatment Services (N-SSATS), 2000; U.S. Bureau of the Census, Population Projections of the United States by Age, Sex, Race, and Hispanic Origin: 1995 to 2050. Population Electronic Product #45.

Table 86. Additions to mental health organizations according to type of service and organization: United States, selected years 1986–98

[Data are based on inventories of mental health organizations]

Service and organization	1986	1990	1992	1994[1]	1998[1]	1986	1990	1992	1994[1]	1998[1]
24-hour hospital and residential treatment[2]	Additions[3] in thousands					Additions per 100,000 civilian population				
All organizations	1,819	2,035	2,092	2,267	2,349	759.9	833.7	830.1	874.6	872.9
State and county mental hospitals	333	276	275	238	206	139.1	113.2	109.3	92.0	76.8
Private psychiatric hospitals	235	407	470	485	489	98.0	166.5	186.4	187.1	181.6
Non-Federal general hospital psychiatric services	849	960	951	1,067	1,154	354.8	393.2	377.4	411.5	428.9
Department of Veterans Affairs medical centers[4]	180	198	181	173	147	75.1	81.2	71.6	66.9	54.7
Residential treatment centers for emotionally disturbed children	25	42	36	47	50	10.2	17.0	14.4	18.0	18.4
All other organizations[5]	198	153	179	257	303	82.7	62.6	70.9	99.0	112.5
Less than 24-hour care[6]										
All organizations	2,955	3,298	3,164	3,516	4,228	1,233.4	1,352.4	1,255.2	1,356.8	1,571.2
State and county mental hospitals	68	48	50	42	42	28.4	19.8	19.7	16.1	15.7
Private psychiatric hospitals	132	163	206	214	237	55.2	66.9	81.8	82.4	87.9
Non-Federal general hospital psychiatric services	533	659	480	498	663	222.4	270.0	190.2	192.0	246.3
Department of Veterans Affairs medical centers[4]	133	184	159	132	149	55.3	75.3	63.1	51.1	55.3
Residential treatment centers for emotionally disturbed children	67	100	121	167	155	28.1	40.8	48.0	64.6	57.6
All other organizations[5]	2,022	2,145	2,149	2,464	2,982	844.0	879.6	852.4	950.7	1,108.4

[1]Beginning in 1994 data for supportive residential clients (moderately staffed housing arrangements such as supervised apartments, group homes, and halfway houses) are included in the totals and all other organizations. This change affects the comparability of trend data prior to 1994 with data for 1994 and later years.
[2]These data exclude mental health care provided in non-psychiatric units of hospitals such as general medical units.
[3]See Appendix II, Addition.
[4]Includes Department of Veterans Affairs (VA) neuropsychiatric hospitals, VA general hospital psychiatric services, and VA psychiatric outpatient clinics.
[5]Includes freestanding psychiatric outpatient clinics, partial care organizations, and multiservice mental health organizations. See Appendix I.
[6]Formerly reported as partial care and outpatient treatment, the survey format was changed in 1994 and the reporting of these services was combined due to similarities in the care provided. These data exclude office-based mental health care (psychiatrists, psychologists, licensed clinical social workers, and psychiatric nurses).

NOTES: Data for 1998 are revised and differ from the previous edition of *Health, United States*.

SOURCE: Manderscheid RW and Henderson MJ. *Mental Health, United States, 2000*. Center for Mental Health Services. DHHS. Washington, DC. 2001.

Table 87. Home health care patients, according to age, sex, and diagnosis: United States, selected years 1992–2000

[Data are based on a survey of current home health care patients]

Age, sex, and diagnosis	1992	1994	1996	1998	2000
	Number of current patients				
Total home health care patients	1,232,200	1,889,327	2,427,483	1,881,768	1,355,290
	Current patients per 10,000 population				
Total	47.8	71.8	90.6	69.6	48.7
Age at time of survey:					
Under 65 years, crude	12.6	21.0	27.8	25.0	16.4
65 years and over, crude	295.4	424.9	526.3	375.7	277.0
65 years and over, age adjusted[1]	315.8	449.6	546.6	381.0	276.5
65–74 years	151.7	209.1	240.1	202.0	130.2
75–84 years	398.3	542.2	753.6	470.3	347.6
85 years and over	775.9	1,206.1	1,253.4	885.4	694.1
Sex:					
Male, total	32.6	47.8	60.9	47.9	35.1
Under 65 years, crude	10.9	17.8	22.1	22.9	15.6
65 years and over, crude	219.2	303.1	386.4	255.2	199.6
65 years and over, age adjusted[1]	255.8	350.0	438.3	277.6	216.4
65–74 years	121.8	169.9	187.0	159.7	100.7
75–84 years	322.0	427.5	598.7	321.4	270.0
85 years and over	635.2	893.1	1,044.3	653.0	553.9
Female, total	62.4	94.7	118.9	90.4	61.8
Under 65 years, crude	14.3	24.2	33.6	27.0	17.2
65 years and over, crude	347.4	508.9	623.9	460.4	332.6
65 years and over, age adjusted[1]	351.5	506.6	615.0	445.8	315.5
65–74 years	175.3	240.6	283.2	236.3	154.6
75–84 years	445.3	614.5	854.0	568.8	400.4
85 years and over	830.7	1,327.6	1,337.0	981.7	754.9
	Percent distribution				
Age at time of survey:[2]					
Under 65 years	23.1	25.7	27.0	31.3	29.5
65 years and over	76.9	74.3	73.0	68.7	70.5
65–74 years	22.6	20.6	18.4	19.7	17.3
75–84 years	33.9	31.2	35.3	29.9	31.3
85 years and over	20.4	22.4	19.4	19.1	21.9
Sex:					
Male	33.2	32.5	32.9	33.6	35.2
Female	66.8	67.5	67.1	66.4	64.8
Primary admission diagnosis:[3]					
Malignant neoplasms	5.7	5.7	4.8	3.8	4.9
Diabetes	7.7	8.1	8.5	6.1	7.8
Diseases of the nervous system and sense organs	6.3	8.0	5.8	7.6	6.1
Diseases of the circulatory system	25.9	27.2	25.6	23.6	23.6
Diseases of heart	12.6	14.3	10.9	12.3	10.9
Cerebrovascular diseases	5.8	6.1	7.8	5.1	7.3
Diseases of the respiratory system	6.6	6.1	7.7	7.9	6.8
Decubitus ulcers	1.9	1.1	1.0	1.2	1.9
Diseases of the musculoskeletal system and connective tissue	9.4	8.3	8.8	8.3	9.8
Osteoarthritis	2.5	2.8	3.2	2.7	3.5
Fractures, all sites	3.8	3.7	3.3	4.0	4.1
Fracture of neck of femur (hip)	1.4	1.7	1.3	1.1	1.5
Other	32.7	31.8	34.6	37.5	34.9

[1]Age adjusted by the direct method to the year 2000 standard population using the following three age groups: 65–74 years, 75–84 years, and 85 years and over. See Appendix II, Age adjustment.
[2]Denominator excludes persons with unknown age.
[3]Denominator excludes persons with unknown diagnosis.

NOTES: Current home health care patients are those who were on the rolls of the agency as of midnight on the day immediately before the date of the survey. Rates are based on the civilian population as of July 1. Population figures are adjusted for net underenumeration using the 1990 National Population Adjustment Matrix from the U.S. Bureau of the Census. Diagnostic categories are based on the *International Classification of Diseases, 9th Revision, Clinical Modification*. For a listing of the code numbers, see Appendix II, table IX.

SOURCE: Centers for Disease Control and Prevention, National Center for Health Statistics, National Home and Hospice Care Survey.

Table 88. Hospice patients, according to age, sex, and diagnosis: United States, selected years 1992–2000

[Data are based on a survey of current hospice patients]

Age, sex, and diagnosis	1992	1994	1996	1998	2000
	Number of current patients				
Total hospice patients.	52,100	60,783	59,363	79,837	105,496
	Current patients per 10,000 population				
Total.	2.0	2.3	2.2	3.0	3.8
Age at time of survey:					
Under 65 years, crude	0.5	0.8	0.5	0.7	0.8
65 years and over, crude.	13.1	12.9	13.9	18.2	24.9
65 years and over, age adjusted[1]	13.7	13.6	14.4	18.4	24.9
65–74 years	7.8	7.3	7.8	9.9	10.1
75–84 years	19.2	16.9	16.9	22.0	31.9
85 years and over.	23.4	30.6	34.7	44.7	67.3
Sex:					
Male, total	1.9	2.1	2.0	2.6	3.3
Under 65 years, crude.	0.5	0.9	0.5	0.7	0.8
65 years and over, crude	13.9	12.5	14.8	18.5	24.8
65 years and over, age adjusted[1]	16.0	14.4	16.1	20.3	26.9
65–74 years	6.3	7.0	10.4	10.2	13.0
75–84 years	25.8	18.2	18.5	25.2	32.6
85 years and over	28.8	34.8	33.9	49.2	69.9
Female, total	2.1	2.5	2.4	3.3	4.3
Under 65 years, crude.	0.4	0.7	0.6	0.8	0.9
65 years and over, crude	12.6	13.2	13.2	18.0	25.0
65 years and over, age adjusted[1]	12.6	13.2	12.9	17.3	23.3
65–74 years	8.9	7.5	5.8	9.6	7.6
75–84 years	15.1	16.1	15.9	19.9	31.5
85 years and over	21.4	29.0	35.0	42.9	66.2
	Percent distribution				
Age at time of survey:[2]					
Under 65 years	19.5	30.1	21.3	21.6	18.6
65 years and over	80.5	69.9	78.7	78.4	81.4
65–74 years	27.3	22.2	24.5	22.7	17.2
75–84 years	38.6	30.1	32.4	32.9	37.0
85 years and over.	14.6	17.6	21.9	22.7	27.3
Sex:					
Male	46.1	44.7	44.9	42.7	42.6
Female	53.9	55.3	55.1	57.3	57.4
Primary admission diagnosis:[3]					
Malignant neoplasms	65.7	57.2	58.3	55.5	51.9
Large intestine and rectum.	9.0	8.0	4.0	6.4	4.9
Trachea, bronchus, and lung	21.1	12.5	15.8	13.0	12.3
Breast	3.9	4.8	6.2	4.9	4.8
Prostate.	6.0	5.9	6.6	6.1	7.7
Diseases of heart.	10.2	9.3	8.3	9.7	12.8
Diseases of the respiratory system.	4.3	6.6	7.3	10.6	6.5
Other	19.8	27.0	26.1	24.3	28.8

[1]Age adjusted by the direct method to the year 2000 standard population using the following three age groups: 65–74 years, 75–84 years, and 85 years and over. See Appendix II, Age adjustment.
[2]Denominator excludes persons with unknown age.
[3]Denominator excludes persons with unknown diagnosis.

NOTES: Current hospice patients are those who were on the rolls of the agency as of midnight on the day immediately before the date of the survey. Rates are based on the civilian population as of July 1. Population figures are adjusted for net underenumeration using the 1990 National Population Adjustment Matrix from the U.S. Bureau of the Census. Diagnostic categories are based on the *International Classification of Diseases, 9th Revision, Clinical Modification*. For a listing of the code numbers, see Appendix II, table IX.

SOURCE: Centers for Disease Control and Prevention, National Center for Health Statistics, National Home and Hospice Care Survey.

[Data are based on household interviews of a sample of the civilian noninstitutionalized population]

Characteristic	Discharges[1]			Days of care[1]			Average length of stay[1]		
	1997	1999	2001	1997	1999	2001	1997	1999	2001
	Number per 1,000 population						Number of days		
Total[2,3]	124.3	119.7	122.0	601.2	555.1	554.2	4.8	4.6	4.5
Age									
Under 18 years	90.8	76.3	78.6	319.0	302.6	312.4	3.5	4.0	4.0
Under 6 years	203.5	183.2	184.6	632.6	664.8	674.0	3.1	3.6	3.7
6–17 years. :	34.0	24.3	27.0	163.1	*126.5	136.5	4.8	*5.2	5.1
18–44 years	96.8	95.8	94.8	358.8	352.8	348.9	3.7	3.7	3.7
45–64 years	124.9	125.6	125.2	631.1	592.5	616.0	5.1	4.7	4.9
45–54 years	99.2	110.1	103.7	527.5	473.9	465.9	5.3	4.3	4.5
55–64 years	164.8	149.6	159.2	792.4	775.5	853.5	4.8	5.2	5.4
65 years and over	274.4	269.7	286.6	1,852.5	1,620.5	1,560.6	6.8	6.0	5.4
65–74 years	249.1	229.8	231.2	1,595.2	1,386.4	1,239.0	6.4	6.0	5.4
75 years and over	307.3	318.5	351.9	2,188.4	1,907.6	1,941.2	7.1	6.0	5.5
Under 65 years of age									
All persons under 65 years of age[2,4]	102.2	97.6	97.8	416.4	398.9	406.6	4.1	4.1	4.2
Sex[4]									
Male	79.1	77.9	76.1	374.9	374.0	372.9	4.7	4.8	4.9
Female	124.7	116.7	119.0	456.6	422.8	439.7	3.7	3.6	3.7
Race[4,5]									
White only	100.8	94.7	93.2	385.8	368.7	369.4	3.8	3.9	4.0
Black or African American only	126.3	122.8	130.3	688.6	638.3	657.2	5.5	5.2	5.0
American Indian and Alaska Native only	111.9	128.3	169.2	*494.3	*570.0	*767.6	*4.4	*4.4	*4.5
Asian only	61.7	78.4	68.0	*268.6	*249.5	228.7	*4.4	*3.2	3.4
Native Hawaiian and Other Pacific Islander only	- - -	*	*	- - -	*	*	- - -	*	*
2 or more races	- - -	139.1	139.5	- - -	*688.8	*586.2	- - -	*5.0	*4.2
Hispanic origin and race[4,5]									
Hispanic or Latino	109.9	90.1	101.5	416.7	389.8	406.3	3.8	4.3	4.0
Not Hispanic or Latino	101.2	98.7	97.5	415.4	401.5	407.9	4.1	4.1	4.2
White only	99.6	95.4	92.6	382.7	368.4	368.2	3.8	3.9	4.0
Black or African American only	125.7	122.7	129.4	692.6	625.5	656.0	5.5	5.1	5.1
Poverty status[4,6]									
Poor	196.8	174.0	167.9	971.0	992.9	857.7	4.9	5.7	5.1
Near poor	125.5	150.3	136.2	553.7	671.4	646.5	4.4	4.5	4.7
Nonpoor	85.6	82.1	86.5	312.1	291.9	316.7	3.6	3.6	3.7
Hispanic origin and race and poverty status[4,5,6]									
Hispanic or Latino:									
Poor	163.9	122.3	167.8	625.1	555.2	723.9	3.8	4.5	4.3
Near poor	93.9	97.0	93.5	421.4	*434.9	362.0	4.5	*4.5	3.9
Nonpoor	95.4	79.2	79.8	297.9	295.4	288.1	3.1	3.7	3.6
Not Hispanic or Latino:									
White only:									
Poor	222.2	181.2	145.7	1,053.4	1,042.5	812.3	4.7	5.8	5.6
Near poor	132.8	166.8	144.3	539.1	683.8	725.4	4.1	4.1	5.0
Nonpoor	85.7	81.5	86.6	306.8	289.7	305.4	3.6	3.6	3.5
Black or African American only:									
Poor	195.9	223.6	230.4	1,260.0	1,424.2	1,243.3	6.4	6.4	5.4
Near poor	142.0	154.1	163.7	819.2	*920.3	732.2	5.8	*6.0	4.5
Nonpoor	92.3	86.7	96.8	389.0	332.7	489.8	4.2	3.8	5.1
Health insurance status[4,7]									
Insured	108.1	101.6	104.3	442.5	416.8	433.2	4.1	4.1	4.2
Private	85.6	80.2	84.4	310.2	287.8	311.8	3.6	3.6	3.7
Medicaid	311.6	332.5	296.2	1,575.3	1,695.5	1,495.1	5.1	5.1	5.0
Uninsured	75.3	75.7	64.2	296.3	304.2	270.9	3.9	4.0	4.2

See footnotes at end of table.

Table 89 (page 2 of 3). Discharges, days of care, and average length of stay in short-stay hospitals, according to selected characteristics: United States, selected years 1997–2001

[Data are based on household interviews of a sample of the civilian noninstitutionalized population]

Characteristic	Discharges[1]			Days of care[1]			Average length of stay[1]		
	1997	1999	2001	1997	1999	2001	1997	1999	2001
Poverty status and health insurance status[4,6]	Number per 1,000 population						Number of days		
Poor:									
Insured	243.9	217.1	210.9	1,272.5	1,294.5	1,123.1	5.2	6.0	5.3
Uninsured	110.0	101.5	90.1	459.4	476.9	366.5	4.2	4.7	4.1
Near poor:									
Insured	149.2	184.3	164.7	663.8	837.5	788.6	4.4	4.5	4.8
Uninsured	73.4	75.2	72.9	302.1	295.5	*333.1	4.1	3.9	*4.6
Nonpoor:									
Insured	88.1	84.1	88.9	316.0	299.7	327.4	3.6	3.6	3.7
Uninsured	59.8	58.8	54.5	*253.5	197.6	166.4	*4.2	3.4	3.1
Geographic region[4]									
Northeast	96.0	85.6	87.5	455.4	381.6	403.9	4.7	4.5	4.6
Midwest	108.7	99.6	100.5	384.4	359.9	400.0	3.5	3.6	4.0
South	111.8	112.8	110.6	466.1	463.9	456.3	4.2	4.1	4.1
West	82.9	80.0	82.5	327.2	348.3	332.4	3.9	4.4	4.0
Location of residence[4]									
Within MSA[8]	99.3	94.0	96.1	411.8	383.0	400.1	4.1	4.1	4.2
Outside MSA[8]	113.2	111.9	104.7	435.9	459.4	432.7	3.8	4.1	4.1
65 years of age and over									
All persons 65 years of age and over[2,9]	276.9	272.1	288.8	1,878.4	1,635.3	1,574.3	6.8	6.0	5.5
Sex[9]									
Male	291.6	280.2	304.4	2,077.4	1,551.7	1,746.2	7.1	5.5	5.7
Female	265.2	264.0	277.1	1,727.4	1,676.5	1,457.2	6.5	6.4	5.3
Hispanic origin and race[5,9]									
Hispanic or Latino	312.7	289.8	304.4	2,512.1	1,882.8	1,568.9	8.0	6.5	5.2
Not Hispanic or Latino	274.6	271.2	287.8	1,846.3	1,618.0	1,574.6	6.7	6.0	5.5
White only	274.8	271.4	287.7	1,808.2	1,586.4	1,525.4	6.6	5.8	5.3
Black or African American only	290.8	300.7	336.7	2,423.5	2,064.8	2,311.8	8.3	6.9	6.9
Poverty status[6,9]									
Poor	357.4	394.7	416.1	2,690.9	2,169.0	2,220.6	7.5	5.5	5.3
Near poor	329.6	328.5	310.7	2,498.3	1,954.8	1,849.7	7.6	6.0	6.0
Nonpoor	256.6	247.3	266.7	1,680.3	1,510.4	1,345.9	6.5	6.1	5.0
Health insurance status[7,9]									
Medicare HMO	217.8	241.9	252.8	1,355.3	1,396.0	1,305.8	6.2	5.8	5.2
Private	271.9	270.9	286.3	1,756.1	1,592.8	1,485.9	6.5	5.9	5.2
Medicaid	539.7	455.0	484.0	3,810.6	3,286.7	2,663.2	7.1	7.2	5.5
Medicare fee-for-service only	252.9	266.0	264.2	1,906.6	1,565.3	1,717.7	7.5	5.9	6.5
Geographic region[9]									
Northeast	265.0	288.0	272.0	1,828.5	1,873.4	1,467.7	6.9	6.5	5.4
Midwest	285.2	244.0	280.0	1,971.1	1,475.3	1,517.9	6.9	6.0	5.4
South	298.1	298.1	312.3	2,140.2	1,783.8	1,757.4	7.2	6.0	5.6
West	237.2	238.5	275.7	1,299.2	1,284.6	1,434.7	5.5	5.4	5.2

See footnotes at end of table.

Table 89 (page 3 of 3). Discharges, days of care, and average length of stay in short-stay hospitals, according to selected characteristics: United States, selected years 1997–2001

[Data are based on household interviews of a sample of the civilian noninstitutionalized population]

	Discharges[1]			Days of care[1]			Average length of stay[1]		
Characteristic	1997	1999	2001	1997	1999	2001	1997	1999	2001
Location of residence[9]	Number per 1,000 population						Number of days		
Within MSA[8]	271.3	265.3	286.8	1,875.9	1,653.3	1,584.1	6.9	6.2	5.5
Outside MSA[8]	295.1	295.3	295.8	1,893.6	1,574.8	1,540.8	6.4	5.3	5.2

* Estimates are considered unreliable. Data preceded by an asterisk have a relative standard error of 20–30 percent. Data not shown have a relative standard error of greater than 30 percent.

- - - Data not available.

[1]See Appendix II, Discharge; Days of care; Average length of stay.

[2]Includes all other races not shown separately, unknown poverty status, and unknown health insurance status.

[3]Estimates for all persons are age adjusted to the year 2000 standard using six age groups: Under 18 years, 18–44 years, 45–54 years, 55–64 years, 65–74 years, and 75 years of age and over. See Appendix II, Age adjustment.

[4]Estimates are for persons under 65 years of age and are age adjusted to the year 2000 standard population using four age groups: Under 18 years, 18–44 years, 45–54 years, and 55–64 years of age. See Appendix II, Age adjustment.

[5]The race groups, white, black, American Indian and Alaska Native (AI/AN), Asian, Native Hawaiian and Other Pacific Islander, and 2 or more races, include persons of Hispanic and non-Hispanic origin. Persons of Hispanic origin may be of any race. Starting with data year 1999 race-specific estimates are tabulated according to 1997 Standards for Federal data on Race and Ethnicity and are not strictly comparable with estimates for earlier years. The five single race categories plus multiple race categories shown in the table conform to 1997 Standards. The 1999 race-specific estimates are for persons who reported only one racial group; the category "2 or more races" includes persons who reported more than one racial group. Prior to data year 1999, data were tabulated according to 1977 Standards with four racial groups and the category "Asian only" included Native Hawaiian and Other Pacific Islander. Estimates for single race categories prior to 1999 included persons who reported one race or, if they reported more than one race, identified one race as best representing their race. The effect of the 1997 Standard on the 1999 estimates can be seen by comparing 1999 data tabulated according to the two Standards: Age-adjusted estimates based on the 1977 Standard of the hospital discharge rate for persons under 65 years of age are: 0.2 percentage points lower for white persons; 0.3 percentage points lower for black persons; 12.4 percentage points lower for AI/AN persons; 1.2 percentage points higher for Asian and Pacific Islander persons; and for persons 65 years of age and older: 0.4 percentage points lower for white persons; and 0.6 percentage points higher for black persons than estimates based on the 1997 Standards. See Appendix II, Race.

[6]Poor persons are defined as below the poverty threshold. Near poor persons have incomes of 100 percent to less than 200 percent of the poverty threshold. Nonpoor persons have incomes of 200 percent or greater than the poverty threshold. See Appendix II, Poverty level; Family income. Poverty status was missing for 20 percent of persons in the sample in 1997, 25 percent in 1998, 28 percent in 1999, 27 percent in 2000, and 28 percent in 2001.

[7]Health insurance categories are mutually exclusive. Persons who reported both Medicaid and private coverage are classified as having private coverage. Persons 65 years of age and over who reported Medicare HMO (health maintenance organization) and some other type of health insurance coverage are classified as having Medicare HMO. Starting in 1997 Medicaid includes state-sponsored health plans and State Children's Health Insurance Program (SCHIP). The category "insured" also includes military, other State, and Medicare coverage. See Appendix II, Health insurance coverage.

[8]MSA is metropolitan statistical area.

[9]Estimates are for persons 65 years of age and over and are age adjusted to the year 2000 standard population using two age groups: 65–74 years and 75 years and over. See Appendix II, Age adjustment.

NOTES: Some numbers in this table for health insurance estimates were revised and differ from previous editions of *Health, United States*. Estimates of hospital utilization presented in *Health, United States* utilize two data sources: the National Health Interview Survey (NHIS) and the National Hospital Discharge Survey (NHDS). Differences in estimates from the two surveys are particularly evident for children and the elderly. See Appendix II, Hospital Utilization. Data for additional years are available (see Appendix III). Standard errors for selected years are available in the spreadsheet version of this table. See www.cdc.gov/nchs/hus.htm.

SOURCE: Centers for Disease Control and Prevention, National Center for Health Statistics, National Health Interview Survey, family core questionnaire.

Table 90 (page 1 of 2). Discharges, days of care, and average length of stay in non-Federal short-stay hospitals, according to selected characteristics: United States, selected years 1980–2001

[Data are based on a sample of hospital records]

Characteristic	1980[1]	1985[1]	1990	1997	1998	1999	2000[2]	2001[3]
	Discharges per 1,000 population							
Total[4]	173.4	151.4	125.2	116.1	117.9	117.8	113.3	115.3
Age								
Under 18 years	75.6	61.4	46.4	40.6	40.4	42.2	40.3	43.4
18–44 years	155.3	128.0	102.7	86.0	88.8	86.4	85.0	87.6
45–54 years	174.8	146.8	112.4	93.7	92.7	94.5	92.1	94.5
55–64 years	215.4	194.8	163.3	149.1	155.1	151.4	141.5	139.3
65 years and over	383.7	369.8	334.1	361.1	365.3	370.4	353.5	354.9
65–74 years	315.8	297.2	261.6	265.9	267.6	270.6	254.6	256.2
75 years and over	489.3	475.6	434.0	474.0	477.4	481.6	462.3	461.4
Sex[4]								
Male	153.2	137.3	113.0	103.0	102.8	103.4	99.1	100.2
Female	195.0	167.3	139.0	130.0	133.3	132.2	127.8	130.9
Geographic region[4]								
Northeast	162.0	142.6	133.2	125.5	127.3	129.0	- - -	- - -
Midwest	192.1	158.1	128.8	115.5	116.4	115.6	- - -	- - -
South	179.7	155.5	132.5	122.4	126.4	124.7	- - -	- - -
West	150.5	145.7	100.7	97.9	97.1	98.5	- - -	- - -
	Days of care per 1,000 population							
Total[4]	1,297.0	997.5	818.9	595.2	598.6	588.8	557.8	563.2
Age								
Under 18 years	341.4	281.2	226.3	169.8	182.4	185.5	179.0	192.7
18–44 years	818.6	619.2	467.7	317.4	328.3	316.9	309.5	323.6
45–54 years	1,314.9	967.8	699.7	460.8	452.9	451.0	437.5	455.9
55–64 years	1,889.4	1,436.9	1,172.3	821.4	836.1	795.1	729.0	732.4
65 years and over	4,098.3	3,228.0	2,895.6	2,285.6	2,264.2	2,256.8	2,112.5	2,067.8
65–74 years	3,147.0	2,437.3	2,087.8	1,599.3	1,596.1	1,578.1	1,438.9	1,450.3
75 years and over	5,578.8	4,381.3	4,009.1	3,099.6	3,030.8	3,012.9	2,853.7	2,734.0
Sex[4]								
Male	1,239.7	973.3	805.8	573.8	576.7	565.4	536.0	535.7
Female	1,365.2	1,033.1	840.5	619.3	622.9	613.6	581.2	592.9
Geographic region[4]								
Northeast	1,400.6	1,113.0	1,026.7	739.2	731.0	733.6	- - -	- - -
Midwest	1,484.8	1,078.6	830.6	556.3	552.5	532.6	- - -	- - -
South	1,262.3	957.7	820.4	629.5	643.9	622.1	- - -	- - -
West	956.9	824.7	575.5	445.3	450.4	461.4	- - -	- - -
	Average length of stay in days							
Total[4]	7.5	6.6	6.5	5.1	5.1	5.0	4.9	4.9
Age								
Under 18 years	4.5	4.6	4.9	4.2	4.5	4.4	4.4	4.4
18–44 years	5.3	4.8	4.6	3.7	3.7	3.7	3.6	3.7
45–54 years	7.5	6.6	6.2	4.9	4.9	4.8	4.8	4.8
55–64 years	8.8	7.4	7.2	5.5	5.4	5.3	5.2	5.3
65 years and over	10.7	8.7	8.7	6.3	6.2	6.1	6.0	5.8
65–74 years	10.0	8.2	8.0	6.0	6.0	5.8	5.7	5.7
75 years and over	11.4	9.2	9.2	6.5	6.3	6.3	6.2	5.9
Sex[4]								
Male	8.1	7.1	7.1	5.6	5.6	5.5	5.4	5.3
Female	7.0	6.2	6.0	4.8	4.7	4.6	4.6	4.5

See footnotes at end of table.

Table 90 (page 2 of 2). Discharges, days of care, and average length of stay in non-Federal short-stay hospitals, according to selected characteristics: United States, selected years 1980–2001

[Data are based on a sample of hospital records]

Characteristic	1980[1]	1985[1]	1990	1997	1998	1999	2000[2]	2001[3]
Geographic region[4]			Average length of stay in days					
Northeast	8.6	7.8	7.7	5.9	5.7	5.7	- - -	- - -
Midwest	7.7	6.8	6.5	4.8	4.7	4.6	- - -	- - -
South	7.0	6.2	6.2	5.1	5.1	5.0	- - -	- - -
West	6.4	5.7	5.7	4.5	4.6	4.7	- - -	- - -

- - - Data not available.

[1]Comparisons of data from 1980–85 with data from later years should be made with caution as estimates of change may reflect improvements in the design rather than true changes in hospital use. See Appendix I, National Hospital Discharge Survey.

[2]The civilian population estimates used to compute rates for 2000 differ from those used in *Health, United States, 2002*. Rates for 2000 were computed using Census 2000 counts, while in the previous edition of *Health, United States*, rates for 2000 were computed using 1990-based postcensal estimates.

[3]Rates for 2001 were computed using 2000-based postcensal estimates.

[4]Estimates are age adjusted to the year 2000 standard population using six age groups: under 18 years, 18–44 years, 45–54 years, 55–64 years, 65–74 years, and 75 years and over. See Appendix II, Age adjustment.

NOTES: Rates are based on the civilian population as of July 1. Rates for 1990–99 use population estimates based on the 1990 census adjusted for net underenumeration using the 1990 National Population Adjustment Matrix from the U.S. Bureau of the Census. Rates for 1990–99 are not strictly comparable with rates for 2000 and 2001 because population estimates for 1990–99 have not been revised to reflect Census 2000. See Appendix I, National Hospital Discharge Survey. Estimates of hospital utilization from the National Health Interview Survey (NHIS) and the National Hospital Discharge Survey (NHDS) may differ because NHIS data are based on household interviews of the civilian noninstitutionalized population, whereas NHDS data are based on hospital discharge records of all persons. See Appendix II, Hospital utilization. Data for additional years are available (see Appendix III).

SOURCE: Centers for Disease Control and Prevention, National Center for Health Statistics, National Hospital Discharge Survey.

Table 91. Discharges, days of care, and average length of stay in non-Federal short-stay hospitals for discharges with the diagnosis of human immunodeficiency virus (HIV) and for all discharges: United States, selected years 1986–2001

[Data are based on a sample of hospital records]

Type of discharge, sex, and age	1986[1]	1987[1]	1990	1995	1997	1998	1999	2000[2]	2001[3]
Discharges in thousands									
HIV discharges............	44	67	146	249	178	189	180	173	185
Male, 20–49 years........	35	51	102	162	107	113	101	88	93
Female, 20–49 years.....	*	*	27	55	46	51	52	48	55
All discharges............	34,256	33,387	30,788	30,722	30,914	31,827	32,132	31,706	32,653
Male, 20–49 years.......	4,300	4,075	3,649	3,360	3,116	3,154	3,149	3,195	3,333
Female, 20–49 years.....	9,027	8,980	8,228	7,593	7,322	7,639	7,396	7,350	7,679
Discharges per 1,000 population									
HIV discharges............	0.18	0.28	0.58	0.94	0.66	0.69	0.65	0.62	0.65
Male, 20–49 years........	0.67	0.96	1.79	2.72	1.77	1.88	1.68	1.43	1.51
Female, 20–49 years.....	*	*	0.47	0.91	0.76	0.84	0.85	0.77	0.89
All discharges............	143.7	138.8	122.3	115.7	114.3	116.5	116.6	112.9	115.1
Male, 20–49 years.......	82.2	76.8	64.2	56.5	51.8	52.6	52.3	52.1	53.9
Female, 20–49 years.....	166.7	163.6	142.2	125.9	120.8	125.2	121.0	118.8	123.4
Days of care in thousands									
HIV discharges............	714	936	2,188	2,326	1,448	1,503	1,310	1,257	1,435
Male, 20–49 years........	573	724	1,645	1,408	855	892	669	723	713
Female, 20–49 years.....	*	*	341	559	364	365	384	299	454
All discharges............	218,496	214,942	197,422	164,627	157,458	160,914	160,128	155,857	159,365
Male, 20–49 years.......	26,488	26,295	22,539	17,984	15,529	16,085	15,278	15,665	16,435
Female, 20–49 years.....	40,620	39,356	34,473	26,596	24,955	25,976	25,415	24,883	26,502
Days of care per 1,000 population									
HIV discharges............	2.99	3.89	8.69	8.76	5.35	5.50	4.75	4.47	5.06
Male, 20–49 years.......	10.95	13.64	28.96	23.70	14.22	14.86	11.11	11.79	11.55
Female, 20–49 years.....	*	*	5.90	9.27	6.00	5.98	6.28	4.83	7.29
All discharges............	916.5	893.6	784.0	620.2	582.3	589.2	581.1	554.8	561.9
Male, 20–49 years.......	506.4	495.2	396.8	302.7	258.3	268.0	253.8	255.4	266.0
Female, 20–49 years.....	750.2	717.1	595.7	441.0	411.7	425.8	415.7	402.1	425.9
Average length of stay in days									
HIV discharges............	16.4	14.1	14.9	9.3	8.1	8.0	7.3	7.3	7.8
Male, 20–49 years.......	16.4	14.1	16.2	8.7	8.0	8.0	6.6	8.2	7.7
Female, 20–49 years.....	*	*	12.6	10.2	7.9	7.1	7.4	6.3	8.2
All discharges............	6.4	6.4	6.4	5.4	5.1	5.1	5.0	4.9	4.9
Male, 20–49 years.......	6.2	6.5	6.2	5.4	5.0	5.1	4.9	4.9	4.9
Female, 20–49 years.....	4.5	4.4	4.2	3.5	3.4	3.4	3.4	3.4	3.5

* Statistics based on fewer than 5,000 estimated discharges are considered unreliable and are not shown. These estimates generally have a relative standard error of more than 30 percent or a sample size of less than 30 discharges.

[1]Comparisons of data from 1986 and 1987 with data from later years should be made with caution as estimates of change may reflect improvements in the design rather than true changes in hospital use. See Appendix I, National Hospital Discharge Survey.

[2]The civilian population estimates used to compute rates for 2000 differ from those used in *Health, United States, 2002*. Rates for 2000 were computed using Census 2000 counts, while in the previous edition of *Health, United States*, rates for 2000 were computed using 1990-based postcensal estimates.

[3]Rates for 2001 were computed using 2000-based postcensal estimates.

NOTES: Excludes newborn infants. Rates are based on the civilian population as of July 1. Rates for 1990–99 use population estimates based on the 1990 census adjusted for net underenumeration using the 1990 National Population Adjustment Matrix from the U.S. Bureau of the Census. Rates for 1990–99 are not strictly comparable with rates for 2000 and 2001 because population estimates for 1990–99 have not been revised to reflect Census 2000. See Appendix I, National Hospital Discharge Survey. Discharges with diagnosis of HIV have at least one HIV diagnosis listed on the face sheet of the medical record and are not limited to the first-listed diagnosis. See Appendix II, Human immunodeficiency virus (HIV) infection. Data for additional years are available (see Appendix III).

SOURCE: Centers for Disease Control and Prevention, National Center for Health Statistics, National Hospital Discharge Survey.

Table 92 (page 1 of 3). Rates of discharges and days of care in non-Federal short-stay hospitals, according to sex, age, and selected first-listed diagnoses: United States, selected years 1990–2001

[Data are based on a sample of hospital records]

Sex, age, and first-listed diagnosis	Discharges			Days of care		
	1990	2000[1]	2001[2]	1990	2000[1]	2001[2]
Both sexes	Number per 1,000 population					
Total[3,4]	125.2	113.3	115.3	818.9	557.8	563.2
Male						
All ages[3,4]	113.0	99.1	100.2	805.8	536.0	535.7
Under 18 years[4]	46.3	40.9	43.8	233.6	195.6	200.7
Pneumonia	5.3	5.4	6.2	22.6	17.3	21.2
Asthma	3.3	3.5	2.0	9.3	7.4	4.8
Injuries and poisoning	6.8	5.0	5.2	30.1	21.4	*21.3
Fracture, all sites	2.2	1.8	1.7	9.3	7.2	6.0
18–44 years[4]	57.9	45.0	46.2	351.7	217.5	225.9
Alcohol and drug[5]	3.7	4.0	4.0	33.1	19.1	*20.4
Serious mental illness[6]	3.4	*5.3	*6.1	47.1	*43.6	*47.7
Diseases of heart	3.0	2.7	2.7	16.3	9.4	10.0
Intervertebral disc disorders	2.6	1.5	1.3	10.7	3.2	3.0
Injuries and poisoning	13.1	7.3	7.4	65.7	33.2	35.7
Fracture, all sites	4.0	2.5	2.7	22.7	12.8	12.7
45–64 years[4]	140.3	112.7	112.2	943.4	570.5	578.0
Malignant neoplasms	10.6	6.2	6.3	99.1	42.1	48.5
Trachea, bronchus, lung	2.7	0.9	0.9	19.1	5.2	*8.0
Diabetes	2.9	3.7	3.4	21.2	22.5	18.7
Alcohol and drug[5]	3.5	3.5	3.7	29.7	15.8	17.1
Serious mental illness[6]	2.5	*4.0	4.7	34.8	*34.6	*43.9
Diseases of heart	31.7	26.4	24.5	185.0	101.5	98.4
Ischemic heart disease	22.6	17.7	15.7	128.2	63.8	57.2
Acute myocardial infarction	7.4	5.9	5.5	55.8	27.8	25.3
Congestive heart failure	3.0	3.3	3.5	19.7	17.2	17.4
Cerebrovascular diseases	4.1	3.8	3.3	40.7	19.8	18.5
Pneumonia	3.5	3.4	3.4	27.4	20.5	18.4
Injuries and poisoning	11.6	8.8	9.8	82.6	49.8	50.0
Fracture, all sites	3.3	2.5	2.7	24.2	16.2	13.3
65–74 years[4]	287.8	264.9	260.9	2,251.5	1,489.6	1,473.0
Malignant neoplasms	27.9	17.6	18.0	277.6	121.2	136.2
Large intestine and rectum	3.0	3.0	2.8	34.2	27.3	24.0
Trachea, bronchus, lung	6.4	2.8	2.8	55.7	19.2	23.0
Prostate	5.1	3.7	3.4	33.1	14.0	*15.4
Diabetes	4.4	4.7	4.9	39.8	29.0	25.1
Serious mental illness[6]	2.5	*3.4	*2.9	43.8	39.9	*
Diseases of heart	69.4	70.6	68.2	487.2	331.9	315.0
Ischemic heart disease	42.0	39.6	38.6	285.2	171.1	169.7
Acute myocardial infarction	14.0	12.5	12.1	122.4	66.5	69.5
Congestive heart failure	11.4	13.4	12.9	90.2	76.8	74.7
Cerebrovascular diseases	13.8	13.2	13.1	114.8	59.0	62.1
Pneumonia	11.4	12.8	13.3	107.8	82.0	75.1
Hyperplasia of prostate	14.4	5.4	4.2	65.0	15.0	10.1
Osteoarthritis	5.0	9.6	7.8	44.9	46.7	35.1
Injuries and poisoning	17.6	17.9	17.3	139.0	105.7	127.5
Fracture, all sites	4.5	4.7	5.0	45.9	29.9	38.5
Fracture of neck of femur (hip)	1.5	*2.0	2.0	*18.1	*15.9	*15.6
75 years and over[4]	478.5	467.8	471.9	4,231.6	2,890.5	2,801.1
Malignant neoplasms	41.0	21.9	24.8	408.3	165.4	171.7
Large intestine and rectum	5.4	4.2	4.3	80.7	44.1	38.8
Trachea, bronchus, lung	5.4	3.0	4.1	53.4	18.3	28.8
Prostate	9.7	3.2	*4.3	65.6	*19.4	*18.0
Diabetes	4.6	6.5	6.1	51.2	43.2	39.6
Serious mental illness[6]	*2.6	2.9	3.1	*40.5	*32.7	*28.3
Diseases of heart	106.2	113.3	115.6	855.7	601.4	584.8
Ischemic heart disease	49.1	53.0	49.5	398.1	276.3	246.4
Acute myocardial infarction	23.1	23.0	21.1	227.5	136.6	136.3
Congestive heart failure	31.0	30.6	33.5	242.3	175.6	171.9
Cerebrovascular diseases	30.2	30.3	24.9	298.3	171.5	129.4
Pneumonia	38.6	37.2	39.5	393.6	233.5	254.5
Hyperplasia of prostate	17.9	6.8	7.2	109.2	21.6	*25.2
Osteoarthritis	5.8	6.2	8.2	60.7	28.8	36.4
Injuries and poisoning	31.2	33.6	31.6	341.3	257.9	206.2
Fracture, all sites	13.7	14.4	13.7	145.1	*119.3	99.4
Fracture of neck of femur (hip)	8.5	8.5	7.9	97.8	63.3	56.6

See footnotes at end of table.

[Data are based on a sample of hospital records]

Sex, age, and first-listed diagnosis	Discharges			Days of care		
	1990	2000[1]	2001[2]	1990	2000[1]	2001[2]
Female	Number per 1,000 population					
All ages[3,4]	139.0	127.8	130.9	840.5	581.2	592.9
Under 18 years[4]	46.4	39.6	43.0	218.7	161.5	184.3
Pneumonia	4.0	4.8	5.0	17.4	17.2	17.1
Asthma	2.2	2.4	1.3	6.8	5.5	2.8
Injuries and poisoning	4.3	3.1	3.4	16.7	*12.0	12.1
Fracture, all sites	1.3	0.9	0.8	6.4	2.3	2.5
18–44 years[4]	146.8	124.9	129.1	582.0	401.3	421.5
Delivery	69.9	64.6	66.3	195.0	160.3	167.0
Alcohol and drug[5]	1.6	*2.1	2.0	14.1	*10.8	*10.4
Serious mental illness[6]	3.7	*5.4	6.1	54.3	*41.1	45.4
Diseases of heart	1.3	1.7	1.8	7.2	6.3	6.3
Intervertebral disc disorders	1.5	1.0	1.0	7.3	2.4	2.7
Injuries and poisoning	6.7	4.3	4.8	36.6	18.1	18.7
Fracture, all sites	1.6	1.0	1.1	10.7	4.5	4.8
45–64 years[4]	131.0	110.2	111.9	886.5	533.7	551.6
Malignant neoplasms	12.7	6.1	6.1	107.4	34.7	37.6
Trachea, bronchus, lung	1.7	0.5	0.8	14.8	3.4	5.2
Breast	2.8	1.3	1.2	12.1	2.6	3.0
Diabetes	2.9	2.9	2.8	25.8	15.0	12.8
Alcohol and drug[5]	1.0	1.5	1.5	8.0	*7.1	*7.0
Serious mental illness[6]	4.0	4.6	5.6	60.5	42.7	58.1
Diseases of heart	16.6	14.6	15.0	101.1	59.5	64.5
Ischemic heart disease	9.9	7.8	8.2	57.4	29.5	32.5
Acute myocardial infarction	2.8	2.0	2.6	21.6	10.0	14.6
Congestive heart failure	2.1	2.9	2.8	15.8	13.6	14.3
Cerebrovascular diseases	3.0	3.5	3.1	32.1	19.5	14.9
Pneumonia	3.4	3.6	3.4	26.5	20.8	18.4
Injuries and poisoning	9.4	7.7	8.5	63.3	41.2	45.9
Fracture, all sites	3.1	2.7	2.5	25.0	13.3	11.5
65–74 years[4]	241.1	246.1	252.3	1,959.3	1,397.1	1,431.5
Malignant neoplasms	20.9	14.1	14.7	189.8	101.0	106.7
Large intestine and rectum	2.4	1.7	2.1	34.9	15.2	19.0
Trachea, bronchus, lung	2.6	2.4	2.3	26.9	*17.5	16.5
Breast	3.9	2.8	2.2	17.6	*	5.4
Diabetes	5.8	4.6	5.9	46.8	26.1	36.4
Serious mental illness[6]	3.9	4.0	4.7	62.8	46.3	60.1
Diseases of heart	45.1	52.1	48.8	316.9	256.0	237.9
Ischemic heart disease	24.4	23.3	22.1	153.8	113.9	108.0
Acute myocardial infarction	7.5	8.0	8.0	58.1	52.8	59.6
Congestive heart failure	9.2	12.7	11.1	81.8	68.4	63.1
Cerebrovascular diseases	11.3	12.3	11.7	96.0	59.4	61.8
Pneumonia	8.7	11.7	11.5	81.8	73.5	74.7
Osteoarthritis	6.9	9.3	10.0	68.9	43.6	46.6
Injuries and poisoning	17.8	18.3	18.9	166.2	109.9	117.9
Fracture, all sites	8.4	7.7	7.9	97.3	43.8	41.9
Fracture of neck of femur (hip)	3.6	3.2	3.4	*59.6	21.1	20.3

See footnotes at end of table.

Table 92 (page 3 of 3). Rates of discharges and days of care in non-Federal short-stay hospitals, according to sex, age, and selected first-listed diagnoses: United States, selected years 1990–2001

[Data are based on a sample of hospital records]

Sex, age, and first-listed diagnosis	Discharges			Days of care		
	1990	2000[1]	2001[2]	1990	2000[1]	2001[2]
Female—Con.	Number per 1,000 population					
75 years and over[4]	409.6	459.0	455.2	3,887.1	2,832.3	2,694.5
Malignant neoplasms	22.1	17.6	18.0	257.3	125.7	136.2
Large intestine and rectum	4.6	3.4	3.2	69.8	28.4	29.6
Trachea, bronchus, lung	2.1	1.9	1.8	20.6	14.0	13.8
Breast	3.9	2.5	2.6	22.0	*8.9	*9.5
Diabetes	4.6	6.3	6.3	55.3	34.0	32.8
Serious mental illness[6]	4.2	4.7	4.2	78.4	49.3	45.7
Diseases of heart	84.6	99.1	94.4	672.8	523.7	476.7
Ischemic heart disease	33.7	35.5	34.0	253.2	185.6	160.0
Acute myocardial infarction	13.1	16.5	16.9	125.9	110.7	101.6
Congestive heart failure	28.0	32.2	31.4	236.6	181.8	175.2
Cerebrovascular diseases	29.6	27.6	28.2	302.0	156.9	146.9
Pneumonia	23.9	30.5	26.7	260.1	209.8	180.8
Osteoarthritis	5.3	8.7	10.0	54.1	40.4	44.0
Injuries and poisoning	46.3	44.7	47.1	489.2	275.6	284.9
Fracture, all sites	31.5	30.0	30.1	352.7	190.1	179.9
Fracture of neck of femur (hip)	18.8	17.9	17.8	236.3	125.3	113.8

* Estimates are considered unreliable. Data preceded by an asterisk have a relative standard error (RSE) of 20–30 percent. Data not shown have a RSE of greater than 30 percent.
[1]The civilian population estimates used to compute rates for 2000 differ from those used in *Health, United States, 2002*. Rates for 2000 were computed using Census 2000 counts, while in the previous edition of *Health, United States*, rates for 2000 were computed using 1990-based postcensal estimates.
[2]Rates for 2001 were computed using 2000-based postcensal estimates.
[3]Estimates are age adjusted to the year 2000 standard population using six age groups: under 18 years, 18–44 years, 45–54 years, 55–64 years, 65–74 years, and 75 years and over. See Appendix II, Age adjustment.
[4]Includes discharges with first-listed diagnoses not shown in table.
[5]Includes abuse, dependence, and withdrawal. These estimates are for non-Federal short-stay hospitals and do not include alcohol and drug discharges from other types of facilities or programs such as the Department of Veterans Affairs or day treatment programs.
[6]These estimates are for non-Federal short-stay hospitals and do not include serious mental illness discharges from other types of facilities or programs such as the Department of Veterans Affairs or long-term hospitals.

NOTES: Excludes newborn infants. Rates are based on the civilian population as of July 1. Diagnostic categories are based on the *International Classification of Diseases, Ninth Revision, Clinical Modification*. For a listing of the code numbers, see Appendix II, table IX. Rates for 1990–99 use population estimates based on the 1990 census adjusted for net underenumeration using the 1990 National Population Adjustment Matrix from the U.S. Bureau of the Census. Rates for 1990–99 are not strictly comparable with rates for 2000 and 2001 because population estimates for 1990–99 have not been revised to reflect Census 2000. See Appendix I, National Hospital Discharge Survey. Data for additional years are available (see Appendix III).

SOURCE: Centers for Disease Control and Prevention, National Center for Health Statistics, National Hospital Discharge Survey.

[Data are based on a sample of hospital records]

Sex, age, and first-listed diagnosis	Discharges			Average length of stay		
	1990	2000	2001	1990	2000	2001
Both sexes	Number in thousands			Number of days		
Total[1,2]	30,788	31,706	32,653	6.5	4.9	4.9
Male						
All ages[1,2]	12,280	12,514	12,852	7.1	5.4	5.3
Under 18 years[2]	1,572	1,515	1,629	5.0	4.8	4.6
Pneumonia	178	199	229	4.3	3.2	3.4
Asthma	111	129	76	2.8	2.1	2.3
Injuries and poisoning	232	185	192	4.4	4.3	*4.1
Fracture, all sites	76	68	63	4.2	3.9	3.5
18–44 years[2]	3,120	2,498	2,573	6.1	4.8	4.9
Alcohol and drug[3]	201	224	225	8.9	4.7	*5.1
Serious mental illness[4]	184	*296	*338	13.8	*8.2	*7.9
Diseases of heart	163	148	150	5.4	3.5	3.7
Intervertebral disc disorders	138	81	74	4.2	2.2	2.2
Injuries and poisoning	704	408	412	5.0	4.5	4.8
Fracture, all sites	217	141	148	5.6	5.0	4.8
45–64 years[2]	3,115	3,424	3,519	6.7	5.1	5.2
Malignant neoplasms	235	188	199	9.4	6.8	7.7
Trachea, bronchus, lung	60	26	28	7.1	6.0	*8.8
Diabetes	65	114	107	7.3	6.0	5.5
Alcohol and drug[3]	77	106	115	8.5	4.5	4.7
Serious mental illness[4]	56	*120	148	13.7	*8.8	*9.3
Diseases of heart	704	802	768	5.8	3.8	4.0
Ischemic heart disease	502	539	492	5.7	3.6	3.6
Acute myocardial infarction	165	178	172	7.5	4.7	4.6
Congestive heart failure	66	101	110	6.7	5.2	5.0
Cerebrovascular diseases	91	116	102	10.0	5.2	5.7
Pneumonia	77	104	108	7.9	6.0	5.4
Injuries and poisoning	257	266	307	7.2	5.7	5.1
Fracture, all sites	74	77	85	7.2	6.4	4.9
65–74 years[2]	2,268	2,199	2,165	7.8	5.6	5.6
Malignant neoplasms	220	146	149	9.9	6.9	7.6
Large intestine and rectum	24	24	23	11.4	9.2	8.7
Trachea, bronchus, lung	50	23	23	8.7	6.8	8.4
Prostate	40	31	28	6.5	3.8	*4.6
Diabetes	34	39	41	9.1	6.2	5.1
Serious mental illness[4]	20	*28	*24	17.4	*11.7	*
Diseases of heart	547	586	566	7.0	4.7	4.6
Ischemic heart disease	331	329	320	6.8	4.3	4.4
Acute myocardial infarction	110	104	100	8.8	5.3	5.8
Congestive heart failure	90	112	107	7.9	5.7	5.8
Cerebrovascular diseases	108	109	109	8.3	4.5	4.7
Pneumonia	90	106	111	9.5	6.4	5.6
Hyperplasia of prostate	113	45	35	4.5	2.8	2.4
Osteoarthritis	39	80	65	9.0	4.9	4.5
Injuries and poisoning	139	149	143	7.9	5.9	7.4
Fracture, all sites	36	39	41	10.2	6.4	7.8
Fracture of neck of femur (hip)	12	*17	17	*11.8	*7.9	*7.8
75 years and over[2]	2,203	2,878	2,966	8.8	6.2	5.9
Malignant neoplasms	189	135	156	10.0	7.6	6.9
Large intestine and rectum	25	26	27	15.0	10.6	9.1
Trachea, bronchus, lung	25	18	26	10.0	6.1	7.1
Prostate	45	20	*27	6.8	*6.1	*4.2
Diabetes	21	40	38	11.0	6.6	6.5
Serious mental illness[4]	*12	18	19	*15.5	*11.2	*9.1
Diseases of heart	489	697	727	8.1	5.3	5.1
Ischemic heart disease	226	326	311	8.1	5.2	5.0
Acute myocardial infarction	106	141	133	9.9	5.9	6.4
Congestive heart failure	143	188	210	7.8	5.7	5.1
Cerebrovascular diseases	139	186	157	9.9	5.7	5.2
Pneumonia	178	229	248	10.2	6.3	6.4
Hyperplasia of prostate	82	42	45	6.1	3.2	*3.5
Osteoarthritis	27	38	52	10.5	4.6	4.4
Injuries and poisoning	144	207	199	10.9	7.7	6.5
Fracture, all sites	63	89	86	10.6	*8.3	7.3
Fracture of neck of femur (hip)	39	52	50	11.5	7.5	7.1

See footnotes at end of table.

[Data are based on a sample of hospital records]

Sex, age, and first-listed diagnosis	Discharges			Average length of stay		
	1990	2000	2001	1990	2000	2001
Female	Number in thousands			Number of days		
All ages[1,2]	18,508	19,192	19,801	6.0	4.5	4.5
Under 18 years[2]	1,500	1,397	1,523	4.7	4.1	4.3
Pneumonia	129	168	176	4.4	3.6	3.5
Asthma	71	85	45	3.1	2.3	2.2
Injuries and poisoning	138	111	120	3.9	*3.8	3.6
Fracture, all sites	42	32	30	5.0	2.5	2.9
18–44 years[2]	8,018	6,941	7,178	4.0	3.2	3.3
Delivery	3,815	3,588	3,685	2.8	2.5	2.5
Alcohol and drug[3]	85	*116	112	9.1	*5.2	*5.2
Serious mental illness[4]	200	*300	338	14.8	*7.6	7.5
Diseases of heart	73	95	99	5.4	3.7	3.5
Intervertebral disc disorders	84	58	55	4.7	2.3	2.7
Injuries and poisoning	366	237	267	5.5	4.2	3.9
Fracture, all sites	85	57	62	6.9	4.4	4.3
45–64 years[2]	3,129	3,534	3,705	6.8	4.8	4.9
Malignant neoplasms	303	195	203	8.5	5.7	6.1
Trachea, bronchus, lung	41	17	28	8.6	6.4	6.2
Breast	67	40	40	4.3	2.1	2.5
Diabetes	70	93	94	8.9	5.2	4.5
Alcohol and drug[3]	23	47	51	8.2	*4.8	*4.5
Serious mental illness[4]	95	146	184	15.2	9.4	10.4
Diseases of heart	397	470	497	6.1	4.1	4.3
Ischemic heart disease	237	251	272	5.8	3.8	4.0
Acute myocardial infarction	68	64	86	7.6	5.0	5.6
Congestive heart failure	51	94	91	7.4	4.6	5.2
Cerebrovascular diseases	72	113	102	10.7	5.5	4.9
Pneumonia	80	117	113	7.9	5.7	5.4
Injuries and poisoning	225	248	280	6.7	5.3	5.4
Fracture, all sites	75	87	83	7.9	4.9	4.6
65–74 years[2]	2,421	2,479	2,527	8.1	5.7	5.7
Malignant neoplasms	210	142	147	9.1	7.2	7.3
Large intestine and rectum	24	17	21	14.5	9.0	8.9
Trachea, bronchus, lung	26	25	23	10.2	*7.1	7.2
Breast	40	29	22	4.5	*	2.4
Diabetes	59	47	59	8.0	5.6	6.1
Serious mental illness[4]	· 39	40	47	16.3	11.7	12.8
Diseases of heart	453	525	489	7.0	4.9	4.9
Ischemic heart disease	245	235	222	6.3	4.9	4.9
Acute myocardial infarction	75	81	80	7.8	6.6	7.4
Congestive heart failure	92	128	111	8.9	5.4	5.7
Cerebrovascular diseases	114	124	118	8.5	4.8	5.3
Pneumonia	87	117	115	9.4	6.3	6.5
Osteoarthritis	69	94	100	10.0	4.7	4.7
Injuries and poisoning	179	185	189	9.3	6.0	6.2
Fracture, all sites	85	77	79	11.5	5.7	5.3
Fracture of neck of femur (hip)	36	32	34	*16.7	6.7	5.9

See footnotes at end of table.

Table 93 (page 3 of 3). Discharges and average length of stay in non-Federal short-stay hospitals, according to sex, age, and selected first-listed diagnoses: United States, selected years 1990–2001

[Data are based on a sample of hospital records]

Sex, age, and first-listed diagnosis	Discharges			Average length of stay		
	1990	2000	2001	1990	2000	2001
Female—Con.	Number in thousands			Number of days		
75 years and over[2]	3,440	4,840	4,867	9.5	6.2	5.9
Malignant neoplasms	185	186	192	11.7	7.1	7.6
Large intestine and rectum.	39	36	34	15.1	8.4	9.3
Trachea, bronchus, lung	18	20	19	9.9	7.3	7.7
Breast	33	27	28	5.7	*3.5	*3.7
Diabetes	39	67	67	11.9	5.4	5.2
Serious mental illness[4]	35	49	45	18.7	10.5	10.9
Diseases of heart	711	1,045	1,010	8.0	5.3	5.0
Ischemic heart disease	283	375	363	7.5	5.2	4.7
Acute myocardial infarction	110	174	181	9.6	6.7	6.0
Congestive heart failure	235	339	336	8.5	5.6	5.6
Cerebrovascular diseases	249	292	301	10.2	5.7	5.2
Pneumonia	201	322	286	10.9	6.9	6.8
Osteoarthritis	45	91	107	10.2	4.7	4.4
Injuries and poisoning	389	472	503	10.6	6.2	6.1
Fracture, all sites.	265	316	322	11.2	6.3	6.0
Fracture of neck of femur (hip)	158	189	190	12.5	7.0	6.4

* Estimates are considered unreliable. Data preceded by an asterisk have a relative standard error (RSE) of 20–30 percent. Data not shown have a RSE of greater than 30 percent.
[1]Average length of stay estimates are age adjusted to the year 2000 standard population using six age groups: under 18 years, 18–44 years, 45–54 years, 55–64 years, 65–74 years, and 75 years and over. See Appendix II, Age adjustment.
[2]Includes discharges with first-listed diagnoses not shown in table.
[3]Includes abuse, dependence, and withdrawal. These estimates are for non-Federal short-stay hospitals and do not include alcohol and drug discharges from other types of facilities or programs such as the Department of Veterans Affairs or day treatment programs.
[4]These estimates are for non-Federal short-stay hospitals and do not include serious mental illness discharges from other types of facilities or programs such as the Department of Veterans Affairs or long-term hospitals.

NOTES: Excludes newborn infants. Diagnostic categories are based on the *International Classification of Diseases, Ninth Revision, Clinical Modification.* For a listing of the code numbers, see Appendix II, table IX. Data for additional years are available (see Appendix III).

SOURCE: Centers for Disease Control and Prevention, National Center for Health Statistics, National Hospital Discharge Survey.

Table 94 (page 1 of 3). Ambulatory and inpatient procedures according to place, sex, age, and type of procedure: United States, selected years 1994–2001

[Data are based on a sample of inpatient and ambulatory surgery records]

Sex, age, and procedure category	Ambulatory[1]			Inpatient[2]					
	1994	1995	1996	1994	1995	1996	1999	2000[3]	2001[4]
Both sexes				Procedures per 1,000 population					
Total[5,6]	107.9	113.6	120.1	157.9	152.7	153.3	151.5	142.8	144.9
Male									
All ages[5,6]	102.5	107.9	115.0	139.1	135.1	136.1	133.4	124.1	124.9
Under 18 years[6]	45.6	43.0	44.7	36.0	37.4	36.3	37.6	34.7	39.9
Myringotomy with insertion of tube	9.1	8.5	8.2	0.4	0.3	0.4	*0.2	0.3	*0.2
Tonsillectomy, with or without adenoidectomy . . .	3.6	4.1	3.6	0.4	0.4	0.4	*0.2	*0.2	0.3
Reduction of fracture.	1.0	1.0	1.2	1.6	1.2	1.5	1.3	1.3	1.4
18–44 years[6]	58.4	61.3	63.7	62.7	59.5	58.1	52.5	49.2	50.0
Cardiac catheterization	0.5	*0.3	0.6	1.1	1.1	1.2	1.2	1.1	1.1
Endoscopy of small or large intestine with or without biopsy . . .	5.2	5.2	5.8	2.0	1.8	1.5	1.5	1.5	1.7
Cholecystectomy	*0.2	*0.3	0.5	0.5	0.5	0.4	0.5	0.4	0.5
Reduction of fracture.	1.0	1.0	1.4	2.3	2.5	2.4	2.2	2.1	2.0
Arthroscopy of the knee	3.5	4.0	3.4	0.5	0.3	*0.2	*	*	*
Excision or destruction of intervertebral disc	*	*	*0.3	1.7	1.5	1.4	1.4	1.3	1.2
Angiocardiography with contrast material.	0.7	0.4	0.6	1.8	1.8	1.8	1.7	1.6	1.5
45–64 years[6]	132.7	146.8	155.9	189.0	180.7	185.9	177.9	165.8	161.5
Coronary angioplasty	*	*	*	5.6	5.6	6.4	7.2	5.7	5.7
Coronary artery bypass graft[7]	–	–	–	6.7	7.6	7.2	6.2	5.6	5.1
Cardiac catheterization	3.3	3.8	5.4	11.7	11.7	12.7	12.6	11.4	10.0
Endoscopy of small or large intestine with or without biopsy . . .	20.2	21.1	21.8	7.2	6.5	6.4	5.8	6.0	6.1
Cholecystectomy	*0.5	*0.7	1.1	2.1	1.8	2.1	1.7	1.6	1.5
Prostatectomy	*	*	*	2.5	2.2	1.9	1.7	1.6	1.8
Reduction of fracture.	*0.6	*0.8	0.8	2.3	2.3	2.0	1.9	1.9	2.0
Arthroscopy of the knee	3.7	4.5	4.4	*0.3	*	*	*	*	*
Excision or destruction of intervertebral disc	*	*	*	2.6	2.2	2.6	2.4	2.2	2.1
Angiocardiography with contrast material.	4.6	5.1	6.4	16.0	15.8	17.7	15.7	14.7	11.9
65–74 years[6]	271.6	282.5	316.4	426.4	419.5	417.7	417.1	388.6	376.3
Coronary angioplasty	*	*	*	10.0	9.4	11.7	12.6	12.2	12.0
Extraction of lens	31.6	33.4	36.9	*	*	*	*	*	*
Insertion of prosthetic lens (pseudophakos).	25.8	26.0	29.6	*	*	*	*	*	*
Coronary artery bypass graft[7]	–	–	–	15.4	18.3	19.2	15.9	13.5	14.2
Cardiac catheterization	5.7	7.1	10.2	22.3	23.6	23.1	24.1	22.4	22.9
Pacemaker insertion or replacement.	*	*	*	5.6	4.8	5.7	5.0	4.4	4.2
Carotid endarterectomy	*	*	*	3.3	4.2	3.9	3.1	3.0	2.7
Endoscopy of small or large intestine with or without biopsy . . .	42.6	42.8	40.2	18.4	16.5	16.6	17.1	16.6	16.8
Cholecystectomy	*	*	*	4.5	4.4	4.0	3.7	3.8	3.6
Prostatectomy	*	*	*1.5	14.2	12.3	10.3	9.1	8.6	7.4
Reduction of fracture.	*	*	*	2.8	2.5	2.4	2.8	2.8	3.0
Total hip replacement	–	-	–	1.7	2.5	2.3	2.5	2.7	1.9
Angiocardiography with contrast material.	9.0	9.3	13.5	31.0	30.5	29.7	30.3	28.0	27.6
75 years and over[6]	339.2	355.1	378.7	584.1	567.2	578.9	593.3	548.1	564.6
Coronary angioplasty	*	*	*	6.5	8.2	7.4	10.9	10.3	12.0
Extraction of lens	61.7	71.5	71.6	*	*	*	*	*	*
Insertion of prosthetic lens (pseudophakos).	47.9	53.6	55.1	*	*	*	*	*	*
Coronary artery bypass graft[7]	–	-	–	10.7	12.5	11.6	11.5	12.4	11.4
Cardiac catheterization	*3.8	4.7	7.1	18.1	19.2	19.7	21.4	21.5	22.5
Pacemaker insertion or replacement.	*	*	*	15.4	15.4	16.4	13.9	14.6	20.0
Carotid endarterectomy	*	–	-	3.6	4.6	4.6	4.2	4.3	4.9
Endoscopy of small or large intestine with or without biopsy . . .	43.2	43.4	48.9	35.9	36.4	35.2	33.6	33.0	38.8
Cholecystectomy	*	*	*	6.2	5.5	5.8	4.5	4.6	5.9
Prostatectomy	*2.1	*2.3	*2.2	16.1	15.3	12.3	10.8	10.2	10.7
Reduction of fracture.	*	*	*	6.4	6.4	6.6	6.3	6.6	6.4
Total hip replacement	–	-	–	2.2	2.1	2.2	2.5	1.8	2.3
Angiocardiography with contrast material.	*3.8	5.5	10.3	24.2	24.0	25.9	25.5	27.0	25.5

See footnotes at end of table.

Table 94 (page 2 of 3). Ambulatory and inpatient procedures according to place, sex, age, and type of procedure: United States, selected years 1994–2001

[Data are based on a sample of inpatient and ambulatory surgery records]

Sex, age, and procedure category	Ambulatory[1]			Inpatient[2]					
	1994	1995	1996	1994	1995	1996	1999	2000[3]	2001[4]
Female	Procedures per 1,000 population								
All ages[5,6]	114.2	120.1	126.1	179.2	172.7	173.0	171.5	163.4	167.0
Under 18 years[6]	35.3	34.3	34.8	40.3	39.0	38.4	38.0	34.6	36.7
Myringotomy with insertion of tube	6.7	6.3	5.6	0.4	0.3	*0.3	*	*0.2	*0.2
Tonsillectomy, with or without adenoidectomy	4.8	4.4	4.7	0.5	0.4	0.3	*0.2	*0.2	*0.1
Reduction of fracture	*0.5	0.7	0.8	0.8	0.7	0.5	0.5	0.7	0.7
18–44 years[6]	94.9	96.9	102.2	203.6	195.4	195.0	185.8	184.0	189.5
Cardiac catheterization	*	*0.2	*0.3	0.5	0.5	0.4	0.6	0.6	0.5
Endoscopy of small or large intestine with or without biopsy	6.6	7.4	8.4	2.1	1.9	1.9	1.7	1.7	1.8
Cholecystectomy	1.4	1.9	2.2	2.2	2.4	2.0	1.8	1.9	2.2
Bilateral destruction or occlusion of fallopian tubes	5.6	6.4	5.7	6.6	5.9	6.2	5.9	5.7	5.8
Hysterectomy[8]	*	*0.3	*0.2	5.4	5.9	5.6	5.7	5.7	5.9
Cesarean section[8]	–	-	–	15.0	13.8	14.6	14.7	15.0	17.0
Repair of current obstetrical laceration	*	*	*	15.7	16.8	18.3	19.4	19.6	20.4
Reduction of fracture	0.4	0.5	0.5	1.1	1.1	1.1	1.1	0.9	1.0
Arthroscopy of the knee	1.8	2.0	2.0	0.2	*0.1	*0.1	*	*	*
Excision or destruction of intervertebral disc	*	*	*	1.2	0.9	1.0	1.0	0.9	0.9
Lumpectomy	2.5	2.0	2.2	*0.1	*0.1	*	*	*	*
Mastectomy	*	*	*	0.3	0.2	0.2	0.2	0.2	0.3
45–64 years[6]	155.5	165.9	173.2	173.4	162.6	162.2	160.9	147.7	151.7
Coronary angioplasty	*	*	*	2.1	2.0	2.0	2.6	2.1	2.1
Coronary artery bypass graft[7]	–	-	–	2.0	1.7	2.0	1.8	1.4	1.8
Cardiac catheterization	2.2	2.0	2.4	6.0	5.4	6.0	6.1	5.4	5.8
Endoscopy of small or large intestine with or without biopsy	22.1	24.3	22.9	6.5	6.2	5.6	5.9	5.4	5.4
Cholecystectomy	1.8	2.3	3.3	3.7	3.5	3.4	2.9	2.5	2.5
Hysterectomy	*	*	*	7.2	7.1	7.9	7.9	7.9	7.8
Reduction of fracture	*0.7	*0.7	0.8	2.2	2.2	2.3	2.0	2.1	2.0
Arthroscopy of the knee	2.8	3.4	3.5	*	*	*	*	*	*
Excision or destruction of intervertebral disc	*	*	*	2.0	1.6	1.8	2.1	1.9	1.9
Lumpectomy	4.9	5.0	4.6	0.5	0.4	0.4	*0.3	0.4	*0.2
Mastectomy	*	*	*0.4	1.6	1.5	1.3	1.1	1.1	1.1
Angiocardiography with contrast material	3.0	2.7	3.3	8.5	8.1	8.4	8.5	7.6	7.5
65–74 years[6]	254.6	272.5	291.9	328.3	326.1	334.4	340.8	318.8	329.8
Coronary angioplasty	*	*	*	4.9	4.6	5.7	6.3	6.3	5.8
Extraction of lens	41.8	48.3	47.8	*	*	*	*	*	*
Insertion of prosthetic lens (pseudophakos)	33.5	35.7	35.9	*	*	*	*	*	*
Coronary artery bypass graft[7]	–	*	–	5.1	6.1	6.7	6.5	5.1	4.7
Cardiac catheterization	3.3	3.6	5.4	12.6	12.4	14.7	15.0	13.5	13.1
Pacemaker insertion or replacement	*	*	*	4.3	3.9	3.7	5.6	3.8	4.3
Carotid endarterectomy	–	-	–	1.7	2.3	2.2	2.6	2.0	2.0
Endoscopy of small or large intestine with or without biopsy	39.0	41.0	45.5	16.1	18.2	14.7	18.2	18.1	18.0
Cholecystectomy	*1.3	*1.6	2.3	5.1	4.6	4.7	4.7	4.6	4.2
Hysterectomy	*	*	*	4.7	4.3	3.7	3.6	3.7	4.0
Reduction of fracture	*	*	*	4.7	4.4	5.0	4.4	4.9	5.2
Total hip replacement	–	-	*	2.6	2.7	2.9	3.3	2.5	2.8
Lumpectomy	4.4	4.7	4.9	*	*	*0.6	*	*0.7	*
Mastectomy	*	*	*	2.8	2.3	2.3	2.1	2.3	2.0
Angiocardiography with contrast material	4.8	5.0	6.9	18.0	17.5	20.3	19.9	17.5	17.9

See footnotes at end of table.

Table 94 (page 3 of 3). Ambulatory and inpatient procedures according to place, sex, age, and type of procedure: United States, selected years 1994–2001

[Data are based on a sample of inpatient and ambulatory surgery records]

Sex, age, and procedure category	Ambulatory[1]			Inpatient[2]					
	1994	1995	1996	1994	1995	1996	1999	2000[3]	2001[4]
Female—Con.	Procedures per 1,000 population								
75 years and over[6]	274.3	304.6	319.3	476.8	468.0	468.4	503.0	467.4	455.7
Coronary angioplasty	*	*	*	4.0	4.2	4.3	6.0	6.0	5.9
Extraction of lens	70.6	82.0	82.6	*	*	*	*	*	*
Insertion of prosthetic lens (pseudophakos)	54.5	61.3	61.4	*	*	*	*	*	*
Coronary artery bypass graft[7]	–	–	–	3.4	4.1	4.6	5.8	4.4	3.8
Cardiac catheterization	*1.5	*1.8	3.5	10.4	11.3	11.6	14.0	13.5	13.9
Pacemaker insertion or replacement	*	*	*1.1	11.5	10.1	11.3	10.4	10.3	10.8
Carotid endarterectomy	–	*	–	2.0	2.0	2.3	2.1	1.9	2.3
Endoscopy of small or large intestine with or without biopsy	34.5	39.3	38.6	36.0	35.0	33.2	38.2	35.8	35.6
Cholecystectomy	*	*	*1.2	4.3	5.5	5.0	5.3	4.1	4.9
Hysterectomy	–	*	*	2.4	2.4	2.7	2.3	2.3	2.1
Reduction of fracture	*	.*	*	13.9	14.6	16.9	16.0	14.4	14.4
Total hip replacement	–	*	*	3.2	3.3	3.5	3.3	2.9	3.9
Lumpectomy	2.7	2.5	2.9	*	*0.7	*	*	*0.6	*
Mastectomy	*	*	*	2.4	2.6	1.8	2.0	2.0	2.0
Angiocardiography with contrast material	2.3	*2.1	5.5	14.5	15.6	15.6	17.8	17.4	18.8

* Estimates are considered unreliable. Rates for inpatient procedures preceded by an asterisk are based on 5,000–8,999 estimated procedures; those based on fewer than 5,000 are not shown. Rates for ambulatory surgery preceded by an asterisk are based on 10,000–19,999 estimated procedures; those based on fewer than 10,000 are not shown. Estimates that are not shown generally have a relative standard error of more than 30 percent.
– Quantity zero.
[1]Data are from the National Survey of Ambulatory Surgery (conducted from 1994–96) and exclude ambulatory surgery procedures for patients who became inpatients. See Appendix II, Ambulatory surgery.
[2]Inpatient data are from the National Hospital Discharge Survey and exclude newborn infants.
[3]The civilian population estimates used to compute rates for 2000 differ from those used in Health, United States, 2002. Rates for 2000 were computed using Census 2000 counts, while in the previous edition of Health, United States, rates for 2000 were computed using 1990-based postcensal estimates.
[4]Rates for 2001 were computed using 2000-based postcensal estimates.
[5]Estimates are age adjusted to the year 2000 standard population using six age groups: under 18 years, 18–44 years, 45–54 years, 55–64 years, 65–74 years, and 75 years and over. See Appendix II, Age adjustment.
[6]Includes procedures not listed in table.
[7]Data in the main body of the table are for all-listed coronary artery bypass grafts. Often, more than one coronary bypass procedure is performed during a single operation. The following table gives additional information based on the number of inpatient discharges with one or more coronary artery bypass grafts.

Sex and age	1994	1995	1996	1997	1998	1999	2000[3]	2001[4]
	Inpatient discharges per 1,000 population							
Male:								
45–64 years	4.1	4.5	4.2	4.0	3.9	3.6	3.3	3.0
65–74 years	9.4	11.2	11.5	11.1	9.2	10.0	8.0	8.3
75 years and over	7.6	8.9	7.6	6.9	8.1	7.5	7.8	6.8
Female:								
45–64 years	1.3	1.0	1.2	1.2	1.0	1.1	0.9	1.1
65–74 years	3.3	3.8	4.1	4.5	3.6	4.4	3.3	2.9
75 years and over	2.3	3.0	3.3	3.4	3.0	3.7	2.8	2.4

[8]Cesarean sections accounted for 22.0 percent of deliveries in 1994, 20.8 percent in 1995, 21.8 percent in 1996, 21.5 percent in 1997, 22.5 percent in 1998, 22.1 percent in 1999, 22.9 percent in 2000, and 25.3 percent in 2001.

NOTES: Data in this table are for up to four procedures for inpatients and up to six procedures for ambulatory surgery patients. See Appendix II, Procedure. Procedure categories are based on the International Classification of Diseases, Ninth Revision, Clinical Modification. For a listing of the code numbers, see Appendix II, table X. Rates are based on the civilian population as of July 1. Rates for 1990–99 use population estimates based on the 1990 census adjusted for net underenumeration using the 1990 National Population Adjustment Matrix from the U.S. Bureau of the Census. Rates for 1990–99 are not strictly comparable with rates for 2000 and 2001 because population estimates for 1990–99 have not been revised to reflect Census 2000. See Appendix I, National Hospital Discharge Survey. Data for additional years are available (see Appendix III).

SOURCES: Centers for Disease Control and Prevention, National Center for Health Statistics, National Hospital Discharge Survey and National Survey of Ambulatory Surgery.

Table 95. Hospital admissions, average length of stay, and outpatient visits, according to type of ownership and size of hospital, and percent outpatient surgery: United States, selected years 1975–2001

[Data are based on reporting by a census of hospitals]

Type of ownership and size of hospital	1975	1980	1990	1995	1999	2000	2001
Admissions			Number in thousands				
All hospitals	36,157	38,892	33,774	33,282	34,181	34,891	35,644
Federal	1,913	2,044	1,759	1,559	1,072	1,034	1,001
Non-Federal[1]	34,243	36,848	32,015	31,723	33,109	33,946	34,644
Community[2]	33,435	36,143	31,181	30,945	32,359	33,089	33,814
Nonprofit	23,722	25,566	22,878	22,557	23,871	24,453	27,983
For profit	2,646	3,165	3,066	3,428	3,905	4,141	4,197
State-local government . . .	7,067	7,413	5,236	4,961	4,583	4,496	4,634
6–24 beds	174	159	95	124	145	141	140
25–49 beds	1,431	1,254	870	944	959	995	1,030
50–99 beds	3,675	3,700	2,474	2,299	2,317	2,355	2,422
100–199 beds	7,017	7,162	5,833	6,288	6,684	6,735	6,778
200–299 beds	6,174	6,596	6,333	6,495	6,389	6,702	6,630
300–399 beds	4,739	5,358	5,091	4,693	5,419	5,135	5,328
400–499 beds	3,689	4,401	3,644	3,413	3,045	3,617	3,779
500 beds or more	6,537	7,513	6,840	6,690	7,400	7,410	7,706
Average length of stay			Number of days				
All hospitals	11.4	9.9	9.1	7.8	7.0	6.8	6.7
Federal	20.3	16.8	14.9	13.1	14.0	12.8	13.2
Non-Federal[1]	10.9	9.6	8.8	7.5	6.8	6.6	6.6
Community[2]	7.7	7.6	7.2	6.5	5.9	5.8	5.7
Nonprofit	7.8	7.7	7.3	6.4	5.8	5.7	5.6
For profit	6.6	6.5	6.4	5.8	5.5	5.4	5.4
State-local government . . .	7.6	7.3	7.7	7.4	6.9	6.7	6.7
6–24 beds	5.6	5.3	5.4	5.5	4.5	4.2	4.0
25–49 beds	6.0	5.8	6.1	5.7	5.2	5.1	5.0
50–99 beds	6.8	6.7	7.2	7.0	6.7	6.4	6.4
100–199 beds	7.1	7.0	7.1	6.4	5.9	5.7	5.7
200–299 beds	7.5	7.4	6.9	6.2	5.7	5.7	5.6
300–399 beds	7.8	7.6	7.0	6.1	5.6	5.5	5.4
400–499 beds	8.1	7.9	7.3	6.3	5.9	5.6	5.6
500 beds or more	9.1	8.7	8.1	7.1	6.3	6.2	6.1
Outpatient visits[3]			Number in thousands				
All hospitals	254,844	262,951	368,184	483,195	573,461	592,673	612,276
Federal	51,957	50,566	58,527	59,934	70,060	63,402	64,035
Non-Federal[1]	202,887	212,385	309,657	423,261	503,401	531,972	548,242
Community[2]	190,672	202,310	301,329	414,345	495,346	521,405	538,480
Nonprofit	131,435	142,156	221,073	303,851	370,784	393,168	404,901
For profit	7,713	9,696	20,110	31,940	39,896	43,378	44,706
State-local government . . .	51,525	50,459	60,146	78,554	84,667	84,858	88,873
6–24 beds	915	1,155	1,471	3,644	4,650	4,555	4,556
25–49 beds	5,855	6,227	10,812	19,465	23,870	27,007	27,941
50–99 beds	16,303	17,976	27,582	38,597	46,156	49,385	51,331
100–199 beds	35,156	36,453	58,940	91,312	110,336	114,183	114,921
200–299 beds	32,772	36,073	60,561	84,080	90,878	99,248	99,596
300–399 beds	29,169	30,495	43,699	54,277	75,849	73,444	75,242
400–499 beds	22,127	25,501	33,394	44,284	43,867	52,205	59,580
500 beds or more	48,375	48,430	64,870	78,685	99,741	101,378	105,314
Outpatient surgery			Percent of total surgeries[4]				
Community hospitals[2]	- - -	16.3	50.5	58.1	62.4	62.7	63.0

- - - Data not available.

[1]The category of non-Federal hospitals comprises psychiatric, tuberculosis and other respiratory diseases hospitals, and long-term and short-term general and other special hospitals. See Appendix II, Hospital.
[2]Community hospitals are non-Federal short-term general and special hospitals whose facilities and services are available to the public. See Appendix II, Hospital.
[3]Outpatient visits include visits to the emergency department, outpatient department, referred visits (pharmacy, EKG, radiology), and outpatient surgery. See Appendix II, Outpatient visit.
[4]The American Hospital Association counts a surgical episode involving more than one surgical procedure as one surgical operation, in contrast to the National Hospital Discharge Survey and the National Survey of Ambulatory Surgery which count up to 4 and 6 procedures that are performed in a single surgical episode as separate surgical operations. See Appendix II, Ambulatory surgery and Outpatient surgery.

NOTE: Data for additional years are available (see Appendix III).

SOURCES: American Hospital Association Annual Survey of Hospitals. Hospital Statistics, 1976, 1981, 1991–2003 Editions. Chicago. (Copyrights 1976, 1981, 1991–2003: Used with the permission of Health Forum LLC, an American Hospital Association Company.)

Table 96. Nursing home residents 65 years of age and over, according to age, sex, and race: United States, 1973–74, 1985, 1995, and 1999

[Data are based on a sample of nursing home residents]

Age, sex, and race	Residents				Residents per 1,000 population			
	1973–74	1985	1995	1999	1973–74	1985	1995	1999
Age								
65 years and over, age adjusted[1]	. . .	. . .	. . .	. . .	58.5	54.0	45.9	43.3
65 years and over, crude	961,500	1,318,300	1,422,600	1,469,500	44.7	46.2	42.4	42.9
65–74 years	163,100	212,100	190,200	194,800	12.3	12.5	10.1	10.8
75–84 years	384,900	509,000	511,900	517,600	57.7	57.7	45.9	43.0
85 years and over	413,600	597,300	720,400	757,100	257.3	220.3	198.6	182.5
Male								
65 years and over, age adjusted[1]	. . .	. . .	. . .	. . .	42.5	38.8	32.8	30.6
65 years and over, crude	265,700	334,400	356,800	377,800	30.0	29.0	26.1	26.5
65–74 years	65,100	80,600	79,300	84,100	11.3	10.8	9.5	10.3
75–84 years	102,300	141,300	144,300	149,500	39.9	43.0	33.3	30.8
85 years and over	98,300	112,600	133,100	144,200	182.7	145.7	130.8	116.5
Female								
65 years and over, age adjusted[1]	. . .	. . .	. . .	. . .	67.5	61.5	52.3	49.8
65 years and over, crude	695,800	983,900	1,065,800	1,091,700	54.9	57.9	53.7	54.6
65–74 years	98,000	131,500	110,900	110,700	13.1	13.8	10.6	11.2
75–84 years	282,600	367,700	367,600	368,100	68.9	66.4	53.9	51.2
85 years and over	315,300	484,700	587,300	612,900	294.9	250.1	224.9	210.5
White[2]								
65 years and over, age adjusted[1]	. . .	. . .	. . .	. . .	61.2	55.5	45.4	41.9
65 years and over, crude	920,600	1,227,400	1,271,200	1,279,600	46.9	47.7	42.3	42.1
65–74 years	150,100	187,800	154,400	157,200	12.5	12.3	9.3	10.0
75–84 years	369,700	473,600	453,800	440,600	60.3	59.1	44.9	40.5
85 years and over	400,800	566,000	663,000	681,700	270.8	228.7	200.7	181.8
Black or African American[2]								
65 years and over, age adjusted[1]	. . .	. . .	. . .	. . .	28.2	41.5	50.4	55.6
65 years and over, crude	37,700	82,000	122,900	145,900	22.0	35.0	45.2	51.1
65–74 years	12,200	22,500	29,700	30,300	11.1	15.4	18.4	18.2
75–84 years	13,400	30,600	47,300	58,700	26.7	45.3	57.2	66.5
85 years and over	12,100	29,000	45,800	56,900	105.7	141.5	167.1	183.1

. . . Category not applicable.

[1]Age adjusted by the direct method to the year 2000 population standard using the following three age groups: 65–74 years, 75–84 years, and 85 years and over.
[2]Beginning in 1999 the instruction for the race item on the Current Resident Questionnaire was changed so that more than one race could be recorded. In previous years only one racial category could be checked. Estimates for racial groups presented in this table are for residents for whom only one race was recorded. Estimates for residents where multiple races were checked are unreliable due to small sample sizes and are not shown.

NOTES: Excludes residents in personal care or domiciliary care homes. Age refers to age at time of interview. Civilian population estimates used to compute rates for the 1990s are 1990-based postcensal estimates, as of July 1. Starting in 1997, population figures are adjusted for net underenumeration using the 1990 National Population Adjustment Matrix from the U.S. Bureau of the Census. Data for additional years are available (see Appendix III).

SOURCES: Hing E, Sekscenski E, Strahan G. The National Nursing Home Survey: 1985 summary for the United States. National Center for Health Statistics. Vital Health Stat 13(97). 1989; and Centers for Disease Control and Prevention, National Center for Health Statistics, National Nursing Home Survey for other data years.

Table 97. Nursing home residents 65 years of age and over, according to selected functional status and age, sex, and race: United States, 1985, 1995, and 1999

[Data are based on a sample of nursing home residents]

Age, sex, and race	Functional status[1]											
	Dependent mobility			Incontinent			Dependent eating			Dependent mobility, eating, and incontinent		
	1985	1995	1999	1985	1995	1999	1985	1995	1999	1985	1995	1999
All persons	Percent											
65 years and over, age adjusted[2]	75.7	79.0	80.3	55.0	63.8	65.7	40.9	44.9	47.3	32.5	36.5	36.9
65 years and over, crude. . . .	74.8	79.0	80.4	54.5	63.8	65.7	40.5	44.9	47.4	32.1	36.5	37.0
65–74 years.	61.2	73.0	73.9	42.9	61.9	58.5	33.5	43.8	43.1	25.7	35.8	31.7
75–84 years.	70.5	76.5	77.8	55.1	62.5	64.2	39.4	45.2	46.6	30.6	35.3	35.4
85 years and over.	83.3	82.4	83.8	58.1	65.3	68.6	43.9	45.0	49.0	35.6	37.5	39.4
Male												
65 years and over, age adjusted[2]	71.2	76.6	76.6	54.2	63.8	66.6	36.0	42.1	45.2	28.0	34.3	35.0
65 years and over, crude. . . .	67.8	75.8	75.9	51.9	63.9	66.0	34.9	42.7	45.1	26.9	34.8	35.0
65–74 years.	55.8	70.6	70.5	38.8	63.4	59.6	32.8	44.2	45.0	24.1	36.9	34.8
75–84 years.	65.7	76.6	76.9	54.4	64.6	68.9	32.6	44.1	44.7	25.5	35.5	35.2
85 years and over.	79.2	78.2	78.1	58.1	63.4	66.8	39.2	40.2	45.7	30.9	32.7	34.9
Female												
65 years and over, age adjusted[2]	77.3	79.7	81.5	55.4	63.6	65.0	42.4	45.6	47.8	33.9	36.9	37.2
65 years and over, crude. . . .	77.1	80.1	81.9	55.4	63.8	65.6	42.4	45.6	48.1	33.8	37.0	37.7
65–74 years.	64.5	74.8	76.4	45.4	60.9	57.7	34.0	43.6	41.6	26.7	35.0	29.3
75–84 years.	72.3	76.5	78.2	55.3	61.7	62.2	42.0	45.7	47.4	32.6	35.2	35.6
85 years and over.	84.3	83.3	85.2	58.1	65.7	69.0	45.0	46.0	49.7	36.7	38.6	40.4
White[3]												
65 years and over, age adjusted[2]	75.2	78.5	79.9	54.6	63.2	64.9	40.4	44.2	46.1	32.1	35.7	35.7
65 years and over, crude. . . .	74.3	78.7	80.2	54.2	63.3	65.1	40.1	44.2	46.2	31.7	35.7	35.8
65–74 years.	60.2	71.4	72.6	42.2	60.2	57.1	32.6	41.9	40.7	24.9	33.8	28.8
75–84 years.	69.6	76.4	77.5	54.2	61.8	63.8	38.9	44.9	45.8	30.1	34.7	34.8
85 years and over.	83.1	81.9	83.6	58.2	65.0	67.8	43.5	44.3	47.7	35.5	36.9	38.1
Black or African American[3]												
65 years and over, age adjusted[2]	83.4	83.2	82.1	61.0	69.3	71.9	49.2	52.2	55.9	38.2	44.0	46.8
65 years and over, crude. . . .	81.1	82.1	81.5	59.9	69.1	70.6	47.9	51.7	54.9	37.7	43.7	45.7
65–74 years.	70.9	79.6	78.7	48.6	68.3	64.6	43.1	51.2	53.3	33.8	43.1	42.6
75–84 years.	82.5	77.8	80.1	70.1	68.9	67.5	47.9	49.5	49.7	40.6	42.3	41.0
85 years and over.	87.4	88.0	84.5	57.9	69.8	77.0	51.7	54.3	61.0	37.6	45.5	52.1

[1]Nursing home residents who are dependent in mobility and eating require the assistance of a person or special equipment. Nursing home residents who are incontinent have difficulty in controlling bowels and/or bladder or have an ostomy or indwelling catheter.
[2]Age adjusted by the direct method to the 1995 National Nursing Home Survey population using the following three age groups: 65–74 years, 75–84 years, and 85 years and over.
[3]Beginning in 1999 the instruction for the race item on the Current Resident Questionnaire was changed so that more than one race could be recorded. In previous years only one racial category could be checked. Estimates for racial groups presented in this table are for residents for whom only one race was recorded. Estimates for residents where multiple races were checked are unreliable due to small sample sizes and are not shown.

NOTES: Age refers to age at time of interview. Excludes residents in personal care or domiciliary care homes. Data for additional years are available (see Appendix III).

SOURCES: Hing E, Sekscenski E, Strahan G. The National Nursing Home Survey: 1985 summary for the United States. National Center for Health Statistics. Vital Health Stat 13(97). 1989; and Centers for Disease Control and Prevention, National Center for Health Statistics, National Nursing Home Survey for other data years.

Table 98. Persons employed in health service sites: United States, selected years 1970–2002

[Data are based on household interviews of a sample of the civilian noninstitutionalized population]

Site	1970	1980	1990	1995[1]	1997	1998	1999	2000[2]	2001	2002
					Number of persons in thousands					
All employed civilians.........	76,805	99,303	117,914	124,900	129,558	131,463	133,488	136,891	136,933	136,485
All health service sites........	4,246	7,339	9,447	10,928	11,525	11,504	11,646	11,742	12,110	12,653
Offices and clinics of physicians............	477	777	1,098	1,512	1,559	1,581	1,624	1,697	1,799	1,907
Offices and clinics of dentists.............	222	415	580	644	662	666	694	676	699	740
Offices and clinics of chiropractors[3].........	19	40	90	99	118	127	142	124	117	138
Hospitals.................	2,690	4,036	4,690	4,961	5,130	5,116	5,117	5,092	5,270	5,340
Nursing and personal care facilities................	509	1,199	1,543	1,718	1,755	1,801	1,786	1,737	1,771	1,942
Other health service sites	330	872	1,446	1,995	2,301	2,213	2,283	2,414	2,454	2,585
					Percent of employed civilians					
All health service sites........	5.5	7.4	8.0	8.7	8.9	8.8	8.7	8.6	8.8	9.3
					Percent distribution					
All health service sites........	100.0	100.0	100.0	100.0	100.0	100.0	100.0	100.0	100.0	100.0
Offices and clinics of physicians............	11.2	10.6	11.6	13.8	13.5	13.7	13.9	14.5	14.9	15.1
Offices and clinics of dentists.............	5.2	5.7	6.1	5.9	5.7	5.8	6.0	5.8	5.8	5.8
Offices and clinics of chiropractors[3].........	0.4	0.5	1.0	0.9	1.0	1.1	1.2	1.1	1.0	1.1
Hospitals.................	63.4	55.0	49.6	45.4	44.5	44.5	43.9	43.4	43.5	42.2
Nursing and personal care facilities................	12.0	16.3	16.3	15.7	15.2	15.7	15.3	14.8	14.6	15.3
Other health service sites	7.8	11.9	15.3	18.3	20.0	19.2	19.6	20.6	20.3	20.4

[1]Data for years prior to 1995 are not strictly comparable with data from 1995 onwards due to a redesign of the Current Population Survey.
[2]Starting in 2000, 2000-based population estimates are used as survey controls. See Appendix I, Current Population Survey.
[3]Data for 1980 are from the American Chiropractic Association; data for all other years are from the U.S. Bureau of Labor Statistics.

NOTES: Employment is full- or part-time work. Totals exclude persons in health-related occupations who are working in nonhealth industries, as classified by the U.S. Bureau of the Census, such as pharmacists employed in drugstores, school nurses, and nurses working in private households. Totals include Federal, State, and county health workers. In 1970–82, employed persons were classified according to the industry groups used in the 1970 Census of Population. In 1983–91, persons were classified according to the system used in the 1980 Census of Population. Beginning in 1992 persons were classified according to the system used in the 1990 Census of Population. Data for additional years are available (see Appendix III).

SOURCES: U.S. Bureau of the Census: 1970 Census of Population, occupation by industry. Subject Reports. Final Report PC(2)–7C. Washington. U.S. Government Printing Office, Oct. 1972; U.S. Bureau of Labor Statistics: Labor Force Statistics Derived from the Current Population Survey: A Databook, Vol. I. Washington. U.S. Government Printing Office, Sept. 1982; Employment and Earnings, January issue 1986, 1991–2003. U.S. Government Printing Office, Jan. 1986, 1991–2003; American Chiropractic Association: Unpublished data.

Table 99 (page 1 of 2). Active non-Federal physicians and doctors of medicine in patient care, according to geographic division and State: United States, 1975, 1985, 1995, and 2001

[Data are based on reporting by physicians]

Geographic division and State	Total physicians[1]				Doctors of medicine in patient care[2]			
	1975	1985	1995[3]	2001[4]	1975	1985	1995	2001
	Number per 10,000 civilian population							
United States	15.3	20.7	24.2	25.5	13.5	18.0	21.3	22.6
New England	19.1	26.7	32.5	35.0	16.9	22.9	28.8	31.2
Maine.	12.8	18.7	22.3	27.3	10.7	15.6	18.2	22.4
New Hampshire.	14.3	18.1	21.5	24.7	13.1	16.7	19.8	22.6
Vermont	18.2	23.8	26.9	33.2	15.5	20.3	24.2	30.1
Massachusetts	20.8	30.2	37.5	39.3	18.3	25.4	33.2	35.2
Rhode Island.	17.8	23.3	30.4	33.4	16.1	20.2	26.7	29.8
Connecticut.	19.8	27.6	32.8	34.4	17.7	24.3	29.5	31.0
Middle Atlantic.	19.5	26.1	32.4	34.0	17.0	22.2	28.0	29.4
New York	22.7	29.0	35.3	36.7	20.2	25.2	31.6	32.9
New Jersey.	16.2	23.4	29.3	31.4	14.0	19.8	24.9	26.9
Pennsylvania.	16.6	23.6	30.1	31.6	13.9	19.2	24.6	25.8
East North Central.	13.9	19.3	23.3	25.0	12.0	16.4	19.8	21.5
Ohio.	14.1	19.9	23.8	25.8	12.2	16.8	20.0	21.9
Indiana	10.6	14.7	18.4	20.6	9.6	13.2	16.6	18.7
Illinois.	14.5	20.5	24.8	26.2	13.1	18.2	22.1	23.3
Michigan.	15.4	20.8	24.8	26.2	12.0	16.0	19.0	20.6
Wisconsin	12.5	17.7	21.5	23.6	11.4	15.9	19.6	21.5
West North Central	13.3	18.3	21.8	23.5	11.4	15.6	18.9	20.4
Minnesota.	14.9	20.5	23.4	25.7	13.7	18.5	21.5	23.7
Iowa.	11.4	15.6	19.2	20.0	9.4	12.4	15.1	15.8
Missouri	15.0	20.5	23.9	24.9	11.6	16.3	19.7	20.8
North Dakota.	9.7	15.8	20.5	22.1	9.2	14.9	18.9	20.4
South Dakota	8.2	13.4	16.7	19.8	7.7	12.3	15.7	18.3
Nebraska	12.1	15.7	19.8	22.4	10.9	14.4	18.3	20.8
Kansas.	12.8	17.3	20.8	21.9	11.2	15.1	18.0	19.0
South Atlantic	14.0	19.7	23.4	24.8	12.6	17.6	21.0	22.3
Delaware	14.3	19.7	23.4	25.1	12.7	17.1	19.7	21.7
Maryland.	18.6	30.4	34.1	35.9	16.5	24.9	29.9	31.7
District of Columbia	39.6	55.3	63.6	62.5	34.6	45.6	53.6	54.6
Virginia.	12.9	19.5	22.5	24.4	11.9	17.8	20.8	22.5
West Virginia.	11.0	16.3	21.0	23.7	10.0	14.6	17.9	20.0
North Carolina.	11.7	16.9	21.1	23.0	10.6	15.0	19.4	21.2
South Carolina.	10.0	14.7	18.9	21.5	9.3	13.6	17.6	19.9
Georgia.	11.5	16.2	19.7	20.4	10.6	14.7	18.0	18.8
Florida	15.2	20.2	22.9	24.0	13.4	17.8	20.3	21.3
East South Central	10.5	15.0	19.2	21.1	9.7	14.0	17.8	19.5
Kentucky.	10.9	15.1	19.2	21.0	10.1	13.9	18.0	19.6
Tennessee	12.4	17.7	22.5	24.0	11.3	16.2	20.8	22.3
Alabama	9.2	14.2	18.4	20.0	8.6	13.1	17.0	18.4
Mississippi	8.4	11.8	13.9	17.1	8.0	11.1	13.0	15.6
West South Central	11.9	16.4	19.5	20.7	10.5	14.5	17.3	18.5
Arkansas	9.1	13.8	17.3	19.0	8.5	12.8	16.0	17.7
Louisiana	11.4	17.3	21.7	24.4	10.5	16.1	20.3	23.1
Oklahoma.	11.6	16.1	18.8	19.2	9.4	12.9	14.7	15.0
Texas	12.5	16.8	19.4	20.4	11.0	14.7	17.3	18.2
Mountain	14.3	17.8	20.2	20.8	12.6	15.7	17.8	18.4
Montana	10.6	14.0	18.4	21.4	10.1	13.2	17.1	19.9
Idaho	9.5	12.1	13.9	16.1	8.9	11.4	13.1	14.8
Wyoming.	9.5	12.9	15.3	18.0	8.9	12.0	13.9	16.5
Colorado.	17.3	20.7	23.7	24.1	15.0	17.7	20.6	21.2
New Mexico	12.2	17.0	20.2	21.3	10.1	14.7	18.0	19.0
Arizona.	16.7	20.2	21.4	20.7	14.1	17.1	18.2	17.7
Utah.	14.1	17.2	19.2	19.9	13.0	15.5	17.6	18.0
Nevada.	11.9	16.0	16.7	18.0	10.9	14.5	14.6	16.1

See footnotes at end of table.

Health, United States, 2003

Table 99 (page 2 of 2). Active non-Federal physicians and doctors of medicine in patient care, according to geographic division and State: United States, 1975, 1985, 1995, and 2001

[Data are based on reporting by physicians]

Geographic division and State	Total physicians[1]				Doctors of medicine in patient care[2]			
	1975	1985	1995[3]	2001[4]	1975	1985	1995	2001
	Number per 10,000 civilian population							
Pacific	17.9	22.5	23.3	24.1	16.3	20.5	21.2	21.9
Washington..............	15.3	20.2	22.5	24.4	13.6	17.9	20.2	22.0
Oregon.................	15.6	19.7	21.6	23.7	13.8	17.6	19.5	21.4
California	18.8	23.7	23.7	24.0	17.3	21.5	21.7	21.9
Alaska	8.4	13.0	15.7	19.3	7.8	12.1	14.2	17.0
Hawaii	16.2	21.5	24.8	27.4	14.7	19.8	22.8	25.0

[1]Includes active non-Federal doctors of medicine and active doctors of osteopathy. See Appendix II, Physician.

[2]Excludes doctors of osteopathy (DO's); States with more than 2,500 active DO's are Pennsylvania, Michigan, Ohio, Florida, New York, and Texas. States with fewer than 100 active DO's are Wyoming, Vermont, North Dakota, South Dakota, Montana, Louisiana, Alaska, Nebraska, and District of Columbia. Excludes doctors of medicine in medical teaching, administration, research, and other nonpatient care activities.

[3]Data for doctors of osteopathy are as of July 1996.

[4]Data for doctors of osteopathy are as of June 2001.

NOTE: Data for doctors of medicine are as of December 31.

SOURCES: American Medical Association (AMA). Physician distribution and medical licensure in the U.S., 1975; Physician characteristics and distribution in the U.S., 1986 edition; 1996–97 edition; 2003–2004 edition; Department of Physician Practice and Communication Information, Division of Survey and Data Resources, AMA. (Copyrights 1976, 1986, 1997, 2003: Used with the permission of the AMA); American Osteopathic Association: 1975–76 Yearbook and Directory of Osteopathic Physicians, 1985–86 Yearbook and Directory of Osteopathic Physicians; American Association of Colleges of Osteopathic Medicine: 2001 Annual Report on Osteopathic Medical Education, 2002.

Table 100. Doctors of medicine, according to activity and place of medical education: United States and outlying U.S. areas, selected years 1975–2001

[Data are based on reporting by physicians]

Activity and place of medical education	1975	1985	1995	1997	1998	1999	2000	2001
	\multicolumn{8}{c}{Number of doctors of medicine}							
Doctors of medicine	393,742	552,716	720,325	756,710	777,859	797,634	813,770	836,156
Professionally active[1]	340,280	497,140	625,443	664,556	667,000	668,949	690,128	709,168
Place of medical education:								
U.S. medical graduates	- - -	392,007	481,137	509,942	509,524	510,738	525,691	537,529
International medical graduates[2]	- - -	105,133	144,306	154,614	157,476	158,211	164,437	171,639
Activity:								
Non-Federal	312,089	475,573	604,364	645,203	648,009	650,899	672,987	693,358
Patient care[3]	287,837	431,527	564,074	603,684	606,425	610,656	631,431	652,328
Office-based practice	213,334	329,041	427,275	458,209	468,788	473,241	490,398	514,016
General and family practice	46,347	53,862	59,932	62,022	64,588	66,246	67,534	70,030
Cardiovascular diseases	5,046	9,054	13,739	15,026	15,112	15,586	16,300	16,991
Dermatology	3,442	5,325	6,959	7,353	7,641	7,788	7,969	8,199
Gastroenterology	1,696	4,135	7,300	7,938	7,948	8,185	8,515	8,905
Internal medicine	28,188	52,712	72,612	81,352	83,270	84,633	88,699	94,674
Pediatrics	12,687	22,392	33,890	36,846	38,359	40,502	42,215	44,824
Pulmonary diseases	1,166	3,035	4,964	4,965	4,927	5,745	6,095	6,596
General surgery	19,710	24,708	24,086	27,865	27,509	26,822	24,475	25,632
Obstetrics and gynecology	15,613	23,525	29,111	30,063	31,194	31,103	31,726	32,582
Ophthalmology	8,795	12,212	14,596	15,118	15,560	15,238	15,598	15,994
Orthopedic surgery	8,148	13,033	17,136	18,482	18,479	16,974	17,367	17,829
Otolaryngology	4,297	5,751	7,139	7,378	7,498	7,282	7,581	7,866
Plastic surgery	1,706	3,299	4,612	5,257	5,303	5,127	5,308	5,545
Urological surgery	5,025	7,081	7,991	8,383	8,424	8,229	8,460	8,636
Anesthesiology	8,970	15,285	23,770	25,569	26,218	26,635	27,624	28,868
Diagnostic radiology	1,978	7,735	12,751	14,142	14,241	14,259	14,622	15,596
Emergency medicine	- - -	- - -	11,700	12,450	13,253	13,932	14,541	15,823
Neurology	1,862	4,691	7,623	8,199	8,458	8,065	8,559	9,156
Pathology, anatomical/clinical	4,195	6,877	9,031	10,229	9,970	10,074	10,267	10,554
Psychiatry	12,173	18,521	23,334	24,541	24,962	24,393	24,955	25,653
Radiology	6,970	7,355	5,994	6,297	6,353	6,523	6,674	6,830
Other specialty	15,320	28,453	29,005	28,734	29,521	29,900	35,314	37,233
Hospital-based practice	74,503	102,486	136,799	145,318	137,637	137,225	141,033	138,312
Residents and interns[4]	53,527	72,159	93,650	95,808	92,332	92,461	95,125	92,935
Full-time hospital staff	20,976	30,327	43,149	49,510	45,305	44,764	45,908	45,377
Other professional activity[5]	24,252	44,046	40,290	41,519	41,584	41,243	41,556	41,118
Federal[6]	28,191	21,567	21,079	19,353	18,991	18,050	19,381	20,017
Patient care	24,100	17,293	18,057	16,947	15,311	14,678	15,999	16,611
Office-based practice	2,095	1,156	. . .	. . .	. . .	. . .	. . .	. . .
Hospital-based practice	22,005	16,137	18,057	16,945	15,311	14,678	15,999	16,611
Residents and interns	4,275	3,252	2,702	4,068	660	375	600	739
Full-time hospital staff	17,730	12,885	15,355	12,877	14,651	14,303	15,399	15,872
Other professional activity[5]	4,091	4,274	3,022	2,406	3,680	3,372	3,382	3,406
Inactive	21,449	38,646	72,326	71,106	69,889	75,893	75,168	81,520
Not classified	26,145	13,950	20,579	20,049	40,032	50,906	45,136	38,314
Unknown address	5,868	2,980	1,977	999	938	886	1,098	2,947

- - - Data not available.
. . . Category not applicable.

[1]Excludes inactive, not classified, and address unknown. See Appendix II, Physician.
[2]International medical graduates received their medical education in schools outside the United States and Canada.
[3]Specialty information based on the physician's self-designated primary area of practice. Categories include generalists and specialists. See Appendix II, Physician specialty.
[4]Beginning in 1990 clinical fellows are included in this category. In prior years clinical fellows were included in other professional activity.
[5]Includes medical teaching, administration, research, and other. Prior to 1990 this category also included clinical fellows.
[6]Beginning in 1993 data collection for Federal physicians was revised.

NOTES: Data for doctors of medicine are as of December 31, except for 1990–94 data, which are as of January 1. Outlying areas include Puerto Rico, Virgin Islands, and the Pacific islands of Canton, Caroline, Guam, Mariana, Marshall, American Samoa, and Wake. Data for additional years are available (see Appendix III).

SOURCES: American Medical Association (AMA). Distribution of physicians in the United States, 1970; Physician distribution and medical licensure in the U.S., 1975; Physician characteristics and distribution in the U.S., 1981, 1986, 1989, 1990, 1992, 1993, 1994, 1995–96, 1996–97, 1997–98, 1999, 2000–2001, 2001–2002, 2002–2003, 2003–2004 editions, Department of Physician Practice and Communications Information, Division of Survey and Data Resources, AMA. (Copyrights 1971, 1976, 1982, 1986, 1989, 1990, 1992, 1993, 1994, 1996, 1997, 1997, 1999, 2000, 2001, 2002, 2003: Used with the permission of the AMA.)

Table 101. Doctors of medicine in primary care, according to specialty: United States and outlying U.S. areas, selected years 1949–2001

[Data are based on reporting by physicians]

Specialty	1949[1]	1960[1]	1970	1980	1990	1995	1997	1998	1999	2000	2001
						Number					
Total doctors of medicine[2]	201,277	260,484	334,028	467,679	615,421	720,325	756,710	777,859	797,634	813,770	836,156
Active doctors of medicine[3]	191,577	247,257	310,845	414,916	547,310	625,443	664,556	667,000	669,949	692,368	713,375
Primary care generalists	113,222	125,359	115,822	146,093	183,294	207,810	216,598	218,421	221,206	227,992	246,714
General/family practice	95,980	88,023	57,948	60,049	70,480	75,976	78,258	79,769	81,487	83,165	88,597
Internal medicine.	12,453	26,209	39,924	58,462	76,295	88,240	93,797	93,227	92,976	96,469	105,229
Pediatrics	4,789	11,127	17,950	27,582	36,519	43,594	44,543	45,425	46,743	48,358	52,888
Primary care specialists	- - -	- - -	2,817	14,949	27,434	35,290	32,918	34,299	37,424	40,675	51,134
Internal medicine.	- - -	- - -	1,948	13,069	22,054	26,928	24,582	25,365	27,140	29,382	37,558
Pediatrics	- - -	- - -	869	1,880	5,380	8,362	8,336	8,934	10,284	11,293	13,576
					Percent of active doctors of medicine						
Primary care generalists	59.1	50.7	37.3	35.2	33.5	33.2	32.6	32.7	33.0	32.9	34.6
General/family practice	50.1	35.6	18.6	14.5	12.9	12.1	11.8	12.0	12.2	12.0	12.4
Internal medicine.	6.5	10.6	12.8	14.1	.13.9	14.1	14.1	14.0	13.9	13.9	14.8
Pediatrics	2.5	4.5	5.8	6.6	6.7	7.0	6.7	6.8	7.0	7.0	7.4
Primary care specialists . . . . :	- - -	- - -	0.9	3.6	5.0	5.6	5.0	5.1	5.6	5.9	7.2
Internal medicine.	- - -	- - -	0.6	3.1	4.0	4.3	3.7	3.8	4.1	4.2	5.3
Pediatrics	- - -	- - -	0.3	0.5	1.0	1.3	1.3	1.3	1.5	1.6	1.9

- - - Data not available.

[1]Estimated by the Bureau of Health Professions, Health Resources Administration. Active doctors of medicine (M.D.'s) include those with address unknown and primary specialty not classified.

[2]Includes M.D.'s engaged in Federal and non-Federal patient care (office-based or hospital-based) and other professional activities.

[3]Beginning in 1970, M.D.'s who are inactive, have unknown address, or primary specialty not classified are excluded. See Appendix II, Physician.

NOTES: See Appendix II, Physician specialty. Data are as of December 31 except for 1990–94 data, which are as of January 1, and 1949 data, which are as of midyear. Outlying areas include Puerto Rico, Virgin Islands, and the Pacific islands of Canton, Caroline, Guam, Mariana, Marshall, American Samoa, and Wake. Data for additional years are available (see Appendix III).

SOURCES: Health Manpower Source Book: Medical Specialists, USDHEW, 1962; American Medical Association (AMA). Distribution of physicians in the United States, 1970; Physician characteristics and distribution in the U.S., 1981, 1992, 1996–97, 1997–98, 1999, 2000–2001, 2001–2002, 2002–2003, 2003–2004 editions, Department of Data Survey and Planning, Division of Survey and Data Resources, AMA. (Copyrights 1971, 1982, 1992, 1996, 1997, 1997, 1999, 2000, 2001, 2002: Used with the permission of the AMA.)

Table 102. Active health personnel according to occupation: United States, selected years 1980–2000

[Data are compiled by the Bureau of Health Professions]

Occupation	1980	1985[1]	1990	1995	1999	2000[2]
	Number of active health personnel					
Chiropractors	25,600	- - -	41,500	47,200	- - -	- - -
Dentists[3].................	121,900	133,500	147,500	158,600	164,700	168,000
Nurses, registered[4]	1,272,900	1,538,100	1,789,600	2,115,800	2,271,300	- - -
Associate and diploma	908,300	1,024,500	1,107,300	1,235,100	1,290,400	- - -
Baccalaureate	297,300	419,900	549,000	673,200	739,000	- - -
Masters and doctorate	67,300	93,700	133,300	207,500	241,900	- - -
Nutritionists/Dieticians	32,000	- - -	67,000	- - -	- - -	97,000
Occupational therapists	25,000	- - -	34,000	- - -	- - -	55,000
Optometrists	22,330	23,900	26,000	28,900	- - -	29,500
Pharmacists	142,780	159,200	161,900	182,300	- - -	208,000
Physical therapists...........	50,000	- - -	92,000	- - -	- - -	144,000
Physicians	427,122	542,653	567,610	672,859	753,176	772,296
Federal	17,642	23,305	20,784	21,153	17,338	19,228
Doctors of medicine[5]	16,585	21,938	19,166	19,830	17,224	19,110
Doctors of osteopathy	1,057	1,367	1,618	1,323	114	118
Non-Federal..............	409,480	519,348	546,826	651,706	735,838	753,068
Doctors of medicine[5]	393,407	497,473	520,450	617,362	693,345	708,463
Doctors of osteopathy	16,073	21,875	26,376	34,344	42,493	44,605
Podiatrists[6]...............	7,000	9,700	10,600	10,300	- - -	- - -
Speech therapists	50,000	- - -	65,000	- - -	- - -	97,000
	Number per 100,000 population					
Chiropractors	11.2	- - -	16.5	17.8	- - -	- - -
Dentists[3].................	54.0	56.5	59.5	60.7	60.7	60.4
Nurses, registered[4]	560.0	641.4	713.7	797.6	832.9	- - -
Associate and diploma	399.9	425.8	441.6	465.5	473.2	- - -
Baccalaureate	130.9	175.6	218.9	253.8	271.0	- - -
Masters and doctorate	29.6	39.9	53.2	78.2	88.7	- - -
Nutritionists/Dieticians	14.0	- - -	26.7	- - -	- - -	35.2
Occupational therapists	10.9	- - -	13.5	- - -	- - -	20.0
Optometrists	9.8	9.9	10.4	10.9	- - -	11.1
Pharmacists	62.5	66.3	64.4	68.9	- - -	75.6
Physical therapists...........	21.8	- - -	36.6	- - -	- - -	52.3
Physicians	189.8	221.3	230.2	255.9	277.4	277.8
Federal	7.8	9.5	8.4	8.0	6.4	6.9
Doctors of medicine[5]	7.4	8.9	7.7	7.5	6.3	6.9
Doctors of osteopathy	0.5	0.6	0.7	0.5	0.1	0.0
Non-Federal..............	182.0	211.8	221.8	247.9	271.0	270.9
Doctors of medicine[5]	174.9	202.9	211.1	234.8	255.4	254.9
Doctors of osteopathy	7.1	8.9	10.7	13.1	15.7	16.0
Podiatrists[6]...............	3.0	4.2	4.2	3.9	- - -	- - -
Speech therapists	21.8	- - -	25.9	- - -	- - -	36.4

- - - Data not available.

[1]Osteopath data are for 1986 and podiatric data are for 1984.

[2]Data for optometrists and speech therapists are for 1996.

[3]Excludes dentists in military service, U.S. Public Health Service, and Department of Veterans Affairs.

[4]See Appendix I, Nurse Supply Estimates.

[5]Excludes physicians with unknown addresses and those who do not practice or practice less than 20 hours per week. From 1989 to 1994 data for doctors of medicine are as of January 1; in other years these data are as of December 31. See Appendix II, Physician.

[6]Podiatrists in patient care.

NOTES: Ratios for physicians and dentists are based on civilian population; ratios for all other health occupations are based on resident population.

SOURCES: Division of Health Professions Analysis, Bureau of Health Professions: Supply and Characteristics of Selected Health Personnel. DHHS Pub. No. (HRA) 81–20. Health Resources Administration. Hyattsville, Md., June 1981 and unpublished data; American Medical Association. Physician characteristics and distribution in the U.S., 1981, 1992, 1996–97, 1999, 2000–2001, and 2001–2002 editions. Chicago, 1982, 1992, 1997, 1999, 2000, and 2001; American Osteopathic Association. 1980–81 Yearbook and Directory of Osteopathic Physicians. Chicago, 1980. American Association of Colleges of Osteopathic Medicine. Annual statistical report, 1990, 1997, 1998, 1999, and 2000 editions. Rockville, Md., 1990, 1997, 1998, 2000 and 2001; Bureau of Labor Statistics: unpublished data.

Table 103. First-year enrollment and graduates of health professions schools and number of schools, according to profession: United States, selected years 1980–2001

[Data are based on reporting by health professions schools]

Profession	1980	1985	1990	1995	1996	1999	2000	2001
First-year enrollment				Number				
Chiropractic[1]	- - -	1,383	1,485	- - -	- - -	- - -	- - -	- - -
Dentistry	6,132	5,047	3,979	4,121	4,237	4,268	4,314	4,327
Medicine (Allopathic)	16,930	16,997	16,756	17,085	17,058	16,790	16,856	16,699
Medicine (Osteopathic)	1,426	1,750	1,844	2,217	2,274	2,745	2,848	2,927
Nursing:								
Licensed practical	56,316	47,034	52,969	57,906	- - -	- - -	- - -	- - -
Registered, total	105,952	118,224	108,580	127,184	119,205	- - -	- - -	- - -
Baccalaureate	35,414	39,573	29,858	43,451	40,048	- - -	- - -	- - -
Associate degree	53,633	63,776	68,634	76,016	72,930	- - -	- - -	- - -
Diploma	16,905	14,875	10,088	7,717	6,227	- - -	- - -	- - -
Optometry	1,202	1,187	1,258	1,390	1,438	1,369	1,410	1,384
Pharmacy	8,035	6,986	8,033	9,157	8,740	8,346	8,382	8,922
Podiatry	718	782	599	652	630	623	606	475
Public Health[2]	3,348	3,836	4,087	5,332	5,342	5,575	5,839	5,895
Graduates								
Chiropractic	2,049	- - -	1,661	- - -	- - -	- - -	- - -	- - -
Dentistry	5,256	5,353	4,233	3,908	3,810	4,095	4,171	4,367
Medicine (Allopathic)	15,113	16,318	15,398	15,888	15,907	15,996	15,704	15,778
Medicine (Osteopathic)	1,059	1,474	1,529	1,843	1,932	2,169	2,304	2,597
Nursing:								
Licensed practical	41,892	36,955	35,417	44,234	41,846	- - -	- - -	- - -
Registered, total	75,523	82,075	66,088	97,052	94,757	76,523	71,392	68,709
Baccalaureate	24,994	24,975	18,571	31,254	32,413	28,107	26,048	24,832
Associate degree	36,034	45,208	42,318	58,749	56,641	45,255	42,665	41,567
Diploma	14,495	11,892	5,199	7,049	5,703	3,161	2,679	2,310
Occupational therapy	- - -	- - -	2,424	3,473	4,270	4,805	- - -	- - -
Optometry	1,073	1,114	1,115	1,219	1,210	1,316	1,315	1,310
Pharmacy	7,432	5,735	6,956	7,837	8,003	7,141	7,260	7,000
Physical therapy	- - -	- - -	- - -	- - -	- - -	4,752	- - -	- - -
Podiatry	577	586	671	558	680	584	583	531
Public Health	3,326	3,047	3,549	4,636	5,064	5,568	5,879	5,747
Schools								
Chiropractic	14	17	17	- - -	- - -	- - -	- - -	- - -
Dentistry	60	60	56	54	54	55	55	54
Medicine (Allopathic)	126	127	126	125	125	125	125	125
Medicine (Osteopathic)	14	15	15	16	17	19	19	19
Nursing:[3]								
Licensed practical	1,299	1,165	1,154	1,210	- - -	- - -	- - -	- - -
Registered, total	1,385	1,473	1,470	1,516	1,508	- - -	- - -	- - -
Baccalaureate	377	441	489	521	523	- - -	- - -	- - -
Associate degree	697	776	829	876	876	- - -	- - -	- - -
Diploma	311	256	152	119	109	- - -	- - -	- - -
Occupational therapy	50	61	69	98	105	130	131	141
Optometry	16	17	17	17	17	17	17	17
Pharmacy	72	72	74	75	79	81	81	83
Physical therapy	- - -	- - -	- - -	- - -	- - -	190	196	200
Podiatry	5	7	7	7	7	7	7	7
Public Health	21	23	25	27	28	28	28	29
Speech therapy	- - -	- - -	194	222	223	223	224	- - -

- - - Data not available.

[1]Chiropractic first-year enrollment data are partial data from eight reporting schools.
[2]Number of students entering Schools of Public Health for the first time.
[3]Some nursing schools offer more than one type of program. Numbers shown for nursing are number of nursing programs.

NOTES: Some numbers in this table for 1999 and 2000 have been revised and differ from previous editions of *Health, United States*. Data on the number of schools are reported as of the beginning of the academic year while data on first-year enrollment and number of graduates are reported as of the end of the academic year. Data on first-year enrollment for occupational, physical, and speech therapy were not available.

SOURCES: Association of American Medical Colleges: AAMC Data Book, Statistical Information Related to Medical Education. Washington, DC. 2001 and unpublished data; Bureau of Health Professions: Health Personnel in the United States, Eighth Report to Congress, 1991. Health Resources and Services Administration. DHHS Pub. No. HRS-P-OD–92–1, Rockville, Maryland. 1992 and unpublished data; National League for Nursing: Nursing Data Review, 1997 and unpublished data; American Nurses Association: Facts About Nursing, 1951 and 1961; American Dental Association: 1999–2000 Survey of predoctoral dental education academic programs, enrollments, and graduates, vol. 1, Chicago. 2001; American Association of Colleges of Osteopathic Medicine. 2001 Annual Report on Osteopathic Medical Education, Chevy Chase, Maryland. 2002; American Chiropractic Association: unpublished data; Association of Schools of Public Health: 2001 Annual Data Report. Washington, DC. 2002; Association of Schools and Colleges of Optometry: unpublished data; American Association of Colleges of Pharmacy: Profile of Pharmacy Students, Fall 2002, and unpublished data; American Association of Colleges of Podiatric Medicine: unpublished data.

Table 104 (page 1 of 2). Total enrollment of minorities in schools for selected health occupations, according to detailed race and Hispanic origin: United States, academic years 1970–71, 1980–81, 1990–91, and 2000–01

[Data are based on reporting by health professions associations]

Occupation, detailed race, and Hispanic origin	1970–71[1]	1980–81	1990–91	2000–01[2]	1970–71[1]	1980–81	1990–91	2000–01[2]
Dentistry[3]	Number of students				Percent distribution of students			
All races	19,187	22,842	15,951	17,242	100.0	100.0	100.0	100.0
Not Hispanic or Latino:								
White[4]	17,531	20,208	11,185	11,106	91.4	88.5	70.1	64.4
Black or African American	872	1,022	940	808	4.5	4.5	5.9	4.7
Hispanic or Latino	185	519	1,254	912	1.0	2.3	7.9	5.3
American Indian	28	53	53	99	0.1	0.2	0.3	0.6
Asian	490	1,040	2,519	4,317	2.6	4.6	15.8	25.0
Medicine (Allopathic)								
All races[4]	40,238	65,189	65,163	66,160	100.0	100.0	100.0	100.0
Not Hispanic or Latino:								
White	37,944	55,434	47,893	42,242	94.3	85.0	73.5	63.8
Black or African American	1,509	3,708	4,241	4,900	3.8	5.7	6.5	7.4
Hispanic or Latino	196	2,761	3,538	4,220	0.5	4.2	5.4	6.4
Mexican.	- - -	951	1,109	1,665	- - -	1.5	1.7	2.5
Mainland Puerto Rican	- - -	329	457	469	- - -	0.5	0.7	0.7
Other Hispanic[5]	- - -	1,481	1,972	2,086	- - -	2.3	3.0	3.2
American Indian	18	221	277	519	0.0	0.3	0.4	0.8
Asian	571	1,924	8,436	13,331	1.4	3.0	12.9	20.1
Medicine (Osteopathic)								
All races	2,304	4,940	6,792	10,817	100.0	100.0	100.0	100.0
Not Hispanic or Latino:								
White[4]	2,241	4,688	5,680	8,230	97.3	94.9	83.6	76.1
Black or African American	27	94	217	400	1.2	1.9	3.2	3.7
Hispanic or Latino	19	52	277	381	0.8	1.1	4.1	3.5
American Indian	6	19	36	72	0.3	0.4	0.5	0.7
Asian	11	87	582	1,734	0.5	1.8	8.6	16.0
Nursing, registered[3,6]								
All races	211,239	230,966	221,170	238,244	- - -	- - -	100.0	100.0
Not Hispanic or Latino:								
White[4]	- - -	- - -	183,102	193,061	- - -	- - -	82.8	81.0
Black or African American	- - -	- - -	23,094	23,611	- - -	- - -	10.4	9.9
Hispanic or Latino	- - -	- - -	6,580	9,227	- - -	- - -	3.0	3.9
American Indian	- - -	- - -	1,803	1,816	- - -	- - -	0.8	0.8
Asian	- - -	- - -	6,591	10,529	- - -	- - -	3.0	4.4
Optometry[3,5]								
All races	3,094	4,540	4,650	5,313	100.0	100.0	100.0	100.0
Not Hispanic or Latino:								
White[4]	2,913	4,148	3,706	3,619	94.1	91.4	79.7	68.1
Black or African American	32	57	134	108	1.0	1.3	2.9	2.0
Hispanic or Latino	30	80	186	269	1.0	1.8	4.0	5.1
American Indian	2	12	21	30	0.1	0.3	0.5	0.6
Asian	117	243	603	1,287	3.8	5.4	13.0	24.2
Pharmacy[7]								
All races[4]	17,909	21,628	22,764	35,885	100.0	100.0	100.0	100.0
Not Hispanic or Latino:								
White	16,222	19,153	18,325	21,088	90.6	88.6	80.5	58.8
Black or African American	659	945	1,301	3,407	3.7	4.4	5.7	9.5
Hispanic or Latino	254	459	945	1,322	1.4	2.1	4.2	3.7
American Indian	29	36	63	179	0.2	0.2	0.3	0.5
Asian	672	1,035	2,130	7,405	3.8	4.8	9.4	20.6

See footnotes at end of table.

Table 104 (page 2 of 2). Total enrollment of minorities in schools for selected health occupations, according to detailed race and Hispanic origin: United States, academic years 1970–71, 1980–81, 1990–91, and 2000–01

[Data are based on reporting by health professions associations]

Occupation, detailed race, and Hispanic origin	1970–71[1]	1980–81	1990–91	2000–01[2]	1970–71[1]	1980–81	1990–91	2000–01[2]
Podiatry	Number of students				Percent distribution of students			
All races	1,268	2,577	2,226	2,258	100.0	100.0	100.0	100.0
Not Hispanic or Latino:								
White[4]	1,228	2,353	1,671	1,576	96.8	91.3	75.1	69.8
Black or African American	27	110	237	192	2.1	4.3	10.6	8.5
Hispanic or Latino	5	39	148	122	0.4	1.5	6.6	5.4
American Indian	1	6	7	10	0.1	0.2	0.3	0.4
Asian	7	69	163	358	0.6	2.7	7.3	15.9

- - - Data not available.

[1]Data for osteopathic medicine, podiatry, and optometry are for 1971–72. Data for pharmacy and registered nurses are for 1972–73.

[2]Data for podiatry exclude New York College of Podiatric Medicine. Data for registered nursing are for 1996–97, optometry are for 1998–99, and dentistry are for 1999–2000.

[3]Excludes Puerto Rican schools.

[4]Includes race and ethnicity unspecified.

[5]Includes Puerto Rican Commonwealth students.

[6]In 1990 the National League for Nursing developed a new system for analyzing minority data. In evaluating the former system, much underreporting was noted. Therefore, race-specific data before 1990 would not be comparable and are not shown. Additional changes in the minority data question were introduced for academic years 1992–93 and 1993–94 resulting in a discontinuity in the trend.

[7]Prior to 1992–93 pharmacy total enrollment data are for students in the final 3 years of pharmacy education. Beginning in 1992–93 pharmacy data are for all students.

NOTES: Total enrollment data are collected at the beginning of the academic year. Data for chiropractic students and occupational, physical, and speech therapy students were not available for this table.

SOURCES: Association of American Medical Colleges: AAMC Data Book: Statistical Information Related to Medical Education. Washington, DC. 2001. AAMC Student Records System, unpublished data; American Association of Colleges of Osteopathic Medicine: 2001 Annual Report on Medical Education. Chevy Chase, Maryland. 2002; Bureau of Health Professions: Minorities and Women in the Health Fields, 1990 Edition; American Dental Association: 1999–2000 Survey of predoctoral dental education, academic programs, enrollments, and graduates, vol. 1, Chicago. 2001; Association of Schools and Colleges of Optometry: unpublished data; American Association of Colleges of Pharmacy: Profile of Pharmacy Students, Fall 2000; American Association of Colleges of Podiatric Medicine: unpublished data; National League for Nursing: Nursing Data Review, 1997; Nursing Databook. New York. 1982.

Table 105. First-year and total enrollment of women in schools for selected health occupations, according to detailed race and Hispanic origin: United States, academic years 1971–72, 1980–81, 1990–91, and 1999–2000

[Data are based on reporting by health professions associations]

Enrollment, occupation, detailed race, and Hispanic origin	Both sexes				Women			
	1971–72[1]	1980–81	1990–91	1999–2000[2]	1971–72[1]	1980–81	1990–91	1999–2000[2]
First-year enrollment	Number of students				Percent of students			
Dentistry	4,705	5,964	3,961	4,314	3.1	19.8	37.9	37.6
Medicine (Allopathic)[3]	12,361	17,186	16,876	16,790	13.7	28.9	38.8	44.4
Not Hispanic or Latino:								
White	- - -	14,262	11,830	10,987	- - -	27.4	37.7	- - -
Black or African American	881	1,128	1,263	1,354	22.7	45.5	55.3	- - -
Hispanic or Latino	- - -	818	933	1,102	- - -	31.5	42.0	- - -
Mexican	118	258	285	453	8.5	30.6	39.3	- - -
Mainland Puerto Rican	40	95	120	116	15.0	43.2	43.3	- - -
Other Hispanic or Latino[4]	- - -	465	528	533	- - -	29.7	43.3	- - -
American Indian	23	67	76	165	34.8	35.8	40.8	- - -
Asian	217	572	2,527	3,182	19.4	31.5	40.3	- - -
Medicine (Osteopathic)	670	1,496	1,950	2,848	4.3	22.0	34.2	42.2
Nurses, registered[5]	93,344	110,201	113,526	119,205	94.5	92.7	89.3	87.5
Optometry[5]	906	1,174	1,207	1,369	5.3	25.3	50.6	55.5
Pharmacy[5,6]	6,532	7,442	8,009	8,123	25.8	48.4	- - -	64.7
Podiatry	399	695	622	606	- - -	- - -	- - -	34.7
Public Health	- - -	3,348	4,289	5,840	- - -	- - -	62.1	69.8
Total enrollment								
Dentistry	16,553	22,842	15,951	17,242	- - -	17.0	34.4	37.8
Medicine (Allopathic)[3]	43,650	65,189	65,163	66,444	10.9	26.5	37.3	43.9
Not Hispanic or Latino:								
White	- - -	55,434	47,893	42,589	- - -	25.0	35.4	41.5
Black or African American	2,055	3,708	4,241	5,051	20.4	44.3	55.8	62.0
Hispanic or Latino	- - -	2,761	3,538	4,322	- - -	30.1	39.0	45.4
Mexican	252	951	1,109	1,746	9.5	26.4	38.5	44.0
Mainland Puerto Rican	76	329	457	482	17.1	35.9	43.1	48.8
Other Hispanic[4]	- - -	1,481	1,972	2,094	- - -	31.1	38.4	45.9
American Indian	42	221	277	574	23.8	28.5	42.6	47.6
Asian	647	1,924	8,436	12,950	17.9	30.4	37.7	44.0
Medicine (Osteopathic)	2,304	4,940	6,792	10,388	3.4	19.7	32.7	40.2
Nurses, registered[5]	211,239	230,966	221,170	238,244	95.5	94.3	- - -	87.9
Optometry[5]	3,094	4,540	4,650	5,313	- - -	- - -	47.3	53.1
Pharmacy[5]	16,476	26,617	29,797	32,537	24.0	47.4	62.4	64.9
Podiatry	1,268	2,577	2,226	2,258	1.2	11.9	- - -	34.7
Public Health	- - -	8,486	11,386	15,839	- - -	55.2	62.5	66.8

- - - Data not available.

[1]Total enrollment for registered nurse students is for 1972–73.

[2]First-year enrollments for allopathic medicine and first-year and total enrollments for registered nurses and optometry are for 1998–99.

[3]Includes race and ethnicity unspecified.

[4]Includes Puerto Rican Commonwealth students.

[5]Excludes Puerto Rican schools.

[6]Pharmacy first-year enrollment is for students in the first year of the final 3 years of pharmacy education.

NOTES: Total enrollment data are collected at the beginning of the academic year while first-year enrollment data are collected during the academic year. Data for chiropractic students and occupational, physical, and speech therapy students were not available for this table.

SOURCES: Association of American Medical Colleges: AAMC Data Book: Statistical Information Related to Medical Education. Washington, DC. 2000 and unpublished data; American Association of Colleges of Osteopathic Medicine: 2000 Annual Statistical Report. Rockville, Maryland. 2001; Bureau of Health Professions: Minorities and women in the health fields, 1990 edition; American Dental Association: 1999–2000 Survey of predoctoral dental education academic programs, enrollments, and graduates vol. 1, Chicago. 2001; Association of Schools and Colleges of Optometry: unpublished data; American Association of Colleges of Pharmacy: Profile of Pharmacy Students, Fall 1999; American Association of Colleges of Podiatric Medicine: unpublished data; National League for Nursing: Nursing Data Review. New York. 1997; Nursing data book. New York. 1982; State-Approved Schools of Nursing-RN. New York. 1973; Association of Schools of Public Health: 2000 Annual Data Report. Washington, DC. 2001.

Table 106. Hospitals, beds, and occupancy rates, according to type of ownership and size of hospital: United States, selected years 1975–2001

[Data are based on reporting by a census of hospitals]

Type of ownership and size of hospital	1975	1980	1990	1995	1998	1999	2000	2001
Hospitals				Number				
All hospitals	7,156	6,965	6,649	6,291	6,021	5,890	5,810	5,801
Federal	382	359	337	299	275	264	245	243
Non-Federal[1]	6,774	6,606	6,312	5,992	5,746	5,626	5,565	5,558
Community[2]	5,875	5,830	5,384	5,194	5,015	4,956	4,915	4,908
Nonprofit	3,339	3,322	3,191	3,092	3,026	3,012	3,003	2,998
For profit	775	730	749	752	771	747	749	754
State-local government . . .	1,761	1,778	1,444	1,350	1,218	1,197	1,163	1,156
6–24 beds	299	259	226	278	293	299	288	281
25–49 beds	1,155	1,029	935	922	900	887	910	916
50–99 beds	1,481	1,462	1,263	1,139	1,085	1,082	1,055	1,070
100–199 beds	1,363	1,370	1,306	1,324	1,304	1,266	1,236	1,218
200–299 beds	678	715	739	718	644	642	656	635
300–399 beds	378	412	408	354	352	365	341	348
400–499 beds	230	266	222	195	183	161	182	191
500 beds or more	291	317	285	264	254	254	247	249
Beds								
All hospitals	1,465,828	1,364,516	1,213,327	1,080,601	1,012,582	993,866	983,628	987,440
Federal	131,946	117,328	98,255	77,079	56,698	55,120	53,067	51,900
Non-Federal[1]	1,333,882	1,247,188	1,115,072	1,003,522	955,884	938,746	930,561	935,540
Community[2]	941,844	988,387	927,360	872,736	839,988	829,575	823,560	825,966
Nonprofit	658,195	692,459	656,755	609,729	587,658	586,673	582,988	585,070
For profit	73,495	87,033	101,377	105,737	112,975	106,790	109,883	108,718
State-local government . . .	210,154	208,895	169,228	157,270	139,355	136,112	130,689	132,178
6–24 beds	5,615	4,932	4,427	5,085	5,351	5,442	5,156	4,964
25–49 beds	41,783	37,478	35,420	34,352	33,510	32,816	33,333	33,263
50–99 beds	106,776	105,278	90,394	82,024	78,035	78,121	75,865	76,924
100–199 beds	192,438	192,892	183,867	187,381	186,118	181,115	175,778	174,024
200–299 beds	164,405	172,390	179,670	175,240	156,978	155,831	159,807	154,420
300–399 beds	127,728	139,434	138,938	121,136	120,512	126,259	117,220	119,753
400–499 beds	101,278	117,724	98,833	86,459	81,247	71,580	80,763	84,745
500 beds or more	201,821	218,259	195,811	181,059	178,237	178,411	175,638	177,873
Occupancy rate[3]				Percent				
All hospitals	76.7	77.7	69.5	65.7	65.4	66.1	66.1	66.7
Federal	80.7	80.1	72.9	72.6	78.9	74.4	68.2	69.8
Non-Federal[1]	76.3	77.4	69.2	65.1	64.6	65.6	65.9	66.5
Community[2]	75.0	75.6	66.8	62.8	62.5	63.4	63.9	64.5
Nonprofit	77.5	78.2	69.3	64.5	64.2	64.9	65.5	65.8
For profit	65.9	65.2	52.8	51.8	53.2	54.8	55.9	57.8
State-local government . . .	70.4	71.1	65.3	63.7	62.7	63.4	63.2	64.1
6–24 beds	48.0	46.8	32.3	36.9	33.2	33.0	31.7	31.3
25–49 beds	56.7	52.8	41.3	42.6	41.2	41.5	41.3	42.5
50–99 beds	64.7	64.2	53.8	54.1	54.7	54.5	54.8	55.5
100–199 beds	71.2	71.4	61.5	58.8	58.4	59.3	60.0	60.7
200–299 beds	77.1	77.4	67.1	63.1	62.9	64.1	65.0	65.5
300–399 beds	79.7	79.7	70.0	64.8	64.7	66.1	65.7	66.4
400–499 beds	81.1	81.2	73.5	68.1	67.3	68.3	69.1	68.9
500 beds or more	80.9	82.1	77.3	71.4	70.9	71.7	72.2	72.8

[1]The category of non-Federal hospitals comprises psychiatric, tuberculosis and other respiratory diseases hospitals, and long-term and short-term general and other special hospitals. See Appendix II, Hospital.
[2]Community hospitals are non-Federal short-term general and special hospitals whose facilities and services are available to the public. See Appendix II, Hospital.
[3]Estimated percent of staffed beds that are occupied. See Appendix II, Occupancy rate.

NOTE: Data for additional years are available (see Appendix III).

SOURCES: American Hospital Association Annual Survey of Hospitals. Hospital Statistics, 1976, 1981, 1991–2003 Editions. Chicago. (Copyrights 1976, 1981, 1991–2003: Used with the permission of Health Forum LLC, an American Hospital Association Company.)

Table 107. Mental health organizations and beds for 24-hour hospital and residential treatment according to type of organization: United States, selected years 1986–98

[Data are based on inventories of mental health organizations]

Type of organization	1986	1990	1992	1994[1]	1998[1]
	Number of mental health organizations				
All organizations.	4,747	5,284	5,498	5,392	5,722
State and county mental hospitals	285	273	273	256	229
Private psychiatric hospitals.	314	462	475	430	348
Non-Federal general hospital psychiatric services . . .	1,351	1,674	1,616	1,612	1,707
Department of Veterans Affairs medical centers[2].	139	141	162	161	145
Residential treatment centers for emotionally disturbed children	437	501	497	459	461
All other organizations[3]	2,221	2,233	2,475	2,474	2,832
	Number of beds				
All organizations.	267,613	272,253	270,867	290,604	266,729
State and county mental hospitals	119,033	98,789	93,058	81,911	63,769
Private psychiatric hospitals.	30,201	44,871	43,684	42,399	34,154
Non-Federal general hospital psychiatric services . . .	45,808	53,479	52,059	52,984	55,145
Department of Veterans Affairs medical centers[2].	26,874	21,712	22,466	21,146	13,742
Residential treatment centers for emotionally disturbed children	24,547	29,756	30,089	32,110	33,997
All other organizations[3]	21,150	23,646	29,511	60,054	65,922
	Beds per 100,000 civilian population				
All organizations.	111.7	111.6	107.5	112.1	99.1
State and county mental hospitals	49.7	40.5	36.9	31.6	23.7
Private psychiatric hospitals.	12.6	18.4	17.3	16.4	12.7
Non-Federal general hospital psychiatric services . . .	19.1	21.9	20.7	20.4	20.5
Department of Veterans Affairs medical centers[2].	11.2	8.9	8.9	8.2	5.1
Residential treatment centers for emotionally disturbed children	10.3	12.2	11.9	12.4	12.6
All other organizations[3]	8.8	9.7	11.7	23.2	24.6

[1]Beginning in 1994 data for supportive residential clients (moderately staffed housing arrangements such as supervised apartments, group homes, and halfway houses) are included in the totals and all other organizations. This change affects the comparability of trend data prior to 1994 with data for 1994 and later years.
[2]Includes Department of Veterans Affairs (VA) neuropsychiatric hospitals, VA general hospital psychiatric services, and VA psychiatric outpatient clinics.
[3]Includes freestanding psychiatric outpatient clinics, partial care organizations, and multiservice mental health organizations.

NOTES: Data for 1998 are revised and differ from the previous edition of *Health, United States*. These data exclude mental health care provided in non-psychiatric units of hospitals such as general medical units.

SOURCE: Manderscheid RW and Henderson MJ. *Mental Health, United States, 2000.* Center for Mental Health Services. DHHS. Washington, DC. 2001.

Table 108. Community hospital beds and average annual percent change, according to geographic division and State: United States, selected years 1960–2001

[Data are based on reporting by a census of hospitals]

Geographic division and State	1960[1,2]	1970[1]	1980[1]	1990[3]	2000[3]	2001[3]	1960–70[1,2]	1970–80[1]	1980–90[4]	1990–2000[3]	2000–01[3]
	Beds per 1,000 resident population[5]						Average annual percent change				
United States	3.6	4.3	4.5	3.7	2.9	2.9	1.8	0.5	−1.9	−2.4	0.0
New England	3.9	4.1	4.1	3.4	2.5	2.5	0.5	0.0	−1.9	−3.0	0.0
Maine	3.4	4.7	4.7	3.7	2.9	3.0	3.3	0.0	−2.4	−2.4	3.4
New Hampshire	4.4	4.0	3.9	3.1	2.3	2.3	−0.9	−0.3	−2.3	−2.9	0.0
Vermont	4.5	4.5	4.4	3.0	2.7	2.8	0.0	−0.2	−3.8	−1.0	3.7
Massachusetts	4.2	4.4	4.4	3.6	2.6	2.6	0.5	0.0	−2.0	−3.2	0.0
Rhode Island	3.7	4.0	3.8	3.2	2.3	2.3	0.8	−0.5	−1.7	−3.2	0.0
Connecticut	3.4	3.4	3.5	2.9	2.3	2.3	0.0	0.3	−1.9	−2.3	0.0
Middle Atlantic	4.0	4.4	4.6	4.1	3.4	3.4	1.0	0.4	−1.1	−1.9	0.0
New York	4.3	4.6	4.5	4.1	3.5	3.5	0.7	−0.2	−0.9	−1.6	0.0
New Jersey	3.1	3.6	4.2	3.7	3.0	2.9	1.5	1.6	−1.3	−2.1	−3.3
Pennsylvania	4.1	4.7	4.8	4.4	3.4	3.4	1.4	0.2	−0.9	−2.5	0.0
East North Central	3.6	4.4	4.7	3.9	2.9	2.9	2.0	0.7	−1.8	−2.9	0.0
Ohio	3.4	4.2	4.7	4.0	3.0	2.9	2.1	1.1	−1.6	−2.8	−3.3
Indiana	3.1	4.0	4.5	3.9	3.2	3.1	2.6	1.2	−1.4	−2.0	−3.1
Illinois	4.0	4.7	5.1	4.0	3.0	3.0	1.6	0.8	−2.4	−2.8	0.0
Michigan	3.3	4.3	4.4	3.7	2.6	2.6	2.7	0.2	−1.7	−3.5	0.0
Wisconsin	4.3	5.2	4.9	3.8	2.9	2.9	1.9	−0.6	−2.5	−2.7	0.0
West North Central	4.3	5.7	5.8	4.9	3.9	3.9	2.9	0.2	−1.7	−2.3	0.0
Minnesota	4.8	6.1	5.7	4.4	3.4	3.3	2.4	−0.7	−2.6	−2.5	−2.9
Iowa	3.9	5.6	5.7	5.1	4.0	3.9	3.7	0.2	−1.1	−2.4	−2.5
Missouri	3.9	5.1	5.7	4.8	3.6	3.4	2.7	1.1	−1.7	−2.8	−5.6
North Dakota	5.2	6.8	7.4	7.0	6.0	5.9	2.7	0.8	−0.6	−1.5	−1.7
South Dakota	4.5	5.6	5.5	6.1	5.7	5.9	2.2	−0.2	1.0	−0.7	3.5
Nebraska	4.4	6.2	6.0	5.5	4.8	4.9	3.5	−0.3	−0.9	−1.4	2.1
Kansas	4.2	5.4	5.8	4.8	4.0	4.2	2.5	0.7	−1.9	−1.8	5.0
South Atlantic	3.3	4.0	4.5	3.7	2.9	2.9	1.9	1.2	−1.9	−2.4	0.0
Delaware	3.7	3.7	3.6	3.0	2.3	2.3	0.0	−0.3	−1.8	−2.6	0.0
Maryland	3.3	3.1	3.6	2.8	2.1	2.1	−0.6	1.5	−2.5	−2.8	0.0
District of Columbia	5.9	7.4	7.3	7.6	5.8	5.9	2.3	−0.1	0.4	−2.7	1.7
Virginia	3.0	3.7	4.1	3.3	2.4	2.3	2.1	1.0	−2.1	−3.1	−4.2
West Virginia	4.1	5.4	5.5	4.7	4.4	4.4	2.8	0.2	−1.6	−0.7	0.0
North Carolina	3.4	3.8	4.2	3.3	2.9	2.9	1.1	1.0	−2.4	−1.3	0.0
South Carolina	2.9	3.7	3.9	3.3	2.9	2.8	2.5	0.5	−1.7	−1.3	−3.4
Georgia	2.8	3.8	4.6	4.0	2.9	2.9	3.1	1.9	−1.4	−3.2	0.0
Florida	3.1	4.4	5.1	3.9	3.2	3.2	3.6	1.5	−2.6	−2.0	0.0
East South Central	3.0	4.4	5.1	4.7	3.8	3.8	3.9	1.5	−0.8	−2.1	0.0
Kentucky	3.0	4.0	4.5	4.3	3.7	3.7	2.9	1.2	−0.5	−1.5	0.0
Tennessee	3.4	4.7	5.5	4.8	3.6	3.6	3.3	1.6	−1.4	−2.8	0.0
Alabama	2.8	4.3	5.1	4.6	3.7	3.7	4.4	1.7	−1.0	−2.2	0.0
Mississippi	2.9	4.4	5.3	5.0	4.8	4.8	4.3	1.9	−0.6	−0.4	0.0
West South Central	3.3	4.3	4.7	3.8	3.0	3.0	2.7	0.9	−2.1	−2.3	0.0
Arkansas	2.9	4.2	5.0	4.6	3.7	3.5	3.8	1.8	−0.8	−2.2	−5.4
Louisiana	3.9	4.2	4.8	4.6	3.9	4.0	0.7	1.3	−0.4	−1.6	2.6
Oklahoma	3.2	4.5	4.6	4.0	3.2	3.2	3.5	0.2	−1.4	−2.2	0.0
Texas	3.3	4.3	4.7	3.5	2.7	2.6	2.7	0.9	−2.9	−2.6	−3.7
Mountain	3.5	4.3	3.8	3.1	2.3	2.3	2.1	−1.2	−2.0	−2.9	0.0
Montana	5.1	5.8	5.9	5.8	4.7	4.9	1.3	0.2	−0.2	−2.1	4.3
Idaho	3.2	4.0	3.7	3.2	2.7	2.6	2.3	−0.8	−1.4	−1.7	−3.7
Wyoming	4.6	5.5	3.6	4.8	3.9	3.9	1.8	−4.1	2.9	−2.1	0.0
Colorado	3.8	4.6	4.2	3.2	2.2	2.1	1.9	−0.9	−2.7	−3.7	−4.5
New Mexico	2.9	3.5	3.1	2.8	1.9	2.0	1.9	−1.2	−1.0	−3.8	5.3
Arizona	3.0	4.1	3.6	2.7	2.1	2.0	3.2	−1.3	−2.8	−2.5	−4.8
Utah	2.8	3.6	3.1	2.6	1.9	2.0	2.5	−1.5	−1.7	−3.1	5.3
Nevada	3.9	4.2	4.2	2.8	1.9	1.9	0.7	0.0	−4.0	−3.8	0.0
Pacific	3.1	3.7	3.5	2.7	2.1	2.1	1.8	−0.6	−2.6	−2.5	0.0
Washington	3.3	3.5	3.1	2.5	1.9	1.9	0.6	−1.2	−2.1	−2.7	0.0
Oregon	3.5	4.0	3.5	2.8	1.9	1.9	1.3	−1.3	−2.2	−3.8	0.0
California	3.0	3.8	3.6	2.7	2.1	2.1	2.4	−0.5	−2.8	−2.5	0.0
Alaska	2.4	2.3	2.7	2.3	2.3	2.3	−0.4	1.6	−1.6	0.0	0.0
Hawaii	3.7	3.4	3.1	2.7	2.5	2.6	−0.8	−0.9	−1.4	−0.8	4.0

[1]Data exclude facilities for the mentally retarded. See Appendix II, Hospital.
[2]1960 data include hospital units of institutions such as prisons and college infirmaries.
[3]Starting with 1990, data exclude hospital units of institutions, facilities for the mentally retarded, and alcoholism and chemical dependency hospitals. See Appendix II, Hospital.
[4]1990 data used in this calculation (not shown in table) exclude only facilities for the mentally retarded, consistent with exclusions from 1980 data.
[5]Civilian population for 1997 and earlier years.

NOTE: Data for additional years are available (see Appendix III).

SOURCES: American Hospital Association (AHA): Hospitals. *JAHA* 35(15):383–430, 1961 (Copyright 1961: Used with permission of AHA); National Center for Health Statistics, Division of Health Care Statistics and AHA Annual Survey of Hospitals for 1970, 1980; Hospital Statistics 1991–92, 2003 Editions. Chicago (Copyrights 1971, 1981, 1991, 2003: Used with permission of Health Forum LLC, an American Hospital Association Company).

Table 109. Occupancy rates in community hospitals and average annual percent change, according to geographic division and State: United States, selected years 1960–2001

[Data are based on reporting by a census of hospitals]

Geographic division and State	1960[1,2]	1970[1]	1980[1]	1990[3]	2000[3]	2001[3]	1960–70[1,2]	1970–80[1]	1980–90[4]	1990–2000[3]	2000–01[3]
	Occupancy rate[5]						Average annual percent change				
United States	75	77	75	67	64	64	0.3	−0.3	−1.1	−0.5	0.0
New England	75	80	80	74	70	71	0.6	0.0	−0.8	−0.6	1.4
Maine	73	73	75	72	64	64	0.0	0.3	−0.4	−1.2	0.0
New Hampshire	67	73	73	67	59	61	0.9	0.0	−0.9	−1.3	3.4
Vermont	69	76	74	67	67	65	1.0	−0.3	−1.0	0.0	−3.0
Massachusetts............	76	80	82	74	71	73	0.5	0.2	−1.0	−0.4	2.8
Rhode Island	76	83	86	79	72	71	0.9	0.4	−0.8	−0.9	−1.4
Connecticut	78	83	80	77	75	74	0.6	−0.4	−0.4	−0.3	−1.3
Middle Atlantic............	78	82	83	81	74	73	0.5	0.1	−0.2	−0.9	−1.4
New York.................	79	83	86	86	79	77	0.5	0.4	0.0	−0.8	−2.5
New Jersey	78	83	83	80	69	69	0.6	0.0	−0.4	−1.5	0.0
Pennsylvania	76	82	80	73	68	68	0.8	−0.2	−0.9	−0.7	0.0
East North Central...........	78	80	77	65	61	61	0.3	−0.4	−1.7	−0.6	0.0
Ohio	81	82	79	65	61	62	0.1	−0.4	−1.9	−0.6	1.6
Indiana	80	80	78	61	56	57	0.0	−0.3	−2.4	−0.9	1.8
Illinois	76	79	75	66	60	61	0.4	−0.5	−1.3	−0.9	1.7
Michigan	81	81	78	66	65	65	0.0	−0.4	−1.7	−0.2	0.0
Wisconsin	74	73	74	65	60	61	−0.1	0.1	−1.3	−0.8	1.7
West North Central	72	74	71	62	60	61	0.3	−0.4	−1.3	−0.3	1.7
Minnesota	72	74	74	67	67	68	0.3	0.0	−1.0	0.0	1.5
Iowa	73	72	69	62	58	59	−0.1	−0.4	−1.1	−0.7	1.7
Missouri.................	76	79	75	62	58	60	0.4	−0.5	−1.9	−0.7	3.4
North Dakota	71	67	69	64	60	58	−0.6	0.3	−0.7	−0.6	−3.3
South Dakota............	66	66	61	62	65	64	0.0	−0.8	0.2	0.5	−1.5
Nebraska................	66	70	67	58	59	60	0.6	−0.4	−1.4	0.2	1.7
Kansas	69	71	69	56	53	53	0.3	−0.3	−2.1	−0.5	0.0
South Atlantic	75	78	76	67	65	65	0.4	−0.3	−1.3	−0.3	0.0
Delaware................	70	79	82	77	75	74	1.2	0.4	−0.6	−0.3	−1.3
Maryland	74	79	84	79	73	73	0.7	0.6	−0.6	−0.8	0.0
District of Columbia	81	78	83	75	74	73	−0.4	0.6	−1.0	−0.1	−1.4
Virginia	78	81	78	67	68	69	0.4	−0.4	−1.5	0.1	1.5
West Virginia	75	79	76	63	61	63	0.5	−0.4	−1.9	−0.3	3.3
North Carolina	74	79	78	73	70	69	0.7	−0.1	−0.7	−0.4	−1.4
South Carolina...........	77	76	77	71	69	71	−0.1	0.1	−0.8	−0.3	2.9
Georgia	72	77	70	66	63	62	0.7	−0.9	−0.6	−0.5	−1.6
Florida..................	74	76	72	62	61	61	0.3	−0.5	−1.5	−0.2	0.0
East South Central	72	78	75	63	59	58	0.8	−0.4	−1.7	−0.7	−1.7
Kentucky................	73	80	77	62	62	61	0.9	−0.4	−2.1	0.0	−1.6
Tennessee...............	76	78	76	64	56	55	0.3	−0.3	−1.7	−1.3	−1.8
Alabama	71	80	73	63	60	59	1.2	−0.9	−1.5	−0.5	−1.7
Mississippi..............	63	74	71	59	59	60	1.6	−0.4	−1.8	0.0	1.7
West South Central	69	73	70	58	58	60	0.6	−0.4	−1.9	0.0	3.4
Arkansas................	70	74	70	62	59	58	0.6	−0.6	−1.2	−0.5	−1.7
Louisiana................	68	74	70	57	56	57	0.8	−0.6	−2.0	−0.2	1.8
Oklahoma	71	73	68	58	56	58	0.3	−0.7	−1.6	−0.4	3.6
Texas	68	73	70	57	59	61	0.7	−0.4	−2.0	0.3	3.4
Mountain	70	71	70	61	61	61	0.1	−0.1	−1.4	0.0	0.0
Montana	60	66	66	61	67	65	1.0	0.0	−0.8	0.9	−3.0
Idaho	56	66	65	56	53	54	1.7	−0.2	−1.5	−0.5	1.9
Wyoming	61	63	57	54	56	54	0.3	−1.0	−0.5	0.4	−3.6
Colorado	81	74	72	64	58	61	−0.9	−0.3	−1.2	−1.0	5.2
New Mexico..............	65	70	66	58	58	58	0.7	−0.6	−1.3	0.0	0.0
Arizona	74	73	74	62	63	64	−0.1	0.1	−1.8	0.2	1.6
Utah	70	74	70	59	56	56	0.6	−0.6	−1.7	−0.5	0.0
Nevada	71	73	69	60	71	68	0.3	−0.6	−1.4	1.7	−4.2
Pacific	71	71	69	64	65	66	0.0	−0.3	−0.7	0.2	1.5
Washington	63	70	72	63	60	60	1.1	0.3	−1.3	−0.5	0.0
Oregon	66	69	69	57	59	60	0.4	0.0	−1.9	0.3	1.7
California................	74	71	69	64	66	67	−0.4	−0.3	−0.7	0.3	1.5
Alaska..................	54	59	58	50	57	58	0.9	−0.2	−1.5	1.3	1.8
Hawaii..................	62	76	75	85	76	74	2.1	−0.1	1.3	−1.1	−2.6

[1]Data exclude facilities for the mentally retarded. See Appendix II, Hospital.
[2]1960 data include hospital units of institutions such as prisons and college infirmaries.
[3]Starting with 1990, data exclude hospital units of institutions, facilities for the mentally retarded, and alcoholism and chemical dependency hospitals. See Appendix II, Hospital.
[4]1990 data used in this calculation (not shown in table) exclude only facilities for the mentally retarded, consistent with exclusions from 1980 data.
[5]Estimated percent of staffed beds that are occupied. See Appendix II, Occupancy rate.

NOTE: Data for additional years are available (see Appendix III).

SOURCES: American Hospital Association (AHA): Hospitals. *JAHA* 35(15):383–430, 1961. (Copyright 1961: Used with permission of AHA); AHA Annual Survey of Hospitals, 1970 and 1980 unpublished; Hospital Statistics 1991–92, 2002, and 2003 Editions. Chicago (Copyrights 1971, 1981, 1991, 2002, 2003: Used with permission of Health Forum LLC, an American Hospital Association Company).

Table 110 (page 1 of 2). Nursing homes, beds, occupancy, and residents, according to geographic division and State: United States, 1995–2001

[Data are based on a census of certified nursing facilities]

Geographic division and State	Nursing homes			Beds		
	1995	2000	2001	1995	2000	2001
United States	16,389	16,886	16,675	1,751,302	1,795,388	1,779,924
New England	1,140	1,137	1,110	115,488	118,562	115,939
Maine	132	126	126	9,243	8,248	8,002
New Hampshire	74	83	83	7,412	7,837	7,883
Vermont	23	44	44	1,862	3,743	3,636
Massachusetts	550	526	506	54,532	56,030	54,514
Rhode Island	94	99	97	9,612	10,271	10,183
Connecticut	267	259	254	32,827	32,433	31,721
Middle Atlantic	1,650	1,796	1,799	244,342	267,772	268,888
New York	624	665	669	107,750	120,514	121,592
New Jersey	300	361	364	43,967	52,195	52,463
Pennsylvania	726	770	766	92,625	95,063	94,833
East North Central	3,171	3,301	3,265	367,879	369,657	364,309
Ohio	943	1,009	998	106,884	105,038	103,974
Indiana	556	564	560	59,538	56,762	56,861
Illinois	827	869	854	103,230	110,766	108,287
Michigan	432	439	434	49,473	50,696	49,535
Wisconsin	413	420	419	48,754	46,395	45,652
West North Central	2,258	2,281	2,247	200,109	193,754	191,091
Minnesota	432	433	427	43,865	42,149	40,836
Iowa	419	467	466	39,959	37,034	36,944
Missouri	546	551	545	52,679	54,829	54,882
North Dakota	87	88	87	7,125	6,954	6,757
South Dakota	114	114	112	8,296	7,844	7,568
Nebraska	231	236	230	18,169	17,877	17,369
Kansas	429	392	380	30,016	27,067	26,735
South Atlantic	2,215	2,418	2,410	243,069	264,147	265,149
Delaware	42	43	42	4,739	4,906	4,736
Maryland	218	255	251	28,394	31,495	30,507
District of Columbia	19	20	21	3,206	3,078	3,136
Virginia	271	278	277	30,070	30,595	31,102
West Virginia	129	139	139	10,903	11,413	11,373
North Carolina	391	410	413	38,322	41,376	42,194
South Carolina	166	178	179	16,682	18,102	18,185
Georgia	352	363	361	38,097	39,817	39,806
Florida	627	732	727	72,656	83,365	84,110
East South Central	1,014	1,071	1,080	99,707	106,250	107,656
Kentucky	288	307	304	23,221	25,341	25,482
Tennessee	322	349	349	37,074	38,593	38,923
Alabama	221	225	228	23,353	25,248	25,797
Mississippi	183	190	199	16,059	17,068	17,454
West South Central	2,264	2,199	2,143	224,695	224,100	220,048
Arkansas	256	255	250	29,952	25,715	25,061
Louisiana	337	337	332	37,769	39,430	38,861
Oklahoma	405	392	379	33,918	33,903	32,776
Texas	1,266	1,215	1,182	123,056	125,052	123,350
Mountain	800	827	806	70,134	75,152	74,034
Montana	100	104	103	7,210	7,667	7,594
Idaho	76	84	84	5,747	6,181	6,368
Wyoming	37	40	39	3,035	3,119	3,098
Colorado	219	225	223	19,912	20,240	20,119
New Mexico	83	80	80	6,969	7,289	7,263
Arizona	152	150	139	16,162	17,458	16,836
Utah	91	93	92	7,101	7,651	7,683
Nevada	42	51	46	3,998	5,547	5,073
Pacific	1,877	1,856	1,815	185,879	175,994	172,810
Washington	285	277	268	28,464	25,905	24,983
Oregon	161	150	145	13,885	13,500	12,977
California	1,382	1,369	1,342	140,203	131,762	129,928
Alaska	15	15	15	814	821	882
Hawaii	34	45	45	2,513	4,006	4,040

See footnotes at end of table.

[Data are based on a census of certified nursing facilities]

Geographic division and State	Residents			Occupancy rate[1]			Resident rate[2]	
	1995	2000	2001	1995	2000	2001	1995	2000
United States	1,479,550	1,480,076	1,469,001	84.5	82.4	82.5	404.5	349.1
New England	105,792	106,308	104,573	91.6	89.7	90.2	474.2	419.5
Maine	8,587	7,298	7,189	92.9	88.5	89.8	417.9	313.0
New Hampshire	6,877	7,158	7,126	92.8	91.3	90.4	434.1	392.6
Vermont	1,792	3,349	3,293	96.2	89.5	90.6	207.0	335.0
Massachusetts	49,765	49,805	48,876	91.3	88.9	89.7	477.3	426.8
Rhode Island	8,823	9,041	8,923	91.8	88.0	87.6	476.9	432.6
Connecticut	29,948	29,657	29,166	91.2	91.4	91.9	541.7	461.4
Middle Atlantic	228,649	242,674	242,784	93.6	90.6	90.3	384.0	354.2
New York	103,409	112,957	114,141	96.0	93.7	93.9	371.8	362.6
New Jersey	40,397	45,837	45,672	91.9	87.8	87.1	351.6	337.0
Pennsylvania	84,843	83,880	82,971	91.6	88.2	87.5	419.2	353.1
East North Central	294,319	289,404	284,563	80.0	78.3	78.1	476.1	414.3
Ohio	79,026	81,946	80,930	73.9	78.0	77.8	499.5	463.5
Indiana	44,328	42,328	41,946	74.5	74.6	73.8	548.9	462.3
Illinois	83,696	83,604	81,749	81.1	75.5	75.5	495.3	435.4
Michigan	43,271	42,615	41,508	87.5	84.1	83.8	345.0	299.1
Wisconsin	43,998	38,911	38,430	90.2	83.9	84.2	518.9	406.9
West North Central	164,660	157,224	154,804	82.3	81.1	81.0	489.6	429.8
Minnesota	41,163	38,813	38,052	93.8	92.1	93.2	537.4	453.4
Iowa	27,506	29,204	28,825	68.8	78.9	78.0	458.0	448.5
Missouri	39,891	38,586	38,706	75.7	70.4	70.5	432.8	391.5
North Dakota	6,868	6,343	6,279	96.4	91.2	92.9	522.0	430.7
South Dakota	7,926	7,059	6,952	95.5	90.0	91.9	543.3	438.8
Nebraska	16,166	14,989	14,492	89.0	83.8	83.4	501.4	441.5
Kansas	25,140	22,230	21,498	83.8	82.1	80.4	528.9	429.4
South Atlantic	217,303	227,818	228,961	89.4	86.2	86.4	335.4	291.9
Delaware	3,819	3,900	3,950	80.6	79.5	83.4	448.7	369.7
Maryland	24,716	25,629	25,361	87.0	81.4	83.1	432.7	383.1
District of Columbia	2,576	2,858	2,863	80.3	92.9	91.3	297.6	318.4
Virginia	28,119	27,091	26,875	93.5	88.5	86.4	385.2	310.4
West Virginia	10,216	10,334	10,304	93.7	90.5	90.6	355.2	325.2
North Carolina	35,511	36,658	37,106	92.7	88.6	87.9	401.1	347.6
South Carolina	14,568	15,739	16,117	87.3	86.9	88.6	366.0	313.1
Georgia	35,933	36,559	36,356	94.3	91.8	91.3	496.0	416.1
Florida	61,845	69,050	70,029	85.1	82.8	83.3	228.2	208.4
East South Central	91,563	96,348	96,598	91.8	90.7	89.7	416.6	385.5
Kentucky	20,696	22,730	22,776	89.1	89.7	89.4	391.9	390.1
Tennessee	33,929	34,714	34,588	91.5	89.9	88.9	479.6	426.1
Alabama	21,691	23,089	23,538	92.9	91.4	91.2	370.1	343.1
Mississippi	15,247	15,815	15,696	94.9	92.7	89.9	405.3	368.7
West South Central	169,047	159,160	156,961	75.2	71.0	71.3	486.1	397.6
Arkansas	20,823	19,317	18,677	69.5	75.1	74.5	508.3	415.5
Louisiana	32,493	30,735	30,127	86.0	77.9	77.5	639.3	523.8
Oklahoma	26,377	23,833	22,640	77.8	70.3	69.1	499.1	416.8
Texas	89,354	85,275	85,517	72.6	68.2	69.3	439.9	358.4
Mountain	58,738	59,379	59,395	83.8	79.0	80.2	335.9	271.2
Montana	6,415	5,973	5,928	89.0	77.9	78.1	491.4	389.5
Idaho	4,697	4,640	4,619	81.7	75.1	72.5	321.7	257.0
Wyoming	2,661	2,605	2,546	87.7	83.5	82.2	468.2	386.8
Colorado	17,055	17,045	16,855	85.7	84.2	83.8	420.6	353.5
New Mexico	6,051	6,503	6,364	86.8	89.2	87.6	332.0	279.0
Arizona	12,382	13,253	13,455	76.6	75.9	79.9	233.3	193.4
Utah	5,832	5,703	5,592	82.1	74.5	72.8	323.5	262.2
Nevada	3,645	3,657	4,036	91.2	65.9	79.6	312.0	215.3
Pacific	149,479	141,761	140,362	80.4	80.5	81.2	302.4	241.3
Washington	24,954	21,158	20,663	87.7	81.7	82.7	362.5	251.6
Oregon	11,673	9,990	9,444	84.1	74.0	72.8	244.9	173.9
California	109,805	106,460	105,923	78.3	80.8	81.5	302.9	250.1
Alaska	634	595	638	77.9	72.5	72.3	348.0	225.9
Hawaii	2,413	3,558	3,694	96.0	88.8	91.4	178.5	202.6

[1] Percent of beds occupied (number of nursing home residents per 100 nursing home beds).
[2] Number of nursing home residents (all ages) per 1,000 resident population 85 years of age and over.

NOTES: Annual numbers of nursing homes, beds, and residents are based on a 15-month OSCAR reporting cycle (see Appendix I). Data for additional years are available (see Appendix III).

SOURCES: Cowles CM, 1995 Nursing Home Statistical Yearbook. 1996 Nursing Home Statistical Yearbook. 1997 Nursing Home Statistical Yearbook. Anacortes, WA: Cowles Research Group, 1995; 1997; 1998; and Cowles CM, 1998 Nursing Home Statistical Yearbook. 1999 Nursing Home Statistical Yearbook. 2000 Nursing Home Statistical Yearbook. Washington, DC: American Association of Homes and Services for the Aging, 1999; 2000; 2001. Based on data from the Centers for Medicare & Medicaid Services' Online Survey Certification and Reporting (OSCAR) database.

This table will be updated with 2001 resident rates on the web. Go to www.cdc.gov/nchs/hus.htm.

Table 111. Total health expenditures as a percent of gross domestic product and per capita health expenditures in dollars: Selected countries and years 1960–2000

[Data compiled by the Organization for Economic Cooperation and Development]

Country	1960	1970	1980	1990	1995	1996	1997	1998	1999	2000[1]
				Health expenditures as a percent of gross domestic product						
Australia	4.3	- - -	7.0	7.8	8.2	8.3	8.4	8.5	8.4	8.3
Austria	4.3	5.3	7.6	7.1	8.6	8.7	8.0	8.0	8.1	8.0
Belgium	- - -	4.0	6.4	7.4	8.7	8.8	8.5	8.5	8.7	8.7
Canada	5.4	7.0	7.1	9.0	9.1	8.9	8.9	9.1	9.2	9.1
Czech Republic	- - -	- - -	- - -	5.0	7.3	7.1	7.1	7.1	7.2	7.2
Denmark	- - -	- - -	9.1	8.5	8.2	8.3	8.2	8.4	8.5	8.3
Finland	3.9	5.6	6.4	7.9	7.5	7.7	7.3	6.9	6.9	6.6
France	- - -	- - -	- - -	8.6	9.6	9.6	9.4	9.3	9.4	9.5
Germany	4.8	6.3	8.8	8.7	10.6	10.9	10.7	10.6	10.7	10.6
Greece	- - -	6.1	6.6	7.5	8.9	8.9	8.7	8.7	8.7	8.3
Hungary	- - -	- - -	- - -	- - -	7.5	7.2	7.0	6.9	6.8	6.8
Iceland	3.3	4.9	6.1	7.9	8.2	8.2	8.0	8.3	8.7	8.9
Ireland	3.6	5.1	8.4	6.6	7.2	7.0	6.9	6.8	6.8	6.7
Italy	3.6	5.1	- - -	8.0	7.4	7.5	7.7	7.7	7.8	8.1
Japan	3.0	4.5	6.4	5.9	7.0	7.0	7.2	7.1	7.4	7.8
Korea	. - - -	- - -	- - -	4.8	4.7	4.9	5.0	5.1	5.6	5.9
Luxembourg	- - -	3.6	5.9	6.1	6.4	6.4	5.9	5.8	6.0	- - -
Mexico	- - -	- - -	- - -	4.4	5.6	5.3	5.3	5.3	5.4	5.4
Netherlands	- - -	- - -	7.5	8.0	8.4	8.3	8.2	8.1	8.2	8.1
New Zealand	- - -	5.1	5.9	6.9	7.2	7.2	7.5	7.9	7.9	8.0
Norway	2.9	4.4	7.0	7.8	8.0	8.0	7.9	8.6	8.8	7.8
Poland	- - -	- - -	- - -	5.3	6.0	6.4	6.1	6.4	6.2	- - -
Portugal	- - -	2.6	5.6	6.2	8.3	8.5	8.6	8.3	8.4	8.2
Slovak Republic	- - -	- - -	- - -	- - -	- - -	- - -	6.1	5.9	5.8	5.9
Spain	1.5	3.6	5.4	6.6	7.7	7.7	7.6	7.6	7.7	7.7
Sweden	4.5	6.9	9.1	8.5	8.1	8.4	8.1	7.9	- - -	- - -
Switzerland	4.9	5.6	7.6	8.5	10.0	10.4	10.4	10.6	10.7	10.7
Turkey	- - -	2.4	3.3	3.6	3.4	3.9	4.2	4.8	- - -	- - -
United Kingdom	3.9	4.5	5.6	6.0	7.0	7.0	6.8	6.8	7.1	7.3
United States	5.1	7.0	8.8	12.0	13.4	13.3	13.1	13.1	13.2	13.3
				Per capita health expenditures[2]						
Australia	$ 87	- - -	$ 658	$1,300	$1,765	$1,854	$1,950	$2,058	$2,141	$2,211
Austria	64	$159	662	1,206	1,831	1,940	1,873	1,968	2,061	2,162
Belgium	- - -	130	577	1,245	1,896	1,982	2,013	2,008	2,144	2,269
Canada	109	260	710	1,676	2,114	2,091	2,181	2,285	2,428	2,535
Czech Republic	- - -	- - -	- - -	576	902	917	930	944	972	1,031
Denmark	- - -	- - -	819	1,453	1,882	2,004	2,100	2,241	2,358	2,420
Finland	54	161	509	1,295	1,415	1,487	1,550	1,529	1,605	1,664
France	- - -	- - -	- - -	1,517	1,980	1,997	2,046	2,109	2,226	2,349
Germany	90	223	824	1,600	2,164	2,341	2,465	2,520	2,616	2,748
Greece	- - -	98	348	712	1,131	1,179	1,224	1,307	1,375	1,399
Hungary	- - -	- - -	- - -	- - -	677	671	693	751	787	841
Iceland	50	137	576	1,376	1,823	1,911	1,988	2,204	2,409	2,608
Ireland	36	99	454	777	1,300	1,318	1,526	1,576	1,752	1,953
Italy	48	151	- - -	1,321	1,486	1,566	1,684	1,774	1,882	2,032
Japan	26	130	522	1,083	1,631	1,699	1,831	1,735	1,852	2,012
Korea	- - -	- - -	- - -	355	535	611	657	630	758	893
Luxembourg	- - -	148	605	1,492	2,122	2,192	2,204	2,361	2,613	- - -
Mexico	- - -	- - -	- - -	260	388	381	411	431	452	490
Netherlands	- - -	- - -	668	1,333	1,787	1,818	1,958	2,040	2,172	2,246
New Zealand	- - -	174	458	937	1,244	1,267	1,364	1,450	1,526	1,623
Norway	46	131	632	1,363	1,865	2,026	2,193	2,439	2,550	2,362
Poland	- - -	- - -	- - -	258	420	469	461	543	558	- - -
Portugal	- - -	40	265	611	1,146	1,211	1,360	1,345	1,402	1,441
Slovak Republic	- - -	- - -	- - -	- - -	- - -	- - -	608	641	649	690
Spain	14	83	328	813	1,184	1,238	1,294	1,384	1,469	1,556
Sweden	89	270	850	1,492	1,622	1,716	1,770	1,748	- - -	- - -
Switzerland	136	288	881	1,836	2,555	2,615	2,841	2,952	3,080	3,222
Turkey	- - -	23	75	171	190	234	272	303	- - -	- - -
United Kingdom	74	144	444	972	1,315	1,422	1,481	1,527	1,666	1,763
United States	143	348	1,067	2,738	3,688	3,847	4,007	4,178	4,392	4,672

- - - Data not available.

[1]Preliminary figures.

[2]Per capita health expenditures for each country have been adjusted to U.S. dollars using gross domestic product purchasing power parities for each year.

NOTE: Some numbers in this table have been revised and differ from previous editions of *Health, United States*.

SOURCES: All countries except United States from the Organization for Economic Cooperation and Development Health Data File 2002, following the annual update, www.oecd.org/els/health; United States data from the Centers for Medicare and Medicaid Services, Office of the Actuary, National Health Statistics Group, National health expenditures, 2001. Internet address: cms.hhs.gov/statistics/nhe.

Health Care Expenditures

Table 112. Gross domestic product, Federal and State and local government expenditures, national health expenditures, and average annual percent change: United States, selected years 1960–2001

[Data are compiled from various sources by the Centers for Medicare & Medicaid Services]

Gross domestic product, government expenditures, and national health expenditures	1960	1970	1980	1990	1995	1998	1999	2000	2001
	Amount in billions								
Gross domestic product (GDP).	$ 527	$1,040	$2,796	$ 5,803	$ 7,400	$ 8,781	$ 9,274	$ 9,825	$ 10,082
Federal government expenditures.	85.8	198.6	576.6	1,228.7	1,575.7	1,705.9	1,755.3	1,827.1	1,936.4
State and local government expenditures	38.1	107.5	307.8	660.8	902.5	1,033.7	1,105.8	1,196.2	1,292.6
National health expenditures	26.7	73.1	245.8	696.0	990.1	1,150.0	1,219.7	1,310.0	1,424.5
Private.	20.1	45.4	140.9	413.5	532.5	628.4	669.7	718.7	777.9
Public.	6.6	27.6	104.8	282.5	457.7	521.6	550.0	591.3	646.7
Federal government	2.8	17.6	71.3	192.7	323.5	368.7	386.2	415.1	454.8
State and local government.	3.8	10.0	33.5	89.8	134.2	152.9	163.8	176.2	191.8
	Amount per capita								
National health expenditures	$ 143	$ 348	$1,067	$ 2,738	$ 3,697	$ 4,178	$ 4,392	$ 4,672	$ 5,035
Private	108	216	612	1,627	1,988	2,283	2,411	2,563	2,749
Public.	35	131	455	1,111	1,709	1,895	1,980	2,109	2,286
	Percent								
National health expenditures as percent of GDP.	5.1	7.0	8.8	12.0	13.4	13.1	13.2	13.3	14.1
Health expenditures as a percent of total government expenditures									
Federal	3.3	8.9	12.4	15.7	20.5	21.6	22.0	22.7	23.5
State and local	9.9	9.3	10.9	13.6	14.9	14.8	14.8	14.7	14.8
	Percent distribution								
National health expenditures	100.0	100.0	100.0	100.0	100.0	100.0	100.0	100.0	100.0
Private	75.2	62.2	57.3	59.4	53.8	54.6	54.9	54.9	54.6
Public.	24.8	37.8	42.7	40.6	46.2	45.4	45.1	45.1	45.4
	Average annual percent change from previous year shown								
Gross domestic product.	. . .	7.0	10.4	7.6	5.0	5.9	5.6	5.9	2.6
Federal government expenditures.	. . .	8.8	11.2	7.9	5.1	2.7	2.9	4.1	6.0
State and local government expenditures	. . .	10.9	11.1	7.9	6.4	4.6	7.0	8.2	8.1
National health expenditures	. . .	10.6	12.9	11.0	7.3	5.1	6.1	7.4	8.7
Private	. . .	8.5	12.0	11.4	5.2	5.7	6.6	7.3	8.2
Public.	. . .	15.4	14.3	10.4	10.1	4.5	5.4	7.5	9.4
Federal government	. . .	20.1	15.0	10.5	10.9	4.5	4.7	7.5	9.6
State and local government.	. . .	10.2	12.8	10.4	8.4	4.4	7.2	7.5	8.9
National health expenditures, per capita	. . .	9.3	11.9	9.9	6.2	4.2	5.1	6.4	7.8
Private	. . .	7.2	11.0	10.3	4.1	4.7	5.6	6.3	7.3
Public.	. . .	14.0	13.2	9.3	9.0	3.5	4.5	6.5	8.4

. . . Category not applicable.

NOTES: These data include revisions in health expenditures and differ from previous editions of *Health, United States*. They reflect U.S. Bureau of the Census resident population estimates as of July 2002. Federal and State and local government total expenditures reflect October 2002 revisions from the Bureau of Economic Analysis.

SOURCE: Centers for Medicare & Medicaid Services, Office of the Actuary, National Health Statistics Group, National health accounts, National health expenditures, 2001. Internet address: www.cms.hhs.gov/statistics/nhe/.

Table 113. Consumer Price Index and average annual percent change for all items, selected items, and medical care components: United States, selected years 1960–2002

[Data are based on reporting by samples of providers and other retail outlets]

Items and medical care components	1960	1970	1980	1990	1995	1999	2000	2001	2002
	Consumer Price Index (CPI)								
All items	29.6	38.8	82.4	130.7	152.4	166.6	172.2	177.1	179.9
All items excluding medical care	30.2	39.2	82.8	128.8	148.6	162.0	167.3	171.9	174.3
All services	24.1	35.0	77.9	139.2	168.7	188.8	195.3	203.4	209.8
Food	30.0	39.2	86.8	132.4	148.4	164.1	167.8	173.1	176.2
Apparel	45.7	59.2	90.9	124.1	132.0	131.3	129.6	127.3	124.0
Housing	- - -	36.4	81.1	128.5	148.5	163.9	169.6	176.4	180.3
Energy	22.4	25.5	86.0	102.1	105.2	106.6	124.6	129.3	121.7
Medical care	22.3	34.0	74.9	162.8	220.5	250.6	260.8	272.8	285.6
Components of medical care									
Medical care services	19.5	32.3	74.8	162.7	224.2	255.1	266.0	278.8	292.9
Professional services	- - -	37.0	77.9	156.1	201.0	229.2	237.7	246.5	253.9
Physicians' services	21.9	34.5	76.5	160.8	208.8	236.0	244.7	253.6	260.6
Dental services	27.0	39.2	78.9	155.8	206.8	247.2	258.5	269.0	281.0
Eye glasses and eye care[1]	- - -	- - -	- - -	117.3	137.0	145.5	149.7	154.5	155.5
Services by other medical professionals[1]	- - -	- - -	- - -	120.2	143.9	158.7	161.9	167.3	171.8
Hospital and related services	- - -	- - -	69.2	178.0	257.8	299.5	317.3	338.3	367.8
Hospital services[2]	- - -	- - -	- - -	- - -	- - -	109.3	115.9	123.6	134.7
Inpatient hospital services[2]	- - -	- - -	- - -	- - -	- - -	107.9	113.8	121.0	131.2
Outpatient hospital services[1]	- - -	- - -	- - -	138.7	204.6	246.0	263.8	281.1	309.8
Hospital rooms	9.3	23.6	68.0	175.4	251.2	- - -	- - -	- - -	- - -
Other inpatient services[1]	- - -	- - -	- - -	142.7	206.8	- - -	- - -	- - -	- - -
Nursing homes and adult day care	- - -	- - -	- - -	- - -	- - -	111.6	117.0	121.8	127.9
Medical care commodities	46.9	46.5	75.4	163.4	204.5	230.7	238.1	247.6	256.4
Prescription drugs and medical supplies	54.0	47.4	72.5	181.7	235.0	273.4	285.4	300.9	316.5
Nonprescription drugs and medical supplies[1]	- - -	- - -	- - -	120.6	140.5	148.5	149.5	150.6	150.4
Internal and respiratory over-the-counter drugs	- - -	42.3	74.9	145.9	167.0	175.9	176.9	178.9	178.8
Nonprescription medical equipment and supplies	- - -	- - -	79.2	138.0	166.3	176.7	178.1	178.2	177.5
	Average annual percent change from previous year shown								
All items	...	2.7	7.8	4.7	3.1	2.3	3.4	2.8	1.6
All items excluding medical care	...	2.6	7.8	4.5	2.9	2.2	3.3	2.7	1.4
All services	...	3.8	8.3	6.0	3.9	2.9	3.4	4.1	3.1
Food	...	2.7	8.3	4.3	2.3	2.5	2.3	3.2	1.8
Apparel	...	2.6	4.4	3.2	1.2	–0.1	–1.3	–1.8	–2.6
Housing	...	- - -	8.3	4.7	2.9	2.5	3.5	4.0	2.2
Energy	...	1.3	12.9	1.7	0.6	0.3	16.9	3.8	–5.9
Medical care	...	4.3	8.2	8.1	6.3	3.3	4.1	4.6	4.7
Components of medical care									
Medical care services	...	5.2	8.8	8.1	6.6	3.3	4.3	4.8	5.1
Professional services	...	- - -	7.7	7.2	5.2	3.3	3.7	3.7	3.0
Physicians' services	...	4.6	8.3	7.7	5.4	3.1	3.7	3.6	2.8
Dental services	...	3.8	7.2	7.0	5.8	4.6	4.6	4.1	4.5
Eye glasses and eye care[1]	...	- - -	- - -	- - -	3.2	1.5	2.9	3.2	0.6
Services by other medical professionals[1]	...	- - -	- - -	- - -	3.7	2.5	2.0	3.3	2.7
Hospital and related services	...	- - -	- - -	9.9	7.7	3.8	5.9	6.6	8.7
Hospital services[2]	...	- - -	- - -	- - -	- - -	- - -	6.0	6.6	9.0
Inpatient hospital services[2]	...	- - -	- - -	- - -	- - -	- - -	5.5	6.3	8.4
Outpatient hospital services[1]	...	- - -	- - -	- - -	8.1	4.7	7.2	6.6	10.2
Hospital rooms	...	9.8	11.2	9.9	7.4	- - -	- - -	- - -	- - -
Other inpatient services[1]	...	- - -	- - -	- - -	7.7	- - -	- - -	- - -	- - -
Nursing homes and adult day care	...	- - -	- - -	- - -	- - -	- - -	4.8	4.1	5.0
Medical care commodities	...	–0.1	5.0	8.0	4.6	3.1	3.2	4.0	3.6
Prescription drugs and medical supplies	...	–1.3	4.3	9.6	5.3	3.9	4.4	5.4	5.2
Nonprescription drugs and medical supplies[1]	...	- - -	- - -	- - -	3.1	1.4	0.7	0.7	–0.1
Internal and respiratory over-the-counter drugs	...	- - -	5.9	6.9	2.7	1.3	0.6	1.1	–0.1
Nonprescription medical equipment and supplies	...	- - -	- - -	5.7	3.8	1.5	0.8	0.1	–0.4

- - - Data not available.
... Category not applicable.
[1]Dec. 1986 = 100.
[2]Dec. 1996 = 100.

NOTE: 1982–84 = 100, except where noted.

SOURCE: U.S. Department of Labor, Bureau of Labor Statistics, Consumer Price Index. Various releases. 2002 data available from the Bureau of Labor Statistics website at www.bls.gov/cpi.

Table 114. Growth in personal health care expenditures and percent distribution of factors affecting growth: United States, 1960–2001

[Data are compiled from various sources by the Centers for Medicare & Medicaid Services]

Period	Average annual percent increase	All factors	Factors affecting growth				
			Inflation[1]				
			Economy-wide	Medical	Population	Intensity[2]
			Percent distribution[3]				
1960–2001	10.2	100	41	17	11	32
1960–65	8.2	100	17	10	18	55
1965–70	12.7	100	34	12	8	46
1970–75	12.3	100	55	1	8	36
1975–80	13.7	100	55	12	7	26
1980–85	11.7	100	46	32	9	13
1980–81	16.1	100	60	18	7	16
1981–82	12.4	100	52	35	9	5
1982–83	10.1	100	40	35	10	14
1983–84	9.7	100	40	39	10	11
1984–85	10.1	100	32	40	10	18
1985–90	10.4	100	33	26	10	32
1985–86	8.7	100	26	31	11	31
1986–87	9.6	100	32	20	10	38
1987–88	11.3	100	31	25	9	35
1988–89	10.6	100	37	29	10	24
1989–90	11.7	100	35	24	10	31
1990–95	7.3	100	36	28	15	21
1990–91	10.3	100	36	20	11	33
1991–92	8.5	100	30	33	14	23
1992–93	6.4	100	38	36	18	9
1993–94	5.2	100	40	32	19	9
1994–95	6.0	100	37	25	17	22
1995–2000	5.5	100	31	17	17	34
1995–96	5.3	100	37	20	17	25
1996–97	5.2	100	38	4	18	40
1997–98	5.3	100	24	19	18	39
1998–99	5.2	100	27	25	17	31
1999–2000	6.4	100	31	19	14	36
2000–2001	8.7	100	28	15	11	46

[1]Total inflation is economy-wide and medical inflation is the medical inflation above economy-wide inflation.
[2]The residual percent of growth which cannot be attributed to price increases or population growth represents changes in use or kinds of services and supplies.
[3]Percents may not sum to 100 due to rounding.

NOTE: These data include revisions in health expenditures and in population back to 1994 and differ from previous editions of *Health, United States*.

SOURCE: Centers for Medicare & Medicaid Services, Office of the Actuary, National Health Statistics Group, National health accounts, National health expenditures, 2001. Internet address: www.cms.hhs.gov/statistics/nhe/.

Table 115 (page 1 of 2). National health expenditures, average annual percent change, and percent distribution, according to type of expenditure: United States, selected years 1960–2001

[Data are compiled from various sources by the Centers for Medicare & Medicaid Services]

Type of national health expenditure	1960	1970	1980	1990	1995	1998	1999	2000	2001
					Amount in billions				
National health expenditures	$26.7	$73.1	$245.8	$696.0	$990.1	$1,150.0	$1,219.7	$1,310.0	$1,424.5
Health services and supplies	25.0	67.3	233.5	669.6	957.5	1,111.8	1,178.7	1,262.3	1,372.6
Personal health care	23.4	63.2	214.6	609.4	865.7	1,009.4	1,064.6	1,137.6	1,236.4
Hospital care	9.2	27.6	101.5	253.9	343.6	378.4	393.7	416.5	451.2
Professional services	8.3	20.7	67.3	216.9	316.5	375.7	396.9	425.0	462.4
Physician and clinical services	5.4	14.0	47.1	157.5	220.5	256.8	270.2	288.8	313.6
Other professional services	0.4	0.7	3.6	18.2	28.5	35.5	36.7	38.8	42.3
Dental services	2.0	4.7	13.3	31.5	44.5	53.2	56.4	60.7	65.6
Other personal health care	0.6	1.3	3.3	9.6	22.9	30.2	33.6	36.7	40.9
Nursing home and home health	0.9	4.4	20.1	65.3	105.1	122.7	121.9	125.5	132.1
Home health care[1]	0.1	0.2	2.4	12.6	30.5	33.6	32.3	31.7	33.2
Nursing home care[1]	0.8	4.2	17.7	52.7	74.6	89.1	89.6	93.8	98.9
Retail outlet sales of medical products	5.0	10.5	25.7	73.3	100.5	132.7	152.1	170.5	190.7
Prescription drugs	2.7	5.5	12.0	40.3	60.8	87.3	104.4	121.5	140.6
Other medical products	2.3	5.0	13.7	33.1	39.7	45.4	47.7	48.9	50.1
Government administration and net cost of private health insurance	1.2	2.8	12.1	40.0	60.4	64.3	73.2	80.7	89.7
Government public health activities[2]	0.4	1.4	6.7	20.2	31.4	38.0	40.9	44.1	46.4
Investment	1.7	5.7	12.3	26.4	32.6	38.2	41.0	47.7	52.0
Research[3]	0.7	2.0	5.5	12.7	17.1	20.5	23.5	29.1	32.8
Construction	1.0	3.8	6.8	13.7	15.5	17.7	17.6	18.6	19.2
				Average annual percent change from previous year shown					
National health expenditures	...	10.6	12.9	11.0	7.3	5.1	6.1	7.4	8.7
Health services and supplies	...	10.4	13.2	11.1	7.4	5.1	6.0	7.1	8.7
Personal health care	...	10.5	13.0	11.0	7.3	5.3	5.5	6.9	8.7
Hospital care	...	11.7	13.9	9.6	6.2	3.3	4.1	5.8	8.3
Professional services	...	9.5	12.5	12.4	7.9	5.9	5.6	7.1	8.8
Physician and clinical services	...	10.1	12.9	12.8	7.0	5.2	5.2	6.9	8.6
Other professional services	...	6.6	17.1	17.5	9.5	7.6	3.3	5.8	9.1
Dental services	...	9.1	11.1	9.0	7.1	6.1	6.1	7.7	8.0
Other personal health care	...	7.2	10.0	11.4	18.9	9.6	11.3	9.1	11.5
Nursing home and home health	...	17.2	16.3	12.5	10.0	5.3	-0.6	3.0	5.2
Home health care[1]	...	14.5	26.9	18.1	19.4	3.2	-3.7	-1.8	4.5
Nursing home care[1]	...	17.4	15.4	11.5	7.2	6.1	0.5	4.7	5.5
Retail outlet sales of medical products	...	7.8	9.4	11.1	6.5	9.7	14.6	12.1	11.9
Prescription drugs	...	7.5	8.2	12.8	8.6	12.8	19.7	16.4	15.7
Other medical products	...	8.1	10.6	9.2	3.8	4.6	4.9	2.7	2.4
Government administration and net cost of private health insurance	...	8.6	15.9	12.7	8.6	2.1	13.7	10.3	11.2
Government public health activities	...	13.2	17.4	11.6	9.2	6.5	7.7	7.7	5.3
Investment	...	12.9	7.9	8.0	4.3	5.5	7.3	16.2	9.0
Research[3]	...	10.9	10.8	8.8	6.2	6.2	14.5	24.1	12.7
Construction	...	14.1	6.1	7.3	2.4	4.6	-0.9	5.8	3.2

See footnotes at end of table.

Table 115 (page 2 of 2). National health expenditures, average annual percent change, and percent distribution, according to type of expenditure: United States, selected years 1960–2001

[Data are compiled from various sources by the Centers for Medicare & Medicaid Services]

Type of national health expenditure	1960	1970	1980	1990	1995	1998	1999	2000	2001
					Percent distribution				
National health expenditures	100.0	100.0	100.0	100.0	100.0	100.0	100.0	100.0	100.0
Health services and supplies	93.6	92.2	95.0	96.2	96.7	96.7	96.6	96.4	96.4
Personal health care	87.6	86.5	87.3	87.6	87.4	87.8	87.3	86.8	86.8
Hospital care	34.4	37.8	41.3	36.5	34.7	32.9	32.3	31.8	31.7
Professional services	31.3	28.3	27.4	31.2	32.0	32.7	32.5	32.4	32.5
Physician and clinical services	20.1	19.1	19.2	22.6	22.3	22.3	22.2	22.0	22.0
Other professional services	1.5	1.0	1.5	2.6	2.9	3.1	3.0	3.0	3.0
Dental services	7.4	6.4	5.4	4.5	4.5	4.6	4.6	4.6	4.6
Other personal health care.	2.4	1.7	1.3	1.4	2.3	2.6	2.8	2.8	2.9
Nursing home and home health	3.4	6.1	8.2	9.4	10.6	10.7	10.0	9.6	9.3
Home health care[1]	0.2	0.3	1.0	1.8	3.1	2.9	2.6	2.4	2.3
Nursing home care[1]	3.2	5.8	7.2	7.6	7.5	7.7	7.3	7.2	6.9
Retail outlet sales of medical products.	18.6	14.3	10.5	10.5	10.2	11.5	12.5	13.0	13.4
Prescription drugs	10.0	7.5	4.9	5.8	6.1	7.6	8.6	9.3	9.9
Other medical products	8.5	6.8	5.6	4.7	4.0	4.0	3.9	3.7	3.5
Government administration and net cost of private health insurance	4.5	3.8	4.9	5.7	6.1	5.6	6.0	6.2	6.3
Government public health activities	1.5	1.9	2.7	2.9	3.2	3.3	3.4	3.4	3.3
Investment	6.4	7.8	5.0	3.8	3.3	3.3	3.4	3.6	3.6
Research[3]	2.6	2.7	2.2	1.8	1.7	1.8	1.9	2.2	2.3
Construction	3.8	5.2	2.8	2.0	1.6	1.5	1.4	1.4	1.3

. . . Category not applicable.
[1]Freestanding facilities only. Additional services of this type are provided in hospital-based facilities and counted as hospital care.
[2]Includes personal care services delivered by government public health agencies.
[3]Research and development expenditures of drug companies and other manufacturers and providers of medical equipment and supplies are excluded from "research expenditures," but are included in the expenditure class in which the product falls in that they are covered by the payment received for that product.

NOTE: These data include revisions in health expenditures and differ from previous editions of *Health, United States.*

SOURCE: Centers for Medicare & Medicaid Services, Office of the Actuary, National Health Statistics Group, National health accounts, National health expenditures, 2001. Internet address: www.cms.hhs.gov/statistics/nhe/.

Table 116 (page 1 of 2). Personal health care expenditures, according to type of expenditure and source of funds: United States, selected years 1960–2001

[Data are compiled from various sources by the Centers for Medicare & Medicaid Services]

Type of personal health care expenditures and source of funds	1960	1970	1980	1990	1995	1998	1999	2000	2001
					Amount				
Per capita.	$ 126	$ 301	$ 931	$2,398	$3,233	$ 3,668	$ 3,833	$ 4,057	$ 4,370
					Amount in billions				
All personal health care expenditures[1].	$ 23.4	$ 63.2	$214.6	$609.4	$865.7	$1,009.4	$1,064.6	$1,137.6	$1,236.4
					Percent distribution				
All sources of funds.	100.0	100.0	100.0	100.0	100.0	100.0	100.0	100.0	100.0
Out-of-pocket payments	55.2	39.7	27.1	22.5	16.9	17.4	17.3	17.1	16.6
Private health insurance	21.4	22.3	28.3	33.4	33.3	33.8	34.4	34.9	35.4
Other private funds	2.0	2.8	4.3	5.0	5.1	5.4	5.3	4.9	4.6
Government	21.4	35.2	40.3	39.0	44.7	43.4	43.0	43.0	43.4
Federal	8.7	22.9	29.3	28.6	34.2	33.2	32.6	32.6	32.9
State and local	12.6	12.3	11.1	10.5	10.5	10.2	10.3	10.4	10.6
					Amount in billions				
Hospital care expenditures[2]	$ 9.2	$ 27.6	$101.5	$253.9	$343.6	$ 378.4	$ 393.7	$ 416.5	$ 451.2
					Percent distribution				
All sources of funds.	100.0	100.0	100.0	100.0	100.0	100.0	100.0	100.0	100.0
Out-of-pocket payments	20.8	9.1	5.2	4.4	3.0	3.1	3.2	3.2	3.1
Private health insurance	35.8	32.6	35.6	38.3	32.3	31.9	32.7	33.4	33.7
Other private funds	1.2	3.3	4.9	4.1	4.3	5.2	5.2	5.3	4.9
Government[3].	42.2	55.1	54.3	53.2	60.3	59.7	58.9	58.1	58.3
Medicaid[4].	. . .	9.6	10.4	10.9	15.9	16.1	16.8	16.8	17.1
Medicare	. . .	19.4	26.0	26.7	31.4	32.1	31.0	30.2	29.9
					Amount in billions				
Physician services expenditures	$ 5.4	$ 14.0	$ 47.1	$157.5	$220.5	$ 256.8	$ 270.2	$ 288.8	$ 313.6
					Percent distribution				
All sources of funds.	100.0	100.0	100.0	100.0	100.0	100.0	100.0	100.0	100.0
Out-of-pocket payments	61.6	46.1	30.2	19.3	11.9	12.0	11.6	11.6	11.2
Private health insurance	29.8	30.1	35.3	43.0	48.6	47.8	47.2	47.6	48.1
Other private funds	1.4	1.6	3.9	7.2	8.0	8.6	8.5	7.5	7.1
Government[3].	7.2	22.2	30.5	30.6	31.5	31.7	32.7	33.3	33.6
Medicaid[4].	. . .	4.6	5.2	4.5	6.7	6.5	6.5	6.6	6.8
Medicare	. . .	11.8	17.4	19.1	18.9	19.9	20.4	20.6	20.4
					Amount in billions				
Nursing home expenditures[5]	$ 0.8	$ 4.2	$ 17.7	$ 52.7	$ 74.6	$ 89.1	$ 89.6	$ 93.8	$ 98.9
					Percent distribution				
All sources of funds.	100.0	100.0	100.0	100.0	100.0	100.0	100.0	100.0	100.0
Out-of-pocket payments	77.9	53.6	40.0	37.5	26.7	28.0	28.3	27.9	27.2
Private health insurance	0.0	0.2	1.2	5.8	7.5	8.3	8.4	7.8	7.6
Other private funds	6.3	4.9	4.5	7.5	6.4	5.1	5.1	4.4	3.7
Government[3].	15.7	41.2	54.2	49.2	59.5	58.7	58.2	59.9	61.5
Medicaid[4].	. . .	22.3	50.2	43.9	47.5	45.0	46.7	47.6	47.5
Medicare	. . .	3.4	1.7	3.2	9.7	11.5	9.3	10.1	11.7

See footnotes at end of table.

[Data are compiled from various sources by the Centers for Medicare & Medicaid Services]

Type of personal health care expenditures and source of funds	1960	1970	1980	1990	1995	1998	1999	2000	2001
	Amount in billions								
Prescription drug expenditures	$ 2.7	$ 5.5	$ 12.0	$ 40.3	$ 60.8	$ 87.3	$104.4	$121.5	$140.6
	Percent distribution								
All sources of funds.	100.0	100.0	100.0	100.0	100.0	100.0	100.0	100.0	100.0
Out-of-pocket payments	96.0	82.4	69.4	59.1	42.7	34.9	32.9	31.4	30.7
Private health insurance	1.3	8.8	16.7	24.4	37.1	43.9	45.8	46.6	47.4
Other private funds	0.0	0.0	0.0	0.0	0.0	0.0	0.0	0.0	0.0
Government[3]	2.7	8.8	13.9	16.6	20.1	21.1	21.3	22.0	21.9
Medicaid[4].	. . .	7.6	11.7	12.6	16.0	16.5	16.5	17.1	17.1
Medicare	. . .	0.0	0.0	0.5	1.3	2.0	2.0	1.9	1.7
	Amount in billions								
All other personal health care expenditures[6]	$ 5.3	$ 11.9	$ 36.3	$104.9	$166.2	$197.9	$206.6	$216.9	$232.1
	Percent distribution								
All sources of funds.	100.0	100.0	100.0	100.0	100.0	100.0	100.0	100.0	100.0
Out-of-pocket payments	84.2	78.6	64.3	49.6	38.3	39.0	39.1	38.6	37.4
Private health insurance	1.6	3.3	15.5	24.7	25.1	26.3	26.2	25.9	25.8
Other private funds	4.2	3.6	4.3	4.7	4.3	4.3	4.2	3.9	3.7
Government[3]	10.1	14.5	16.0	20.9	32.3	30.4	30.5	31.5	33.1
Medicaid[4].	. . .	3.3	3.9	6.5	12.5	14.0	14.9	15.6	16.8
Medicare	. . .	1.1	3.8	7.1	13.3	10.0	9.0	9.0	9.3

. . . Category not applicable.

[1]Includes all expenditures for specified health services and supplies other than expenses for program administration, net cost of private health insurance, and government public health activities.

[2]Includes expenditures for hospital-based nursing home care and home health agency care.

[3]Includes other government expenditures for these health care services, for example, Medicaid State Children's Health Insurance Program (SCHIP) expansion and SCHIP, care funded by the Department of Veterans Affairs, and State and locally financed subsidies to hospitals.

[4]Excludes Medicaid SCHIP expansion and SCHIP.

[5]Includes expenditures for care in freestanding nursing homes. Expenditures for care in facility-based nursing homes are included with hospital care.

[6]Includes expenditures for dental services, other professional services, home health care, nonprescription drugs and other medical nondurables, vision products and other medical durables, and other personal health care, not shown separately.

NOTE: These data include revisions in health expenditures and differ from previous editions of Health, United States.

SOURCE: Centers for Medicare & Medicaid Services, Office of the Actuary, National Health Statistics Group, National health accounts, National health expenditures, 2001. Internet address: www.cms.hhs.gov/statistics/nhe/.

Table 117 (page 1 of 2). Expenditures for health care and prescribed medicine according to selected population characteristics: United States, selected years 1987–99

[Data are based on household interviews of a sample of the noninstitutionalized population and a sample of medical providers]

| | Total expenses[1] | | | | | | | | | | |
| | Population in millions[2] | | | Percent of persons with expense | | | | Mean annual expense per person with expense | | | |
Characteristic	1997	1998	1999	1987	1997	1998	1999	1987	1997	1998	1999
All ages	271.3	273.5	276.4	84.5	84.1	83.8	84.3	$1,562	$2,424	$2,444	$2,557
Under 65 years:											
Total	237.1	239.2	241.7	83.2	82.5	82.2	82.8	$1,216	$1,838	$1,810	$1,939
Under 6 years	23.8	23.7	23.8	88.9	88.0	87.6	87.9	1,033	858	905	995
6–17 years	48.1	48.7	48.8	80.2	81.7	80.6	81.5	681	963	888	1,022
18–44 years	108.9	108.8	109.0	81.5	78.3	78.0	78.9	1,069	1,666	1,734	1,855
45–64 years	56.3	58.0	60.1	87.0	89.2	89.2	88.9	2,070	3,226	2,996	3,125
Sex											
Male	118.0	119.3	120.0	78.8	77.6	77.4	77.8	1,147	1,661	1,665	1,691
Female	119.1	119.9	121.8	87.5	87.4	87.0	87.7	1,275	1,994	1,938	2,155
Hispanic origin and race											
Hispanic or Latino	29.4	30.2	31.2	71.0	69.5	68.9	68.7	970	1,530	1,536	1,508
Not Hispanic or Latino:											
White	166.2	167.4	168.3	86.9	87.2	87.1	87.5	1,220	1,972	1,877	2,039
Black or African American . .	31.3	31.6	31.9	72.2	72.1	71.8	72.0	1,471	1,474	1,716	1,837
Other	10.2	10.0	10.3	72.8	75.8	74.0	81.1	807	1,222	1,555	1,555
Insurance status[3]											
Any private insurance	174.0	176.0	183.1	86.5	86.5	86.8	86.8	1,166	1,873	1,769	1,882
Public insurance only	29.8	31.0	28.6	82.4	83.3	83.7	84.5	1,956	2,234	2,501	2,819
Uninsured all year	33.3	32.3	30.1	61.8	61.1	55.6	56.4	760	1,098	1,156	1,214
65 years and over	34.2	34.3	34.7	93.7	95.2	95.2	95.3	$3,858	$5,947	$6,264	$6,299
Sex											
Male	14.6	14.3	14.6	92.0	94.5	94.2	94.9	3,948	6,683	5,333	6,615
Female	19.6	20.0	20.1	94.9	95.7	95.9	95.6	3,795	5,405	6,917	6,070
Hispanic origin and race											
Hispanic or Latino	1.7	1.8	1.8	82.5	94.2	93.5	94.3	3,674	6,223	5,488	6,518
Not Hispanic or Latino:											
White	28.8	29.0	29.1	94.9	95.9	95.8	95.9	3,798	5,977	6,250	6,400
Black or African American . .	2.8	2.9	2.9	88.5	92.2	92.1	92.9	4,650	5,857	6,703	5,584
Other	*	*	0.8	*	*	*	*	*	*	*	*
Insurance status[4]											
Medicare only	8.8	10.4	11.3	85.9	92.1	94.0	93.7	3,039	5,479	6,252	5,752
Medicare and private insurance	21.7	19.5	19.5	95.4	97.0	96.3	97.3	3,817	5,800	5,931	6,133
Medicare and other public coverage	3.2	3.9	3.4	94.4	93.2	95.0	90.5	5,928	8,382	8,004	9,515

See footnotes at end of table.

Table 117 (page 2 of 2). Expenditures for health care and prescribed medicine according to selected population characteristics: United States, selected years 1987–99

[Data are based on household interviews of a sample of the noninstitutionalized population and a sample of medical providers]

	Prescribed medicine expenses[5]							
	Percent of persons with expense				Mean annual out-of-pocket expense per person with expense			
Characteristic	1987	1997	1998	1999	1987	1997	1998	1999
All ages	57.3	62.1	61.8	62.4	$92	$202	$221	$252
Under 65 years:								
Total	54.0	58.7	58.1	58.7	$68	$143	155	175
Under 6 years.	61.8	61.3	59.0	58.5	24	35	35	36
6–17 years	44.3	48.2	46.4	46.2	45	54	60	67
18–44 years	51.3	55.9	55.6	56.4	53	122	129	146
45–64 years	65.3	71.8	72.4	73.1	129	266	283	314
Sex								
Male	46.5	51.5	50.6	51.6	63	127	128	157
Female	61.4	65.8	65.7	65.7	72	155	175	188
Hispanic origin and race								
Hispanic or Latino	41.6	47.7	47.6	45.9	49	95	107	140
Not Hispanic or Latino:								
White	57.7	63.1	62.9	63.7	71	155	159	184
Black or African American . .	44.1	50.0	47.7	48.1	60	115	177	158
Other	41.1	44.8	42.9	48.7	50	124	145	133
Insurance status[3]								
Any private insurance	56.5	61.6	61.3	61.8	70	136	135	156
Public insurance only	56.5	62.0	61.2	61.8	47	141	212	252
Uninsured all year	35.1	40.2	38.1	37.2	75	206	238	245
65 years and over	81.6	86.0	87.5	88.0	$212	$483	$531	$614
Sex								
Male	78.0	82.8	85.8	86.1	197	435	463	531
Female	84.0	88.3	88.7	89.3	221	516	577	673
Hispanic origin and race								
Hispanic or Latino	74.7	87.5	85.6	85.9	*280	394	394	463
Not Hispanic or Latino:								
White	82.3	86.7	87.8	88.7	216	499	553	633
Black or African American . .	79.5	85.3	88.0	85.4	166	401	385	554
Other	*	*	*	*	*	*	*	*
Insurance status[4]								
Medicare only	70.6	82.1	86.8	86.2	234	558	648	733
Medicare and private insurance.	83.4	88.1	88.4	89.9	220	490	511	592
Medicare and other public coverage	88.2	85.0	86.8	84.4	80	270	303	394

* Estimates are considered unreliable. Data not shown are based on fewer than 100 sample cases. Data preceded by an asterisk have a relative standard error equal to or greater than 30 percent.

[1]Includes expenses for inpatient hospital and physician services, ambulatory physician and nonphysician services, prescribed medicines, home health services, dental services, and other medical equipment, supplies, and services that were purchased or rented during the year. Over-the-counter medications, alternative care services, phone contacts with health providers, and premiums for health insurance are excluded.

[2]Includes persons who were in the civilian noninstitutionalized population for all or part of the year. Expenditures for persons who were only in this population for part of the year are restricted to those incurred during periods of eligibility (e.g., expenses incurred during periods of institutionalization and military service are not included in estimates).

[3]Any private insurance includes individuals with insurance that provided coverage for hospital and physician care at any time during the year, other than Medicare, Medicaid, or other public coverage for hospital or physician services. Public insurance only includes individuals who were not covered by private insurance at any time during the year but were covered by Medicare, Medicaid, other public coverage for hospital or physician services, and/or CHAMPUS/CHAMPVA (TRICARE) at any point during the year. Uninsured includes persons not covered by either private or public insurance throughout the entire year or period of eligibility for the survey.

[4]Populations do not add to total because uninsured persons and persons with unknown insurance status were excluded.

[5]Includes expenses for all prescribed medications that were purchased or refilled during the survey year.

NOTES: 1987 estimates are based on the National Medical Expenditure Survey (NMES) while 1996–99 estimates are based on the Medical Expenditure Panel Survey (MEPS). Because expenditures in NMES were based primarily on charges while those for MEPS were based on payments, data for NMES were adjusted to be more comparable to MEPS using estimated charge to payment ratios for 1987. Overall, this resulted in an approximate 11 percent reduction from the unadjusted 1987 NMES expenditure estimates. For a detailed explanation of this adjustment, see Zuvekas S and Cohen S. A guide to comparing health care estimates in the 1996 Medical Expenditure Panel Survey to the 1987 National Medical Expenditure Survey. Inquiry. vol. 39. Spring 2002. Persons of Hispanic origin may be of any race. Data for additional years are available (see Appendix III).

SOURCE: Agency for Healthcare Research and Quality, Center for Cost and Financing Studies, 1987 National Medical Expenditure Survey and 1996–99 Medical Expenditure Panel Surveys.

Table 118 (page 1 of 2). Sources of payment for health care according to selected population characteristics: United States, selected years 1987–99

[Data are based on household interviews of a sample of the noninstitutionalized population and a sample of medical providers]

		Sources of payment for health care							
		Out of pocket				Private insurance[1]			
Characteristic	All sources	1987	1997	1998	1999	1987	1997	1998	1999
		Percent distribution							
All ages	100.0	24.8	19.4	19.3	19.2	36.6	40.3	38.4	39.9
Under 65 years:									
Total	100.0	26.2	21.1	21.6	20.7	46.6	53.1	52.7	53.9
Under 6 years.	100.0	18.5	14.2	11.4	13.8	39.5	49.3	57.9	45.2
6–17 years.	100.0	35.7	29.0	28.3	27.2	47.3	53.2	55.2	53.4
18–44 years	100.0	27.4	21.1	21.8	19.5	46.8	52.9	51.1	55.7
45–64 years	100.0	24.0	20.1	21.1	21.3	47.8	53.6	52.9	53.4
Sex									
Male	100.0	24.5	21.3	20.4	20.5	44.6	50.3	50.8	51.8
Female	100.0	27.5	21.0	22.5	20.9	48.1	55.1	54.1	55.3
Hispanic origin and race									
Hispanic or Latino	100.0	22.0	18.8	17.9	19.3	36.1	42.3	39.7	44.2
Not Hispanic or Latino:									
White.	100.0	28.2	21.8	23.0	22.1	50.1	55.8	56.7	56.9
Black or African American . .	100.0	15.5	17.1	15.8	13.2	30.0	42.3	34.0	43.8
Other.	100.0	27.2	21.2	18.4	16.9	46.7	45.2	55.0	40.2
Insurance status									
Any private insurance[2]	100.0	29.0	21.6	22.2	21.4	60.0	67.6	69.1	69.7
Public insurance only[3].	100.0	8.9	10.6	10.7	10.3	. . .	. . .	. . .	. . .
Uninsured all year[4].	100.0	40.6	41.3	47.7	45.7	. . .	. . .	. . .	. . .
65 years and over	100.0	22.0	16.3	15.3	16.4	15.8	16.5	13.5	13.9
Sex									
Male.	100.0	21.7	14.2	15.8	14.0	17.6	20.1	17.2	13.7
Female	100.0	22.2	18.1	15.0	18.3	14.4	13.2	11.5	14.1
Hispanic origin and race									
Hispanic or Latino	100.0	*13.5	13.6	11.2	10.1	*4.7	5.9	5.8	*10.8
Not Hispanic or Latino:									
White.	100.0	23.7	17.0	16.3	17.0	16.7	17.9	14.6	14.4
Black or African American . .	100.0	11.2 ·	11.4	8.9	13.5	*11.9	8.8	6.0	10.9
Other.	100.0	*	*	*	*	*	*	*	*
Insurance status									
Medicare only	100.0	29.8	19.8	17.1	19.7	. . .	. . .	. . .	. . .
Medicare and private insurance.	100.0	23.4	17.3	16.8	17.4	18.9	25.7	23.5	23.9
Medicare and other public coverage	100.0	*6.2	5.2	5.6	5.4	. . .	. . .	. . .	. . .

See footnotes at end of table.

[Data are based on household interviews of a sample of the noninstitutionalized population and a sample of medical providers]

| | Sources of payment for health care | | | | | | | |
| | Public coverage[5] | | | | Other[6] | | | |
Characteristic	1987	1997	1998	1999	1987	1997	1998	1999
	Percent distribution							
All ages	34.1	34.4	36.5	35.7	4.5	5.9	5.9	5.1
Under 65 years:								
Total	21.3	18.1	18.6	19.2	6.0	7.7	7.1	6.2
Under 6 years...........	35.8	25.4	24.9	31.1	6.2	11.2	5.8	*9.9
6–17 years.............	11.8	14.1	12.8	14.7	5.2	3.7	3.6	4.7
18–44 years............	19.4	15.7	17.3	18.1	6.4	10.3	9.7	6.7
45–64 years............	22.4	20.3	20.3	19.8	5.8	6.0	5.6	5.6
Sex								
Male	23.9	19.5	18.7	19.8	7.1	8.9	10.1 .	7.9
Female	19.2	17.0	18.5	18.8	5.2	6.8	4.9	5.0
Hispanic origin and race								
Hispanic or Latino	35.8	28.9	29.3	26.6	6.0	10.0	13.1	9.9
Not Hispanic or Latino:								
White..................	15.9	15.3	13.9	15.0	5.8	7.1	6.3	5.9
Black or African American ..	47.2	30.7	41.1	37.4	7.3	9.9	9.0	5.7
Other..................	21.0	23.7	23.4	*37.5	5.1	9.9	3.1	*5.4
Insurance status								
Any private insurance[2]	6.2	6.6	5.0	5.1	4.8	4.2	3.6	3.8
Public insurance only[3]........	87.2	80.7	79.0	82.1	3.9	8.7	*10.3	7.6
Uninsured all year[4].........	28.6	7.5	6.7	*16.1	30.9	51.1	45.6	38.2
65 years and over	60.8	64.8	67.6	66.6	1.5	2.5	3.6	3.1
Sex								
Male	58.8	63.4	62.8	69.4	*1.9	2.3	4.1	2.8
Female	62.3	65.9	70.2	64.3	1.1	2.7	3.3	*3.3
Hispanic origin and race								
Hispanic or Latino	80.2	77.8	81.2	76.5	*1.6	*2.7	*1.9	*2.7
Not Hispanic or Latino:								
White..................	58.0	62.6	65.6	65.3	1.6	2.5	3.5	3.3
Black or African American ..	76.3	77.6	79.8	73.5	0.6	2.2	5.3	2.1
Other..................	*	*	*	*	*	*	*	*
Insurance status								
Medicare only	68.8	72.4	73.9	73.0	1.4	7.7	9.0	7.4
Medicare and private insurance...............	56.1	56.3	58.8	57.5	1.6	0.6	0.9	*1.1
Medicare and other public coverage	92.9	92.7	92.0	92.2	1.0	*2.1	*2.4	*2.4

. . . Category not applicable.

* Estimates are considered unreliable. Data not shown are based on fewer than 100 sample cases. Data preceded by an asterisk have a relative standard error equal to or greater than 30 percent.

[1]Private insurance—Includes any type of private insurance payments reported for people with private health insurance coverage during the year.

[2]Includes individuals with insurance that provided coverage for hospital and physician care at any time during the year, other than Medicare, Medicaid, or other public coverage for hospital or physician services.

[3]Includes individuals who were not covered by private insurance at any time during the year but were covered by Medicare, Medicaid, other public coverage for hospital or physician services, and/or CHAMPUS/CHAMPVA (TRICARE) at any point during the year.

[4]Includes individuals not covered by either private or public insurance throughout the entire year or period of eligibility for the survey. However, a portion of expenses for the uninsured were paid by sources that were not defined as health insurance coverage such as the Department of Veterans Affairs, community and neighborhood clinics, the Indian Health Service, State and local health departments, State programs other than Medicaid, Workers' Compensation, and other unclassified sources (e.g., automobile, homeowner's, liability insurance).

[5]Public coverage—Includes payments made by Medicare, Medicaid, the Department of Veterans Affairs, other Federal sources (e.g., Indian Health Service, military treatment facilities, and other care provided by the Federal Government), and various State and local sources (e.g., community and neighborhood clinics, State and local health departments, and State programs other than Medicaid).

[6]Other sources—Includes Workers' Compensation, unclassified sources (automobile, homeowner's, or liability insurance, and other miscellaneous or unknown sources), Medicaid payments reported for people who were not enrolled in the program at any time during the year, and any type of private insurance payments reported for people without private health insurance coverage during the year as defined in the survey.

NOTES: 1987 estimates are based on the National Medical Expenditure Survey (NMES) while 1996–99 estimates are based on the Medical Expenditure Panel Survey (MEPS). Because expenditures in NMES were based primarily on charges while those for MEPS were based on payments, data for NMES were adjusted to be more comparable to MEPS using estimated charge to payment ratios for 1987. Overall, this resulted in an approximate 11 percent reduction from the unadjusted 1987 NMES expenditure estimates. For a detailed explanation of this adjustment, see Zuvekas S and Cohen S. A guide to comparing health care estimates in the 1996 Medical Expenditure Panel Survey to the 1987 National Medical Expenditure Survey. Inquiry. vol. 39. Spring 2002. Persons of Hispanic origin may be of any race. Data for additional years are available (see Appendix III).

SOURCE: Agency for Healthcare Research and Quality, Center for Cost and Financing Studies, 1987 National Medical Expenditure Survey and 1996–99 Medical Expenditure Panel Surveys.

Table 119. Health care expenses paid out of pocket for persons with medical expenses by age: United States 1987, 1998, and 1999

[Data are based on household interviews for a sample of the noninstitutionalized population and a sample of medical providers]

Age and year	Percent of persons with expense	Total	Amount paid out of pocket for persons with expense[1]					
			$0	$1–124	$125–249	$250–499	$500–999	$1,000+
All ages			Percent distribution					
1987......................	84.5	100.0	10.4	29.2	16.6	17.4	13.3	13.1
1998......................	83.8	100.0	7.7	36.5	15.8	16.1	12.2	11.8
1999......................	84.3	100.0	7.4	35.9	15.5	15.6	12.8	12.7
Under 6 years								
1987......................	88.9	100.0	19.2	38.7	18.9	14.7	5.3	3.2
1998......................	87.6	100.0	17.4	60.1	12.4	6.8	2.3	0.9
1999......................	87.9	100.0	17.7	60.5	12.2	5.9	2.6	1.1
6–17 years								
1987......................	80.2	100.0	15.5	37.9	18.2	12.4	8.5	7.6
1998......................	80.6	100.0	16.3	47.0	15.0	11.1	5.6	5.1
1999......................	81.5	100.0	15.0	46.6	15.4	11.2	6.0	5.8
18–44 years								
1987......................	81.5	100.0	10.1	32.3	17.7	18.2	11.9	9.8
1998......................	78.0	100.0	6.4	40.2	17.9	17.0	10.7	7.7
1999......................	78.9	100.0	6.4	40.2	17.6	16.6	11.1	8.1
45–64 years								
1987......................	87.0	100.0	5.7	20.4	15.6	20.7	18.8	18.8
1998......................	89.2	100.0	2.9	25.6	16.2	20.1	17.7	17.5
1999......................	88.9	100.0	2.7	24.0	16.4	19.7	19.0	18.2
65–74 years								
1987......................	92.8	100.0	5.3	15.4	11.6	18.5	22.1	27.1
1998......................	94.3	100.0	2.0	17.8	13.3	20.7	20.6	25.6
1999......................	95.3	100.0	1.4	16.1	11.3	17.9	23.7	29.6
75 years or more								
1987......................	95.1	100.0	5.6	12.9	10.0	17.1	21.2	33.2
1998......................	96.3	100.0	3.0	14.3	11.6	17.7	22.2	31.3
1999......................	95.3	100.0	2.6	14.5	10.2	18.6	20.2	33.8

[1]1987 dollars were converted to 1998 dollars using the national Consumer Price Index (CPI).

NOTES: Out-of-pocket expenses include inpatient hospital and physician services, ambulatory physician and nonphysician services, prescribed medicines, home health services, dental services, and various other medical equipment, supplies, and services that were purchased or rented during the year. Out-of-pocket expenses for over-the-counter medications, alternative care services, phone contacts with health providers, and premiums for health insurance policies are not contained in these estimates. 1987 estimates are based on the National Medical Expenditure Survey (NMES) while estimates for other years are based on the Medical Expenditure Panel Survey (MEPS). Because expenditures in NMES were based primarily on charges while those for MEPS were based on payments, data for the NMES were adjusted to be more comparable to MEPS using estimated charge to payment ratios for 1987. Overall this resulted in an approximate 11 percent reduction from the unadjusted 1987 NMES expenditure estimates. For a detailed explanation of this adjustment, see Zuvekas S and Cohen S. A guide to comparing health care estimates in the 1996 Medical Expenditure Panel Survey to the 1987 National Medical Expenditure Survey. Inquiry. vol 39. Spring 2002.

SOURCES: Agency for Healthcare Research and Quality, Center for Cost and Financing Studies. 1987 National Medical Expenditure Survey and 1998 and 1999 Medical Expenditure Panel Surveys.

Table 120 (page 1 of 2). Expenditures for health services and supplies and percent distribution, by type of payer: United States, selected calendar years 1987–2000

[Data are compiled from various sources by the Centers for Medicare & Medicaid Services]

Type of payer	1987	1993	1994	1995	1996	1997	1998	1999	2000
					Amount in billions				
Total[1]	$477.8	$856.3	$904.8	$957.7	$1,005.7	$1,053.9	$1,111.5	$1,175.0	$1,255.5
Private	331.5	548.8	573.0	607.3	633.4	666.3	716.4	754.8	806.3
Private business	123.3	223.7	237.8	251.2	265.5	270.2	288.1	307.6	334.5
Employer contribution to private health insurance premiums	85.3	163.9	172.6	183.4	194.9	197.0	210.5	224.3	246.2
Private employer contribution to Medicare hospital insurance trust fund[2]	24.6	35.8	40.5	43.1	45.8	49.6	53.6	57.4	61.4
Workers compensation and temporary disability insurance	11.7	21.1	21.6	21.4	21.4	20.0	20.2	22.0	22.7
Industrial inplant health services	1.7	2.8	3.1	3.3	3.4	3.6	3.8	4.0	4.2
Household	185.8	288.9	297.5	314.4	323.2	347.7	376.5	393.9	418.8
Employee contribution to private health insurance premiums and individual policy premiums	41.3	86.4	88.6	95.6	96.8	107.0	116.1	120.0	126.4
Employee and self-employment contributions and voluntary premiums paid to Medicare hospital insurance trust fund[2]	29.4	43.7	50.6	55.9	59.2	62.9	68.8	74.8	81.5
Premiums paid by individuals to Medicare supplementary medical insurance trust fund	6.2	11.9	14.4	16.4	15.1	15.4	17.0	14.8	16.3
Out-of-pocket health spending	108.9	146.9	143.9	146.5	152.1	162.3	174.5	184.4	194.5
Other private revenues	22.4	36.2	37.7	41.7	44.7	48.5	51.8	53.3	53.0
Public	146.2	307.5	331.8	350.4	372.3	387.6	395.1	420.2	449.3
Federal Government	75.1	175.5	184.9	196.6	213.0	218.9	214.9	223.7	237.1
Employer contributions to private health insurance premiums	4.9	11.5	11.9	11.3	11.3	11.4	11.4	13.2	14.3
Medicaid[3]	28.1	78.1	83.1	88.1	94.2	97.1	101.9	110.8	120.8
Other[4]	42.1	85.8	90.0	97.2	107.4	110.4	101.6	99.6	102.0
State and local government	71.1	132.0	146.9	153.8	159.3	168.7	180.3	196.5	212.1
Employer contributions to private health insurance premiums	16.4	36.3	39.0	39.8	41.8	44.1	45.2	52.0	56.9
Medicaid[3]	22.8	45.8	53.7	59.2	61.5	66.4	73.4	80.1	86.1
Other[5]	32.0	49.9	54.2	54.7	56.0	58.2	61.6	64.5	69.1
					Percent distribution				
Total	100.0	100.0	100.0	100.0	100.0	100.0	100.0	100.0	100.0
Private	69.4	64.1	63.3	63.4	63.0	63.2	64.5	64.2	64.2
Private business	25.8	26.1	26.3	26.2	26.4	25.6	25.9	26.2	26.6
Employer contribution to private health insurance premiums	17.9	19.1	19.1	19.2	19.4	18.7	18.9	19.1	19.6
Private employer contribution to Medicare hospital insurance trust fund[2]	5.2	4.2	4.5	4.5	4.6	4.7	4.8	4.9	4.9
Workers compensation and temporary disability insurance	2.4	2.5	2.4	2.2	2.1	1.9	1.8	1.9	1.8
Industrial inplant health services	0.4	0.3	0.3	0.3	0.3	0.3	0.3	0.3	0.3
Household	38.9	33.7	32.9	32.8	32.1	33.0	33.9	33.5	33.4
Employee contribution to private health insurance premiums and individual policy premiums	8.7	10.1	9.8	10.0	9.6	10.2	10.4	10.2	10.1
Employee and self-employment contributions and voluntary premiums paid to Medicare hospital insurance trust fund[2]	6.1	5.1	5.6	5.8	5.9	6.0	6.2	6.4	6.5
Premiums paid by individuals to Medicare supplementary medical insurance trust fund	1.3	1.4	1.6	1.7	1.5	1.5	1.5	1.3	1.3
Out-of-pocket health spending	22.8	17.2	15.9	15.3	15.1	15.4	15.7	15.7	15.5
Other private revenues	4.7	4.2	4.2	4.4	4.4	4.6	4.7	4.5	4.2

See footnotes at end of table.

Table 120 (page 2 of 2). Expenditures for health services and supplies and percent distribution, by type of payer: United States, selected calendar years 1987–2000

[Data are compiled from various sources by the Centers for Medicare & Medicaid Services]

Type of payer	1987	1993	1994	1995	1996	1997	1998	1999	2000
	Percent distribution								
Public	30.6	35.9	36.7	36.6	37.0	36.8	35.5	35.8	35.8
Federal Government	15.7	20.5	20.4	20.5	21.2	20.8	19.3	19.0	18.9
Employer contributions to private health insurance premiums	1.0	1.3	1.3	1.2	1.1	1.1	1.0	1.1	1.1
Medicaid[3]	5.9	9.1	9.2	9.2	9.4	9.2	9.2	9.4	9.6
Other[4]	8.8	10.0	9.9	10.1	10.7	10.5	9.1	8.5	8.1
State and local government	14.9	15.4	16.2	16.1	15.8	16.0	16.2	16.7	16.9
Employer contributions to private health insurance premiums	3.4	4.2	4.3	4.2	4.2	4.2	4.1	4.4	4.5
Medicaid[3]	4.8	5.3	5.9	6.2	6.1	6.3	6.6	6.8	6.9
Other[5]	6.7	5.8	6.0	5.7	5.6	5.5	5.5	5.5	5.5

[1]Excludes research and construction.
[2]Includes one-half of self-employment contribution to Medicare hospital insurance trust fund.
[3]Includes Medicaid buy-in premiums for Medicare.
[4]Includes expenditures for Medicare with adjustments for contributions by employers and individuals and premiums paid to the Medicare insurance trust fund and maternal and child health, vocational rehabilitation, Substance Abuse and Mental Health Services Administration, Indian Health Service, Federal workers' compensation, and other miscellaneous general hospital and medical programs, public health activities, Department of Defense, and Department of Veterans Affairs.
[5]Includes other public and general assistance, maternal and child health, vocational rehabilitation, public health activities, hospital subsidies, and employer contributions to Medicare hospital insurance trust fund.

NOTES: This table disaggregates health expenditures according to four classes of payers: businesses, households (individuals), Federal Government, and State and local governments with a small amount of revenue coming from non-patient revenue sources such as philanthropy. Where businesses or households pay dedicated funds into government health programs (for example, Medicare) or employers and employees share in the cost of health premiums, these costs are assigned to businesses or households accordingly. This results in a lower share of expenditures being assigned to the Federal Government than for tabulations of expenditures by source of funds. Estimates of national health expenditure by source of funds aim to track government-sponsored health programs over time and do not delineate the role of business employers in paying for health care. Figures may not sum to totals due to rounding.

SOURCE: Centers for Medicare & Medicaid Services, Office of the Actuary, National Health Statistics Group. The Burden of Health Care Costs: Business, Households, and Government, 2000. Health Care Financing Review vol 23, no 2. Washington. Winter 2001.

Table 121. Employers' costs per employee-hour worked for total compensation, wages and salaries, and health insurance, according to selected characteristics: United States, selected years 1991–2002

[Data are based on surveys of employers]

Characteristic	Total compensation					Wages and salaries				
	1991	1994	2000	2001	2002	1991	1994	2000	2001	2002
	Amount per employee-hour worked									
State and local government.......	$22.31	$25.27	$29.05	$30.06	$31.29	$15.52	$17.57	$20.57	$21.34	$22.14
Total private industry............	15.40	17.08	19.85	20.81	21.71	11.14	12.14	14.49	15.18	15.80
Industry:										
Goods producing	18.48	20.85	23.55	24.40	25.44	12.70	13.87	16.25	16.86	17.47
Service producing	14.31	15.82	18.72	19.74	20.66	10.58	11.56	13.95	14.68	15.33
Manufacturing	18.22	20.72	23.41	24.30	25.20	12.40	13.69	16.01	16.66	17.19
Nonmanufacturing	14.67	16.19	19.12	20.12	21.06	10.81	11.76	14.18	14.89	15.55
Occupation:										
White collar................	18.15	20.26	24.19	25.34	26.43	13.40	14.72	17.91	18.71	19.48
Blue collar.................	15.15	16.92	18.73	19.35	20.15	10.37	11.31	12.99	13.48	14.01
Service	7.82	8.38	9.72	10.32	10.95	5.96	6.33	7.57	8.00	8.42
Census region:										
Northeast	17.56	20.03	22.67	23.91	25.00	12.65	14.13	16.37	17.22	17.97
Midwest ....:..	15.05	16.26	19.22	20.47	21.25	10.70	11.34	13.91	14.69	15.29
South	13.68	15.05	17.81	18.59	19.49	10.03	10.85	13.09	13.71	14.34
West....................	15.97	18.08	20.88	21.86	22.68	11.62	13.01	15.45	16.19	16.68
Union status:										
Union	19.76	23.26	25.88	27.80	29.42	13.02	14.76	16.87	18.36	19.33
Nonunion	14.54	16.04	19.07	19.98	20.79	10.78	11.70	14.18	14.81	15.38
Establishment employment size:										
1–99 employees	13.38	14.58	17.16	17.86	18.51	10.00	10.72	12.95	13.41	13.88
100 or more	17.34	19.45	22.81	24.19	25.48	12.23	13.48	16.19	17.20	18.07
100–499	14.31	15.88	19.30	20.97	21.99	10.32	11.37	14.05	15.21	15.87
500 or more.............	20.60	23.35	26.93	28.17	29.79	14.28	15.79	18.70	19.67	20.79

Characteristic	Health insurance					Health insurance as a percent of total compensation				
	1991	1994	2000	2001	2002	1991	1994	2000	2001	2002
	Amount per employee-hour worked									
State and local government.......	$1.54	$2.06	$2.27	$2.56	$2.69	6.9	8.2	7.8	8.5	8.6
Total private industry............	0.92	1.14	1.09	1.28	1.29	6.0	6.7	5.5	6.2	5.9
Industry:										
Goods producing	1.28	1.70	1.62	1.85	1.84	6.9	8.1	6.9	7.6	7.2
Service producing	0.79	0.95	0.92	1.11	1.13	5.5	6.0	4.9	5.6	5.5
Manufacturing	1.37	1.79	1.69	1.93	1.92	7.5	8.6	7.2	7.9	7.6
Nonmanufacturing	0.80	0.98	0.96	1.15	1.17	5.5	6.0	5.0	5.7	5.6
Occupation:										
White collar................	1.02	1.25	1.21	1.43	1.42	5.6	6.2	5.0	5.6	5.4
Blue collar.................	1.06	1.35	1.28	1.45	1.48	7.0	8.0	6.8	7.5	7.3
Service	0.36	0.45	0.42	0.52	0.56	4.6	5.4	4.3	5.0	5.1
Census region:										
Northeast	1.08	1.37	1.27	1.50	1.48	6.2	6.9	5.6	6.3	5.9
Midwest	0.95	1.19	1.12	1.35	1.35	6.3	7.3	5.8	6.6	6.4
South	0.76	0.95	0.96	1.16	1.14	5.5	6.3	5.4	6.2	5.8
West....................	0.92	1.10	1.05	1.19	1.26	5.8	6.1	5.0	5.4	5.6
Union status:										
Union	1.63	2.28	2.17	2.48	2.57	8.2	9.8	8.4	8.9	8.7
Nonunion	0.78	0.94	0.95	1.14	1.13	5.4	5.9	5.0	5.7	5.4
Establishment employment size:										
1–99 employees	0.68	0.84	0.82	0.94	0.96	5.1	5.7	4.8	5.3	5.2
100 or more	1.14	1.42	1.38	1.66	1.67	6.6	7.3	6.0	6.9	6.6
100–499	0.90	1.03	1.09	1.38	1.40	6.3	6.5	5.6	6.6	6.4
500 or more.............	1.40	1.84	1.73	2.00	1.99	6.8	7.9	6.4	7.1	6.7

NOTES: Costs are calculated from March survey data each year. Total compensation includes wages and salaries, and benefits. Data for additional years are available (see Appendix III).

SOURCES: U.S. Department of Labor, Bureau of Labor Statistics, National Compensation Survey, Employer Costs for Employee Compensation, March release; *News* pub nos 91–292, 94–290, 00–186, 01–194, and 02–346. June 19, 1991; June 16, 1994; June 29, 2000; June 29, 2001; and June 19, 2002. Washington.

Table 122. Hospital expenses, according to type of ownership and size of hospital: United States, selected years 1980–2001

[Data are based on reporting by a census of hospitals]

Type of ownership and size of hospital	1980	1990	1995	1998	1999	2000	2001	1980–90	1990–95	1995–2001
Total expenses				Amount in billions					Average annual percent change	
All hospitals.	$ 91.9	$234.9	$320.3	$355.5	$372.9	$395.4	$426.8	9.8	6.4	4.9
Federal	7.9	15.2	20.2	22.6	23.7	23.9	27.5	6.8	5.9	5.3
Non-Federal[1]	84.0	219.6	300.0	332.9	349.2	371.5	399.4	10.1	6.4	4.9
Community[2]	76.9	203.7	285.6	318.8	335.2	356.6	383.7	10.2	7.0	5.0
Nonprofit.	55.8	150.7	209.6	238.0	251.5	267.1	287.3	10.4	6.8	5.4
For profit	5.8	18.8	26.7	31.7	31.2	35.0	37.3	12.5	7.3	5.7
State-local government	15.2	34.2	49.3	49.1	52.5	54.5	59.1	8.4	7.6	3.1
6–24 beds	0.2	0.5	1.1	1.4	1.7	1.5	1.6	9.6	17.1	6.4
25–49 beds	1.7	4.0	7.2	8.8	9.3	10.4	11.4	8.9	12.5	8.0
50–99 beds	5.4	12.6	17.8	20.0	21.0	22.3	24.0	8.8	7.2	5.1
100–199 beds	12.5	33.3	50.7	59.4	60.8	63.4	66.4	10.3	8.8	4.6
200–299 beds	13.4	38.7	55.8	57.1	61.1	67.1	68.9	11.2	7.6	3.6
300–399 beds	11.5	33.1	43.3	49.6	55.5	54.3	59.0	11.2	5.5	5.3
400–499 beds	10.5	25.3	33.7	36.4	33.9	41.3	47.3	9.2	5.9	5.8
500 beds or more.	21.6	56.2	76.1	86.0	92.0	96.3	105.1	10.0	6.3	5.5
Expenses per inpatient day				Amount						
Community[2]	$ 245	$ 687	$ 968	$1,067	$1,103	$1,149	$1,217	10.9	7.1	3.9
Nonprofit.	246	692	994	1,111	1,140	1,182	1,255	10.9	7.5	4.0
For profit	257	752	947	968	999	1,057	1,121	11.3	4.7	2.9
State-local government	239	634	878	949	1,007	1,064	1,114	10.2	6.7	4.0
6–24 beds	203	526	678	823	955	896	1,020	10.0	5.2	7.0
25–49 beds	197	489	696	817	846	891	907	9.5	7.3	4.5
50–99 beds	191	493	647	699	717	745	786	9.9	5.6	3.3
100–199 beds	215	585	796	877	897	925	974	10.5	6.4	3.4
200–299 beds	239	665	943	1,035	1,077	1,122	1,174	10.8	7.2	3.7
300–399 beds	248	731	1,070	1,176	1,215	1,277	1,338	11.4	7.9	3.8
400–499 beds	215	756	1,135	1,256	1,285	1,353	1,492	13.4	8.5	4.7
500 beds or more.	239	825	1,212	1,353	1,404	1,468	1,549	13.2	8.0	4.2
Expenses per inpatient stay										
Community[2]	$1,851	$4,947	$6,216	$6,386	$6,512	$6,649	$6,980	10.3	4.7	2.0
Nonprofit.	1,902	5,001	6,279	6,526	6,608	6,717	7,052	10.2	4.7	2.0
For profit	1,676	4,727	5,425	5,262	5,350	5,642	5,972	10.9	2.8	1.6
State-local government	1,750	4,838	6,445	6,612	6,923	7,106	7,400	10.7	5.9	2.3
6–24 beds	1,072	2,701	3,578	3,757	4,098	3,652	3,826	9.7	5.8	1.1
25–49 beds	1,138	2,967	3,797	4,106	4,226	4,381	4,557	10.1	5.1	3.1
50–99 beds	1,271	3,461	4,427	4,734	4,677	4,760	4,943	10.5	5.0	1.9
100–199 beds	1,512	4,109	5,103	5,219	5,290	5,305	5,595	10.5	4.4	1.5
200–299 beds	1,767	4,618	5,851	6,012	6,174	6,392	6,590	10.1	4.8	2.0
300–399 beds	1,881	5,096	6,512	6,642	6,811	6,988	7,240	10.5	5.0	1.8
400–499 beds	2,090	5,500	7,164	7,431	7,595	7,629	8,436	10.2	5.4	2.8
500 beds or more.	2,517	6,667	8,531	8,670	8,853	9,149	9,453	10.2	5.1	1.7

[1]The category of non-Federal hospitals comprises psychiatric, tuberculosis and other respiratory diseases hospitals, and long-term and short-term general and other special hospitals. See Appendix II, Hospital.

[2]Community hospitals are non-Federal short-term general and special hospitals whose facilities and services are available to the public. See Appendix II, Hospital.

NOTES: In 2001 employee payroll and benefit expenses comprised 51 percent of expenses in community hospitals and 60 percent in Federal hospitals. Data for additional years are available (see Appendix III).

SOURCES: American Hospital Association Annual Survey of Hospitals. Hospital Statistics, 1981, 1991–2003 Editions. Chicago, 1981, 1991–2003 (Copyrights 1981, 1991–2003: Used with the permission of the Health Forum LLC, an American Hospital Association Company); and unpublished data.

Table 123. Nursing home average monthly charges per resident and percent of residents, according to selected facility and resident characteristics: United States, 1977, 1985, 1995, 1997, and 1999

[Data are based on reporting by a sample of nursing homes]

Facility and resident characteristic	Average monthly charge[1]					Percent of residents				
	1977	1985	1995	1997	1999	1977	1985	1995	1997	1999
Facility characteristic										
All facilities....................	$689	$1,456	$3,135	$3,609	$ 3,891	100.0	100.0	100.0	100.0	100.0
Ownership:										
Proprietary	670	1,379	3,047	3,508	3,698	68.2	68.7	63.6	65.5	64.4
Nonprofit and government	732	1,624	3,288	3,792	4,225	31.8	31.3	36.4	34.5	35.6
Certification:										
Both Medicare and Medicaid......	- - -	- - -	3,317	3,765	4,060	- - -	- - -	78.4	84.9	86.9
Medicare only	- - -	- - -	4,211	4,221	4,437	- - -	- - -	3.0	2.9	2.3
Medicaid only	- - -	- - -	2,169	2,436	2,508	- - -	- - -	15.8	9.7	8.8
Neither......................	- - -	- - -	2,323	2,422	*2,360	- - -	- - -	2.8	2.4	*2.0
Bed size:										
Less than 50 beds.............	546	1,036	4,978	3,521	3,808	12.9	8.9	4.5	3.9	3.6
50–99 beds...................	643	1,335	2,691	3,178	3,627	30.5	27.6	24.9	24.7	25.5
100–199 beds.................	706	1,478	3,028	3,592	3,867	38.8	43.2	51.1	51.9	50.8
200 beds or more	837	1,759	3,560	4,211	4,281	17.9	20.2	19.5	19.5	20.1
Geographic region:										
Northeast	918	1,781	3,904	4,589	4,852	22.4	23.6	22.8	23.3	23.5
Midwest	640	1,399	2,740	3,203	3,474	34.5	32.5	32.3	31.0	30.6
South........................	585	1,256	2,752	3,225	3,263	27.2	29.4	32.0	32.6	32.6
West	653	1,458	3,710	3,791	4,725	15.9	14.5	12.9	13.1	13.2
Resident characteristic										
All residents	689	1,456	3,135	3,609	3,891	100.0	100.0	100.0	100.0	100.0
Age:										
Under 65 years	585	1,379	3,662	3,760	4,158	13.6	11.6	8.0	8.5	9.7
65–74 years	669	1,372	3,409	3,877	4,134	16.2	14.2	12.0	12.8	12.0
75–84 years	710	1,468	3,138	3,595	3,960	35.7	34.1	32.5	32.8	31.8
85 years and over	719	1,497	2,974	3,521	3,731	34.5	40.0	47.5	45.9	46.5
Sex:										
Male........................	652	1,438	3,345	3,758	4,043	28.8	28.4	26.6	27.8	28.1
Female......................	705	1,463	3,059	3,553	3,833	71.2	71.6	73.4	72.2	71.9

- - - Data not available.

* Starting in 1997 data preceded by an asterisk have a relative standard error of 20–30 percent and are considered unreliable.

[1] Includes life-care residents and no-charge residents.

NOTE: Data for additional years are available (see Appendix III).

SOURCES: Van Nostrand JF, Zappolo A, Hing E, et al. The National Nursing Home Survey, 1977 summary for the United States. National Center for Health Statistics. Vital Health Stat 13(43). 1979; Hing E, Sekscenski E, Strahan G. The National Nursing Home Survey: 1985 summary for the United States. National Center for Health Statistics. Vital Health Stat 13(97). 1989; and Centers for Disease Control and Prevention, National Center for Health Statistics, National Nursing Home Survey for other data years.

Table 124. Nursing home average monthly charges per resident and percent of residents, according to primary source of payments and selected facility characteristics: United States, 1985, 1995, and 1999

[Data are based on reporting by a sample of nursing homes]

Facility characteristic	All sources 1999	Own income or family support[1] 1985	Own income or family support[1] 1995	Own income or family support[1] 1999	Medicare 1985	Medicare 1995	Medicare 1999	Medicaid 1985	Medicaid 1995	Medicaid 1999
	Average monthly charge[2]									
All facilities	$3,891	$1,450	$3,081	$3,947	$2,141	$5,546	$5,764	$1,504	$2,769	$3,505
Ownership										
Proprietary	3,698	1,444	3,190	3,984	2,058	5,668	5,275	1,363	2,560	3,312
Nonprofit and government	4,225	1,462	2,967	3,903	*	5,304	6,548	1,851	3,201	3,918
Certification										
Both Medicare and Medicaid	4,060	- - -	3,365	4,211	- - -	5,472	5,887	- - -	2,910	3,626
Medicare only	4,437	- - -	3,344	3,873	- - -	*	*	. . .	. . .	. . .
Medicaid only	2,508	- - -	2,352	2,533	. . .	. . .	. . .	- - -	2,069	2,501
Neither	2,360	- - -	2,390	2,685	. . .	. . .	. . .	. . .	. . .	. . .
Bed size										
Less than 50 beds	3,808	886	3,377	3,358	*	*	*	1,335	2,990	3,533
50–99 beds	3,627	1,388	2,849	3,698	1,760	4,929	*	1,323	2,335	3,121
100–199 beds	3,867	1,567	3,138	4,160	2,192	4,918	5,318	1,413	2,659	3,487
200 beds or more	4,281	1,701	3,316	4,029	2,767	4,523	5,912	1,919	3,520	4,011
Geographic region										
Northeast	4,852	1,645	4,117	5,300	2,109	4,883	6,368	2,035	3,671	4,397
Midwest	3,474	1,398	2,650	3,413	2,745	5,439	4,726	1,382	2,478	3,239
South	3,263	1,359	2,945	3,467	2,033	4,889	4,859	1,200	2,333	2,943
West	4,725	1,498	3,666	4,868	1,838	8,825	*	1,501	2,848	3,865
	Percent of residents									
All facilities	100.0	41.6	27.8	23.7	1.4	9.9	14.7	50.4	60.2	58.7
Ownership										
Proprietary	100.0	40.1	24.1	20.2	1.6	10.4	14.2	52.1	63.8	62.9
Nonprofit and government	100.0	44.9	34.3	30.2	*	9.2	15.5	46.6	54.0	51.1
Certification										
Both Medicare and Medicaid	100.0	- - -	23.1	21.5	- - -	11.6	15.5	- - -	63.9	60.4
Medicare only	100.0	- - -	71.2	71.4	- - -	16.2	*21.0	. . .	. . .	. . .
Medicaid only	100.0	- - -	32.1	21.9	. . .	. . .	. . .	- - -	63.0	69.5
Neither	100.0	- - -	91.0	73.6	. . .	. . .	. . .	. . .	. . .	. . .
Bed size										
Less than 50 beds	100.0	53.1	35.3	40.3	*	13.1	*15.9	33.8	49.9	42.5
50–99 beds	100.0	49.5	34.5	28.3	*	6.2	12.4	42.9	57.6	56.9
100–199 beds	100.0	39.6	26.2	21.8	1.5	10.6	15.0	55.2	61.5	61.0
200 beds or more	100.0	30.1	22.0	20.1	*	12.1	16.3	57.7	62.4	58.1
Geographic region										
Northeast	100.0	34.8	18.2	18.0	1.7	14.0	16.4	52.9	64.9	62.3
Midwest	100.0	49.1	36.3	32.9	*	6.7	13.3	45.9	55.8	51.1
South	100.0	39.4	26.1	19.2	*	10.1	14.9	53.8	62.2	63.5
West	100.0	40.4	27.9	23.9	*	10.5	13.9	49.2	57.9	57.8

* Estimates are considered unreliable. Data not shown have a relative standard error greater than 30 percent. After 1995 data preceded by an asterisk have a relative standard error of 20–30 percent.
- - - Data not available.
. . . Category not applicable.
[1] Includes private health insurance.
[2] Includes life-care residents and no-charge residents.

NOTE: Data for additional years are available (see Appendix III).

SOURCES: Hing E, Sekscenski E, Strahan G. The National Nursing Home Survey: 1985 summary for the United States. National Center for Health Statistics. Vital Health Stat 13(97). 1989; and Centers for Disease Control and Prevention, National Center for Health Statistics, National Nursing Home Survey for other data years.

Table 125. Mental health expenditures, percent distribution, and per capita expenditures, according to type of mental health organization: United States, selected years 1975–98

[Data are based on inventories of mental health organizations]

Type of organization	1975	1979	1983	1986	1990	1992	1994[1]	1998
	Amount in millions							
All organizations	$6,564	$8,764	$14,432	$18,458	$28,410	$29,765	$33,136	$38,596
State and county psychiatric hospitals	3,185	3,757	5,491	6,326	7,774	7,970	7,825	7,180
Private psychiatric hospitals	467	743	1,712	2,629	6,101	5,302	6,468	4,120
Non-Federal general hospital psychiatric services	621	723	2,176	2,878	4,662	5,193	5,344	5,589
Department of Veterans Affairs medical centers[2]	699	848	1,316	1,338	1,480	1,530	1,386	1,690
Residential treatment centers for emotionally disturbed children	279	436	573	978	1,969	2,167	2,360	3,557
All other organizations[3]	1,313	2,256	3,164	4,310	6,424	7,603	9,753	16,460
	Percent distribution							
All organizations	100.0	100.0	100.0	100.0	100.0	100.0	100.0	100.0
State and county psychiatric hospitals	48.5	42.9	38.0	34.3	27.4	26.8	23.6	18.6
Private psychiatric hospitals	7.1	8.5	11.9	14.2	21.5	17.8	19.5	10.7
Non-Federal general hospital psychiatric services	9.5	8.2	15.1	15.6	16.4	17.4	16.1	14.5
Department of Veterans Affairs medical centers[2]	10.6	9.7	9.1	7.2	5.2	5.1	4.2	4.4
Residential treatment centers for emotionally disturbed children	4.2	5.0	4.0	5.3	6.9	7.3	7.1	9.2
All other organizations[3]	20.0	25.7	21.9	23.3	22.6	25.5	29.4	42.6
	Amount per capita[4]							
All organizations	$ 31	$ 40	$ 62	$ 77	$ 116	$ 117	$ 128	$ 141
State and county psychiatric hospitals	15	17	24	26	32	31	30	26
Private psychiatric hospitals	2	3	7	11	25	21	25	15
Non-Federal general hospital psychiatric services	3	3	9	12	19	20	21	20
Department of Veterans Affairs medical centers[2]	3	4	6	6	6	6	5	6
Residential treatment centers for emotionally disturbed children	1	2	2	4	8	9	9	13
All other organizations[3]	6	10	14	18	26	30	38	60

[1]Beginning in 1994 data for supportive residential clients (moderately staffed housing arrangements such as supervised apartments, group homes, and halfway houses) are included in the totals and all other organizations. This change affects the comparability of trend data prior to 1994 with data for 1994 and later years.
[2]Includes Department of Veterans Affairs neuropsychiatric hospitals, general hospital psychiatric services, and psychiatric outpatient clinics.
[3]Includes freestanding psychiatric outpatient clinics, partial care organizations, multiservice mental health organizations, residential treatment centers for adults, substance abuse organizations, and in 1975 and 1979 Federally funded community mental health centers.
[4]Civilian population as of July 1 each year.

NOTES: Changes in reporting procedures and definitions may affect the comparability of data prior to 1980 with those of later years. Mental health expenditures include salaries, other operating expenditures, and capital expenditures. These data exclude mental health care provided in nonpsychiatric units of hospitals such as general medical units.

SOURCES: Substance Abuse and Mental Health Services Administration, Center for Mental Health Services, Division of State and Community Systems Development, Survey and Analysis Branch. Manderscheid RW, Henderson MJ. *Mental health, United States, 2000.* U.S. Government Printing Office, 2000; unpublished data from the 1998 inventory of mental health organizations and general hospital mental health services.

Table 126. Federal spending for human immunodeficiency virus (HIV)-related activities, according to agency and type of activity: United States, selected fiscal years 1985–2002

[Data are compiled from Federal Government appropriations]

Agency and type of activity	1985	1990	1995	1998	1999	2000	2001	2002[1]
Agency				Amount in millions				
All Federal spending	$209	$3,070	$7,019	$9,689	$10,779	$12,025	$14,184	$14,988
Department of Health and Human Services, total	201	2,372	5,200	7,537	8,494	9,621	11,406	12,039
Department of Health and Human Services discretionary spending, total[2]	109	1,592	2,700	3,537	4,094	4,546	5,226	5,789
National Institutes of Health	66	908	1,334	1,603	1,793	2,004	2,247	2,499
Substance Abuse and Mental Health Services Administration	–	50	24	66	92	110	157	169
Centers for Disease Control and Prevention	33	443	590	625	657	687	859	931
Food and Drug Administration	9	57	73	77	70	76	76	76
Health Resources and Services Administration	–	113	661	1,155	1,416	1,599	1,815	1,917
Ricky Ray Hemophilia Relief Fund[3]	...	...	...	...	...	75	580	...
Agency for Healthcare Research and Quality	–	8	9	2	2	2	3	3
Office of the Secretary[4]	–	10	6	7	12	13	15	14
Indian Health Service	–	3	4	4	4	4	4	4
Emergency Fund	...	...	...	...	50	50	50	50
Global AIDS Trust Fund	...	...	...	...	...	...	...	125
Centers for Medicare & Medicaid Services	75	780	2,500	4,000	4,400	5,000	5,600	6,250
Social Security Administration[5]	17	...	...	...	...	...	...	...
Social Security Administration[5]	...	239	881	1,092	1,158	1,240	1,259	1,351
Department of Veterans Affairs	8	220	317	378	401	345	405	391
Department of Defense	–	124	110	95	86	97	108	96
Agency for International Development	–	71	120	121	139	200	430	510
Department of Housing and Urban Development	–	–	171	204	225	232	257	277
Office of Personnel Management	–	37	212	253	266	279	292	297
Other departments	–	7	8	9	10	11	27	27
Activity								
Research	75	1,013	1,460	1,727	1,900	2,125	2,368	2,614
Department of Health and Human Services discretionary spending[2]	75	974	1,417	1,682	1,869	2,085	2,328	2,580
Department of Veterans Affairs	–	6	5	7	7	7	7	8
Department of Defense	–	33	38	38	24	33	33	26
Education and prevention	33	591	770	807	902	998	1,396	1,629
Department of Health and Human Services discretionary spending[2]	33	460	604	641	719	751	950	1,091
Department of Veterans Affairs	–	29	31	32	30	33	35	35
Department of Defense	–	28	12	10	10	10	17	17
Agency for International Development	–	71	120	121	139	200	380	473
Other	–	3	3	3	4	4	14	13
Medical care	83	1,227	3,738	5,858	6,595	7,356	8,324	9,117
Centers for Medicare & Medicaid Services: Medicaid (Federal share)	70	670	1,500	2,600	2,900	3,300	3,700	4,200
Medicare	5	110	1,000	1,400	1,500	1,700	1,900	2,050
Department of Health and Human Services discretionary spending[2]	–	158	680	1,213	1,507	1,711	1,948	2,118
Department of Veterans Affairs	8	185	281	339	364	305	363	348
Department of Defense	–	63	60	47	52	54	58	53
Agency for International Development	–	–	–	–	–	–	50	38
Office of Personnel Management	–	37	212	253	266	279	292	297
Other	–	4	5	6	6	7	13	14
Cash assistance	17	239	1,052	1,296	1,383	1,547	2,096	1,628
Social Security Administration: Disability Insurance	12	184	631	787	828	870	919	961
Supplemental Security Income	5	55	250	305	330	370	340	390
Department of Housing and Urban Development	–	–	171	204	225	232	257	277
Ricky Ray Hemophilia Relief Fund[3]	–	–	–	–	–	75	580	–

– Quantity zero.   ... Category not applicable.   [1]Preliminary figures.
[2]Department of Health and Human Services discretionary spending is spending that is not entitlement spending. Medicare and Medicaid are examples of entitlement spending.
[3]The Ricky Ray Hemophilia Relief Fund was established by the U.S. Congress in 1998 to make compassionate payments to certain individuals who were treated with anti-hemophilic factor between July 1, 1982 and December 31, 1987, and who contracted HIV. Some family members may also be covered by the Fund. $75 million was appropriated in fiscal year 2000 and $580 million in fiscal year 2001.
[4]The Office of the Assistant Secretary for Health prior to FY 1996.
[5]Prior to 1995 the Social Security Administration was part of the Department of Health and Human Services.

NOTE: These data include revisions and differ from previous editions of Health, United States.

SOURCE: Office of the Assistant Secretary for Budget, Technology, and Finance, Office of the Secretary, Department of Health and Human Services. Unpublished data.

Table 127 (page 1 of 3). Private health insurance coverage among persons under 65 years of age, according to selected characteristics: United States, selected years 1984–2001

[Data are based on household interviews of a sample of the civilian noninstitutionalized population]

Characteristic	1984	1989	1995	1996	1997[1]	1998	1999	2000	2001
	Number in millions								
Total[2]	157.5	162.7	164.2	165.6	165.8	170.8	174.3	173.0	174.1
	Percent of population								
Total, age adjusted[2,3]	77.1	76.2	71.6	71.5	70.9	72.3	72.9	71.7	71.5
Total, crude[2]	76.8	75.9	71.3	71.2	70.7	72.1	72.8	71.7	71.5
Age									
Under 18 years	72.6	71.8	65.2	66.2	66.1	68.4	68.8	67.0	66.7
Under 6 years	68.1	67.9	59.5	60.8	61.3	64.7	64.7	63.1	63.4
6–17 years	74.9	74.0	68.3	68.9	68.5	70.2	70.9	68.9	68.3
18–44 years	76.5	75.5	70.9	70.5	69.4	71.1	72.0	70.9	70.6
18–24 years	67.4	64.5	60.8	60.3	59.3	61.5	63.2	60.9	60.9
25–34 years	77.4	75.9	70.1	69.4	68.1	70.6	71.2	70.6	70.8
35–44 years	83.9	82.7	77.7	77.4	76.4	76.9	77.9	77.1	76.3
45–64 years	83.3	82.5	80.1	79.4	79.0	79.0	79.3	78.7	78.6
45–54 years	83.3	83.4	80.9	80.4	80.4	80.0	80.4	80.0	79.4
55–64 years	83.3	81.6	79.0	78.0	76.9	77.3	77.7	76.6	77.3
Sex[3]									
Male	77.7	76.5	72.1	71.9	71.2	72.5	73.0	72.1	71.7
Female	76.5	75.9	71.1	71.1	70.6	72.1	72.8	71.4	71.3
Race[3,4]									
White only	80.1	79.3	74.7	74.5	74.3	75.9	76.8	75.8	75.2
Black or African American only	59.2	58.7	54.9	55.9	56.1	55.9	58.1	56.9	57.4
American Indian and Alaska Native only	#	#	#	#	#	#	41.3	44.2	49.4
Asian only	70.9	71.6	68.4	68.3	68.2	72.2	73.2	71.9	72.1
Native Hawaiian and Other Pacific Islander only	- - -	- - -	- - -	- - -	- - -	- - -	*	*	*
2 or more races	- - -	- - -	- - -	- - -	- - -	- - -	63.5	63.1	62.6
Hispanic origin and race[3,4]									
Hispanic or Latino	57.1	53.2	48.0	48.2	47.9	49.9	50.3	49.0	47.6
Mexican	54.9	48.5	44.3	44.3	43.9	45.6	48.0	46.6	45.0
Puerto Rican	51.0	46.8	48.9	52.4	48.2	52.7	51.4	52.6	51.5
Cuban	72.1	70.0	63.4	65.6	70.7	71.7	71.4	63.6	66.1
Other Hispanic or Latino	62.0	62.4	52.9	53.2	51.2	52.8	53.4	51.6	50.5
Not Hispanic or Latino	78.9	78.6	74.6	74.6	74.1	75.5	76.3	75.1	75.2
White only	82.4	82.5	78.6	78.6	78.0	79.6	80.3	79.3	79.2
Black or African American only	59.4	58.8	55.3	56.3	56.3	56.1	58.2	57.0	57.6
Age and percent of poverty level[5]									
All ages:[3]									
Below 100 percent	33.0	27.5	23.0	21.8	23.4	24.1	26.1	25.8	25.6
100–149 percent	61.8	54.2	47.9	46.6	42.0	43.3	40.1	39.5	39.6
150–199 percent	77.2	70.6	65.2	65.8	63.6	61.4	59.4	58.4	57.0
200 percent or more	91.6	91.0	88.4	88.4	87.6	88.3	88.7	87.2	87.1
Under 18 years:									
Below 100 percent	28.7	22.3	16.9	17.0	17.3	18.9	19.5	18.9	16.7
100–149 percent	66.2	59.6	48.5	48.5	42.5	45.8	40.4	37.9	39.4
150–199 percent	80.9	75.9	67.4	72.1	66.8	66.5	61.6	59.8	56.9
200 percent or more	92.3	92.7	89.5	89.8	88.9	89.9	90.4	88.0	88.4
Geographic region[3]									
Northeast	80.7	82.1	75.5	75.4	74.3	76.4	77.1	76.5	76.5
Midwest	80.9	81.7	77.5	78.7	77.3	79.1	80.2	78.9	78.1
South	74.5	71.7	67.1	66.5	67.5	67.8	68.0	67.0	66.3
West	72.3	71.8	68.1	67.7	65.8	67.8	68.9	67.1	68.6
Location of residence[3]									
Within MSA[6]	77.8	76.8	72.5	72.9	71.5	73.2	74.3	72.7	72.6
Outside MSA[6]	75.5	74.0	68.1	66.3	68.5	68.9	67.8	67.7	66.9

See footnotes at end of table.

Table 127 (page 2 of 3). Private health insurance coverage among persons under 65 years of age, according to selected characteristics: United States, selected years 1984–2001

[Data are based on household interviews of a sample of the civilian noninstitutionalized population]

| Characteristic | \multicolumn{9}{c}{Private insurance obtained through workplace[7]} |
	1984	1989	1995	1996	1997[1]	1998	1999	2000	2001
	\multicolumn{9}{c}{Number in millions}
Total[2]	141.8	146.3	150.7	151.1	155.6	159.3	162.6	161.6	163.1
	\multicolumn{9}{c}{Percent of population}
Total, age adjusted[2,3]	69.2	68.4	65.6	65.2	66.5	67.4	68.1	67.0	67.0
Total, crude[2]	69.1	68.3	65.4	65.0	66.3	67.3	68.0	67.0	67.0
Age									
Under 18 years	66.5	65.8	60.4	60.8	62.7	64.1	64.6	63.1	63.2
Under 6 years	62.1	62.3	55.1	56.2	58.2	60.9	60.8	59.2	59.6
6–17 years	68.7	67.7	63.3	63.2	64.9	65.7	66.5	65.0	64.9
18–44 years	69.6	68.4	65.3	64.6	65.5	66.5	67.7	66.5	66.3
18–24 years	58.7	55.3	53.5	52.2	54.7	55.7	57.8	55.5	55.8
25–34 years	71.2	69.5	65.0	64.3	64.5	66.7	67.2	66.6	66.7
35–44 years	77.4	76.2	72.7	71.9	72.6	72.5	73.8	72.8	72.2
45–64 years	71.8	71.6	72.2	71.4	72.6	72.7	72.7	72.5	72.5
45–54 years	74.6	74.4	74.7	73.9	75.4	75.1	75.1	75.3	74.5
55–64 years	69.0	68.3	68.4	67.5	68.3	69.1	69.2	68.1	69.4
Sex[3]									
Male	70.1	68.9	66.3	65.7	66.9	67.6	68.1	67.4	67.1
Female	68.4	67.9	65.0	64.7	66.1	67.2	68.0	66.6	66.8
Race[3,4]									
White only	72.0	71.2	68.5	67.8	69.6	70.8	71.6	70.8	70.3
Black or African American only	53.3	53.6	51.1	52.7	53.9	53.2	55.4	54.1	55.1
American Indian and Alaska Native only	#	#	#	#	#	#	38.4	42.0	47.3
Asian only	64.4	60.2	59.8	59.4	61.7	63.8	65.3	64.9	65.7
Native Hawaiian and Other Pacific Islander only	- - -	- - -	- - -	- - -	- - -	- - -	*	*	*
2 or more races	- - -	- - -	- - -	- - -	- - -	- - -	59.9	61.2	58.6
Hispanic origin and race[3,4]									
Hispanic or Latino	52.9	48.6	44.6	44.4	45.1	46.8	47.3	46.1	45.0
Mexican	51.7	45.6	42.3	41.3	42.1	43.4	45.4	44.3	43.1
Puerto Rican	48.3	43.4	45.6	49.8	46.1	50.2	48.3	50.6	48.4
Cuban	57.6	56.3	53.8	54.7	58.1	60.3	63.7	53.5	56.7
Other Hispanic or Latino	57.7	55.7	47.7	48.2	48.2	49.4	50.0	48.0	48.0
Not Hispanic or Latino	70.7	70.5	68.3	67.9	69.4	70.3	71.1	70.1	70.4
White only	74.0	74.0	72.1	71.5	73.1	74.2	74.8	73.9	74.0
Black or African American only	53.4	53.7	51.5	53.1	54.1	53.4	55.5	54.2	55.3
Age and percent of poverty level[5]									
All ages:[3]									
Below 100 percent	23.8	19.7	17.6	16.7	19.9	19.8	22.2	21.2	22.0
100–149 percent	51.1	45.0	41.7	40.4	37.3	38.5	35.9	35.0	35.0
150–199 percent	68.6	61.9	58.6	58.9	59.0	55.7	53.9	53.6	52.3
200 percent or more	85.0	83.9	82.4	81.8	83.6	83.7	84.5	83.1	82.9
Under 18 years:									
Below 100 percent	23.2	17.5	13.6	13.9	15.5	16.5	16.7	15.9	14.8
100–149 percent	58.3	52.5	43.6	43.0	38.9	41.8	37.4	34.8	35.9
150–199 percent	75.8	70.1	61.8	66.8	63.8	62.1	57.2	56.4	53.9
200 percent or more	86.9	86.7	84.4	83.6	85.5	85.3	86.5	84.3	84.7

See footnotes at end of table.

Table 127 (page 3 of 3). Private health insurance coverage among persons under 65 years of age, according to selected characteristics: United States, selected years 1984–2001

[Data are based on household interviews of a sample of the civilian noninstitutionalized population]

Characteristic	Private insurance obtained through workplace[7]								
	1984	1989	1995	1996	1997[1]	1998	1999	2000	2001
Geographic region[3]	Percent of population								
Northeast	74.1	75.1	69.9	69.1	71.0	73.0	73.5	72.2	73.0
Midwest	72.1	73.4	71.4	72.5	72.6	73.7	75.4	74.7	73.7
South	66.2	63.8	62.0	60.8	63.0	63.3	63.7	62.4	61.8
West	64.9	64.2	60.8	60.1	60.9	61.6	61.9	61.1	62.8
Location of residence[3]									
Within MSA[6]	71.0	69.8	66.9	66.9	67.4	68.5	69.6	68.1	68.3
Outside MSA[6]	65.3	63.5	60.8	58.9	62.8	63.0	62.0	62.3	61.6

#Estimates calculated upon request.

* Estimates are considered unreliable. Data not shown have a relative standard error of greater than 30 percent.

- - - Data not available.

[1]In 1997 the National Health Interview Survey (NHIS) was redesigned, including changes to the questions on health insurance coverage. See Appendix I, National Health Interview Survey and Appendix II, Health insurance coverage.

[2]Includes all other races not shown separately and unknown poverty level.

[3]Estimates are for persons under 65 years of age and are age adjusted to the year 2000 standard using three age groups: under 18 years, 18–44 years, and 45–64 years. See Appendix II, Age adjustment.

[4]The race groups, white, black, American Indian and Alaska Native (AI/AN), Asian, Native Hawaiian and Other Pacific Islander, and 2 or more races, include persons of Hispanic and non-Hispanic origin. Persons of Hispanic origin may be of any race. Starting with data year 1999 race-specific estimates are tabulated according to 1997 Standards for Federal data on Race and Ethnicity and are not strictly comparable with estimates for earlier years. The five single race categories plus multiple race categories shown in the table conform to 1997 Standards. The 1999 and later race-specific estimates are for persons who reported only one racial group; the category "2 or more races" includes persons who reported more than one racial group. Prior to data year 1999, data were tabulated according to 1977 Standards with four racial groups and the category "Asian only" included Native Hawaiian and Other Pacific Islander. Estimates for single race categories prior to 1999 included persons who reported one race or, if they reported more than one race, identified one race as best representing their race. The effect of the 1997 Standard on the 1999 estimates can be seen by comparing 1999 data tabulated according to the two Standards: Age-adjusted estimates based on the 1977 Standards of the percent with private health insurance are: 0.1 percentage points lower for the white group; 0.1 percentage points higher for the black group; 0.9 percentage points lower for the Asian and Pacific Islander group; and 0.2 percentage points higher for the AI/AN group than estimates based on the 1997 Standards. See Appendix II, Race.

[5]Missing family income data were imputed for 15–17 percent of the sample under 65 years of age in 1994–96. Percent of poverty level was unknown for 19 percent of sample persons under 65 in 1997, 24 percent in 1998, 27 percent in 1999, and 26 percent in 2000 and 2001. See Appendix II, Family income; Poverty level.

[6]MSA is metropolitan statistical area.

[7]Private insurance originally obtained through a present or former employer or union. Starting in 1997 also includes private insurance obtained through workplace, self-employment, or professional association.

SOURCES: Centers for Disease Control and Prevention, National Center for Health Statistics, National Health Interview Survey, health insurance supplements (1984, 1989, 1994–1996). Starting in 1997 data are from the family core questionnaires.

Table 128 (page 1 of 2). Medicaid coverage among persons under 65 years of age, according to selected characteristics: United States, selected years 1984–2001

[Data are based on household interviews of a sample of the civilian noninstitutionalized population]

Characteristic	1984	1989	1995	1996	1997[1]	1998	1999	2000	2001
					Number in millions				
Total[2]	14.0	15.4	26.6	25.8	22.9	21.1	21.9	22.9	25.2
					Percent of population				
Total, age adjusted[2,3]	6.7	7.1	11.3	10.9	9.6	8.8	9.0	9.4	10.3
Total, crude[2]	6.8	7.2	11.5	11.1	9.7	8.9	9.1	9.5	10.4
Age									
Under 18 years	11.9	12.6	21.5	20.7	18.4	17.1	18.1	19.4	21.2
Under 6 years	15.5	15.7	29.3	28.2	24.7	22.4	23.5	24.3	25.8
6–17 years	10.1	10.9	17.4	16.9	15.2	14.5	15.5	17.0	19.0
18–44 years	5.1	5.2	7.8	7.6	6.6	5.8	5.7	5.6	6.3
18–24 years	6.4	6.8	10.4	9.7	8.8	8.0	8.1	8.1	8.4
25–34 years	5.3	5.2	8.2	7.8	6.8	5.7	5.7	5.5	6.2
35–44 years	3.5	4.0	5.9	6.2	5.2	4.6	4.3	4.3	5.1
45–64 years	3.4	4.3	5.6	5.3	4.6	4.5	4.4	4.5	4.7
45–54 years	3.2	3.8	5.1	4.9	4.0	4.1	3.9	4.2	4.4
55–64 years	3.6	4.9	6.4	5.9	5.6	5.0	5.3	4.9	5.2
Sex[3]									
Male	5.2	5.6	9.2	8.9	8.1	7.5	7.7	8.0	8.9
Female	8.0	8.6	13.3	12.8	11.0	10.1	10.4	10.8	11.6
Race[3,4]									
White only	4.6	5.1	8.8	8.7	7.5	6.7	6.9	7.2	8.1
Black or African American only	18.9	17.8	26.0	23.0	20.5	19.6	18.7	19.4	20.4
American Indian and Alaska Native only	#	#	#	#	#	#	41.3	44.2	15.5
Asian only	9.1	11.3	10.7	*11.5	9.4	6.7	8.4	7.8	8.8
Native Hawaiian and Other Pacific Islander only	- - -	- - -	- - -	- - -	- - -	- - -	*	*	*
2 or more races	- - -	- - -	- - -	- - -	- - -	- - -	15.8	15.6	14.6
Hispanic origin and race[3,4]									
Hispanic or Latino	12.2	12.7	19.8	18.5	16.0	14.1	14.1	14.2	16.0
Mexican	11.1	11.5	18.8	17.6	15.3	12.6	12.4	12.5	14.6
Puerto Rican	28.6	26.9	31.1	31.3	28.9	24.5	27.0	27.6	28.5
Cuban	4.8	7.8	13.8	*13.1	8.2	*9.1	8.3	9.7	12.2
Other Hispanic or Latino	7.4	10.4	16.9	15.0	13.9	13.9	13.8	14.1	15.0
Not Hispanic or Latino	6.2	6.6	10.2	9.7	8.7	8.0	8.2	8.6	9.3
White only	3.7	4.2	7.1	7.0	6.2	5.7	6.0	6.3	7.0
Black or African American only	19.1	17.8	25.6	22.7	20.3	19.4	18.7	19.3	20.3
Age and percent of poverty level[5]									
All ages:[3]									
Below 100 percent	30.5	35.3	44.7	42.9	38.8	37.9	36.8	37.2	39.0
100–149 percent	7.5	11.0	18.0	17.4	17.5	16.0	18.6	20.3	23.5
150–199 percent	3.1	5.0	7.9	8.0	7.4	7.2	9.8	10.8	13.3
200 percent or more	0.6	1.1	1.8	1.7	1.7	1.8	2.0	2.3	2.6
Under 18 years:									
Below 100 percent	43.1	47.8	66.0	65.2	59.7	58.7	59.9	60.9	64.3
100–149 percent	9.0	12.3	27.2	26.6	30.2	25.9	33.5	37.1	41.4
150–199 percent	4.4	6.1	13.1	12.2	12.2	12.8	18.0	21.5	26.5
200 percent or more	0.8	1.6	3.3	2.8	2.9	3.2	3.7	4.7	5.3

See footnotes at end of table.

Table 128 (page 2 of 2). Medicaid coverage among persons under 65 years of age, according to selected characteristics: United States, selected years 1984–2001

[Data are based on household interviews of a sample of the civilian noninstitutionalized population]

Characteristic	1984	1989	1995	1996	1997[1]	1998	1999	2000	2001
Geographic region[3]				Percent of population					
Northeast	8.5	6.8	11.7	11.5	11.2	9.8	10.1	10.5	10.8
Midwest	7.2	7.5	10.3	8.7	8.2	7.5	7.3	7.9	9.0
South	5.0	6.4	11.1	11.1	8.6	8.6	8.9	9.4	10.7
West	6.9	8.2	12.4	12.4	11.4	9.7	10.3	10.2	10.6
Location of residence[3]									
Within MSA[6]	7.1	7.0	11.1	10.4	9.5	8.5	8.4	8.8	9.8
Outside MSA[6]	5.9	7.8	12.0	12.7	9.9	9.8	11.5	11.9	12.4

\# Estimates calculated upon request.

* Estimates are considered unreliable. Data preceded by an asterisk have a relative standard error of 20–30 percent. Data not shown have a relative standard error of greater than 30 percent.

- - - Data not available.

[1]In 1997 the National Health Interview Survey (NHIS) was redesigned, including changes to the questions on health insurance coverage. See Appendix I, National Health Interview Survey and Appendix II, Health insurance coverage.

[2]Includes all other races not shown separately and unknown poverty level.

[3]Estimates are for persons under 65 years of age and are age adjusted to the year 2000 standard using three age groups: under 18 years, 18–44 years, and 45–64 years. See Appendix II, Age adjustment.

[4]The race groups, white, black, American Indian and Alaska Native (AI/AN), Asian, Native Hawaiian and Other Pacific Islander, and 2 or more races, include persons of Hispanic and non-Hispanic origin. Persons of Hispanic origin may be of any race. Starting with data year 1999 race-specific estimates are tabulated according to 1997 Standards for Federal data on Race and Ethnicity and are not strictly comparable with estimates for earlier years. The five single race categories plus multiple race categories shown in the table conform to 1997 Standards. The 1999 and later race-specific estimates are for persons who reported only one racial group; the category "2 or more races" includes persons who reported more than one racial group. Prior to data year 1999, data were tabulated according to 1977 Standards with four racial groups and the category "Asian only" included Native Hawaiian and Other Pacific Islander. Estimates for single race categories prior to 1999 included persons who reported one race or, if they reported more than one race, identified one race as best representing their race. The effect of the 1997 Standard on the 1999 estimates can be seen by comparing 1999 data tabulated according to the two Standards: Age-adjusted estimates based on the 1977 Standards of the percent with Medicaid are: 0.1 percentage points higher for the white group; 0.1 percentage points lower for the black group; 0.8 percentage points higher for the Asian and Pacific Islander group; and 0.8 percentage points higher for the AI/AN group than estimates based on the 1997 Standards. See Appendix II, Race.

[5]Missing family income data were imputed for 15–17 percent of the sample under 65 years of age in 1994–96. Percent of poverty level was unknown for 19 percent of sample persons under 65 in 1997, 24 percent in 1998, 27 percent in 1999, and 26 percent in 2000 and 2001. See Appendix II, Family income; Poverty level.

[6]MSA is metropolitan statistical area.

NOTES: Medicaid includes other public assistance through 1996. Starting in 1997 includes state-sponsored health plans. Starting in 1999 includes State Children's Health Insurance Program (SCHIP). In 2001, 7.9 percent were covered by Medicaid, 1.2 percent by state-sponsored health plans, and 1.2 percent by SCHIP.

SOURCES: Centers for Disease Control and Prevention, National Center for Health Statistics, National Health Interview Survey, health insurance supplements (1984, 1989, 1994–1996). Starting in 1997 data are from the family core questionnaires.

Table 129 (page 1 of 2). No health insurance coverage among persons under 65 years of age, according to selected characteristics: United States, selected years 1984–2001

[Data are based on household interviews of a sample of the civilian noninstitutionalized population]

Characteristic	1984	1989	1995	1996	1997[1]	1998	1999	2000	2001
					Number in millions				
Total[2]	29.8	33.4	37.1	38.6	41.0	39.2	38.5	40.5	39.2
					Percent of population				
Total, age adjusted[2,3]	14.3	15.3	15.9	16.5	17.4	16.5	16.1	16.8	16.2
Total, crude[2]	14.5	15.6	16.1	16.6	17.5	16.6	16.1	16.8	16.1
Age									
Under 18 years	13.9	14.7	13.4	13.2	14.0	12.7	11.9	12.4	11.0
Under 6 years	14.9	15.1	11.8	11.7	12.5	11.5	11.0	11.7	9.7
6–17 years.	13.4	14.5	14.3	13.9	14.7	13.3	12.3	12.8	11.7
18–44 years	17.1	18.4	20.4	21.1	22.4	21.4	21.0	22.0	21.7
18–24 years.	25.0	27.1	28.0	29.3	30.1	29.0	27.4	29.7	29.3
25–34 years.	16.2	18.3	21.1	22.4	23.8	22.2	22.1	22.7	22.3
35–44 years.	11.2	12.3	15.1	15.2	16.7	16.4	16.3	16.8	16.7
45–64 years	9.6	10.5	10.9	12.1	12.4	12.2	12.2	12.7	12.3
45–54 years. . . . . : . .	10.5	11.0	11.6	12.4	12.8	12.6	12.8	12.8	13.0
55–64 years.	8.7	10.0	9.9	11.6	11.8	11.4	11.4	12.5	11.0
Sex[3]									
Male.	15.0	16.4	17.2	17.8	18.5	17.5	17.2	17.8	17.2
Female	13.6	14.3	14.6	15.2	16.2	15.5	15.0	15.8	15.1
Race[3,4]									
White only.	13.4	14.2	15.3	15.8	16.3	15.2	14.6	15.2	14.7
Black or African American only	20.0	21.4	18.2	19.6	20.2	20.7	19.5	20.0	19.3
American Indian and Alaska Native only. . .	#	#	#	#	#	#	38.3	38.2	33.4
Asian only.	18.0	18.5	18.2	19.0	19.3	18.1	16.4	17.3	17.1
Native Hawaiian and Other Pacific Islander only	- - -	- - -	- - -	- - -	- - -	- - -	*	*	*
2 or more races.	- - -	- - -	- - -	- - -	- - -	- - -	16.8	18.4	18.6
Hispanic origin and race[3,4]									
Hispanic or Latino	29.1	32.4	31.5	32.4	34.3	34.0	33.9	35.4	34.8
Mexican.	33.2	38.8	36.2	37.5	39.2	40.0	38.0	39.9	39.0
Puerto Rican	18.1	23.3	18.3	15.1	19.4	19.4	19.8	16.4	16.0
Cuban	21.6	20.9	22.1	18.8	20.5	18.4	19.7	25.2	19.2
Other Hispanic or Latino	27.5	25.2	29.7	30.5	32.9	31.1	30.8	32.7	33.1
Not Hispanic or Latino	13.0	13.5	14.0	14.5	15.1	14.1	13.5	14.1	13.4
White only	11.8	11.9	12.9	13.3	13.7	12.5	12.1	12.5	11.9
Black or African American only.	19.7	21.3	18.1	19.5	20.1	20.7	19.4	20.0	19.2
Age and percent of poverty level[5]									
All ages:[3]									
Below 100 percent	34.7	35.8	31.7	34.5	34.4	34.6	34.4	34.2	33.3
100–149 percent.	27.0	31.3	31.7	33.3	36.1	36.5	35.8	36.5	32.4
150–199 percent.	17.4	21.8	24.0	24.3	25.9	26.7	27.7	27.3	26.4
200 percent or more	5.8	6.8	8.6	8.6	8.8	8.0	7.7	8.7	8.4
Under 18 years:									
Below 100 percent	28.9	31.6	20.0	21.0	22.4	21.5	21.6	20.4	19.8
100–149 percent.	22.8	26.1	24.8	25.0	26.1	28.0	24.9	25.6	18.5
150–199 percent.	12.7	15.8	18.0	16.0	19.7	17.3	18.8	16.8	16.1
200 percent or more	4.2	4.4	6.4	6.1	6.1	5.0	4.4	5.5	4.5

See footnotes at end of table.

Table 129 (page 2 of 2). No health insurance coverage among persons under 65 years of age, according to selected characteristics: United States, selected years 1984–2001

[Data are based on household interviews of a sample of the civilian noninstitutionalized population]

Characteristic	1984	1989	1995	1996	1997[1]	1998	1999	2000	2001
Geographic region[3]				Percent of population					
Northeast	10.1	10.7	13.1	13.5	13.4	12.3	12.2	12.1	11.6
Midwest	11.1	10.5	12.1	12.2	13.1	11.9	11.5	12.3	11.7
South	17.4	19.4	19.2	20.0	20.7	20.0	19.8	20.4	20.0
West.	17.8	18.4	17.7	18.6	20.4	19.9	18.6	20.2	18.6
Location of residence[3]									
Within MSA[6]	13.3	14.9	15.2	15.6	16.7	15.8	15.3	16.3	15.6
Outside MSA[6]	16.4	16.9	18.7	19.7	19.9	19.2	18.9	18.8	18.5

#Estimates calculated upon request.

* Estimates are considered unreliable. Data not shown have a relative standard error of greater than 30 percent.

- - - Data not available.

[1]In 1997 the National Health Interview Survey (NHIS) was redesigned, including changes to the questions on health insurance coverage. See Appendix I, National Health Interview Survey and Appendix II, Health insurance coverage.

[2]Includes all other races not shown separately and unknown poverty level.

[3]Estimates are for persons under 65 years of age and are age adjusted to the year 2000 standard using three age groups: under 18 years, 18–44 years, and 45–64 years. See Appendix II, Age adjustment.

[4]The race groups, white, black, American Indian and Alaska Native (AI/AN), Asian, Native Hawaiian and Other Pacific Islander, and 2 or more races, include persons of Hispanic and non-Hispanic origin. Persons of Hispanic origin may be of any race. Starting with data year 1999 race-specific estimates are tabulated according to 1997 Standards for Federal data on Race and Ethnicity and are not strictly comparable with estimates for earlier years. The five single race categories plus multiple race categories shown in the table conform to 1997 Standards. The 1999 and later race-specific estimates are for persons who reported only one racial group; the category "2 or more races" includes persons who reported more than one racial group. Prior to data year 1999, data were tabulated according to 1977 Standards with four racial groups and the category "Asian only" included Native Hawaiian and Other Pacific Islander. Estimates for single race categories prior to 1999 included persons who reported one race or, if they reported more than one race, identified one race as best representing their race. The effect of the 1997 Standard on the 1999 estimates can be seen by comparing 1999 data tabulated according to the two Standards: Age-adjusted estimates based on the 1977 Standards of the percent with no health insurance coverage are: 0.1 percentage points higher for the white group; identical for the black group; 0.1 percentage points lower for the Asian and Pacific Islander group; and 1.5 percentage points higher for the AI/AN group than estimates based on the 1997 Standards. See Appendix II, Race.

[5]Missing family income data were imputed for 15–17 percent of the sample under 65 years of age in 1994–96. Percent of poverty level was unknown for 19 percent of sample persons under 65 in 1997, 24 percent in 1998, 27 percent in 1999, and 26 percent in 2000 and 2001. See Appendix II, Family income; Poverty level.

[6]MSA is metropolitan statistical area.

NOTES: Persons not covered by private insurance, Medicaid, State Children's Health Insurance Program (SCHIP), public assistance (through 1996), state-sponsored or other government-sponsored health plans (starting in 1997), Medicare, or military plans are included. See Appendix II, Health insurance coverage.

SOURCES: Centers for Disease Control and Prevention, National Center for Health Statistics, National Health Interview Survey, health insurance supplements (1984, 1989, 1994–1996). Starting in 1997 data are from the family core questionnaires.

Table 130 (page 1 of 4). Health insurance coverage for persons 65 years of age and over, according to type of coverage and selected characteristics: United States, selected years 1989–2001

[Data are based on household interviews of a sample of the civilian noninstitutionalized population]

Characteristic	Private insurance[1]						Private insurance obtained through workplace[1,2]					
	1989	1995	1998	1999	2000	2001	1989	1995	1998	1999	2000	2001
	Number in millions											
Total[3]	22.4	23.5	21.5	20.8	20.6	20.6	11.2	12.4	12.0	11.3	11.7	11.9
	Percent of population											
Total, age adjusted[3,4]	76.1	74.5	66.7	64.0	63.1	62.7	37.3	38.9	37.1	34.6	35.6	36.0
Total, crude[3]	76.5	74.6	66.7	64.1	63.1	62.7	38.4	39.5	37.3	34.9	35.8	36.1
Age												
65–74 years.	78.2	75.1	66.6	64.5	62.7	63.0	43.7	43.3	40.4	38.6	39.4	39.7
75 years and over	73.9	73.9	66.8	63.5	63.6	62.4	30.2	34.1	33.5	30.3	31.4	31.9
75–84 years	75.9	75.7	68.1	64.6	64.6	63.9	32.0	36.0	35.7	32.3	33.1	33.3
85 years and over	65.5	67.3	61.8	59.6	59.5	57.0	22.8	27.3	25.3	23.2	24.7	26.7
Sex[4]												
Male	77.4	76.6	68.5	64.5	64.3	63.8	42.1	43.3	41.4	38.6	39.7	40.1
Female	75.4	73.2	65.5	63.8	62.2	61.9	34.0	35.8	34.0	31.8	32.5	33.0
Race[4,5]												
White only	79.8	78.3	70.3	67.6	66.9	66.4	38.7	40.4	38.5	35.8	37.2	37.4
Black or African American only.	42.3	40.3	40.3	39.9	35.6	37.6	23.7	24.6	27.4	27.5	25.0	27.9
American Indian and Alaska Native only.	*	*	*37.9	*35.2	*	*31.8	*	*	*	*33.3	*	*
Asian only	#	#	40.8	33.1	43.3	40.9	#	#	28.3	21.4	23.2	23.5
Native Hawaiian and Other Pacific Islander only	- - -	- - -	- - -	*	*	*	- - -	- - -	- - -	*	*	*
2 or more races	- - -	- - -	- - -	56.0	63.1	50.0	- - -	- - -	- - -	*26.9	48.4	32.3
Hispanic origin and race[4,5]												
Hispanic or Latino	42.3	39.8	29.1	26.9	23.4	24.0	22.2	18.4	17.9	17.4	15.1	16.2
Mexican	33.5	31.8	26.5	27.4	20.3	24.8	20.2	15.9	17.5	16.9	12.8	16.8
Not Hispanic or Latino	77.2	76.2	68.7	66.2	65.5	65.2	37.7	39.9	38.2	35.7	36.8	37.2
White only	81.0	80.3	72.3	69.7	69.1	68.8	39.3	41.7	39.5	36.8	38.3	38.6
Black or African American only . . .	42.4	40.1	40.5	40.1	35.6	37.6	23.7	24.4	27.6	27.6	25.0	28.0
Percent of poverty level[4,6]												
Below 100 percent	46.1	40.0	32.8	28.3	29.9	27.8	11.6	13.8	10.2	8.8	10.8	11.9
100–149 percent	67.7	67.6	48.7	44.6	44.2	45.7	22.2	26.7	19.3	14.7	16.1	20.6
150–199 percent	81.1	76.0	65.6	62.0	63.1	63.1	39.0	38.7	31.4	27.2	29.8	28.1
200 percent or more	85.5	85.3	78.6	75.5	74.4	74.2	49.4	49.3	49.8	45.4	47.3	46.8
Geographic region[4]												
Northeast.	76.1	76.2	72.0	66.0	66.7	66.1	42.2	44.6	43.9	39.7	38.7	38.8
Midwest.	81.9	82.3	78.3	77.0	75.9	72.4	40.0	44.7	41.6	38.5	41.2	40.5
South	73.0	70.7	62.0	60.2	58.4	60.2	32.0	33.7	33.3	31.0	31.9	34.1
West.	74.7	68.8	54.9	51.5	51.5	51.7	37.1	33.6	30.9	30.6	31.7	30.6
Location of residence[4]												
Within MSA[7]	76.6	74.7	65.5	62.8	61.4	61.2	39.9	40.9	38.7	36.0	36.9	36.5
Outside MSA[7]	74.8	73.9	70.6	68.2	68.5	68.1	30.2	32.2	31.8	30.0	31.5	34.1

See footnotes at end of table.

Table 130 (page 2 of 4). **Health insurance coverage for persons 65 years of age and over, according to type of coverage and selected characteristics: United States, selected years 1989–2001**

[Data are based on household interviews of a sample of the civilian noninstitutionalized population]

Characteristic	Medicare fee-for-service only[1,8]						Medicare health maintenance organization[1,9]					
	1989	1995	1998	1999	2000	2001	1989	1995	1998	1999	2000	2001
	Number in millions											
Total[3]	4.5	4.6	4.7	5.1	5.5	5.9	- - -	- - -	4.7	5.2	5.0	4.2
	Percent of population											
Total, age adjusted[3,4]	15.7	14.8	14.5	15.8	16.8	17.9	- - -	- - -	14.4	16.0	15.2	12.9
Total, crude[3]	15.4	14.7	14.5	15.8	16.8	17.9	- - -	- - -	14.5	16.0	15.2	12.9
Age												
65–74 years	13.8	14.4	13.7	15.6	16.4	17.4	- - -	- - -	15.3	16.1	15.8	12.8
75 years and over	17.8	15.2	15.4	15.9	17.4	18.4	- - -	- - -	13.5	15.9	14.6	13.1
75–84 years	16.2	14.1	14.2	15.2	16.0	17.0	- - -	- - -	13.7	16.5	15.5	13.4
85 years and over	24.9	19.2	19.7	18.4	22.7	23.7	- - -	- - -	12.8	13.7	11.1	11.9
Sex[4]												
Male	14.9	14.3	13.2	15.4	16.1	17.4	- - -	- - -	14.7	16.5	15.6	12.5
Female	16.2	15.0	15.4	16.0	17.4	18.2	- - -	- - -	14.2	15.6	15.0	13.3
Race[4,5]												
White only	13.9	13.5	13.3	14.4	15.5	16.5	- - -	- - -	14.0	15.8	15.2	13.0
Black or African American only	34.9	29.0	26.7	28.0	29.6	30.5	- - -	- - -	17.6	16.5	14.7	11.2
American Indian and Alaska Native only	*	*	*26.6	*39.1	*	*37.9	- - -	- - -	*	*	*	*
Asian only	#	#	*12.6	22.0	21.4	19.8	- - -	- - -	17.0	18.9	16.0	13.4
Native Hawaiian and Other Pacific Islander only	- - -	- - -	- - -	*	*	*	- - -	- - -	- - -	*	*	*
2 or more races	- - -	- - -	- - -	*19.1	*	*21.7	- - -	- - -	- - -	*21.8	*29.8	*16.3
Hispanic origin and race[4,5]												
Hispanic or Latino	22.7	23.6	20.6	22.8	20.8	23.9	- - -	- - -	24.4	25.7	25.0	20.1
Mexican	#	#	21.5	26.3	22.7	29.3	- - -	- - -	23.3	26.0	24.5	18.9
Not Hispanic or Latino	15.5	14.3	14.2	15.3	16.6	17.5	- - -	- - -	13.9	15.4	14.6	12.5
White only	13.6	12.9	12.9	13.9	15.3	16.1	- - -	- - -	13.5	15.2	14.5	12.5
Black or African American only	34.9	29.1	26.7	28.0	29.6	30.5	- - -	- - -	17.5	16.5	14.7	11.2
Percent of poverty level[4,6]												
Below 100 percent	26.4	23.4	21.9	24.8	23.6	23.3	- - -	- - -	11.0	13.8	14.4	8.6
100–149 percent	20.7	18.6	22.2	23.1	22.0	24.5	- - -	- - -	16.6	17.7	17.0	12.5
150–199 percent	13.6	16.8	14.3	17.1	16.6	16.6	- - -	- - -	18.6	20.4	16.0	15.0
200 percent or more	11.0	10.8	8.0	10.3	11.4	11.5	- - -	- - -	15.2	15.7	16.7	14.5
Geographic region[4]												
Northeast	17.4	15.3	12.3	13.8	17.1	17.6	- - -	- - -	12.7	17.5	12.5	13.5
Midwest	13.8	11.0	12.9	11.7	13.5	16.1	- - -	- - -	7.7	9.0	8.4	7.5
South	16.6	15.9	17.5	20.3	19.6	19.7	- - -	- - -	12.5	12.2	13.2	10.2
West	14.4	17.2	13.7	14.9	15.7	17.3	- - -	- - -	28.2	31.0	30.6	23.8
Location of residence[4]												
Within MSA[7]	15.9	14.9	13.4	14.9	16.4	17.6	- - -	- - -	17.7	19.7	18.7	15.8
Outside MSA[7]	15.5	14.2	18.2	18.7	18.2	19.0	- - -	- - -	3.5	3.4	4.4	3.1

See footnotes at end of table.

Table 130 (page 3 of 4). Health insurance coverage for persons 65 years of age and over, according to type of coverage and selected characteristics: United States, selected years 1989–2001

[Data are based on household interviews of a sample of the civilian noninstitutionalized population]

Characteristic	Medicaid[1,10]					
	1989	1995	1998	1999	2000	2001
	Number in millions					
Total[3]	2.0	3.0	2.6	2.4	2.5	2.7
	Percent of population					
Total, age adjusted[3,4]	7.2	9.6	8.1	7.4	7.6	8.1
Total, crude[3]	7.0	9.4	8.1	7.3	7.6	8.1
Age						
65–74 years.................	6.3	8.4	7.8	6.6	7.7	7.8
75 years and over	8.2	10.9	8.4	8.1	7.5	8.5
75–84 years	7.9	9.9	7.8	7.2	7.2	8.1
85 years and over	9.7	14.3	10.5	11.4	8.6	10.3
Sex[4]						
Male	5.2	5.8	6.2	5.3	5.5	6.1
Female	8.6	12.2	9.5	8.8	9.2	9.7
Race[4,5]						
White only.................	5.6	7.4	6.4	5.6	5.6	6.2
Black or African American only.....	21.2	28.4	18.0	18.2	19.6	20.0
American Indian and Alaska Native only..................	*	*	*	*	*35.8	*
Asian only	#	#	33.4	28.2	21.3	23.7
Native Hawaiian and Other Pacific Islander only	- - -	- - -	- - -	*	*	*
2 or more races	- - -	- - -	- - -	*	*	*19.9
Hispanic origin and race[4,5]						
Hispanic or Latino	26.4	32.7	27.2	24.0	29.6	30.1
Mexican...................	#	#	29.0	17.5	28.1	25.6
Not Hispanic or Latino	6.6	8.5	7.1	6.4	6.3	6.8
White only	4.9	6.1	5.4	4.7	4.6	4.9
Black or African American only ...	21.1	28.5	18.0	18.1	19.5	20.0
Percent of poverty level[4,6]						
Below 100 percent	28.2	36.4	36.7	35.7	35.0	38.8
100–149 percent	9.0	12.8	14.1	15.3	16.2	18.6
150–199 percent	4.7	5.9	6.1	4.2	4.7	7.1
200 percent or more...........	2.4	2.4	3.5	2.9	2.8	3.1
Geographic region[4]						
Northeast..................	5.4	8.9	7.5	7.3	7.4	7.9
Midwest...................	3.7	5.8	4.9	5.7	4.5	5.1
South	9.7	11.8	9.6	8.2	9.4	9.3
West.....................	9.4	11.5	10.2	8.2	8.6	10.0
Location of residence[4]						
Within MSA[7]	6.5	8.9	8.0	6.9	7.2	8.1
Outside MSA[7]	8.8	11.7	8.4	8.8	9.0	8.3

See footnotes at end of table.

[Data are based on household interviews of a sample of the civilian noninstitutionalized population]

* Estimates are considered unreliable. Data preceded by an asterisk have a relative standard error of 20–30 percent. Data not shown have a relative standard error of greater than 30 percent.

Estimates calculated upon request.

- - - Data not available.

[1]Almost all persons 65 years of age and over are covered by Medicare also. In 2001, 90 percent of older persons with private insurance also had Medicare.

[2]Private insurance originally obtained through a present or former employer or union. Starting in 1997 also includes private insurance obtained through workplace, self-employed, or professional association.

[3]Includes all other races not shown separately and unknown poverty level.

[4]Estimates are for persons 65 years of age and older and are age adjusted to the year 2000 standard using two age groups: 65–74 years and 75 years and over. See Appendix II, Age adjustment.

[5]The race groups, white, black, American Indian and Alaska Native (AI/AN), Asian, Native Hawaiian and Other Pacific Islander, and 2 or more races, include persons of Hispanic and non-Hispanic origin. Persons of Hispanic origin may be of any race. Starting with data year 1999 race-specific estimates are tabulated according to 1997 Standards for Federal data on Race and Ethnicity and are not strictly comparable with estimates for earlier years. The five single race categories plus multiple race categories shown in the table conform to 1997 Standards. The 1999 and later race-specific estimates are for persons who reported only one racial group; the category "2 or more races'" includes persons who reported more than one racial group. Prior to data year 1999, data were tabulated according to 1977 Standards with four racial groups and the category "Asian only" included Native Hawaiian and Other Pacific Islander. Estimates for single race categories prior to 1999 included persons who reported one race or, if they reported more than one race, identified one race as best representing their race. The effect of the 1997 Standard on the 1999 estimates can be seen by comparing 1999 data tabulated according to the two Standards: Age-adjusted estimates based on the 1977 Standards of the percent with private health insurance are: 0.1 percentage points lower for the white group; 0.3 percentage points higher for the black group; and 1 percentage point higher for the Asian and Pacific Islander group than estimates based on the 1997 Standards. See Appendix II, Race.

[6]Missing family income data were imputed for 22–25 percent of the sample 65 years of age and over in 1994–96. Percent of poverty level was unknown for 29 percent of sample persons 65 or older in 1997, 34 percent in 1998, 38 percent in 1999, 39 percent in 2000, and 40 percent in 2001. See Appendix II, Family income; Poverty level.

[7]MSA is metropolitan statistical area.

[8]Medicare fee-for-service only includes persons who are not covered by private health insurance, Medicaid, or a Medicare health maintenance organization.

[9]Persons reporting Medicare coverage are considered to have HMO coverage if they responded yes when asked if they were under a Medicare managed care arrangement such as an HMO.

[10]Includes public assistance through 1996. Starting in 1997 includes State-sponsored health plans. In 2001 the age-adjusted percent of the population 65 years of age and over covered by Medicaid was 7.6 percent, and 0.5 percent were covered by State-sponsored health plans.

NOTES: In 1997 the National Health Interview Survey (NHIS) was redesigned, including changes to the questions on health insurance coverage. See Appendix I, National Health Interview Survey and Appendix II, Health insurance coverage. Percents do not add to 100 because elderly persons with more than one type of insurance in addition to Medicare appear in more than one column, and because the percent of elderly persons without health insurance (1.3 percent in 2001) is not shown. Data for additional years are available (see Appendix III).

SOURCES: Centers for Disease Control and Prevention, National Center for Health Statistics, National Health Interview Survey, health insurance supplements (1984, 1989, 1994–1996). Starting in 1997 data are from the family core questionnaires.

Table 131 (page 1 of 2). **Health maintenance organization (HMO) coverage among persons under 65 years of age by private insurance and Medicaid, according to selected characteristics: United States, 1998–2001**

[Data are based on household interviews of a sample of the civilian noninstitutionalized population]

Characteristic	Private[1] and Medicaid[2]				Private[1]				Medicaid[2]			
	1998	1999	2000	2001	1998	1999	2000	2001	1998	1999	2000	2001
	Number of persons in millions											
Total under age 65 years[3]............	83.2	85.5	82.2	78.0	72.3	74.6	71.3	68.0	10.7	10.6	10.8	9.8
	Percent of population											
Total under age 65 years[3]............	35.2	35.7	34.1	32.0	30.5	31.2	29.5	27.9	4.5	4.4	4.5	4.0
Age												
Under 18 years....................	39.4	39.7	37.5	35.4	30.1	30.4	28.4	27.1	9.4	9.3	9.3	8.5
Under 6 years	41.7	42.2	39.7	37.5	29.2	29.5	27.7	26.5	12.7	12.7	12.2	11.1
6–17 years..................	38.3	38.5	36.5	34.4	30.5	30.9	28.7	27.4	7.7	7.7	7.9	7.2
18–44 years	33.4	34.0	32.5	30.3	30.6	31.3	29.9	27.8	2.8	2.6	2.7	2.5
18–24 years.................	28.8	30.1	28.4	26.2	25.0	26.2	24.4	22.9	3.9	3.9	4.0	3.3
25–34 years.................	34.8	34.2	34.0	31.1	31.8	31.6	31.4	28.6	2.9	2.6	2.6	2.5
35–44 years.................	34.9	36.1	33.7	32.2	32.7	34.0	31.8	30.2	2.0	1.9	1.9	2.0
45–64 years	33.0	34.0	32.7	31.0	31.0	31.8	30.4	29.1	1.6	1.7	1.8	1.6
45–54 years.................	34.3	35.3	33.4	32.2	32.5	33.4	31.4	30.4	1.6	1.6	1.9	1.7
55–64 years.................	31.1	32.0	31.4	29.1	28.7	29.5	28.9	27.1	1.7	1.8	1.8	1.5
Sex												
Male...........................	34.2	35.0	33.1	31.3	30.4	31.1	29.3	27.8	3.7	3.7	3.8	3.4
Female.........................	36.1	36.5	35.0	32.7	30.7	31.2	29.8	28.0	5.3	5.2	5.1	4.6
Race[4]												
White only......................	33.9	34.6	33.0	30.8	30.6	31.4	29.7	27.8	3.2	3.1	3.2	2.9
Black or African American only	40.9	41.6	40.0	37.2	29.1	30.4	29.3	28.0	11.6	10.9	10.6	9.2
American Indian and Alaska Native only...	30.3	21.7	22.2	22.2	21.9	13.3	14.6	15.1	*8.2	*8.7	*7.0	*7.0
Asian only......................	41.6	40.7	39.6	37.5	37.5	36.6	36.3	33.7	4.0	*3.9	*3.2	*3.6
Native Hawaiian and Other Pacific Islander only	- - -	*	*	*	- - -	*	*	*	- - -	*	*	*
2 or more races..................	- - -	40.5	39.8	36.0	- - -	29.6	29.6	27.1	- - -	10.9	10.3	8.9
Hispanic origin and race[4]												
Hispanic or Latino	34.6	35.7	34.1	32.2	26.8	27.9	26.3	25.0	7.7	7.7	7.8	7.2
Mexican...................	31.6	32.6	31.6	30.5	24.9	25.7	24.2	23.0	6.6	6.9	7.5	7.4
Puerto Rican	44.8	46.1	44.0	42.0	27.9	29.3	29.2	29.5	16.2	16.5	14.8	12.1
Cuban.....................	42.0	44.3	40.3	41.4	36.5	41.3	35.3	37.3	*	*	*4.3	*4.0
Other Hispanic or Latino	35.3	38.9	35.7	31.5	28.4	31.8	29.9	26.6	6.9	7.0	5.9	4.9
Not Hispanic or Latino	35.2	35.7	34.1	32.0	31.1	31.7	30.0	28.4	4.1	4.0	4.0	3.6
White only	34.0	34.5	32.7	30.7	31.2	31.8	30.0	28.3	2.7	2.6	2.7	2.4
Black or African American only........	40.6	41.7	39.9	37.3	29.1	30.5	29.4	28.0	11.3	10.9	10.5	9.2
Percent of poverty level[5]												
Below 100 percent..................	32.4	31.2	31.0	28.2	9.3	9.9	10.0	8.9	22.9	21.1	21.0	19.3
100–149 percent	26.8	26.2	26.9	27.0	18.4	16.5	16.9	17.2	8.5	9.1	9.6	9.5
150–199 percent	30.7	30.4	31.3	28.1	27.3	25.3	25.8	23.4	3.2	5.0	5.6	4.9
200 percent or more................	38.9	39.8	37.9	35.7	38.1	38.9	37.1	35.0	0.8	0.8	0.8	0.7
Geographic region												
Northeast	44.4	46.6	44.7	42.8	39.7	42.2	40.8	39.7	4.8	4.4	3.9	3.1
Midwest	29.9	29.6	26.6	26.4	25.8	26.3	23.5	22.8	4.0	3.3	3.0	3.6
South	30.7	31.0	30.5	26.9	26.2	26.0	25.3	22.6	4.3	4.8	5.1	4.2
West...........................	40.7	41.2	39.4	37.3	35.4	35.7	33.8	32.1	5.1	5.3	5.5	5.1

See footnotes at end of table.

Table 131 (page 2 of 2). Health maintenance organization (HMO) coverage among persons under 65 years of age by private insurance and Medicaid, according to selected characteristics: United States, 1998–2001

[Data are based on household interviews of a sample of the civilian noninstitutionalized population]

Characteristic	Private[1] and Medicaid[2]				Private[1]				Medicaid[2]			
	1998	1999	2000	2001	1998	1999	2000	2001	1998	1999	2000	2001
Location of residence	Percent of population											
Within MSA[6]	38.4	39.2	36.9	34.8	33.7	34.7	32.5	30.8	4.5	4.3	4.3	4.0
Outside MSA[6]	22.9	22.3	22.4	20.6	18.4	17.4	17.2	16.3	4.5	5.0	5.1	4.2

- - - Data not available.

* Estimates are considered unreliable. Data preceded by an asterisk have a relative standard error of 20–30 percent. Data not shown have a relative standard error of greater than 30 percent.

[1]Persons reporting private health insurance coverage are considered to have health maintenance organization (HMO) coverage if they responded HMO or Individual Practice Association (IPA) when asked their plan type.

[2]Persons reporting Medicaid coverage are considered to have HMO coverage if they must choose from a book or list of doctors or the doctor is assigned or if they are required to sign up with a certain primary care doctor, group of doctors, or certain clinic for all routine care.

[3]Includes all other races not shown separately and unknown poverty level.

[4]The race groups, white, black, American Indian and Alaska Native (AI/AN), Asian, Native Hawaiian and Other Pacific Islander, and 2 or more races, include persons of Hispanic and non-Hispanic origin. Persons of Hispanic origin may be of any race. Starting with data year 1999 race-specific estimates are tabulated according to 1997 Standards for Federal data on Race and Ethnicity and are not strictly comparable with estimates for earlier years. The five single race categories plus multiple race categories shown in the table conform to 1997 Standards. The 1999 and later race-specific estimates are for persons who reported only one racial group; the category "2 or more races" includes persons who reported more than one racial group. Prior to data year 1999, data were tabulated according to 1977 Standards with four racial groups and the category "Asian only" included Native Hawaiian and Other Pacific Islander. Estimates for single race categories prior to 1999 included persons who reported one race or, if they reported more than one race, identified one race as best representing their race. The effect of the 1997 Standard on the 1999 estimates can be seen by comparing 1999 data tabulated according to the two Standards: Estimates based on the 1977 Standards of the percent with HMO coverage among those under 65 years are: identical for the white group; 0.1 percentage points higher for the black group; 0.4 percentage points higher for the Asian and Pacific Islander group; and 0.1 percentage points higher for the AI/AN group than estimates based on the 1997 Standards. See Appendix II, Race.

[5]Missing family income data were imputed for 15–17 percent of the sample under 65 years of age in 1994–96. Percent of poverty level was unknown for 19 percent of sample persons under 65 in 1997, 24 percent in 1998, 27 percent in 1999, and 26 percent in 2000 and 2001. See Appendix II, Family income; Poverty level.

[6]MSA is metropolitan statistical area.

SOURCE: Centers for Disease Control and Prevention, National Center for Health Statistics, National Health Interview Survey. Data are from the family core questionnaires.

Table 132. Health maintenance organizations (HMOs) and enrollment, according to model type, geographic region, and Federal program: United States, selected years 1976–2002

[Data are based on a census of health maintenance organizations]

Plans and enrollment	1976	1980	1990	1995	1997	1998	1999	2000	2001	2002
Plans					Number					
All plans	174	235	572	562	652	651	643	568	541	500
Model type:[1]										
Individual practice association[2]	41	97	360	332	284	317	309	278	257	229
Group[3]	122	138	212	108	98	116	123	101	104	100
Mixed	- - -	- - -	- - -	122	258	212	208	188	180	171
Geographic region:										
Northeast	29	55	115	100	110	107	110	98	96	87
Midwest	52	72	160	157	184	185	179	161	190	140
South	23	45	176	196	236	237	239	203	158	178
West	70	63	121	109	121	122	115	106	97	95
Enrollment[1]					Number of persons in millions					
Total	6.0	9.1	33.0	50.9	66.8	76.6	81.3	80.9	79.5	76.1
Model type:[1]										
Individual practice association[2]	0.4	1.7	13.7	20.1	26.7	32.6	32.8	33.4	33.1	31.6
Group[3]	5.6	7.4	19.3	13.3	11.0	13.8	15.9	15.2	15.6	15.0
Mixed	- - -	- - -	- - -	17.6	29.0	30.1	32.6	32.3	30.9	29.6
Federal program:[4]										
Medicaid[5]	- - -	0.3	1.2	3.5	5.6	7.8	10.4	10.8	11.4	12.8
Medicare	- - -	0.4	1.8	2.9	4.8	5.7	6.5	6.6	6.1	5.4
					Percent of HMO enrollees					
Model type:[1]										
Individual practice association[2]	6.6	18.7	41.6	39.4	39.9	42.6	40.3	41.3	41.6	41.5
Group[3]	93.4	81.3	58.4	26.0	16.5	18.0	19.6	18.9	19.5	19.4
Mixed	- - -	- - -	- - -	34.5	43.4	39.2	40.1	39.9	38.8	38.8
Federal program:[4]										
Medicaid[5]	- - -	2.9	3.5	6.9	8.2	10.2	12.7	13.3	14.3	16.9
Medicare	- - -	4.3	5.4	5.7	7.2	7.4	8.0	8.1	7.7	7.1
					Percent of population enrolled in HMOs					
Total	2.8	4.0	13.4	19.4	25.2	28.6	30.1	30.0	28.3	26.4
Geographic region:										
Northeast	2.0	3.1	14.6	24.4	32.4	37.8	36.7	36.5	35.1	33.4
Midwest	1.5	2.8	12.6	16.4	19.5	22.7	23.3	23.2	21.7	20.6
South	0.4	0.8	7.1	12.4	17.9	21.0	23.9	22.6	21.0	19.8
West	9.7	12.2	23.2	28.6	36.4	39.1	41.4	41.7	40.7	38.2

- - - Data not available.

[1] Enrollment or number of plans may not equal total because some plans did not report these characteristics.

[2] An HMO operating under an individual practice association model contracts with an association of physicians from various settings (a mixture of solo and group practices) to provide health services.

[3] Group includes staff, group, and network model types. See Appendix II, Health maintenance organization.

[4] Federal program enrollment in HMOs refers to enrollment by Medicaid or Medicare beneficiaries, where the Medicaid or Medicare program contracts directly with the HMO to pay the appropriate annual premium.

[5] Data for 1990 and later include enrollment in managed care health insuring organizations.

NOTES: Data as of June 30 in 1976–80, and January 1 from 1990 onwards. Open-ended enrollment in HMO plans, amounting to 8 million on Jan. 1, 2002, is included from 1994 onwards. See Appendix II, Health maintenance organization. HMOs in Guam are included starting in 1994; HMOs in Puerto Rico, starting in 1998. In 2002 HMO enrollment in Guam was 34,000 and in Puerto Rico, 1,825,000. Data for additional years are available (see Appendix III).

SOURCES: The InterStudy Edge, 1990, vol. 2; Competitive Edge, vols. 1–12, 1991–2002; Excelsior, Minnesota (Copyrights 1985–2002: Used with the permission of InterStudy); Office of Health Maintenance Organizations: Summary of the National HMO census of prepaid plans—June 1976 and National HMO Census 1980. Public Health Service. Washington. U.S. Government Printing Office. DHHS Pub. No. (PHS) 80–50159; InterStudy: National HMO Census: Annual Report on the Growth of HMOs in the U.S., 1984–1985 Editions; Population estimates used for calculations from the U.S. Bureau of the Census at www.census.gov.

Table 133 (page 1 of 2). Medical care benefits for employees of private establishments by size of establishment and occupation: United States, selected years 1990–97

[Data are based on a survey of employers]

Size of establishment and type of benefit	All			Professional, technical, and related			Clerical and sales			Blue-collar and service		
	1990	1994	1996	1990	1994	1996	1990	1994	1996	1990	1994	1996
Small private establishments[1]	Percent of all employees											
Participation in medical care benefit:												
Full-time employees	69	66	64	82	80	76	75	70	69	60	57	56
Part-time employees	6	7	6	6	11	14	7	9	9	6	5	3
Type of medical care benefit among participating full-time employees	Percent of participating full-time employees											
Fee arrangement	100	100	100	100	100	100	100	100	100	100	100	100
Traditional fee-for-service	74	55	36	69	53	31	77	55	34	73	57	41
Preferred provider organization (PPO)	13	24	35	16	27	41	13	24	36	11	23	32
Health maintenance organization (HMO)	14	19	27	15	20	27	10	19	28	15	20	25
Other	0	1	2	0	0	1	0	2	2	0	0	2
Individual coverage:												
Employee contributions not required	58	47	48	56	49	49	53	44	46	62	48	48
Employee contributions required	42	53	52	44	51	51	47	56	54	38	52	51
Family coverage:												
Employee contributions not required	32	19	24	28	17	21	29	15	20	37	23	29
Employee contributions required	68	81	75	72	83	78	71	85	80	63	77	70
	Average monthly contribution											
Individual coverage:												
Average monthly employee contribution:												
Total	$ 25	$ 41	$ 43	$ 24	$ 47	$ 41	$ 24	$ 41	$ 42	$ 27	$ 38	$ 44
Non-HMO	25	39	43	24	46	40	24	38	43	28	36	45
HMO	25	49	41	24	48	42	27	50	42	25	47	41
Family coverage:												
Average monthly employee contribution:												
Total	109	160	182	112	181	190	106	160	181	111	149	177
Non-HMO	104	151	181	110	173	192	102	155	181	101	137	175
HMO	135	190	182	118	204	183	134	178	183	145	191	182

See footnotes at end of table.

Table 133 (page 2 of 2). Medical care benefits for employees of private establishments by size of establishment and occupation: United States, selected years 1990–97

[Data are based on a survey of employers]

Size of establishment and type of benefit	All			Professional, technical, and related			Clerical and sales			Blue-collar and service		
	1991	1995	1997	1991	1995	1997	1991	1995	1997	1991	1995	1997
Medium and large private establishments[2]	Percent of all employees											
Participation in medical care benefit:												
Full-time employees.................	83	77	76	85	80	79	81	76	78	84	75	74
Part-time employees	28	19	21	42	31	29	26	20	20	26	15	19
Type of medical care benefit among participating full-time employees	Percent of participating full-time employees											
Fee arrangement	100	100	100	100	100	100	100	100	100	100	100	100
Traditional fee-for-service	67	37	27	62	29	20	59	30	22	73	45	33
Preferred provider organization (PPO)	16	34	40	19	36	40	21	36	42	12	33	39
Health maintenance organization (HMO) ...	17	27	33	18	33	40	19	32	36	14	21	28
Other	0	1	1	1	1	0	0	2	0	0	1	0
Individual coverage:												
Employee contributions not required	49	33	31	45	21	20	43	24	24	55	44	40
Employee contributions required	51	67	69	55	79	80	57	76	76	45	56	60
Family coverage:												
Employee contributions not required	31	22	20	25	11	10	27	15	14	37	33	29
Employee contributions required	69	78	80	75	89	90	73	85	86	63	67	71
	Average monthly contribution											
Individual coverage:												
Average monthly employee contribution:												
Total	$ 27	$ 34	$ 39	$ 26	$ 35	$ 37	$ 28	$ 36	$ 39	$ 26	$ 32	$ 40
Non-HMO	26	33	42	26	33	40	27	34	41	25	32	43
HMO...........................	29	36	34	29	38	33	32	39	36	28	32	34
Family coverage:												
Average monthly employee contribution:												
Total	97	118	130	96	120	125	108	127	135	91	112	131
Non-HMO	92	112	132	93	116	128	104	120	134	84	106	134
HMO...........................	118	133	126	110	128	120	121	141	138	122	130	124

[1]Less than 100 employees in all private nonfarm industries.
[2]100 or more employees in all private nonfarm industries.

NOTE: In 1992–93, 88 percent of full-time employees in private establishments were offered health care plans by their employers (96 percent in medium and large private establishments and 80 percent in small private establishments). In 1999 the National Compensation Survey was redesigned. Starting in 1999, only participation rates in medical care benefits for full-time and part-time employees are available for this table, but not details on type of coverage or employee contributions. In 2000 in medium and large private establishments, the participation rate in health benefits was 67 percent for full-time employees and 28 percent for part-time employees; in small private establishments, 56 percent of full-time and 6 percent of part-time employees received health benefits through their employers.

SOURCES: U.S. Department of Labor, Bureau of Labor Statistics, National Compensation Survey; Employee benefits in small private establishments, 1990 Bulletin 2388, September 1991, 1994 Bulletin 2475, April 1996, and 1996 Bulletin 2507, April 1999. Employee benefits in medium and large private establishments, 1991 Bulletin 2422, May 1993, 1997 Bulletin 2517, Sept. 1999, and news release USDL 97–246. July 25, 1997. Blostin AP and Pfuntner JN. Employee medical care contributions on the rise. Compensation and Working Conditions, Spring 1998.

Table 134 (page 1 of 2). Medicare enrollees and expenditures and percent distribution, according to type of service: United States and other areas, selected years 1970–2001

[Data are compiled from various sources by the Centers for Medicare & Medicaid Services]

Type of service	1970	1980	1990	1995	1997	1998	1999	2000	2001[1]
Enrollees				Number in millions					
Total[2]	20.4	28.4	34.3	37.6	38.5	38.9	39.2	39.7	40.0
Hospital insurance	20.1	28.0	33.7	37.2	38.1	38.5	38.8	39.3	39.6
Supplementary medical insurance	19.5	27.3	32.6	35.6	36.4	36.8	37.0	37.3	37.6
Expenditures				Amount in billions					
Total	$ 7.5	$ 36.8	$111.0	$184.2	$213.6	$213.4	$212.9	$221.8	$244.8
Total hospital insurance (HI)	5.3	25.6	67.0	117.6	139.5	135.8	130.6	131.1	143.4
HI payments to managed care organizations[3]	- - -	0.0	2.7	6.7	16.3	19.0	20.9	21.4	20.8
HI payments for fee-for-service utilization	5.3	25.6	64.3	110.9	123.1	116.8	109.8	109.7	122.6
Inpatient hospital	4.8	24.1	56.9	82.3	89.2	87.4	86.5	87.3	95.6
Skilled nursing facility	0.2	0.4	2.5	9.1	12.5	13.1	10.9	10.9	13.4
Home health agency	0.1	0.5	3.7	16.2	17.5	11.6	7.3	3.9	4.2
Home health agency transfer[4]	- - -	- - -	- - -	- - -	- - -	0.5	0.6	1.7	3.1
Hospice	- - -	- - -	0.3	1.9	2.1	2.2	2.6	3.0	3.7
Administrative expenses[5]	0.2	0.5	0.9	1.4	1.9	2.0	2.0	2.9	2.5
Total supplementary medical insurance (SMI)	2.2	11.2	44.0	66.6	74.1	77.6	82.3	90.7	101.4
SMI payments to managed care organizations[3]	0.0	0.2	2.8	6.6	11.0	15.3	17.7	18.4	17.6
SMI payments for fee-for-service utilization[6]	2.2	11.0	41.2	60.0	63.2	62.3	64.6	72.3	83.8
Physician/supplies[7]	1.8	8.2	29.6	- - -	- - -	- - -	- - -	- - -	- - -
Outpatient hospital[8]	0.1	1.9	8.5	- - -	- - -	- - -	- - -	- - -	- - -
Independent laboratory[9]	0.0	0.1	1.5	- - -	- - -	- - -	- - -	- - -	- - -
Physician fee schedule	- - -	- - -	- - -	31.7	31.9	32.4	33.4	37.0	42.0
Durable medical equipment	- - -	- - -	- - -	3.7	4.2	4.0	4.3	4.7	5.4
Laboratory[10]	- - -	- - -	- - -	4.3	3.9	3.6	3.8	4.0	4.5
Other[11]	- - -	- - -	- - -	9.9	12.2	12.3	12.2	13.7	16.9
Hospital[12]	- - -	- - -	- - -	8.7	9.4	8.7	8.8	8.5	11.9
Home health agency	0.0	0.2	0.1	0.2	0.2	0.2	1.2	4.4	4.3
Home health agency transfer[4]	- - -	- - -	- - -	- - -	- - -	-0.5	-0.6	-1.7	-3.1
Administrative expenses[5]	0.2	0.6	1.5	1.6	1.4	1.5	1.6	1.8	1.7
				Percent distribution of expenditures					
Total hospital insurance (HI)	100.0	100.0	100.0	100.0	100.0	100.0	100.0	100.0	100.0
HI payments to managed care organizations[3]	- - -	0.0	4.0	5.7	11.7	14.0	16.0	16.3	14.5
HI payments for fee-for-service utilization	100.0	100.0	96.0	94.3	88.2	86.0	84.1	83.7	85.5
Inpatient hospital	90.6	94.1	84.9	70.0	63.9	64.4	66.2	66.6	66.7
Skilled nursing facility	3.8	1.6	3.7	7.8	9.0	9.6	8.3	8.3	9.3
Home health agency	1.9	2.0	5.5	13.8	12.5	8.5	5.5	3.0	2.9
Home health agency transfer[4]	- - -	- - -	- - -	- - -	- - -	0.4	0.5	1.3	2.2
Hospice	- - -	- - -	0.4	1.6	1.5	1.6	2.0	2.3	2.6
Administrative expenses[5]	3.8	2.0	1.3	1.2	1.4	1.5	1.5	2.2	1.7

See footnotes at end of table.

Table 134 (page 2 of 2). Medicare enrollees and expenditures and percent distribution, according to type of service: United States and other areas, selected years 1970–2001

[Data are compiled from various sources by the Centers for Medicare & Medicaid Services]

Type of service	1970	1980	1990	1995	1997	1998	1999	2000	2001[1]
				Percent distribution of expenditures					
Total supplementary medical insurance (SMI)....	100.0	100.0	100.0	100.0	100.0	100.0	100.0	100.0	100.0
SMI payments to managed care organizations[3].	0.0	1.8	6.4	9.9	14.8	19.7	21.5	20.3	17.4
SMI payments for fee-for-service utilization[6] ...	100.0	98.2	93.6	90.1	85.3	80.3	78.5	79.7	82.6
Physician/supplies[7]...................	81.8	73.2	67.3	- - -	- - -	- - -	- - -	- - -	- - -
Outpatient hospital[8]...................	4.5	17.0	19.3	- - -	- - -	- - -	- - -	- - -	- - -
Independent laboratory[9]................	0.0	0.9	3.4	- - -	- - -	- - -	- - -	- - -	- - -
Physician fee schedule	- - -	- - -	- - -	47.6	43.0	41.8	40.6	40.8	41.4
Durable medical equipment	- - -	- - -	- - -	5.6	5.7	5.2	5.2	5.2	5.3
Laboratory[10].........................	- - -	- - -	- - -	6.5	5.3	4.6	4.6	4.4	4.4
Other[11].............................	- - -	- - -	- - -	14.9	16.5	15.9	14.8	15.1	16.7
Hospital[12]..........................	- - -	- - -	- - -	13.0	12.7	11.2	10.7	9.4	11.7
Home health agency	0.0	1.8	0.2	0.3	0.3	0.3	1.5	4.9	4.2
Home health agency transfer[4]	- - -	- - -	- - -	- - -	- - -	−0.6	−0.7	−1.9	−3.1
Administrative expenses[5]..............	9.1	5.4	3.4	2.4	1.9	1.9	1.9	2.0	1.7

- - - Data not available.

0.0 Quantity greater than 0 but less than 0.05.

[1]Preliminary figures.

[2]Average number enrolled in the hospital insurance (HI) and/or supplementary medical insurance (SMI) programs for the period. See Appendix II, Medicare.

[3]Medicare-approved managed care organizations.

[4]Reflects annual home health HI to SMI transfer amounts for 1998 and later.

[5]Includes research, costs of experiments and demonstration projects, and peer review activity.

[6]Type of service reporting categories for fee-for-service reimbursement differ before and after 1991.

[7]Includes payment for physicians, practitioners, durable medical equipment, and all suppliers other than Independent laboratory, which is shown separately through 1990. Beginning in 1991, those physician services subject to the Physician fee schedule are so broken out. Payments for laboratory services paid under the Laboratory fee schedule and performed in a physician office are included under "Laboratory" beginning in 1991. Payments for durable medical equipment are broken out and so labeled beginning in 1991. The remaining services from the "Physician" category are included in "Other."

[8]Includes payments for hospital outpatient department services, for skilled nursing facility outpatient services, for Part B services received as an inpatient in a hospital or skilled nursing facility setting, and for other types of outpatient facilities. Beginning 1991, payments for hospital outpatient department services, except for laboratory services, are listed under "Hospital." Hospital outpatient laboratory services are included in the "Laboratory" line.

[9]Beginning in 1991 those independent laboratory services that were paid under the Laboratory fee schedule (most of independent lab) are included in the "Laboratory" line; the remaining services are included in "Physician fee schedule" and "Other" lines.

[10]Payments for laboratory services paid under the Laboratory fee schedule performed in a physician office, independent lab, or in a hospital outpatient department.

[11]Includes payments for physician-administered drugs, free-standing ambulatory surgical center facility services; ambulance services; supplies; free-standing end-stage renal disease (ESRD) dialysis facility services; rural health clinics; outpatient rehabilitation facilities; psychiatric hospitals; and federally qualified health centers.

[12]Includes the hospital facility costs for Medicare Part B services that are predominantly in the outpatient department, with the exception of hospital outpatient laboratory services, which are included on the "Laboratory" line. The physician reimbursement is included on the "Physician fee schedule" line.

NOTES: Table includes service disbursements as of January 2003 for Medicare enrollees residing in Puerto Rico, Virgin Islands, Guam, other outlying areas, foreign countries, and unknown residence. Totals do not necessarily equal the sum of rounded components. Some numbers in this table have been revised and differ from previous editions of *Health, United States*. Data for additional years are available (see Appendix III).

SOURCE: Centers for Medicare & Medicaid Services, Office of the Actuary, Medicare and Medicaid Cost Estimates Group, Medicare Administrative Data.

Table 135. Medicare enrollees and program payments among fee-for-service Medicare beneficiaries, according to sex and age: United States and other areas, 1994–2000

[Data are compiled from administrative data by the Centers for Medicare & Medicaid Services]

Sex and age	1994	1995	1996	1997	1998	1999	2000
	Fee-for-service enrollees in thousands						
Total.	34,076	34,062	33,704	33,009	32,349	32,179	32,740
Sex							
Male.	14,533	14,563	14,440	14,149	13,902	13,872	14,195
Female.	19,543	19,499	19,264	18,860	18,477	18,307	18,545
Age							
Under 65 years	4,031	4,239	4,413	4,498	4,617	4,742	4,907
65–74 years	16,713	16,373	15,810	15,099	14,433	14,072	14,230
75–84 years	9,845	9,911	9,915	9,847	9,722	9,748	9,919
85 years and over	3,486	3,540	3,566	3,565	3,577	3,618	3,684
	Fee-for-service program payments in millions						
Total.	$146,549	$158,980	$167,063 `	$175,423	$168,164	$166,687	$174,261
Sex							
Male.	63,907	68,758	71,011	75,357	72,883	73,171	76,230
Female.	82,642	90,222	95,052	100,066	95,281	93,516	98,031
Age							
Under 65 years	18,835	21,029	24,160	25,798	23,746	24,262	25,773
65–74 years	55,147	58,093	58,737	59,067	57,342	56,031	57,494
75–84 years	50,719	55,256	58,058	61,708	59,745	59,518	62,685
85 years and over	21,847	24,602	26,108	28,231	27,331	26,875	28,309
	Percent distribution of fee-for-service program payments						
Total.	100.0	100.0	100.0	100.0	100.0	100.0	100.0
Sex							
Male.	43.6	43.2	42.5	43.0	43.3	43.9	43.7
Female.	56.4	56.8	56.9	57.0	56.7	56.1	56.3
Age							
Under 65 years	12.9	13.2	14.5	14.7	14.1	14.6	14.8
65–74 years	37.6	36.5	35.2	34.0	34.1	33.6	33.0
75–84 years	34.6	34.8	34.8	35.2	35.5	35.7	36.0
85 years and over	14.9	15.5	15.6	16.1	16.3	16.1	16.2
	Average fee-for-service payment per enrollee						
Total.	$ 4,301	$ 4,667	$ 4,957	$ 5,314	$ 5,198	$ 5,180	$ 5,323
Sex							
Male.	4,397	4,721	4,918	5,326	5,243	5,275	5,370
Female.	4,229	4,627	4,934	5,306	5,165	5,108	5,286
Age							
Under 65 years	4,673	4,960	5,475	5,735	5,143	5,117	5,252
65–74 years	3,300	3,548	3,715	3,953	3,973	3,982	4,040
75–84 years	5,152	5,576	5,856	6,267	6,145	6,106	6,320
85 years and over	6,267	6,950	7,321	7,919	7,641	7,428	7,684

NOTES: Table includes data for Medicare enrollees residing in Puerto Rico, Virgin Islands, Guam, other outlying areas, foreign countries, and unknown residence. Some 1999 numbers in this table have been revised and differ from the previous edition of *Health, United States*.

SOURCE: Centers for Medicare & Medicaid Services, Office of Research, Development, and Information. Health Care Financing Review: Medicare and Medicaid Statistical Supplements for years 1996 to 2002. Website: www.cms.hhs.gov/review/supp/.

Table 136 (page 1 of 2). Medicare beneficiaries by race and ethnicity, according to selected characteristics: United States, 1992 and 1999

[Data are based on household interviews of a sample of current Medicare beneficiaries and Medicare administrative records]

	All		Not Hispanic or Latino — White		Not Hispanic or Latino — Black or African American		Hispanic or Latino	
Characteristic	1992	1999	1992	1999	1992	1999	1992	1999
	Number of beneficiaries in millions							
All Medicare beneficiaries	36.8	40.4	30.9	32.4	3.3	3.6	1.9	2.8
	Percent distribution of beneficiaries							
All Medicare beneficiaries	100.0	100.0	84.2	80.6	8.9	8.9	5.2	6.9
Medical care use	Percent of beneficiaries with at least one service							
All Medicare beneficiaries:								
Long-term care facility stay . . .	7.7	9.2	8.0	9.8	6.2	9.0	4.2	4.4
Community-only residents:								
Inpatient hospital	17.9	19.4	18.1	19.5	18.4	22.3	16.6	16.9
Outpatient hospital	57.9	68.5	57.8	69.2	61.1	69.9	53.1	61.8
Physician/supplier[1]	92.4	94.6	93.0	95.5	89.1	91.1	87.9	89.8
Dental	40.4	43.4	43.1	47.1	23.5	23.5	29.1	32.3
Prescription medicine	85.2	89.8	85.5	90.2	83.1	88.4	84.6	89.0
Expenditures[2]	Expenditures per beneficiary							
All Medicare beneficiaries:								
Total	$6,716	$9,593	$6,816	$9,705	$7,043	$11,176	$5,784	$7,536
Long-term care facility	1,581	2,128	1,674	2,276	1,255	2,188	*758	887
Community-only residents:								
Total personal health care	5,054	7,228	4,988	7,222	5,530	8,633	4,938	6,400
Inpatient hospital	2,098	2,528	2,058	2,528	2,493	3,262	1,999	2,048
Outpatient hospital	504	859	478	800	668	1,396	511	834
Physician/supplier[1]	1,524	2,180	1,525	2,197	1,398	2,286	1,587	2,100
Dental	142	252	153	276	70	121	97	171
Prescription medicine	468	983	481	1,004	417	951	389	878
Long-term care facility residents only:								
Long-term care facility	23,054	29,889	23,177	30,072	21,272	30,234	*25,026	*25,601
Sex	Percent distribution of beneficiaries							
Both sexes	100.0	100.0	100.0	100.0	100.0	100.0	100.0	100.0
Male	42.9	43.7	42.7	43.5	42.0	40.7	46.7	47.4
Female	57.1	56.3	57.3	56.5	58.0	59.3	53.3	52.6
Eligibility criteria and age								
All Medicare beneficiaries[3]	100.0	100.0	100.0	100.0	100.0	100.0	100.0	100.0
Disabled	10.2	13.3	8.6	11.3	19.1	23.5	16.5	20.3
Under 45 years	3.5	3.8	2.9	3.2	7.6	7.9	6.9	5.2
45–64 years	6.5	9.5	5.8	8.1	11.5	15.6	9.6	15.1
Aged	89.8	86.8	91.4	88.7	81.0	76.6	83.5	79.7
65–74 years	51.5	45.9	52.0	45.7	48.0	43.3	49.4	48.2
75–84 years	28.8	29.9	29.5	31.6	24.0	23.6	27.1	22.6
85 years and over	9.7	10.9	9.9	11.4	9.0	9.7	6.9	8.9
Living arrangement								
All living arrangements	100.0	100.0	100.0	100.0	100.0	100.0	100.0	100.0
Alone	27.0	29.4	27.5	30.0	27.7	31.8	20.2	22.6
With spouse	51.2	49.3	53.3	51.2	33.3	31.6	50.4	48.5
With children	9.1	9.3	7.7	7.5	16.8	17.8	16.6	16.3
With others	7.6	7.3	6.2	6.4	18.1	13.4	10.8	10.7
Long-term care facility	5.1	4.8	5.3	5.0	4.0	5.4	*2.0	*1.9

See footnotes at end of table.

Table 136 (page 2 of 2). Medicare beneficiaries by race and ethnicity, according to selected characteristics: United States, 1992 and 1999

[Data are based on household interviews of a sample of current Medicare beneficiaries and Medicare administrative records]

| | | | | | Not Hispanic or Latino | | | |
| | All | | White | | Black or African American | | Hispanic or Latino | |
Characteristic	1992	1999	1992	1999	1992	1999	1992	1999
Age and limitation of activity[4]				Percent distribution of beneficiaries				
Disabled	100.0	100.0	100.0	100.0	100.0	100.0	100.0	100.0
None	22.7	29.2	21.8	27.9	26.2	39.9	21.2	23.6
IADL only	39.0	35.3	38.9	36.4	35.8	32.0	46.1	36.4
1 or 2 ADL	21.2	21.2	21.5	20.9	21.2	18.8	*20.9	*23.7
3–5 ADL	17.2	14.3	17.9	14.9	*16.8	*9.3	*11.9	*16.3
65–74 years	100.0	100.0	100.0	100.0	100.0	100.0	100.0	100.0
None	67.0	71.3	68.7	72.9	55.1	59.6	59.2	68.9
IADL only	17.8	15.7	17.0	15.2	22.9	20.4	*20.9	16.1
1 or 2 ADL	10.4	8.7	9.6	8.2	14.4	11.8	*15.7	*10.6
3–5 ADL	4.8	4.4	4.6	3.7	*7.6	*8.2	*4.2	*4.3
75–84 years	100.0	100.0	100.0	100.0	100.0	100.0	100.0	100.0
None	46.6	52.9	47.5	53.7	42.0	46.9	44.3	50.2
IADL only	23.9	21.3	23.6	21.1	26.7	19.8	*27.8	26.6
1 or 2 ADL	16.5	14.7	16.8	14.5	15.3	16.7	*14.9	*12.4
3–5 ADL	13.0	11.1	12.2	10.7	*15.9	16.6	*13.0	*10.8
85 years and over	100.0	100.0	100.0	100.0	100.0	100.0	100.0	100.0
None	19.9	24.5	20.2	25.0	*19.6	*21.6	*19.7	*23.2
IADL only	20.9	21.5	20.2	21.1	*22.1	*22.3	*24.7	*26.2
1 or 2 ADL	23.5	21.6	23.5	22.5	*24.3	*14.7	*23.7	*23.6
3–5 ADL	35.8	32.3	36.1	31.5	*34.0	41.5	*31.8	*27.0

* Estimates are considered unreliable. Cell is based on 50 persons or fewer or the estimate has a relative standard error of 30 percent or higher.
[1]Physician/supplier services include medical and osteopathic doctor and health practitioner visits; diagnostic laboratory and radiology services; medical and surgical services; durable medical equipment and nondurable medical supplies.
[2]Total health care expenditures by Medicare beneficiaries, including expenses paid by Medicare and all other sources of payment for the following services: inpatient hospital, outpatient hospital, physician/supplier, dental, prescription medicine, home health and hospice care. Does not include health insurance premiums.
[3]Medicare beneficiaries with end-stage renal disease (ESRD) are included within the subgroups "Aged" and "Disabled".
[4]See Appendix II for definitions of Activities of Daily Living (ADL) and Instrumental Activities of Daily Living (IADL). Includes data for both community and long-term care facility residents.

NOTE: Data for additional years are available (see Appendix III).

SOURCE: Centers for Medicare & Medicaid Services, Medicare Current Beneficiary Survey, Health and Health Care of the Medicare Population; www.cms.hhs.gov/mcbs.

Table 137. Medicaid recipients and medical vendor payments, according to basis of eligibility, and race and ethnicity: United States, selected fiscal years 1972–2000

[Data are compiled by the Centers for Medicare & Medicaid Services from the Medicaid Data System]

Basis of eligibility and race and ethnicity	1972	1980	1990	1995	1996	1997	1998[1]	1999[2]	2000
Recipients					Number in millions				
All recipients	17.6	21.6	25.3	36.3	36.1	34.9	40.6	40.1	42.8
					Percent of recipients				
Basis of eligibility:[3]									
Aged (65 years and over)	18.8	15.9	12.7	11.4	11.9	11.3	9.8	9.4	8.7
Blind and disabled	9.8	13.5	14.7	16.1	17.2	17.6	16.3	16.7	16.1
Adults in families with dependent children[4]	17.8	22.6	23.8	21.0	19.7	19.5	19.5	18.7	20.5
Children under age 21[5]	44.5	43.2	44.4	47.3	46.3	45.3	46.7	46.9	46.1
Other Title XIX[6]	9.0	6.9	3.9	1.7	1.8	6.3	7.8	8.4	8.6
Race and ethnicity:[7]									
White	- - -	- - -	42.8	45.5	44.8	44.4	41.3	- - -	- - -
Black or African American	- - -	- - -	25.1	24.7	23.9	23.5	24.2	- - -	- - -
American Indian or Alaska Native	- - -	- - -	1.0	0.8	0.8	1.0	0.8	- - -	- - -
Asian or Pacific Islander	- - -	- - -	2.0	2.2	2.1	1.9	2.5	- - -	- - -
Hispanic or Latino	- - -	- - -	15.2	17.2	17.5	14.3	15.6	- - -	- - -
Unknown	- - -	- - -	14.0	9.6	10.9	14.9	15.5	- - -	- - -
Vendor payments[8]					Amount in billions				
All payments	$ 6.3	$ 23.3	$ 64.9	$120.1	$121.7	$124.4	$ 142.3	$ 153.5	$ 168.3
					Percent distribution				
Total	100.0	100.0	100.0	100.0	100.0	100.0	100.0	100.0	100.0
Basis of eligibility:									
Aged (65 years and over)	30.6	37.5	33.2	30.4	30.4	30.3	28.5	27.7	26.4
Blind and disabled	22.2	32.7	37.6	41.1	42.8	43.5	42.4	42.9	43.2
Adults in families with dependent children[4]	15.3	13.9	13.2	11.2	10.1	9.9	10.4	10.3	10.6
Children under age 21[5]	18.1	13.4	14.0	15.0	14.4	14.1	16.0	15.7	15.9
Other Title XIX[6]	13.9	2.6 ·	1.6	1.2	1.2	2.2	2.6	3.4	3.9
Race and ethnicity:[7]									
White	- - -	- - -	53.4	54.3	54.1	55.0	54.3	- - -	- - -
Black or African American	- - -	- - -	18.3	19.2	18.7	18.5	19.6	- - -	- - -
American Indian or Alaska Native	- - -	- - -	0.6	0.5	0.6	0.6	0.8	- - -	- - -
Asian or Pacific Islander	- - -	- - -	1.0	1.2	1.1	0.9	1.4	- - -	- - -
Hispanic or Latino	- - -	- - -	5.3	7.3	7.4	6.8	8.2	- - -	- - -
Unknown	- - -	- - -	21.3	17.6	18.1	18.2	15.7	- - -	- - -
Vendor payments per recipient[8]					Amount				
All recipients	$ 358	$1,079	$2,568	$3,311	$3,369	$3,568	$ 3,501	$ 3,819	$ 3,936
Basis of eligibility:									
Aged (65 years and over)	580	2,540	6,717	8,868	8,622	9,538	10,242	11,268	11,929
Blind and disabled	807	2,618	6,564	8,435	8,369	8,832	9,095	9,832	10,559
Adults in families with dependent children[4]	307	662	1,429	1,777	1,722	1,809	1,876	2,104	2,030
Children under age 21[5]	145	335	811	1,047	1,048	1,111	1,203	1,282	1,358
Other Title XIX[6]	555	398	1,062	2,380	2,152	1,242	1,166	1,532	1,778
Race and ethnicity:[7]									
White	- - -	- - -	3,207	3,953	4,074	4,421	4,609	- - -	- - -
Black or African American	- - -	- - -	1,878	2,568	2,631	2,798	2,836	- - -	- - -
American Indian or Alaska Native	- - -	- - -	1,706	2,142	2,298	2,500	3,297	- - -	- - -
Asian or Pacific Islander	- - -	- - -	1,257	1,713	1,767	1,610	1,924	- - -	- - -
Hispanic or Latino	- - -	- - -	903	1,400	1,428	1,699	1,842	- - -	- - -
Unknown	- - -	- - -	3,909	6,099	5,603	4,356	3,531	- - -	- - -

- - - Data not available.

[1]Prior to 1998 recipient counts exclude those individuals who only received coverage under prepaid health care and for whom no direct vendor payments were made during the year. Prior to 1998 vendor payments exclude payments to health maintenance organizations and other prepaid health plans ($19.3 billion in 1998 and $18 billion in 1997). The total number of persons who were Medicaid eligible and enrolled was 41.4 million in 1998, 41.6 million in 1997, and 41.2 million in 1996 (HCFA Medicaid Statistics, Program and Financial Statistics FY1996, FY1997, and FY1998, unpublished).
[2]Starting in 1999, the Medicaid data system was changed (see Appendix I, Medicaid Data System).
[3]In 1980 and 1985 recipients included in more than one category. In 1990–96, 0.2–2.5 percent of recipients have unknown basis of eligibility. From 1997 onwards, unknowns are included in Other Title XIX.
[4]Includes adults in the Aid to Families with Dependent Children (AFDC) program. From 1997 onwards includes adults in the Temporary Assistance for Needy Families (TANF) program.
[5]Includes children in the AFDC program. From 1997 onwards includes children and foster care children in the TANF program.
[6]Includes some participants in the Supplemental Security Income program and other people deemed medically needy in participating States. From 1997 onwards excludes foster care and includes unknown eligibility.
[7]Race and ethnicity as determined on initial Medicaid application. Categories are mutually exclusive.
[8]Vendor payments exclude disproportionate share hospital payments ($15 billion in 1999 and 2000).

NOTES: 1972 data are for fiscal year ending June 30. All other years are for fiscal year ending September 30. Data for additional years are available (see Appendix III).

SOURCE: Centers for Medicare & Medicaid Services, Office of Information Services, Enterprise Databases Group, Division of Information Distribution, Medicaid Data System. Before 1999 Medicaid Statistical Report HCFA–2082. From 1999 onwards Medicaid Statistical Information System, MSIS. www.cms.hhs.gov/medicaid/msis/mstats.asp.

Table 138 (page 1 of 2). Medicaid recipients and medical vendor payments, according to type of service: United States, selected fiscal years 1972–2000

[Data are compiled by the Centers for Medicare & Medicaid Services from the Medicaid Data System]

Type of service	1972	1980	1990	1995	1996	1997	1998[1]	1999[2]	2000
Recipients					Number in millions				
All recipients............................	17.6	21.6	25.3	36.3	36.1	34.9	40.6	40.2	42.8
					Percent of recipients				
Inpatient hospital	16.1	17.0	18.2	15.3	14.8	13.6	10.5	11.2	11.5
Mental health facility	0.2	0.3	0.4	0.2	0.3	0.3	0.3	0.2	0.2
Mentally retarded intermediate care facility ...	- - -	0.6	0.6	0.4	0.4	0.4	0.3	0.3	0.3
Nursing facility	- - -	- - -	- - -	4.6	4.4	4.6	4.0	4.0	4.0
Skilled	3.1	2.8	2.4	- - -	- - -	- - -	- - -	- - -	- - -
Intermediate care..................	- - -	3.7	3.4	- - -	- - -	- - -	- - -	- - -	- - -
Physician.............................	69.8	63.7	67.6	65.6	63.3	60.7	45.6	45.7	44.7
Dental................................	13.6	21.5	18.0	17.6	17.2	17.0	12.2	14.0	13.8
Other practitioner	9.1	15.0	15.3	15.2	14.8	14.7	10.7	9.9	11.1
Outpatient hospital	29.6	44.9	49.0	46.1	44.0	39.1	29.9	30.9	30.9
Clinic................................	2.8	7.1	11.1	14.7	14.0	13.5	13.0	16.8	17.9
Laboratory and radiological	20.0	14.9	35.5	36.0	34.9	31.8	23.1	25.4	26.6
Home health..........................	0.6	1.8	2.8	4.5	4.8	5.3	3.0	2.0	2.3
Prescribed drugs	63.3	63.4	68.5	65.4	62.5	60.1	47.6	49.4	48.0
Family planning	. . .	5.2	6.9	6.9	6.6	6.0	4.9	- - -	- - -
Early and periodic screening	. . .	. . .	11.7	18.2	18.2	18.5	15.2	- - -	- - -
Rural health clinic....................	. . .	. . .	0.9	3.4	3.9	4.1	- - -	- - -	- - -
Capitated payment services.............	- - -	- - -	- - -	- - -	- - -	- - -	49.7	51.5	49.7
Primary care case management...........	- - -	- - -	- - -	- - -	- - -	- - -	- - -	9.7	13.0
Personal support	- - -	- - -	- - -	- - -	- - -	- - -	- - -	10.1	10.6
Other care	14.4	11.9	20.3	31.5	36.3	35.5	36.0	21.6	21.4
Vendor payments[3]					Amount in billions				
All payments	$ 6.3	$ 23.3	$ 64.9	$120.1	$121.7	$124.4	$142.3	$153.5	$168.3
					Percent distribution				
Total	100.0	100.0	100.0	100.0	100.0	100.0	100.0	100.0	100.0
Inpatient hospital	40.6	27.5	25.7	21.9	20.7	18.6	15.1	14.5	14.4
Mental health facility	1.8	3.3	2.6	2.1	1.7	1.6	2.0	1.1	1.1
Mentally retarded intermediate care facility ...	- - -	8.5	11.3	8.6	7.9	7.9	6.7	6.1	5.6
Nursing facility	- - -	- - -	- - -	24.2	24.3	24.5	22.4	21.7	20.5
Skilled	23.3	15.8	12.4	- - -	- - -	- - -	- - -	- - -	- - -
Intermediate care..................	- - -	18.0	14.9	- - -	- - -	- - -	- - -	- - -	- - -
Physician.............................	12.6	8.0	6.2	6.1	5.9	5.7	4.3	4.3	4.0
Dental................................	2.7	2.0	0.9	0.8	0.8	0.8	0.6	0.8	0.8
Other practitioner	0.9	0.8	0.6	0.8	0.9	0.8	0.4	0.3	0.4
Outpatient hospital	5.8	4.7	5.1	5.5	5.3	5.0	4.0	4.0	4.2
Clinic................................	0.7	1.4	2.6	3.6	3.5	3.4	2.8	3.8	3.7
Laboratory and radiological	1.3	0.5	1.1	1.0	1.0	0.8	0.7	0.8	0.8
Home health..........................	0.4	1.4	5.2	7.8	8.9	9.8	1.9	1.9	1.9
Prescribed drugs	8.1	5.7	6.8	8.1	8.8	9.6	9.5	10.8	11.9
Family planning	. . .	0.3	0.4	0.4	0.4	0.3	0.3	- - -	- - -
Early and periodic screening	. . .	. . .	0.3	1.0	1.1	1.3	0.9	- - -	- - -
Rural health clinic....................	. . .	. . .	0.1	0.2	0.2	0.2	- - -	- - -	- - -
Capitated payment services.............	- - -	- - -	- - -	- - -	- - -	- - -	13.6	14.0	14.5
Primary care case management...........	- - -	- - -	- - -	- - -	- - -	- - -	- - -	0.3	0.1
Personal support	- - -	- - -	- - -	- - -	- - -	- - -	- - -	6.9	6.9
Other care	1.8	1.9	3.7	7.7	8.4	8.9	13.6	8.6	8.8

See footnotes at end of table.

Table 138 (page 2 of 2). Medicaid recipients and medical vendor payments, according to type of service: United States, selected fiscal years 1972–2000

[Data are compiled by the Centers for Medicare & Medicaid Services from the Medicaid Data System]

Type of service	1972	1980	1990	1995	1996	1997	1998[1]	1999[2]	2000
Vendor payments per recipient[3]					Amount				
Total payment per recipient	$ 358	$ 1,079	$ 2,568	$ 3,311	$ 3,369	$ 3,568	$ 3,501	$ 3,819	$ 3,936
Inpatient hospital	903	1,742	3,630	4,735	4,696	4,877	5,031	4,943	4,919
Mental health facility	2,825	11,742	18,548	29,847	21,873	22,990	20,701	18,094	17,800
Mentally retarded intermediate care facility . . .	- - -	16,438	50,048	68,613	68,232	72,033	74,960	76,443	79,330
Nursing facility	- - -	- - -	- - -	17,424	18,589	19,029	19,379	20,568	20,220
Skilled	2,665	6,081	13,356	- - -	- - -	- - -	- - -	- - -	- - -
Intermediate care.	- - -	5,326	11,236	- - -	- - -	- - -	- - -	- - -	- - -
Physician.	65	136	235	309	317	333	327	357	356
Dental	71	99	130	160	166	175	182	214	238
Other practitioner	37	61	96	178	205	190	135	118	139
Outpatient hospital	70	113	269	397	409	453	474	491	533
Clinic.	82	209	602	804	833	902	742	860	805
Laboratory and radiological	23	38	80	90	96	93	100	114	113
Home health.	229	847	4,733	5,740	6,293	6,575	2,206	3,571	3,135
Prescribed drugs	46	96	256	413	474	571	699	837	975
Family planning	. . .	72	151	206	200	200	223	- - -	- - -
Early and periodic screening	. . .	. . .	67	177	212	251	216	- - -	- - -
Rural health clinic	. . .	. . .	154	174	215	213	- - -	- - -	- - -
Capitated payment services.	- - -	- - -	- - -	- - -	- - -	- - -	955	1,040	1,148
Primary care case management.	- - -	- - -	- - -	- - -	- - -	- - -	- - -	119	30
Personal support	- - -	- - -	- - -	- - -	- - -	- - -	- - -	2,583	2,543
Other care	44	172	465	807	782	891	1,331	1,508	1,600

- - - Data not available.
. . . Category not applicable.

[1]Prior to 1998 recipient counts exclude those individuals who only received coverage under prepaid health care and for whom no direct vendor payments were made during the year. Prior to 1998 vendor payments exclude payments to health maintenance organizations and other prepaid health plans ($19.3 billion in 1998 and $18 billion in 1997). The total number of persons who were Medicaid eligible and enrolled was 41.4 million in 1998, 41.6 million in 1997, and 41.2 million in 1996 (HCFA Medicaid Statistics, Program and Financial Statistics FY1996, FY1997, and FY1998, unpublished).
[2]Starting in 1999, the Medicaid data system was changed (see Appendix I, Medicaid Data System).
[3]Payments exclude disproportionate share hospital payments ($15 billion in 1999 and 2000).

NOTES: 1972 data are for fiscal year ending June 30. All other years are for fiscal year ending September 30. Unknown services are included in the total but not shown separately (0.4 percent of recipients and 0.6 percent of payments in 2000). Data for additional years are available (see Appendix III).

SOURCE: Centers for Medicare & Medicaid Services, Office of Information Services, Enterprise Databases Group, Division of Information Distribution, Medicaid Data System. Before 1999 Medicaid Statistical Report HCFA–2082. From 1999 onwards Medicaid Statistical Information System, MSIS. www.cms.hhs.gov/medicaid/msis/mstats.asp.

Table 139. Department of Veterans Affairs health care expenditures and use, and persons treated according to selected characteristics: United States, selected fiscal years 1970–2002

[Data are compiled from patient records and enrollment information by the Department of Veterans Affairs]

	1970	1980	1990	1995	1998	1999	2000	2001	2002
Health care expenditures	Amount in millions								
All expenditures[1]	$1,689	$ 5,981	$11,500	$16,126	$17,441	$17,876	$19,327	$21,316	$23,003
	Percent distribution								
All services	100.0	100.0	100.0	100.0	100.0	100.0	100.0	100.0	100.0
Inpatient hospital	71.3	64.3	57.5	49.0	38.3	38.8	37.3	34.7	33.6
Outpatient care	14.0	19.1	25.3	30.2	41.8	44.0	45.7	48.0	48.8
Nursing home care	5.5	7.1	9.5	10.0	10.2	8.5	8.2	8.1	8.0
All other[2]	9.1	9.6	7.7	10.8	9.9	8.7	8.8	9.2	9.6
Health care use	Number in thousands								
Inpatient hospital stays[3]	787	1,248	1,029	879	617	611	579	584	590
Outpatient visits	7,312	17,971	22,602	27,527	34,972	36,928	38,370	42,901	46,058
Nursing home stays[4]	47	57	75	79	98	92	91	93	87
Inpatients[5]									
Total	- - -	- - -	598	527	380	447	417	426	436
	Percent distribution								
Total	- - -	- - -	100.0	100.0	100.0	100.0	100.0	100.0	100.0
Veterans with service-connected disability	- - -	- - -	38.9	39.3	38.2	33.8	34.4	34.6	35.2
Veterans without service-connected disability	- - -	- - -	60.3	59.9	60.8	65.3	64.7	64.5	63.9
Low income	- - -	- - -	54.8	56.2	55.4	44.8	41.7	41.4	40.9
Veterans receiving aid and attendance or housebound benefits or who are catastrophically disabled[6]			- - -	- - -	- - -	12.8	16.0	15.7	13.6
Veterans receiving medical care subject to copayments[7]	- - -	- - -	2.8	2.8	3.8	4.7	5.2	6.0	7.7
Other and unknown[8]	- - -	- - -	2.7	0.9	1.6	3.0	1.8	1.4	1.7
Nonveterans	- - -	- - -	0.8	0.8	1.0	0.9	0.9	0.9	0.9
Outpatients[5]	Number in thousands								
Total	- - -	- - -	2,564	2,790	3,235	3,400	3,657	4,072	4,456
	Percent distribution								
Total	- - -	- - -	100.0	100.0	100.0	100.0	100.0	100.0	100.0
Veterans with service-connected disability	- - -	- - -	38.3	37.5	38.7	30.5	30.7	30.0	29.5
Veterans without service-connected disability	- - -	- - -	49.8	50.5	52.9	60.6	60.8	62.5	63.9
Low income	- - -	- - -	41.1	42.2	41.3	38.8	37.6	36.6	34.1
Veterans receiving aid and attendance or housebound benefits or who are catastrophically disabled[6]			- - -	- - -	- - -	3.2	3.8	3.7	3.3
Veterans receiving medical care subject to copayments[7]	- - -	- - -	3.6	4.2	8.4	11.7	15.4	19.9	23.6
Other and unknown[8]	- - -	- - -	5.1	4.1	3.2	6.9	4.0	2.3	2.9
Nonveterans	- - -	- - -	11.8	12.0	10.4	8.9	8.5	7.5	6.6

- - - Data not available.

[1]Health care expenditures exclude construction, medical administration, and miscellaneous operating expenses at Department of Veterans Affairs headquarters.

[2]Includes miscellaneous benefits and services, contract hospitals, education and training, subsidies to State veterans hospitals, nursing homes and domiciliaries, and the Civilian Health and Medical Program of the Department of Veterans Affairs.

[3]One-day dialysis patients were included in 1980. Interfacility transfers were included beginning in 1990.

[4]Includes Department of Veterans Affairs nursing home and domiciliary stays, and community nursing home care stays.

[5]Individuals. The inpatient and outpatient totals are not additive since almost all inpatients are also treated as outpatients.

[6]Veterans who are receiving aid and attendance or housebound benefits; veterans who have been determined by the Department of Veterans Affairs to be catastrophically disabled.

[7]Financial means-tested veterans who receive medical care subject to copayments according to income level.

[8]Prisoner of war, exposed to Agent Orange, and so forth. Prior to fiscal year 1994, veterans who reported exposure to Agent Orange were classified as exempt. Beginning in fiscal year 1994 those veterans reporting Agent Orange exposure but not treated for it were means tested and placed in the low income or other group depending on income.

NOTES: Figures may not add to totals due to rounding. In 1970 and 1980, the fiscal year ended June 30; for years 1990 and later the fiscal year ended September 30. The veteran population was estimated at 25.6 million in 2002 with 38 percent age 65 or over, compared with 11 percent in 1980. Nineteen percent had served during World War II, 15 percent during the Korean conflict, 32 percent during the Vietnam era, 14 percent during the Persian Gulf War, and 24 percent during peacetime. These percentages add to more than 100 due to veterans serving during more than one war. Beginning in fiscal year 1995 categories for health care expenditures and health care use were revised. In fiscal year 1999 a new priority system for reporting data was introduced and starting in 1999, data reflect the new categories. 1999 data have been revised and differ from the previous edition of *Health, United States*. Data for additional years are available (see Appendix III).

SOURCE: Department of Veterans Affairs, Office of Policy and Planning and Preparedness, Policy Analysis Service, National Patient Care Database and National Enrollment Database, unpublished data.

Table 140 (page 1 of 2). Personal health care per capita expenditures, by geographic region and State: United States, selected years 1991–98

[Data are compiled from various sources by the Centers for Medicare & Medicaid Services]

Geographic region and State[1]	1991	1994	1995	1996	1997	1998	1991–98	1998
							Average annual percent change	Ratio to U.S. per capita expenditures
			Per capita expenditures					
United States	$2,685	$3,193	$3,334	$3,472	$3,606	$3,759	4.9	1.00
New England	3,115	3,745	3,945	4,092	4,303	4,540	5.5	1.21
Connecticut	3,338	3,900	4,138	4,250	4,442	4,656	4.9	1.24
Maine	2,464	3,018	3,256	3,512	3,755	4,025	7.3	1.07
Massachusetts	3,334	4,056	4,200	4,347	4,556	4,810	5.4	1.28
New Hampshire	2,511	3,029	3,264	3,441	3,650	3,840	6.3	1.02
Rhode Island	2,943	3,569	3,867	3,978	4,235	4,497	6.2	1.20
Vermont	2,393	2,890	3,133	3,273	3,455	3,654	6.2	0.97
Mideast[2]	3,108	3,748	3,905	4,063	4,209	4,386	5.0	1.17
Delaware	2,878	3,565	3,737	3,847	4,083	4,258	5.8	1.13
Maryland	2,796	3,291	3,401	3,573	3,696	3,848	4.7	1.02
New Jersey	2,966	3,622	3,830	4,009	4,080	4,197	5.1	1.12
New York	3,288	3,997	4,162	4,346	4,486	4,706	5.3	1.25
Pennsylvania	2,988	3,547	3,683	3,791	4,003	4,168	4.9	1.11
Great Lakes	2,666	3,172	3,318	3,467	3,606	3,733	4.9	0.99
Illinois	2,743	3,259	3,394	3,535	3,653	3,801	4.8	1.01
Indiana	2,508	3,052	3,156	3,196	3,416	3,566	5.2	0.95
Michigan	2,643	3,114	3,289	3,457	3,602	3,676	4.8	0.98
Ohio	2,709	3,209	3,353	3,542	3,635	3,747	4.7	1.00
Wisconsin	2,610	3,138	3,306	3,476	3,654	3,845	5.7	1.02
Plains	2,544	3,115	3,271	3,436	3,592	3,797	5.9	1.01
Iowa	2,524	3,014	3,165	3,368	3,519	3,765	5.9	1.00
Kansas	2,574	3,067	3,249	3,412	3,573	3,707	5.3	0.99
Minnesota	2,606	3,246	3,439	3,614	3,791	3,986	6.3	1.06
Missouri	2,555	3,159	3,262	3,390	3,531	3,754	5.6	1.00
Nebraska	2,383	2,947	3,083	3,287	3,407	3,627	6.2	0.96
North Dakota	2,555	3,155	3,420	3,540	3,680	3,881	6.2	1.03
South Dakota	2,394	2,880	3,068	3,253	3,453	3,650	6.2	0.97
Southeast	2,557	3,081	3,241	3,400	3,557	3,686	5.4	0.98
Alabama	2,561	3,059	3,234	3,422	3,626	3,630	5.1	0.97
Arkansas	2,408	2,840	3,012	3,177	3,355	3,540	5.7	0.94
Florida	2,976	3,523	3,632	3,774	3,875	4,046	4.5	1.08
Georgia	2,527	3,007	3,170	3,291	3,412	3,505	4.8	0.93
Kentucky	2,424	2,898	3,098	3,300	3,519	3,711	6.3	0.99
Louisiana	2,619	3,243	3,376	3,496	3,639	3,742	5.2	1.00
Mississippi	2,190	2,686	2,933	3,145	3,286	3,474	6.8	0.92
North Carolina	2,271	2,854	3,040	3,232	3,420	3,535	6.5	0.94
South Carolina	2,276	2,839	2,985	3,131	3,399	3,529	6.5	0.94
Tennessee	2,594	3,186	3,415	3,569	3,728	3,808	5.6	1.01
Virginia	2,378	2,743	2,858	3,009	3,155	3,284	4.7	0.87
West Virginia	2,568	3,233	3,442	3,649	3,858	4,044	6.7	1.08
Southwest	2,373	2,794	2,934	3,075	3,194	3,339	5.0	0.89
Arizona	2,407	2,729	2,769	2,862	2,935	3,100	3.7	0.82
New Mexico	2,211	2,609	2,744	2,943	3,058	3,209	5.5	0.85
Oklahoma	2,336	2,819	3,014	3,188	3,268	3,397	5.5	0.90
Texas	2,387	2,821	2,975	3,117	3,255	3,397	5.2	0.90
Rocky Mountains	2,267	2,608	2,751	2,874	3,010	3,145	4.8	0.84
Colorado	2,481	2,835	2,977	3,071	3,202	3,331	4.3	0.89
Idaho	2,082	2,436	2,580	2,765	2,883	3,035	5.5	0.81
Montana	2,304	2,655	2,876	2,917	3,114	3,314	5.3	0.88
Utah	1,960	2,250	2,349	2,506	2,638	2,731	4.8	0.73
Wyoming	2,234	2,658	2,850	3,046	3,185	3,381	6.1	0.90

See footnotes at end of table.

Table 140 (page 2 of 2). Personal health care per capita expenditures, by geographic region and State: United States, selected years 1991–98

[Data are compiled from various sources by the Centers for Medicare & Medicaid Services]

Geographic region and State[1]	1991	1994	1995	1996	1997	1998	1991–98	1998
							Average annual percent change	Ratio to U.S. per capita expenditures
			Per capita expenditures					
Far West.	2,634	3,028	3,109	3,183	3,255	3,414	3.8	0.91
Alaska.	2,459	2,811	3,050	3,227	3,340	3,442	4.9	0.92
California.	2,690	3,071	3,132	3,200	3,265	3,429	3.5	0.91
Hawaii.	2,638	3,248	3,462	3,656	3,664	3,770	5.2	1.00
Nevada	2,393	2,829	2,881	2,949	3,028	3,147	4.0	0.84
Oregon	2,337	2,780	2,924	3,019	3,160	3,334	5.2	0.89
Washington	2,545	2,946	3,075	3,142	3,225	3,382	4.1	0.90

[1]Data are shown for Bureau of Economic Analysis (BEA) regions that are constructed to show economically interdependent states. These BEA geographic regions differ from Bureau of the Census geographic divisions shown in some *Health, United States* tables. See Appendix II, Geographic region and division.

[2]The Mideast region includes spending in the District of Columbia (DC), although it is not listed separately. Per capita spending in DC is substantially higher than per capita spending in most states. Most of this higher spending comes from spending on hospital care. One contributing factor to higher spending is the concentration of several higher-cost academic medical centers in a very small geographic area populated with a small number of people. Another factor could be the inability of current data sources and methods to accurately portray spending flows between providers located in DC and beneficiary resident locations. As a result, per capita spending in DC is not shown.

NOTES: Personal health care includes the following types of services: hospital care, physician and other professional services, nursing home care and home health care, drugs and nondurable products, dental services, durable products, and other personal health care not otherwise specified. Per capita expenditures for each category except the last three are shown in tables 141–144. Services not shown separately accounted for 6 percent of personal health care expenditures in 1991 and 10 percent in 1998. Data for additional years are available (see Appendix III). Some numbers have been revised and differ from the previous edition of *Health, United States*.

SOURCE: Centers for Medicare & Medicaid Services, Office of the Actuary, National Health Statistics Group, National Health Accounts, State Health Expenditures. www.cms.hhs.gov/statistics/nhe/state-estimates-residence/.

Table 141 (page 1 of 2). Hospital care per capita expenditures, by geographic region and State: United States, selected years 1991–98

[Data are compiled from various sources by the Centers for Medicare & Medicaid Services]

Geographic region and State[1]	1991	1994	1995	1996	1997	1998	1991–98 Average annual percent change	1998 Ratio to U.S. per capita expenditures
				Per capita expenditures				
United States	$1,109	$1,279	$1,310	$1,344	$1,372	$1,405	3.4	1.00
New England	1,253	1,438	1,463	1,503	1,562	1,613	3.7	1.15
Connecticut	1,206	1,345	1,343	1,387	1,423	1,478	2.9	1.05
Maine	1,015	1,204	1,296	1,385	1,441	1,501	5.7	1.07
Massachusetts	1,416	1,636	1,635	1,675	1,738	1,807	3.5	1.29
New Hampshire	987	1,123	1,180	1,187	1,235	1,234	3.2	0.88
Rhode Island	1,191	1,368	1,473	1,498	1,632	1,626	4.5	1.16
Vermont	948	1,135	1,244	1,259	1,304	1,328	4.9	0.95
Mideast[2]	1,320	1,553	1,575	1,616	1,645	1,656	3.3	1.18
Delaware	1,187	1,457	1,513	1,467	1,565	1,581	4.2	1.13
Maryland	1,158	1,312	1,360	1,424	1,457	1,486	3.6	1.06
New Jersey	1,187	1,430	1,424	1,509	1,467	1,481	3.2	1.05
New York	1,380	1,646	1,672	1,726	1,754	1,769	3.6	1.26
Pennsylvania	1,332	1,520	1,548	1,538	1,610	1,599	2.6	1.14
Great Lakes	1,134	1,317	1,361	1,405	1,455	1,471	3.8	1.05
Illinois	1,238	1,416	1,455	1,491	1,531	1,558	3.3	1.11
Indiana	1,048	1,239	1,273	1,228	1,365	1,413	4.4	1.01
Michigan	1,129	1,318	1,393	1,444	1,474	1,489	4.0	1.06
Ohio	1,132	1,325	1,366	1,434	1,459	1,437	3.5	1.02
Wisconsin	998	1,151	1,173	1,266	1,336	1,377	4.7	0.98
Plains	1,069	1,269	1,317	1,365	1,415	1,460	4.6	1.04
Iowa	1,095	1,269	1,325	1,406	1,455	1,520	4.8	1.08
Kansas	1,083	1,278	1,333	1,369	1,412	1,428	4.0	1.02
Minnesota	933	1,060	1,104	1,156	1,249	1,254	4.3	0.89
Missouri	1,170	1,437	1,464	1,476	1,494	1,566	4.3	1.11
Nebraska	1,043	1,258	1,316	1,419	1,433	1,507	5.4	1.07
North Dakota	1,062	1,357	1,466	1,532	1,647	1,741	7.3	1.24
South Dakota	1,106	1,269	1,370	1,436	1,499	1,534	4.8	1.09
Southeast	1,085	1,253	1,297	1,343	1,378	1,409	3.8	1.00
Alabama	1,109	1,284	1,376	1,445	1,473	1,432	3.7	1.02
Arkansas	1,028	1,167	1,228	1,320	1,354	1,430	4.8	1.02
Florida	1,130	1,267	1,290	1,317	1,322	1,371	2.8	0.98
Georgia	1,089	1,249	1,270	1,299	1,309	1,329	2.9	0.95
Kentucky	1,067	1,220	1,266	1,340	1,411	1,479	4.8	1.05
Louisiana	1,207	1,453	1,502	1,520	1,563	1,601	4.1	1.14
Mississippi	1,025	1,231	1,365	1,456	1,443	1,551	6.1	1.10
North Carolina	972	1,169	1,246	1,306	1,366	1,373	5.1	0.98
South Carolina	1,073	1,303	1,326	1,345	1,467	1,480	4.7	1.05
Tennessee	1,122	1,311	1,296	1,346	1,379	1,375	3.0	0.98
Virginia	1,016	1,113	1,167	1,212	1,258	1,286	3.4	0.92
West Virginia	1,186	1,381	1,452	1,562	1,635	1,693	5.2	1.20
Southwest	992	1,137	1,157	1,191	1,205	1,255	3.4	0.89
Arizona	920	1,000	998	1,012	1,022	1,085	2.4	0.77
New Mexico	1,051	1,213	1,218	1,267	1,313	1,389	4.1	0.99
Oklahoma	1,000	1,152	1,210	1,275	1,282	1,307	3.9	0.93
Texas	1,001	1,159	1,179	1,211	1,225	1,274	3.5	0.91
Rocky Mountains	921	1,013	1,067	1,097	1,131	1,164	3.4	0.83
Colorado	986	1,067	1,114	1,111	1,139	1,147	2.2	0.82
Idaho	848	933	978	1,073	1,094	1,163	4.6	0.83
Montana	983	1,111	1,232	1,206	1,333	1,440	5.6	1.02
Utah	781	882	917	978	995	1,016	3.8	0.72
Wyoming	1,038	1,142	1,238	1,341	1,380	1,439	4.8	1.02

See footnotes at end of table.

Table 141 (page 2 of 2). Hospital care per capita expenditures, by geographic region and State: United States, selected years 1991–98

[Data are compiled from various sources by the Centers for Medicare & Medicaid Services]

Geographic region and State[1]	1991	1994	1995	1996	1997	1998	1991–98 Average annual percent change	1998 Ratio to U.S. per capita expenditures
			Per capita expenditures					
Far West.................	974	1,093	1,099	1,098	1,088	1,146	2.3	0.82
Alaska..................	1,118	1,306	1,447	1,496	1,502	1,496	4.3	1.06
California...............	998	1,106	1,103	1,092	1,076	1,145	2.0	0.81
Hawaii.................	1,074	1,318	1,371	1,462	1,413	1,391	3.8	0.99
Nevada.................	879	1,013	1,001	1,021	1,027	1,033	2.3	0.74
Oregon	822	964	1,001	1,021	1,049	1,112	4.4	0.79
Washington	904	1,038	1,061	1,078	1,085	1,116	3.1	0.79

[1]Data are shown for Bureau of Economic Analysis (BEA) regions that are constructed to show economically interdependent states. These BEA geographic regions differ from Bureau of the Census geographic divisions shown in some *Health, United States* tables. See Appendix II, Geographic region and division.

[2]The Mideast region includes spending in the District of Columbia (DC), although it is not listed separately. Per capita spending in DC is substantially higher than per capita spending in most states. Most of this higher spending comes from spending on hospital care. One contributing factor to higher spending is the concentration of several higher-cost academic medical centers in a very small geographic area populated with a small number of people. Another factor could be the inability of current data sources and methods to accurately portray spending flows between providers located in DC and beneficiary resident locations. As a result, per capita spending in DC is not shown.

NOTES: Data for additional years are available (see Appendix III). Some numbers have been revised and differ from the previous edition of *Health, United States*.

SOURCE: Centers for Medicare & Medicaid Services, Office of the Actuary, National Health Statistics Group, National Health Accounts, State Health Expenditures. www.cms.hhs.gov/statistics/nhe/state-estimates-residence/.

Table 142. Physician and other professional services per capita expenditures, by geographic region and State: United States, selected years 1991–98

[Data are compiled from various sources by the Centers for Medicare & Medicaid Services]

Geographic region and State[1]	1991	1994	1995	1996	1997	1998	1991–98	1998
							Average annual percent change	Ratio to U.S. per capita expenditures
			Per capita expenditures					
United States	$ 795	$ 932	$ 972	$1,003	$1,043	$1,095	4.7	1.00
New England	823	980	1,045	1,080	1,163	1,246	6.1	1.14
Connecticut	945	1,072	1,182	1,188	1,249	1,304	4.7	1.19
Maine	621	736	796	847	929	1,020	7.4	0.93
Massachusetts	845	1,035	1,073	1,117	1,224	1,316	6.5	1.20
New Hampshire	726	881	964	1,039	1,101	1,189	7.3	1.09
Rhode Island	751	890	974	974	1,022	1,128	6.0	1.03
Vermont	634	752	796	838	911	988	6.5	0.90
Mideast[2]	812	982	1,027	1,044	1,079	1,136	4.9	1.04
Delaware.................	843	1,002	1,011	1,024	1,084	1,123	4.2	1.03
Maryland	871	1,056	1,060	1,080	1,099	1,140	3.9	1.04
New Jersey	879	1,052	1,153	1,155	1,193	1,225	4.9	1.12
New York................	758	936	982	1,006	1,044	1,112	5.6	1.01
Pennsylvania	806	954	980	998	1,034	1,103	4.6	1.01
Great Lakes	747	882	914	944	963	1,015	4.5	0.93
Illinois..................	751	901	929	970	991	1,046	4.9	0.95
Indiana	681	820	828	860	883	944	4.8	0.86
Michigan	744	855	889	918	937	973	3.9	0.89
Ohio	776	882	911	943	941	992	3.6	0.91
Wisconsin	751	955	1,030	1,033	1,083	1,151	6.3	1.05
Plains....................	690	852	892	937	983	1,051	6.2	0.96
Iowa	662	798	823	856	888	956	5.4	0.87
Kansas	757	879	940	969	993	1,039	4.6	0.95
Minnesota	775	1,020	1,107	1,189	1,260	1,347	8.2	1.23
Missouri.................	649	781	787	822	869	938	5.4	0.86
Nebraska................	580	723	724	750	790	839	5.4	0.77
North Dakota.............	671	826	915	911	880	914	4.5	0.83
South Dakota.............	590	733	764	815	908	998	7.8	0.91
Southeast.................	765	899	936	969	1,018	1,059	4.8	0.97
Alabama	777	902	913	941	1,020	1,075	4.7	0.98
Arkansas................	707	808	842	836	903	941	4.2	0.86
Florida..................	1,033	1,182	1,178	1,201	1,235	1,273	3.0	1.16
Georgia.................	767	883	966	1,007	1,066	1,091	5.2	1.00
Kentucky	656	783	862	898	935	976	5.8	0.89
Louisiana................	702	829	844	867	917	968	4.7	0.88
Mississippi...............	564	661	719	757	838	879	6.5	0.80
North Carolina	627	782	811	854	891	941	6.0	0.86
South Carolina	571	705	747	784	846	896	6.7	0.82
Tennessee...............	720	877	999	1,052	1,112	1,149	6.9	1.05
Virginia	716	822	827	865	894	928	3.8	0.85
West Virginia	682	862	896	923	983	1,040	6.2	0.95
Southwest.................	718	809	856	887	935	989	4.7	0.90
Arizona	856	920	918	949	982	1,037	2.8	0.95
New Mexico..............	591	689	735	810	843	878	5.8	0.80
Oklahoma	656	765	804	841	886	948	5.4	0.87
Texas	711	803	861	887	941	995	4.9	0.91
Rocky Mountains............	678	764	796	830	877	925	4.5	0.84
Colorado	788	897	929	964	1,007	1,058	4.3	0.97
Idaho	618	693	739	767	813	852	4.7	0.78
Montana	609	639	696	730	777	825	4.4	0.75
Utah	557	629	637	675	726	763	4.6	0.70
Wyoming	594	693	746	760	811	896	6.0	0.82
Far West..................	977	1,108	1,148	1,181	1,212	1,261	3.7	1.15
Alaska..................	701	740	792	866	902	953	4.5	0.87
California................	1,039	1,184	1,221	1,259	1,290	1,340	3.7	1.22
Hawaii..................	799	1,012	1,118	1,214	1,235	1,311	7.3	1.20
Nevada	898	960	993	1,000	1,035	1,085	2.7	0.99
Oregon	737	854	899	911	963	1,001	4.5	0.91
Washington	831	914	957	969	988	1,037	3.2	0.95

[1]Data are shown for Bureau of Economic Analysis (BEA) regions that are constructed to show economically interdependent states. These BEA geographic regions differ from Bureau of the Census geographic divisions shown in some *Health, United States* tables. See Appendix II, Geographic region and division.
[2]The Mideast region includes spending in the District of Columbia (DC), although it is not listed separately.

NOTE: Data for additional years are available (see Appendix III).

SOURCE: Centers for Medicare & Medicaid Services, Office of the Actuary, National Health Statistics Group, National Health Accounts, State Health Expenditures. www.cms.hhs.gov/statistics/nhe/state-estimates-residence/.

Table 143. Nursing home care and home health care per capita expenditures, by geographic region and State: United States, selected years 1991–98

[Data are compiled from various sources by the Centers for Medicare & Medicaid Services]

Geographic region and State[1]	1991	1994	1995	1996	1997	1998	1991–98 Average annual percent change	1998 Ratio to U.S. per capita expenditures
			Per capita expenditures					
United States	$290	$374	$398	$420	$430	$433	5.9	1.00
New England	492	618	656	688	693	702	5.2	1.62
Connecticut	578	734	780	827	847	860	5.8	1.99
Maine	384	492	516	525	532	538	4.9	1.24
Massachusetts	534	664	702	735	733	739	4.7	1.71
New Hampshire	268	375	419	450	465	470	8.3	1.08
Rhode Island	443	541	571	587	574	606	4.6	1.40
Vermont	316	357	378	403	412	411	3.9	0.95
Mideast[2]	447	548	578	609	623	648	5.5	1.50
Delaware	328	417	455	492	495	520	6.8	1.20
Maryland	247	323	344	354	369	395	7.0	0.91
New Jersey	309	425	474	499	513	514	7.5	1.19
New York . . . . '.	628	730	749	784	789	827	4.0	1.91
Pennsylvania	353	452	489	530	559	582	7.4	1.34
Great Lakes	306	381	405	425	442	445	5.5	1.03
Illinois	286	359	379	391	403	409	5.2	0.94
Indiana	331	426	443	459	470	464	4.9	1.07
Michigan	246	295	316	339	374	342	4.8	0.79
Ohio	341	438	468	500	511	549	7.1	1.27
Wisconsin	360	424	454	466	480	478	4.2	1.10
Plains	327	404	425	453	465	474	5.5	1.09
Iowa	326	400	424	461	476	502	6.4	1.16
Kansas	289	357	374	404	420	421	5.5	0.97
Minnesota	412	490	502	505	496	503	2.9	1.16
Missouri	285	371	401	443	473	476	7.6	1.10
Nebraska	289	378	397	431	441	459	6.8	1.06
North Dakota	378	405	423	442	455	470	3.2	1.09
South Dakota	274	345	359	387	391	401	5.6	0.93
Southeast	240	340	368	396	406	404	7.7	0.93
Alabama	213	303	333	357	369	360	7.8	0.83
Arkansas	251	332	359	376	410	415	7.4	0.96
Florida	282	404	439	464	465	471	7.6	1.09
Georgia	201	288	303	311	308	308	6.3	0.71
Kentucky	253	345	377	411	446	458	8.8	1.06
Louisiana	265	389	424	471	470	431	7.2	1.00
Mississippi	210	307	327	367	382	366	8.3	0.84
North Carolina	242	355	381	413	433	430	8.5	0.99
South Carolina	197	274	304	337	340	349	8.5	0.81
Tennessee	286	410	448	478	491	474	7.5	1.09
Virginia	177	236	247	271	289	296	7.6	0.68
West Virginia	237	329	375	411	414	414	8.3	0.96
Southwest	205	287	318	346	358	340	7.5	0.79
Arizona	162	247	248	257	251	242	5.9	0.56
New Mexico	149	190	221	239	242	238	6.9	0.55
Oklahoma	257	363	412	440	426	402	6.6	0.93
Texas	209	291	327	361	381	362	8.2	0.84
Rocky Mountains	193	248	260	274	283	277	5.3	0.64
Colorado	203	254	266	289	307	307	6.1	0.71
Idaho	176	254	266	279	281	272	6.4	0.63
Montana	249	336	346	331	322	317	3.5	0.73
Utah	166	189	203	213	218	202	2.9	0.47
Wyoming	173	266	281	301	308	296	8.0	0.68
Far West	173	226	236	240	242	245	5.1	0.57
Alaska	95	121	127	99	97	90	–0.8	0.21
California	155	208	218	224	228	232	5.9	0.54
Hawaii	160	189	195	206	215	223	4.8	0.51
Nevada	143	249	229	218	207	203	5.1	0.47
Oregon	246	267	275	288	299	300	2.8	0.69
Washington	256	321	344	329	323	326	3.5	0.75

[1]Data are shown for Bureau of Economic Analysis (BEA) regions that are constructed to show economically interdependent states. These BEA geographic regions differ from Bureau of the Census geographic divisions shown in some *Health, United States* tables. See Appendix II, Geographic region and division.
[2]The Mideast region includes spending in the District of Columbia (DC), although it is not listed separately.

NOTE: Data for additional years are available (see Appendix III).

SOURCE: Centers for Medicare & Medicaid Services, Office of the Actuary, National Health Statistics Group, National Health Accounts, State Health Expenditures. www.cms.hhs.gov/statistics/nhe/state-estimates-residence/.

Table 144. Drugs and other nondurables per capita expenditures, by geographic region and State: United States, selected years 1991–98

[Data are compiled from various sources by the Centers for Medicare & Medicaid Services]

Geographic region and State[1]	1991	1994	1995	1996	1997	1998	1991–98	1998
							Average annual percent change	Ratio to U.S. per capita expenditures
			Per capita expenditures					
United States	$260	$313	$337	$370	$406	$451	8.2	1.00
New England	265	323	348	380	418	479	8.8	1.06
Connecticut	280	344	375	410	448	521	9.3	1.15
Maine	225	277	301	342	398	449	10.4	1.00
Massachusetts	267	323	347	375	410	469	8.4	1.04
New Hampshire	261	314	336	366	402	455	8.2	1.01
Rhode Island	281	343	373	413	451	511	8.9	1.13
Vermont	230	277	298	321	351	401	8.2	0.89
Mideast[2]	274	337	365	405	449	506	9.1	1.12
Delaware	267	324	349	395	456	524	10.1	1.16
Maryland	274	306	319	356	406	449	7.3	0.99
New Jersey	304	381	416	455	498	562	9.2	1.25
New York	262	326	356	399	437	492	9.4	1.09
Pennsylvania	274	337	366	404	452	513	9.4	1.14
Great Lakes	261	319	345	381	413	453	8.2	1.00
Illinois	255	310	335	368	393	430	7.7	0.95
Indiana	264	331	361	389	422	449	7.9	1.00
Michigan	279	341	371	418	458	498	8.6	1.10
Ohio	260	313	338	371	407	448	8.1	0.99
Wisconsin	245	298	320	352	379	434	8.5	0.96
Plains	246	298	320	348	379	429	8.3	0.95
Iowa	240	292	316	348	375	426	8.6	0.94
Kansas	245	292	312	344	379	413	7.7	0.92
Minnesota	233	286	309	340	372	424	8.9	0.94
Missouri	263	316	336	355	387	442	7.7	0.98
Nebraska	257	319	345	380	414	476	9.2	1.06
North Dakota	237	286	307	332	358	392	7.4	0.87
South Dakota	220	264	280	302	323	363	7.4	0.81
Southeast	268	328	356	392	434	482	8.8	1.07
Alabama	271	327	351	385	432	471	8.2	1.04
Arkansas	266	322	346	388	418	464	8.3	1.03
Florida	285	359	395	444	488	552	9.9	1.22
Georgia	255	308	333	364	403	441	8.1	0.98
Kentucky	275	335	363	399	444	499	8.9	1.11
Louisiana	272	330	357	381	415	456	7.6	1.01
Mississippi	253	304	325	355	396	444	8.4	0.98
North Carolina	251	305	331	366	411	452	8.8	1.00
South Carolina	240	298	325	364	412	449	9.4	0.99
Tennessee	286	348	376	408	453	507	8.5	1.12
Virginia	254	307	333	360	393	434	7.9	0.96
West Virginia	287	357	392	422	477	524	9.0	1.16
Southwest	258	309	332	362	392	433	7.7	0.96
Arizona	254	313	342	371	400	443	8.3	0.98
New Mexico	228	268	284	312	332	363	6.9	0.80
Oklahoma	246	304	333	362	384	424	8.1	0.94
Texas	264	313	333	364	397	439	7.5	0.97
Rocky Mountains	231	280	301	328	353	390	7.7	0.86
Colorado	231	281	304	325	347	389	7.8	0.86
Idaho	226	275	297	325	352	386	7.9	0.86
Montana	236	289	311	338	358	397	7.7	0.88
Utah	236	282	302	336	369	394	7.6	0.87
Wyoming	222	259	275	304	332	370	7.5	0.82
Far West	243	274	288	308	339	374	6.4	0.83
Alaska	228	257	275	301	323	360	6.7	0.80
California	239	264	275	292	323	355	5.8	0.79
Hawaii	314	353	372	388	407	431	4.7	0.96
Nevada	256	329	362	391	429	472	9.1	1.05
Oregon	238	294	316	349	378	422	8.5	0.94
Washington	252	290	308	335	369	416	7.4	0.92

[1]Data are shown for Bureau of Economic Analysis (BEA) regions that are constructed to show economically interdependent states. These BEA geographic regions differ from Bureau of the Census geographic divisions shown in some *Health, United States* tables. See Appendix II, Geographic region and division.
[2]The Mideast region includes spending in the District of Columbia (DC), although it is not listed separately.

NOTE: Data for additional years are available (see Appendix III).

SOURCE: Centers for Medicare & Medicaid Services, Office of the Actuary, National Health Statistics Group, National Health Accounts, State Health Expenditures. www.cms.hhs.gov/statistics/nhe/state-estimates-residence/.

Table 145. Medicare expenditures as a percent of total personal health care expenditures by geographic region and State: United States, 1991–98

[Data are compiled from various sources by the Centers for Medicare & Medicaid Services]

Geographic region and State[1]	1991	1992	1993	1994	1995	1996	1997	1998
					Percent			
United States	17.3	17.9	18.3	19.5	20.5	21.0	21.2	20.6
New England	16.5	17.4	18.1	19.1	20.3	21.2	21.0	20.2
Connecticut	15.5	16.5	17.4	18.5	19.7	20.6	20.5	20.5
Maine	16.4	16.6	16.8	18.2	19.1	19.5	19.6	19.0
Massachusetts	17.4	18.4	19.2	20.1	21.7	22.6	22.1	20.7
New Hampshire	13.9	14.5	14.5	15.8	16.4	16.9	16.7	16.6
Rhode Island	17.9	18.5	18.8	20.1	20.5	22.4	22.8	22.0
Vermont	15.0	15.4	15.6	16.5	17.2	17.6	17.3	16.6
Mideast	17.5	18.2	18.6	19.3	20.1	20.6	21.1	21.1
Delaware	15.1	15.9	16.0	16.3	16.5	17.4	16.9	17.4
District of Columbia	13.1	12.3	12.6	13.2	14.0	15.2	16.1	16.9
Maryland	16.3	17.2	17.4	17.9	18.1	18.3	18.8	19.2
New Jersey	16.8	18.5	18.8	19.1	19.7	19.8	21.1	21.4
New York	16.1	16.6	17.0	17.8	18.9	19.3	19.8	19.6
Pennsylvania	21.2	21.6	22.3	23.0	24.1	24.9	24.9	24.8
Great Lakes	17.0	17.6	17.7	18.8	19.8	20.0	20.1	20.0
Illinois	16.9	17.3	17.5	18.7	19.4	19.5	19.5	19.2
Indiana	16.8	17.5	17.6	18.6	19.9	20.5	20.4	19.8
Michigan	17.7	18.6	18.9	20.2	21.4	21.7	21.8	22.0
Ohio	17.5	18.1	18.1	19.1	20.2	20.3	20.9	21.1
Wisconsin	15.2	15.6	15.3	16.0	16.6	16.8	16.8	16.2
Plains	17.0	17.4	17.4	17.9	18.7	18.8	18.9	18.1
Iowa	17.5	18.0	17.7	18.1	18.7	18.6	18.8	17.8
Kansas	17.4	17.9	18.0	18.8	19.8	19.8	20.4	19.6
Minnesota	14.4	14.6	14.3	14.4	15.0	15.2	15.1	14.7
Missouri	19.1	20.0	20.3	21.2	22.4	22.4	22.4	21.1
Nebraska	15.9	15.7	15.7	16.4	17.2	17.4	18.0	17.2
North Dakota	16.4	16.4	16.7	17.1	17.3	17.0	17.2	16.7
South Dakota	16.5	17.0	16.7	17.2	17.8	17.8	17.7	17.3
Southeast	19.3	20.0	20.3	21.8	22.9	23.3	23.3	22.5
Alabama	19.6	20.8	21.3	22.6	23.6	23.7	23.4	22.6
Arkansas	21.8	21.7	21.3	22.7	23.7	23.9	23.8	23.1
Florida	23.3	24.2	25.1	27.2	28.6	28.8	29.0	28.1
Georgia	15.9	17.0	16.6	17.5	18.3	18.5	18.4	17.3
Kentucky	18.8	19.2	19.5	20.8	21.2	21.4	21.2	20.2
Louisiana	19.4	20.1	20.5	22.9	24.9	26.5	26.9	26.3
Mississippi	21.0	22.5	22.4	24.1	25.4	26.7	27.0	25.1
North Carolina	17.5	17.4	17.3	18.1	19.4	19.6	19.4	19.3
South Carolina	15.1	15.9	16.3	18.6	19.4	20.2	19.8	19.7
Tennessee	18.7	19.4	19.9	21.1	21.7	22.1	21.6	20.6
Virginia	14.9	15.8	15.9	17.1	17.9	18.3	18.5	18.0
West Virginia	20.5	21.3	20.5	21.7	22.5	23.7	23.9	23.1
Southwest	16.4	16.8	17.3	19.4	21.1	21.9	22.3	21.0
Arizona	19.7	19.6	19.3	20.4	21.7	22.2	22.6	21.1
New Mexico	14.7	14.6	14.6	16.1	17.2	17.4	17.5	16.9
Oklahoma	19.1	19.7	20.0	22.4	24.3	25.0	25.5	24.0
Texas	15.4	15.9	16.6	19.0	20.8	21.6	22.0	20.9
Rocky Mountains	13.9	14.6	15.1	16.2	17.2	17.4	17.2	16.4
Colorado	13.4	14.0	14.6	15.8	16.9	17.4	17.1	16.5
Idaho	15.1	15.9	15.9	17.3	18.3	18.3	18.6	17.7
Montana	17.1	17.9	18.4	19.1	18.9	19.1	19.1	18.4
Utah	12.4	13.2	13.8	14.7	16.1	16.1	15.8	14.7
Wyoming	14.3	15.2	16.2	17.2	18.1	17.3	17.1	16.1
Far West	16.1	16.2	17.0	18.2	19.2	19.7	20.1	19.3
Alaska	6.5	6.9	7.1	7.8	8.7	9.0	9.3	9.1
California	16.5	16.5	17.5	18.9	20.1	20.7	21.1	20.1
Hawaii	12.1	12.6	12.8	13.0	13.6	13.4	14.3	14.1
Nevada	16.3	16.7	18.1	19.1	20.2	20.9	21.7	20.7
Oregon	17.2	17.5	17.4	18.3	19.0	19.4	19.5	19.1
Washington	15.0	15.3	15.2	15.8	16.3	16.5	17.0	16.7

[1]Data are shown for Bureau of Economic Analysis (BEA) regions that are constructed to show economically interdependent states. These BEA geographic regions differ from Bureau of the Census geographic divisions shown in some *Health, United States* tables. See Appendix II, Geographic region and division.

NOTE: Some numbers have been revised and differ from the previous edition of *Health, United States*.

SOURCE: Centers for Medicare & Medicaid Services, Office of the Actuary, National Health Statistics Group, National Health Accounts, State Health Expenditures. www.cms.hhs.gov/statistics/nhe/state-estimates-residence/.

Table 146. Medicaid expenditures as a percent of total personal health care expenditures by geographic region and State: United States, 1991–98

[Data are compiled from various sources by the Centers for Medicare & Medicaid Services]

Geographic region and State[1]	1991	1992	1993	1994	1995	1996	1997	1998
					Percent			
United States	13.2	13.7	14.7	15.2	15.6	15.9	15.7	15.7
New England	17.0	16.7	16.6	18.0	18.8	17.8	18.6	18.8
Connecticut	15.7	14.8	15.9	17.0	18.0	17.7	18.5	17.5
Maine	18.3	19.0	21.3	22.1	21.1	21.1	21.9	21.1
Massachusetts	18.1	17.3	16.2	18.0	19.2	17.3	18.3	19.3
New Hampshire	11.7	12.4	13.2	14.5	15.6	15.1	15.7	15.6
Rhode Island	18.6	21.5	20.9	21.2	20.7	20.6	21.4	21.6
Vermont	15.6	15.2	15.6	16.7	17.0	17.6	17.3	18.0
Mideast	18.1	18.5	19.3	20.1	21.0	21.7	21.5	22.2
Delaware	10.2	10.4	11.0	11.4	12.7	14.3	12.6	12.5
District of Columbia	19.2	18.5	20.5	21.7	20.9	20.9	22.5	20.5
Maryland	11.7	12.2	12.5	13.2	13.5	13.5	13.8	12.7
New Jersey	13.1	12.3	13.6	13.9	14.0	13.9	14.6	14.0
New York	26.4	26.5	27.5	28.4	29.8	30.7	29.7	31.5
Pennsylvania	10.4	12.3	12.0	13.3	14.0	15.4	16.1	16.3
Great Lakes	12.2	13.3	14.4	14.3	14.4	14.8	14.6	14.5
Illinois	9.1	11.8	13.2	13.5	14.2	15.1	15.1	14.8
Indiana	14.0	14.9	16.4	14.0	12.0	13.2	12.1	12.0
Michigan	12.2	12.6	14.2	14.6	15.0	15.1	15.3	14.9
Ohio	14.0	14.5	15.0	15.2	15.6	15.4	15.4	15.6
Wisconsin	14.1	14.0	14.0	14.0	13.7	13.6	13.5	13.4
Plains	12.1	13.0	13.4	13.8	13.9	13.9	13.8	14.3
Iowa	11.9	12.0	12.5	12.8	12.8	13.0	12.8	15.4
Kansas	9.7	10.3	11.3	11.4	10.7	10.7	10.8	10.8
Minnesota	15.5	15.2	16.0	16.7	16.9	16.5	15.4	15.4
Missouri	10.3	13.0	12.7	13.2	13.6	13.5	14.3	14.4
Nebraska	11.4	11.8	12.9	12.8	12.6	13.2	13.4	14.4
North Dakota	14.9	14.1	14.5	14.0	13.6	14.3	14.2	13.8
South Dakota	12.7	13.0	13.7	13.8	13.7	13.8	13.1	13.4
Southeast	11.7	12.2	13.4	14.0	14.4	14.2	14.1	14.0
Alabama	8.8	10.1	10.8	11.5	12.2	12.7	13.1	13.0
Arkansas	13.6	14.9	15.4	15.3	15.5	15.6	15.3	15.5
Florida	8.5	9.1	9.9	10.2	10.6	10.4	10.7	10.4
Georgia	12.1	11.8	12.8	14.0	13.8	13.5	12.8	12.2
Kentucky	13.8	15.4	16.2	16.6	16.1	16.6	17.7	16.9
Louisiana	17.8	17.7	22.1	24.3	23.1	20.0	18.9	19.1
Mississippi	14.8	14.7	15.4	16.4	16.8	16.8	16.8	15.8
North Carolina	12.9	13.3	14.3	14.8	16.7	17.3	17.2	16.9
South Carolina	14.8	15.3	15.9	16.5	16.7	16.6	16.0	16.6
Tennessee	12.6	13.9	14.1	15.6	17.1	16.3	16.4	17.4
Virginia	8.9	9.0	9.8	9.8	10.1	10.1	10.2	9.9
West Virginia	15.3	17.5	19.7	19.5	18.6	17.7	17.0	17.3
Southwest	11.1	12.1	13.0	13.7	13.5	13.6	13.2	12.6
Arizona	8.6	11.0	11.3	12.0	11.8	12.2	12.2	12.0
New Mexico	12.1	13.1	14.3	15.5	16.5	18.3	17.9	17.7
Oklahoma	12.3	12.5	12.2	11.2	11.0	10.9	10.9	11.8
Texas	11.4	12.2	13.4	14.3	14.1	14.0	13.5	12.5
Rocky Mountains	10.2	10.9	11.4	11.8	11.8	12.2	11.9	11.9
Colorado	9.1	10.1	10.5	11.1	11.3	11.6	11.5	11.4
Idaho	10.7	11.1	11.3	11.3	11.3	12.1	12.2	12.1
Montana	13.5	13.7	15.2	15.2	14.4	15.4	14.3	13.8
Utah	10.8	11.3	11.7	11.8	11.8	12.0	11.4	11.8
Wyoming	10.1	11.3	11.8	12.7	12.6	12.9	12.7	12.3
Far West	10.9	10.9	12.4	12.8	13.3	14.3	14.0	13.3
Alaska	13.8	14.7	17.3	16.3	15.9	17.1	17.5	16.9
California	10.8	10.7	12.3	12.6	12.9	14.1	13.7	12.7
Hawaii	9.1	8.7	10.0	12.5	16.0	13.9	13.4	14.2
Nevada	7.7	8.7	9.2	8.7	9.2	9.0	9.0	9.1
Oregon	10.4	10.8	11.8	13.2	14.8	15.2	14.5	15.3
Washington	12.9	13.1	14.3	14.8	15.3	16.3	16.3	16.2

[1]Data are shown for Bureau of Economic Analysis (BEA) regions that are constructed to show economically interdependent states. These BEA geographic regions differ from Bureau of the Census geographic divisions shown in some *Health, United States* tables. See Appendix II, Geographic region and division.

NOTE: Some numbers have been revised and differ from the previous edition of *Health, United States*.

SOURCE: Centers for Medicare & Medicaid Services, Office of the Actuary, National Health Statistics Group, National Health Accounts, State Health Expenditures. www.cms.hhs.gov/statistics/nhe/state-estimates-residence/.

Table 147 (page 1 of 2). State mental health agency per capita expenditures for mental health services and average annual percent change by geographic region and State: United States, selected fiscal years 1981–2001

[Data are based on reporting by State mental health agencies]

Geographic region and State[1]	1981	1983	1985	1987	1990	1993	1997	2001	1981–90	1990–2001
					Amount per capita				Average annual percent change	
United States	$ 27	$31	$35	$ 38	$ 48	$ 54	$ 64	$ 81	6.6	4.9
New England:										
Connecticut[2]	32	39	44	56	73	82	99	129	9.6	5.3
Maine	25	32	36	42	67	70	88	107	11.6	4.3
Massachusetts	32	36	46	62	84	83	90	107	11.3	2.2
New Hampshire	35	39	42	36	63	78	99	112	6.7	5.4
Rhode Island[2]	36	32	35	41	50	61	63	88	3.7	5.3
Vermont	32	40	44	44	54	74	92	130	6.0	8.3
Mideast:										
Delaware[2]	44	51	46	41	55	56	73	93	2.5	4.9
District of Columbia[3]	- - -	23	28	130	268	315	337	398	- - -	3.7
Maryland	33	37	40	49	61	64	76	127	7.1	6.9
New Jersey	26	31	36	43	57	68	69	90	9.1	4.2
New York.	67	74	90	99	118	131	113	176	6.5	3.7
Pennsylvania[4]	41	47	52	50	57	68	68	152	3.7	9.3
Great Lakes:										
Illinois	18	21	24	25	34	36	51	64	7.3	5.9
Indiana	19	23	27	31	47	39	40	65	10.6	3.0
Michigan	33	39	49	61	74	75	87	90	9.4	1.8
Ohio	25	29	30	34	41	47	52	61	5.7	3.7
Wisconsin	22	27	28	31	37	35	44	72	5.9	6.2
Plains:										
Iowa	8	10	11	12	17	13	29	73	8.7	14.2
Kansas	18	22	27	28	35	48	59	60	7.7	5.0
Minnesota[5]	17	30	32	42	54	69	87	105	8.8	6.2
Missouri.	24	25	28	32	35	41	56	60	4.3	5.0
Nebraska.	17	19	21	21	29	34	39	51	6.1	5.3
North Dakota	39	42	36	42	40	43	48	79	0.3	6.4
South Dakota.	17	21	22	27	25	47	54	61	4.4	8.4
Southeast:										
Alabama	20	24	28	29	38	43	47	57	7.4	3.8
Arkansas[4]	17	20	24	24	26	30	30	28	4.8	0.7
Florida[4]	20	23	26	25	37	31	44	35	7.1	−0.5
Georgia.	25	26	23	32	51	49	47	46	8.2	−0.9
Kentucky	15	17	19	23	23	25	35	49	4.9	7.1
Louisiana.	19	23	26	25	28	39	43	45	4.4	4.4
Mississippi.	14	16	24	22	34	41	56	87	10.4	8.9
North Carolina	24	29	38	41	46	50	62	76	7.5	4.7
South Carolina	31	33	33	45	51	56	64	74	5.7	3.4
Tennessee.	18	20	23	24	29	37	23	69	5.4	8.2
Virginia	23	29	32	35	45	40	49	65	7.7	3.4
West Virginia	20	20	22	23	24	22	23	26	2.0	0.7
Southwest:										
Arizona	10	10	12	16	27	60	68	89	11.7	11.5
New Mexico[4]	24	25	25	24	23	24	31	33	−0.5	3.3
Oklahoma	22	33	31	30	36	38	41	39	5.6	0.7
Texas	13	16	17	19	23	31	39	38	6.5	4.7
Rocky Mountains:										
Colorado	24	25	28	30	34	41	57	64	3.9	5.9
Idaho	13	15	15	17	20	26	29	46	4.9	7.9
Montana	25	28	29	28	28	34	93	124	1.3	14.5
Utah[4]	13	16	17	19	21	25	28	33	5.5	4.2
Wyoming	23	28	31	30	35	42	43	61	4.8	5.2

See notes at end of table.

Table 147 (page 2 of 2). State mental health agency per capita expenditures for mental health services and average annual percent change by geographic region and State: United States, selected fiscal years 1981–2001

[Data are based on reporting by State mental health agencies]

Geographic region and State[1]	1981	1983	1985	1987	1990	1993	1997	2001	1981–90	1990–2001
	Amount per capita								Average annual percent change	
Far West:										
Alaska[4]	38	41	45	50	72	86	79	81	7.4	1.1
California	28	29	34	30	42	50	58	92	4.6	7.4
Hawaii	19	22	23	26	38	71	85	175	8.0	14.9
Nevada	22	25	26	28	33	32	45	57	4.6	5.1
Oregon	21	21	25	28	41	60	68	97	7.7	8.1
Washington	18	24	30	37	43	66	79	88	10.2	6.7

- - - Data not available.

[1]Data are shown for Bureau of Economic Analysis (BEA) regions that are constructed to show economically interdependent states. These BEA geographic divisions differ from Bureau of the Census geographic divisions shown in some *Health, United States* tables. See Appendix II, Geographic region and division.
[2]In 2001 children's mental health expenditures were not included.
[3]Transfer of St. Elizabeths Hospital from the National Institute of Mental Health to the District of Columbia Office of Mental Health took place over the years 1985–93.
[4]In 2001 Medicaid revenues for community programs were not included.
[5]Data for 1981 not comparable with later years' data for Minnesota. Average annual percent change is for 1983–90.

NOTES: Expenditures are for mental illness, excluding mental retardation and substance abuse. Starting in 1990 data for Puerto Rico, and starting in 1993 data for Guam are included in the U.S. total. In 2001, 20 states included funds for mental health services in jails or prisons and twelve states included some part of publicly supported housing expenses for adults and children with mental illness. State data omissions and inclusions are likely to be consistent across years.

SOURCES: National Association of State Mental Health Program Directors and the National Association of State Mental Health Program Directors Research Institute, Inc.: Final Report: Funding sources and expenditures of State mental health agencies: Revenue/expenditure study results, fiscal year 1990. Nov. 1992; Supplemental report fiscal year 1993. March 1996; Fiscal year 1997: Final report. July 1999; Fiscal year 2001: Final report. April 2003; Website: www.nri-inc.org.

Table 148 (page 1 of 2). Medicare enrollees, enrollees in managed care, payments per enrollee, and short-stay hospital utilization by geographic region and State: United States, 1994 and 2000

[Data are compiled by the Centers for Medicare & Medicaid Services]

Geographic division and State[1]	Enrollment in thousands[2]	Percent of enrollees in managed care[3]		Payments per fee-for-service enrollee		Short-stay hospital utilization			
						Discharges per 1,000 enrollees[4]		Average length of stay in days[4]	
	2000	1994	2000	1994	2000	1994	2000	1994	2000
United States[5].............	38,782	7.9	17.8	$4,375	$5,423	345	368	7.5	6.0
New England:									
Connecticut..............	518	2.6	20.3	4,426	5,926	287	243	8.1	6.2
Maine.................	216	0.1	0.9	3,464	4,554	322	324	7.6	5.6
Massachusetts...........	961	6.1	24.7	5,147	6,235	350	269	7.6	5.7
New Hampshire..........	169	0.2	1.6	3,414	4,382	281	279	7.6	5.6
Rhode Island............	170	7.0	33.1	4,148	5,687	312	222	8.1	6.2
Vermont...............	89	0.1	0.2	3,182	4,533	283	296	7.6	5.7
Mideast:									
Delaware...............	115	0.2	4.9	4,712	5,449	326	321	8.1	6.4
District of Columbia	75	3.9	9.2	5,655	6,761	376	369	10.1	7.9
Maryland...............	646	1.4	10.8	4,997	6,385	362	339	7.5	5.8
New Jersey.............	1,212	2.6	14.2	4,531	6,554	354	318	10.2	7.5
New York...............	2,695	6.2	18.3	4,855	6,392	334	290	11.2	8.2
Pennsylvania............	2,091	3.3	28.4	5,212	5,883	379	296	8.0	6.1
Great Lakes:									
Illinois................	1,626	5.5	11.7	4,324	5,352	374	360	7.3	5.7
Indiana................	848	2.6	4.1	3,945	4,752	345	344	6.9	5.7
Michigan...............	1,402	0.7	5.9	4,307	5,596	328	334	7.6	6.1
Ohio..................	1,706	2.4	17.4	3,982	5,228	350	318	7.1	5.6
Wisconsin..............	776	2.0	6.0	3,246	4,316	310	310	6.8	5.4
Plains:									
Iowa..................	475	3.1	3.7	3,080	4,315	322	347	6.6	5.4
Kansas................	386	3.3	7.9	3,847	4,822	348	350	6.5	5.5
Minnesota..............	655	19.6	13.3	3,394	4,195	334	297	5.7	5.0
Missouri................	859	3.4	15.6	4,191	4,976	349	329	7.3	5.7
Nebraska...............	254	2.2	4.2	2,926	4,269	281	300	6.3	5.2
North Dakota............	102	0.6	0.7	3,218	4,073	327	333	6.3	5.1
South Dakota............	118	0.1	0.4	2,952	4,041	356	352	6.1	5.2
Southeast:									
Alabama...............	686	0.8	8.7	4,454	5,140	413	403	7.0	5.5
Arkansas...............	434	0.2	4.3	3,719	4,774	366	378	7.0	5.9
Florida................	2,827	13.8	26.8	5,027	6,190	326	268	7.1	5.8
Georgia................	928	0.4	6.2	4,402	5,065	378	348	6.9	5.8
Kentucky...............	618	2.3	5.5	3,862	4,764	396	399	7.2	5.6
Louisiana...............	600	0.4	17.9	5,468	6,657	399	381	7.2	5.9
Mississippi..............	419	0.1	1.5	4,189	5,419	423	458	7.4	6.4
North Carolina...........	1,131	0.5	4.2	3,465	4,718	314	352	8.0	6.0
South Carolina...........	570	0.1	0.3	3,777	5,029	319	379	8.3	6.2
Tennessee..............	830	0.3	5.9	4,441	5,181	375	367	7.1	5.9
Virginia................	896	1.5	3.9	3,748	4,648	348	339	7.3	6.1
West Virginia............	338	8.3	7.5	3,798	4,853	420	402	7.1	5.8
Southwest:									
Arizona................	676	24.8	35.8	4,442	4,656	292	196	5.9	5.0
New Mexico.............	234	13.6	19.0	3,110	3,993	301	230	6.0	5.2
Oklahoma..............	507	2.5	10.7	4,098	5,266	355	370	7.0	5.8
Texas	2,268	4.1	17.4	4,703	6,003	333	320	7.2	5.9
Rocky Mountains:									
Colorado...............	470	17.2	34.5	3,935	4,790	302	200	6.0	5.0
Idaho	167	2.5	10.3	3,045	4,251	274	287	5.2	4.6
Montana...............	137	0.4	0.4	3,114	4,097	306	324	5.9	4.8
Utah..................	209	9.4	3.3	3,443	4,072	238	245	5.4	4.8
Wyoming...............	66	3.3	2.6	3,537	4,408	315	335	5.6	5.0

See footnotes at end of table.

Table 148 (page 2 of 2). Medicare enrollees, enrollees in managed care, payments per enrollee, and short-stay hospital utilization by geographic region and State: United States, 1994 and 2000

[Data are compiled by the Centers for Medicare & Medicaid Services]

Geographic division and State[1]	Enrollment in thousands[2]	Percent of enrollees in managed care[3]		Payments per fee-for-service enrollee		Short-stay hospital utilization			
						Discharges per 1,000 enrollees[4]		Average length of stay in days[4]	
	2000	1994	2000	1994	2000	1994	2000	1994	2000
Far West:									
Alaska.................	42	0.6	0.7	3,687	5,003	269	305	6.3	5.8
California...............	3,922	30.0	40.4	5,219	5,992	366	193	6.1	6.0
Hawaii.................	168	29.8	32.1	3,069	3,771	301	153	9.1	8.0
Nevada................	246	19.0	33.1	4,306	4,960	291	191	7.0	6.0
Oregon................	496	27.7	37.5	3,285	4,274	305	190	5.2	4.6
Washington	736	12.5	24.8	3,401	4,463	269	207	5.3	4.9

[1]Data are shown for Bureau of Economic Analysis (BEA) regions that are constructed to show economically interdependent States. These BEA geographic regions differ from Bureau of the Census geographic divisions shown in some *Health, United States* tables.

[2]Total persons enrolled in hospital insurance, supplementary medical insurance, or both, as of July 1. Includes fee-for-service and managed care enrollees.

[3]Includes enrollees in Medicare-approved managed care organizations.

[4]Data are for fee-for-service enrollees only.

[5]Includes residents of any of the 50 States and the District of Columbia. Excludes Puerto Rico, Guam, Virgin Islands, residence unknown, foreign countries, and other outlying areas not shown separately.

NOTES: The distribution of enrollment by State and type of delivery (that is, fee-for-service and managed care) and program payments per fee-for-service enrollee are based on the enrollment and claims information for a 5-percent sample of Medicare enrollees. The short-stay hospital utilization data are based on the claims for a 20-percent sample of Medicare enrollees. Figures may not sum to totals due to rounding. Data for additional years are available (see Appendix III).

SOURCE: Centers for Medicare & Medicaid Services, Office of Research, Development, and Information. Health Care Financing Review: Medicare and Medicaid Statistical Supplements 1996; 2002. Website: www.cms.hhs.gov/review/supp/.

Table 149 (page 1 of 2). Medicaid recipients, recipients in managed care, payments per recipient, and recipients per 100 persons below the poverty level by geographic region and State: United States, selected fiscal years 1989–2000

[Data are compiled from Medicaid administrative records by the Centers for Medicare & Medicaid Services]

Geographic region and State[1]	Recipients in thousands		Percent of recipients in managed care		Payments per recipient			Recipients per 100 persons below the poverty level	
	1996	2000[2]	1996	2000	1990	1996	2000[2]	1989–90	1999–2000
United States	36,118	42,763	40	56	$ 2,568	$3,369	$3,936	75	131
New England:									
Connecticut	329	420	61	72	4,829	6,179	6,762	167	184
Maine	167	192	1	35	3,248	4,321	6,820	88	155
Massachusetts[3]	715	1,047	70	64	4,622	5,285	5,153	103	153
New Hampshire	100	97	16	6	5,423	5,496	6,712	53	119
Rhode Island	130	179	63	69	[4]3,778	5,280	5,982	[4]163	187
Vermont	102	139	–	47	2,530	2,954	3,451	108	208
Mideast:									
Delaware.	82	115	78	79	3,004	3,773	4,584	68	147
District of Columbia	143	139	55	66	2,629	4,955	5,715	86	179
Maryland	399	665	64	81	3,300	5,138	5,396	74	170
New Jersey	714	822	43	59	4,054	5,217	5,724	83	128
New York.	3,281	3,420	23	25	5,099	6,811	7,646	95	128
Pennsylvania	1,168	1,492	53	73	2,449	3,993	4,266	88	141
Great Lakes:									
Illinois	1,454	1,516	13	10	2,271	3,689	5,150	69	115
Indiana	594	705	31	67	3,859	4,130	4,224	45	148
Michigan	1,172	1,352	73	100	2,094	2,867	3,611	85	135
Ohio	1,478	1,305	32	21	2,566	3,729	5,434	98	103
Wisconsin	434	577	32	44	3,179	4,384	5,039	95	113
Plains:									
Iowa	308	314	41	90	2,589	3,534	4,707	80	149
Kansas	251	263	32	56	2,524	3,425	4,670	71	94
Minnesota	455	559	33	63	3,709	5,342	5,857	70	178
Missouri.	636	890	35	40	2,002	3,171	3,673	63	157
Nebraska.	191	229	27	77	2,595	3,548	4,185	61	136
North Dakota	61	61	55	55	3,955	4,889	5,852	58	87
South Dakota.	77	102	65	93	3,368	4,114	3,935	51	155
Southeast:									
Alabama	546	619	11	60	1,731	2,675	3,860	43	88
Arkansas.	363	489	39	57	2,267	3,375	3,086	55	113
Florida.	1,638	2,360	64	60	2,273	2,851	3,114	55	136
Georgia.	1,185	1,290	32	96	3,190	2,604	2,774	64	136
Kentucky	641	771	53	81	2,089	3,014	3,780	81	158
Louisiana.	778	761	6	6	2,247	3,154	3,456	58	95
Mississippi.	510	605	7	39	1,354	2,633	2,987	67	139
North Carolina	1,130	1,209	37	68	2,531	3,255	3,996	66	122
South Carolina.	503	685	1	6	2,343	3,026	3,900	52	157
Tennessee.	1,409	1,568	100	100	1,896	2,049	2,226	67	211
Virginia	623	627	68	59	2,596	2,849	3,960	53	115
West Virginia	395	335	30	35	1,443	2,855	4,154	80	129
Southwest:									
Arizona[5]	528	681	86	92	- - -	- - -	3,100	- - -	113
New Mexico.	318	376	45	64	2,120	2,757	3,325	39	110
Oklahoma	358	507	19	69	2,516	2,852	3,163	56	106
Texas	2,572	2,603	4	34	1,928	2,672	3,487	47	85
Rocky Mountains:									
Colorado	271	381	80	90	2,705	3,815	4,747	45	107
Idaho	119	131	37	30	2,973	3,402	4,530	36	75
Montana	101	104	59	61	2,793	3,478	4,173	47	73
Utah	152	224	82	90	2,279	2,775	4,277	72	132
Wyoming.	51	46	1	–	2,036	3,571	4,609	[4]59	84

See footnotes at end of table.

Table 149 (page 2 of 2). Medicaid recipients, recipients in managed care, payments per recipient, and recipients per 100 persons below the poverty level by geographic region and State: United States, selected fiscal years 1989–2000

[Data are compiled from Medicaid administrative records by the Centers for Medicare & Medicaid Services]

Geographic region and State[1]	Recipients in thousands		Percent of recipients in managed care		Payments per recipient			Recipients per 100 persons below the poverty level	
	1996	2000[2]	1996	2000	1990	1996	2000[2]	1989–90	1999–2000
Far West:									
Alaska.................	69	96	–	–	3,562	4,027	4,876	70	180
California...............	5,107	7,915	23	50	1,795	2,178	2,155	88	162
Hawaii.................	41	204	80	74	2,252	6,574	2,626	73	83
Nevada...............	109	138	41	39	3,161	3,361	3,733	37	70
Oregon	450	542	91	83	2,283	2,915	3,135	74	132
Washington :...........	621	895	100	100	2,128	2,242	2,717	98	155

– Quantity zero.

- - - Data not available.

[1]Data are shown for Bureau of Economic Analysis (BEA) regions that are constructed to show economically interdependent States. These BEA geographic regions differ from Bureau of the Census geographic divisions shown in some *Health, United States* tables. See Appendix II, Geographic region and division.

[2]Prior to 1998 recipient counts exclude those individuals who only received coverage under prepaid health care and for whom no direct vendor payments were made during the year. Prior to 1998 vendor payments exclude payments to health maintenance organizations and other prepaid health plans ($19.3 billion in 1998 and $18 billion in 1997). The total number of persons who were Medicaid eligible and enrolled was 41.4 million in 1998, 41.6 million in 1997, and 41.2 million in 1996 (CMS Medicaid Statistics, Program and Financial Statistics FY1996, FY1997, and FY1998, unpublished).

[3]Data for categorically eligible blind Medicaid recipients in 1990 are estimated by the Bureau of Data Management and Strategy, CMS.

[4]Data are estimated by the Bureau of Data Management and Strategy, CMS.

[5]Arizona has a limited Medicaid program, with care financed largely on a capitated basis.

NOTES: Payments exclude disproportionate share hospital payments ($15 billion in 1999 and 2000). Data for additional years are available (see Appendix III).

SOURCES: Centers for Medicare & Medicaid Services, Office of Information Services, Enterprise Databases Group, Division of Information Distribution, Medicaid Data System; Department of Commerce, Bureau of the Census, Housing and Household Economic Statistics Division.

Table 150. Persons enrolled in health maintenance organizations (HMOs) by geographic region and State: United States, selected years 1980–2002

[Data are based on a census of health maintenance organizations]

Geographic region and State[1]	2002	1980	1985	1990	1995	1999	2000	2001	2002
	Number in thousands	Percent of population							
United States[2]	76,121	4.0	7.9	13.5	19.4	30.1	30.0	27.9	26.4
New England:									
Connecticut	1,311	2.4	7.1	19.9	21.2	38.8	44.6	39.7	38.3
Maine	308	0.4	0.3	2.6	7.0	20.2	22.3	27.9	23.9
Massachusetts	2,702	2.9	13.7	26.5	39.0	52.9	53.0	44.3	42.4
New Hampshire	381	1.2	5.6	9.6	18.5	34.9	33.7	39.3	30.3
Rhode Island	369	3.7	9.1	20.6	19.6	40.5	38.1	35.0	34.8
Vermont	64	–	–	6.4	12.5	4.0	4.6	4.2	10.5
Mideast:									
Delaware	183	–	3.9	17.5	18.4	45.7	22.0	22.8	23.0
District of Columbia[3]	178	- - -	- - -	- - -	- - -	33.7	35.2	31.0	31.2
Maryland	1,865	2.0	4.8	14.2	29.5	46.0	43.9	38.4	34.7
New Jersey	2,622	2.0	5.6	12.3	14.7	29.5	30.9	31.7	30.9
New York	6,390	5.5	8.0	15.1	26.6	38.2	35.8	35.0	33.6
Pennsylvania	3,838	1.2	5.0	12.5	21.5	33.6	33.9	33.4	31.2
Great Lakes:									
Illinois	2,246	1.9	7.1	12.6	17.2	20.8	21.0	19.2	18.0
Indiana	654	0.5	3.6	6.1	8.3	13.2	12.4	11.7	10.7
Michigan	2,551	2.4	9.9	15.2	20.5	27.0	27.1	26.7	25.5
Ohio	2,461	2.2	6.7	13.3	16.3	25.4	25.1	23.4	21.6
Wisconsin	1,585	8.5	17.8	21.7	24.0	30.9	30.2	29.6	29.3
Plains:									
Iowa	150	0.2	4.8	10.1	4.5	4.9	7.4	6.5	5.1
Kansas	356	–	3.3	7.9	4.7	16.8	17.9	16.1	13.2
Minnesota	1,336	9.9	22.2	16.4	26.5	30.4	29.9	28.2	26.9
Missouri	1,758	2.3	6.0	8.2	18.5	34.2	35.2	31.0	31.2
Nebraska	149	1.1	1.8	5.1	8.6	18.4	11.2	9.9	8.7
North Dakota	2	0.4	2.5	1.7	1.2	2.5	2.5	1.3	0.4
South Dakota	87	–	–	3.3	2.8	6.1	6.7	9.7	11.5
Southeast:									
Alabama	209	0.3	0.9	5.3	7.3	10.0	7.2	6.5	4.7
Arkansas	208	–	0.1	2.2	3.8	12.3	10.4	10.5	7.7
Florida	4,886	1.5	5.6	10.6	18.8	32.9	31.4	29.8	29.8
Georgia	1,275	0.1	2.9	4.8	7.6	16.2	17.4	15.9	15.2
Kentucky	1,294	0.9	1.6	5.7	16.1	32.5	31.5	30.4	31.8
Louisiana	627	0.6	0.9	5.4	7.2	17.7	17.0	15.6	14.0
Mississippi	40	–	–	–	0.7	3.2	1.1	0.9	1.4
North Carolina	1,210	0.6	1.6	4.8	8.3	18.8	17.8	16.3	14.8
South Carolina	324	0.2	1.0	1.9	5.5	10.0	9.9	9.5	8.0
Tennessee	1,066	–	1.8	3.7	12.2	37.7	33.0	33.0	18.6
Virginia	1,142	–	1.1	6.1	7.7	19.6	18.5	16.2	15.9
West Virginia	180	0.7	1.7	3.9	5.8	10.5	10.3	10.9	10.0
Southwest:									
Arizona	1,367	6.0	10.3	16.2	25.8	32.0	30.9	32.4	25.8
New Mexico	531	1.4	2.0	12.7	15.1	38.1	37.7	27.9	29.0
Oklahoma	513	–	2.1	5.5	7.6	14.2	14.7	13.9	14.8
Texas	3,180	0.6	3.4	6.9	12.0	18.6	18.5	17.5	14.9
Rocky Mountains:									
Colorado	1,455	6.9	10.8	20.0	23.3	39.4	39.5	36.4	32.9
Idaho	39	1.2	–	1.8	1.4	6.4	7.9	4.3	2.9
Montana	52	–	–	1.0	2.4	6.6	7.0	7.7	5.8
Utah	726	0.6	8.8	13.9	25.1	35.2	35.3	35.5	32.0
Wyoming	10	–	–	–	–	1.2	1.4	1.7	2.0
Far West:									
Alaska	–	–	–	–	–	–	–	–	–
California	17,420	16.8	22.5	30.7	36.0	52.1	53.5	53.4	50.5
Hawaii	402	15.3	18.1	21.6	21.0	33.7	30.0	31.8	32.8
Nevada	472	–	5.8	8.5	15.9	23.5	23.5	20.4	22.4
Oregon	1,046	12.0	14.0	24.7	40.0	43.3	41.1	35.5	30.1
Washington	1,042	9.4	8.7	14.6	18.7	17.3	15.2	15.3	17.4

– Quantity zero. - - - Data not available.

[1]Data are shown for Bureau of Economic Analysis (BEA) regions that are constructed to show economically interdependent states. These BEA geographic regions differ from Bureau of the Census geographic regions and divisions shown in some *Health, United States* tables. See Appendix II, Geographic region and division.
[2]HMOs in Guam included starting 1994; HMOs in Puerto Rico, starting 1998. In 2002 HMO enrollment in Guam was 34,000 and in Puerto Rico, 1,825,000.
[3]Data for District of Columbia (DC) not included for 1980–96 because data not adjusted for high proportion of enrollees of DC-based HMOs living in Maryland and Virginia.

NOTES: Data for 1980–90 are for pure HMO enrollment at midyear. Data for 1994–2002 are for pure and open-ended enrollment as of January 1. In 1990 open-ended enrollment accounted for 3 percent of HMO enrollment compared with 11 percent in 2002. See Appendix II, Health maintenance organization. Data for additional years are available (see Appendix III).

SOURCE: InterStudy National Health Maintenance Organization Census. The InterStudy Edge, Managed care: A decade in review 1980–1990. The InterStudy Competitive Edge, vols 5–12, 1995–2002. St. Paul, Minnesota (Copyrights 1991, 1995–2002: Used with the permission of InterStudy).

Table 151. Persons under 65 years of age without health insurance coverage by State: United States, selected years 1987–2001

[Data are based on household interviews of a sample of the civilian noninstitutionalized population]

Geographic region and State	2001	1987	1990	1995	1996	1997[1]	1998	1999[2]	2000	2001
	Number in thousands	Percent of population								
United States	40,935	14.4	15.7	17.3	17.6	18.2	18.4	16.2	16.1	16.5
New England:										
Connecticut.	342	7.4	8.0	10.3	12.4	13.8	14.3	10.4	11.3	11.7
Maine	132	9.9	12.6	15.4	13.9	17.1	14.6	12.4	12.8	12.3
Massachusetts.	515	7.0	10.2	12.5	14.1	14.3	11.6	10.4	9.9	9.3
New Hampshire	119	11.4	11.1	11.4	10.9	13.3	12.5	10.3	9.6	11.0
Rhode Island	79	7.8	13.1	15.4	12.0	12.3	7.6	7.1	8.7	9.0
Vermont	58	11.1	10.5	14.5	12.4	10.8	11.0	12.3	9.9	10.8
Mideast:										
Delaware.	73	11.9	15.6	17.2	14.8	15.1	17.1	11.1	10.6	10.5
District of Columbia	70	17.1	21.3	19.3	16.8	18.3	19.2	15.7	16.0	14.2
Maryland.	650	10.9	14.2	17.2	12.8	14.9	18.9	12.5	11.8	13.8
New Jersey	1,100	9.0	11.3	16.2	19.1	18.4	18.0	13.3	14.0	15.1
New York	2,898	13.1	13.6	17.2	19.1	20.0	19.7	17.1	18.5	17.7
Pennsylvania.	1,109	8.4	11.8	11.6	11.1	11.7	12.1	9.7	10.0	10.6
Great Lakes:										
Illinois.	1,669	10.9	12.2	12.3	12.5	13.9	16.6	14.5	15.5	15.3
Indiana	708	15.2	12.3	14.6	12.2	12.8	16.1	10.6	12.8	13.6
Michigan	1,022	9.4	10.4	11.0	10.1	13.2	14.9	11.2	10.3	11.7
Ohio	1,248	10.3	11.7	13.5	13.1	13.1	11.7	11.6	12.8	12.8
Wisconsin	406	7.4	7.8	8.1	9.5	9.1	13.2	11.0	8.5	8.8
Plains:										
Iowa	215	8.3	9.4	12.9	13.1	13.6	10.9	8.7	10.3	8.7
Kansas	301	11.6	12.3	14.2	13.1	13.6	12.2	13.3	12.6	13.5
Minnesota	391	7.4	9.9	9.0	11.2	10.2	10.3	8.1	9.0	8.8
Missouri	564	11.8	14.2	16.7	15.3	14.7	12.1	7.8	10.7	11.6
Nebraska	160	11.0	9.6	10.3	12.9	12.2	10.2	11.5	10.3	10.8
North Dakota	60	8.7	7.2	9.4	11.2	11.7	16.5	13.4	13.2	11.2
South Dakota	69	15.4	13.5	10.8	11.1	13.7	16.3	12.3	12.9	10.9
Southeast:										
Alabama	573	17.9	19.3	15.7	14.9	18.0	19.5	15.1	14.9	14.9
Arkansas.	425	23.5	20.1	20.5	24.8	28.1	21.7	16.6	16.7	18.8
Florida	2,822	20.5	21.5	21.7	22.7	23.6	21.1	21.5	21.0	20.6
Georgia.	1,371	14.5	17.1	20.0	19.6	19.3	19.4	16.5	15.7	18.1
Kentucky.	491	16.8	15.1	16.8	17.6	16.9	16.0	14.9	15.3	14.1
Louisiana	839	18.9	22.1	22.9	23.2	22.0	21.3	24.1	20.4	21.7
Mississippi.	458	19.3	22.1	22.3	20.5	22.6	22.9	17.9	15.5	18.4
North Carolina	1,163	15.0	15.6	16.4	18.0	17.6	17.0	16.2	15.3	16.3
South Carolina.	491	12.4	18.1	16.0	18.7	18.7	17.4	18.0	13.7	14.1
Tennessee.	640	16.6	15.4	16.4	17.1	15.2	14.3	11.4	12.2	12.6
Virginia	765	11.4	17.3	15.2	13.8	14.1	15.8	14.8	13.0	12.2
West Virginia	233	15.9	16.0	18.3	17.9	20.5	20.8	18.7	16.5	15.8
Southwest:										
Arizona.	943	20.4	18.1	23.2	27.5	27.7	26.9	22.7	18.7	20.0
New Mexico	372	25.3	24.6	28.3	24.7	25.2	24.0	27.6	27.2	23.9
Oklahoma	619	20.4	21.2	22.1	19.6	20.2	21.2	19.1	21.9	20.9
Texas	4,920	23.0	23.2	27.0	26.7	26.7	26.9	24.4	25.4	25.9
Rocky Mountains:										
Colorado.	687	15.6	16.3	15.9	17.8	16.4	16.4	16.6	15.8	17.2
Idaho	209	17.2	16.9	15.9	18.6	19.9	19.7	20.6	17.3	17.9
Montana	121	17.3	15.7	14.8	15.4	22.0	21.9	20.1	19.2	15.9
Utah	335	13.4	9.8	13.0	13.3	14.8	15.1	14.2	13.6	16.0
Wyoming.	77	12.7	13.7	17.6	15.0	17.4	18.8	17.0	17.8	18.1
Far West:										
Alaska	99	17.0	16.1	12.9	13.8	18.9	17.9	19.2	20.0	16.6
California.	6,659	18.5	21.1	22.6	22.2	23.7	24.4	21.0	20.4	21.3
Hawaii	114	8.5	7.8	9.9	9.7	8.7	11.3	11.4	10.6	10.8
Nevada.	341	17.4	18.3	21.1	17.6	19.9	23.7	20.2	18.8	17.9
Oregon	442	17.2	14.6	13.9	17.4	14.8	16.0	15.6	14.4	14.2
Washington	772	14.4	12.7	13.7	14.8	12.4	13.4	15.3	15.3	14.8

[1]Beginning with data for 1997, people with no coverage other than access to the Indian Health Service are no longer considered covered by health insurance. The effect of this change on the number uninsured is negligible.
[2]Starting in 1999 estimates reflect the results of follow-up verification questions. In 1999 the use of verification questions decreased the percent uninsured by 1.2 percentage points.

NOTES: Data are shown for Bureau of Economic Analysis (BEA) regions that are constructed to show economically interdependent States. These BEA geographic regions differ from Bureau of the Census geographic divisions shown in some *Health, United States* tables. See Appendix II, Geographic region and division. Methodology and sample size changed in 1992, 1993, 1994, and 2000. See Appendix I, Current Population Survey. Data for additional years are available (see Appendix III).

SOURCES: U.S. Bureau of the Census, Current Population Survey, March; Health insurance historical table 6. Health insurance coverage status and type of coverage by State—people under 65: 1987–2001. www.census.gov/hhes/hlthins/historic/hihistt6.html. Sept. 2, 2002.

Appendix Contents

Appendix I

Data Sources

This report consolidates the most current data on the health of the population of the United States, the availability and use of health resources, and health care expenditures. The information was obtained from the data files and/or published reports of many Federal Government and private and global agencies and organizations. In each case, the sponsoring agency or organization collected data using its own methods and procedures. Therefore, the data in this report vary considerably with respect to source, method of collection, definitions, and reference period.

Although a detailed description and comprehensive evaluation of each data source are beyond the scope of this appendix, users should be aware of the general strengths and weaknesses of the different data collection systems. For example, population-based surveys obtain socioeconomic data, data on family characteristics, and information on the impact of an illness, such as days lost from work or limitation of activity. These data are limited by the amount of information a respondent remembers or is willing to report. A respondent may not know detailed medical information, such as precise diagnoses or the types of operations performed, and therefore cannot report it. Health care providers, such as physicians and hospitals, usually have good diagnostic information but little or no information about the socioeconomic characteristics of individuals or the impact of illnesses on individuals.

The populations covered by different data collection systems may not be the same, and understanding the differences is critical to interpreting the data. Data on vital statistics and national expenditures cover the entire population. Most data on morbidity and utilization of health resources cover only the civilian noninstitutionalized population. Such statistics do not include data for military personnel who are usually young, for institutionalized people who may be any age, or for nursing home residents who are usually old.

All data collection systems are subject to error, and records may be incomplete or contain inaccurate information. People may not remember essential information, a question may not mean the same thing to different respondents, and some

institutions or individuals may not respond at all. It is not always possible to measure the magnitude of these errors or their impact on the data. Where possible, table notes describe the universe and method of data collection, to enable the user to place his or her own evaluation on the data quality.

Some information is collected in more than one survey and estimates of the same statistic may vary among surveys because of different survey methodologies, sampling frames, questionnaires, definitions, and tabulation categories. For example, cigarette use is measured by the National Health Interview Survey, the National Household Survey on Drug Abuse, the Monitoring the Future Survey, and the Youth Risk Behavior Survey using slightly different questions of persons of differing ages, interviewed in different settings (at school versus at home), so estimates will differ.

Overall estimates generally have relatively small sampling errors, but estimates for certain population subgroups may be based on small numbers and have relatively large sampling errors. Numbers of births and deaths from the vital statistics system represent complete counts (except for births in those States where data are based on a 50-percent sample for certain years). Therefore, they are not subject to sampling error. However, when the figures are used for analytical purposes, such as the comparison of rates over a period, the number of events that actually occurred may be considered as one of a large series of possible results that could have arisen under the same circumstances. When the number of events is small and the probability of such an event is rare, considerable caution must be observed in interpreting the conditions described by the figures. Estimates that are unreliable because of large sampling errors or small numbers of events are noted with asterisks in selected tables. The criteria used to designate unreliable estimates are indicated in notes to the applicable tables.

Descriptive summaries of the data sets that follow provide a general overview of study design, methods of data collection, and reliability and validity of the data. The agency or organization that sponsored the data collection is specified. More complete and detailed discussions are in the publications and Web sites listed at the end of each summary. The entries are listed alphabetically by dataset name.

Government Sources

Abortion Surveillance

Centers for Disease Control and Prevention

National Center for Chronic Disease Prevention and Health Promotion

In 1969 CDC's National Center for Chronic Disease Prevention and Health Promotion (NCCDPHP) began abortion surveillance to document the number and characteristics of women obtaining legal induced abortions, monitor unintended pregnancy, and assist efforts to identify and reduce preventable causes of morbidity and mortality associated with abortions. For each year from 1973–97 abortion data from central health agencies have been available from 52 reporting areas: 50 States, the District of Columbia, and New York City. Beginning in 1998, abortion data are available from only 46 States (excluding Alaska, California, New Hampshire, and Oklahoma), the District of Columbia, and New York City. While the total number of legal induced abortions is available for those 48 reporting areas, not all areas collect information on the characteristics of women who obtain abortions. Furthermore the number of areas reporting each characteristic and the number of areas with complete data for each characteristic varies from year to year. For example, in 1999, the number of areas reporting different characteristics ranged from 26 areas reporting Hispanic ethnicity and 37 areas reporting race and marital status to 47 areas reporting age. Reporting area data with more than 15 percent unknown for a given characteristic are excluded from the analysis of that characteristic.

For 48 reporting areas, data concerning the number and characteristics of women who obtain legal induced abortions are provided by central health agencies such as State health departments and the health departments of New York City and the District of Columbia. In general the procedures are reported by the State in which the procedure is performed. However, two reporting areas (the District of Columbia and Wisconsin) report characteristics of abortions only for area/State residents; characteristics for out-of-area/State residents are unavailable.

Between 1989 and 1997, the total number of abortions reported to CDC was about 10 percent less than the total estimated independently by the Alan Guttmacher Institute

(AGI), a not-for-profit organization for reproductive health research, policy analysis, and public education. Beginning in 1998, the total number of abortions reported to CDC was about 33 percent less than the total estimated by AGI. The four reporting areas (the largest of which was California) that did not report abortions to CDC in 1998 accounted for 18 percent of all abortions tallied by AGI's 1995–96 survey. See *Alan Guttmacher Institute Abortion Survey*.

For more information, see Centers for Disease Control and Prevention, CDC Surveillance Summaries, November 2002. *Morbidity and Mortality Weekly Report* 2002;51 (NoSS-9), Abortion Surveillance—United States, 1999; or contact: Director, Division of Reproductive Health, NCCDPHP, CDC, Atlanta, GA 30341; or visit the NCCDPHP surveillance and research Web site at www.cdc.gov/nccdphp/drh/surveil.htm.

Aerometric Information Retrieval System (AIRS)

Environmental Protection Agency

The Environmental Protection Agency's Aerometric Information Retrieval System (AIRS) compiles data on ambient air levels of particulate matter smaller than 10 microns (PM-10), lead, carbon monoxide, sulphur dioxide, nitrogen dioxide, and tropospheric ozone. These pollutants were identified in the Clean Air Act of 1970 and in its 1977 and 1990 amendments because they pose significant threats to public health. The National Ambient Air Quality Standards (NAAQS) define for each pollutant the maximum concentration level (micrograms per cubic meter) that cannot be exceeded during specific time intervals. Data shown in this publication reflect percent of the population living in areas that exceed the NAAQS for a pollutant in a calendar year (such areas are called nonattainment areas) and population data from the U.S. Bureau of the Census. For 1996 and later years, estimates of the population in the year 2000 are used for this calculation.

Nonattainment areas may include single counties, multiple counties, parts of counties, municipalities, or combinations of the preceding jurisdictions. When an area is designated as "nonattainment," it retains this status for 3 years, regardless of annual changes in air quality. Nonattainment areas may also include jurisdictions in which the source of the pollutants is located, even if that jurisdiction meets all NAAQS. The areas monitored may change over time to reflect changes in air quality or the pollutants being monitored.

The EPA's ambient air quality monitoring program is carried out by State and local agencies and consists of three major categories of monitoring stations, State and Local Air Monitoring Stations (SLAMS), National Air Monitoring Stations (NAMS), and Special Purpose Monitoring Stations (SPMS), that measure the criteria pollutants. Additionally, a fourth category of a monitoring station, the Photochemical Assessment Monitoring Stations (PAMS), which measures ozone precursors (approximately 60 volatile hydrocarbons and carbonyl), has been required by the 1990 Amendments to the Clean Air Act.

The SLAMS consist of a network of about 4,000 monitoring stations whose size and distribution is largely determined by the needs of State and local air pollution control agencies to meet their respective State implementation plan requirements. The NAMS (1,080 stations) are a subset of the SLAMS network with emphasis being given to urban and multi-source areas. In effect they are key sites under SLAMS, with emphasis on areas of maximum concentrations and high population density. The SPMS provide for special studies needed by the State and local agencies to support State implementation plans and other air program activities. The SPMS are not permanently established and can be adjusted easily to accommodate changing needs and priorities. The SPMS are used to supplement the fixed monitoring network as circumstances require and resources permit.

For more information, write: Office of Air Quality Planning and Standards, Environmental Protection Agency, Research Triangle Park, NC 27711; or visit the EPA Office of Air Quality Planning and Standards Web site at www.epa.gov/oar/oaqps.

AIDS Surveillance

Centers for Disease Control and Prevention

National Center for HIV, STD, and TB Prevention

Acquired immunodeficiency syndrome (AIDS) surveillance is conducted by health departments in each State, territory, and the District of Columbia. Although surveillance activities range from passive to active, most areas employ multifaceted active surveillance programs, which include four major reporting sources of AIDS information: hospitals and hospital-based physicians, physicians in nonhospital practice, public and private clinics, and medical record systems (death certificates, tumor registries, hospital discharge abstracts, and

communicable disease reports). Using a standard confidential case report form, the health departments collect information that is then transmitted electronically to CDC without personal identifiers.

AIDS surveillance data are used to detect epidemiologic trends, to identify unusual cases requiring followup, and for semiannual publication in the *HIV/AIDS Surveillance Report*. Studies to determine the completeness of reporting of AIDS cases meeting the national surveillance definition suggest reporting at greater than or equal to 90 percent.

Decreases in AIDS incidence and in the number of AIDS deaths, first noted in 1996, have been ascribed to the effect of new treatments, which prevent or delay the onset of AIDS and premature death among HIV-infected persons, and result in an increase in the number of persons living with HIV and AIDS. A growing number of States require confidential reporting of persons with HIV infection and participate in CDC's integrated HIV/AIDS surveillance system that compiles information on the population of persons newly diagnosed and living with HIV infection.

For more information on AIDS surveillance, see: Centers for Disease Control and Prevention. *HIV/AIDS Surveillance Report*, published semiannually; or contact: Chief, Surveillance Branch, Division of HIV/AIDS Prevention— Surveillance and Epidemiology, National Center for HIV, STD, and TB Prevention (NCHSTP), Centers for Disease Control and Prevention, Atlanta, GA 30333; or visit the NCHSTP Web site at www.cdc.gov/nchstp/od/nchstp.html.

Census of Fatal Occupational Injuries (CFOI)

Bureau of Labor Statistics

The Census of Fatal Occupational Injuries (CFOI), administered by the Bureau of Labor Statistics (BLS) in conjunction with participating State agencies, has compiled comprehensive and timely information on fatal work injuries occurring in the 50 States and the District of Columbia since 1992. To compile counts that are as complete as possible, the BLS census uses diverse sources to identify, verify, and profile fatal work injuries. Key information about each workplace fatality (occupation and other worker characteristics, equipment or machinery involved, and circumstances of the event) is obtained by cross-referencing the source records. For a fatality to be included in the census, the decedent must have been employed (that is, working for pay, compensation, or profit) at the time of the event, engaged in a legal work activity, or present at the site of the incident as a requirement of his or her job. These criteria are generally broader than those used by Federal and State agencies administering specific laws and regulations. Fatalities that occur during a person's commute to or from work are excluded from the census counts.

Data for the CFOI are compiled from various Federal, State, and local administrative sources—including death certificates, workers' compensation reports and claims, reports to various regulatory agencies, medical examiner reports, and police reports—as well as news reports. Diverse sources are used because studies have shown that no single source captures all job-related fatalities. Source documents are matched so that each fatality is counted only once. To ensure that a fatality occurred while the decedent was at work, information is verified from two or more independent source documents or from a source document and a followup questionnaire.

The number of occupational fatalities and fatality rates shown in this report are revised, except for the most recent year, and may differ from original data published by CFOI. States have up to 1 year to update their initial published State counts. States may identify additional fatal work injuries after data collection closeout for a reference year. In addition, other fatalities excluded from the published count because of insufficient information to determine work relationship may subsequently be verified as work related. Increases in the published counts based on additional information have averaged less than 100 fatalities per year, or less than 1.5 percent of the total.

For more information, see: Bureau of Labor Statistics, *National Census of Fatal Occupational Injuries, 2001.* Washington, DC. U.S. Department of Labor. August 2002; or visit the CFOI Web site at www.bls.gov/iif/oshcfoi1.htm.

Consumer Price Index (CPI)

Bureau of Labor Statistics

The Consumer Price Index (CPI) is a monthly measure of the average change in the prices paid by urban consumers for a fixed market basket of goods and services. The all-urban index (CPI-U) introduced in 1978 covers residents of metropolitan areas as well as residents of urban parts of nonmetropolitan areas (about 87 percent of the U.S. population in 2000).

In calculating the index, price changes for the various items in each location were averaged together with weights that represent their importance in the spending of all urban consumers. Local data were then combined to obtain a U.S. city average.

The index measures price changes from a designated reference date, 1982–84, which equals 100. An increase of 22 percent, for example, is shown as 122. Change can also be expressed in dollars as follows: the price of a base period "market basket" of goods and services bought by all urban consumers has risen from $100 in 1982–84 to $179.9 in 2002.

The current revision of the CPI, completed in 2000, reflects spending patterns based on the Survey of Consumer Expenditures from 1993 to 1995, the 1990 Census of Population, and the ongoing Point-of-Purchase Survey. Using an improved sample design, prices for the goods and services required to calculate the index are collected in urban areas throughout the country and from retail and service establishments. Data on rents are collected from tenants of rented housing and residents of owner-occupied housing units. Food, fuels, and other goods and services are priced monthly in urban locations. Price information is obtained through visits or calls by trained BLS field representatives using computer-assisted telephone interviews.

The earlier 1987 revision changed the treatment of health insurance in the cost-weight definitions for medical care items. This change has no effect on the final index result but provides a clearer picture of the role of health insurance in the CPI. As part of the revision, three new indexes have been created by separating previously combined items, for example, eye care from other professional services and inpatient and outpatient treatment from other hospital and medical care services.

Effective January 1997 the hospital index was restructured by combining the three categories—room, inpatient services, and outpatient services—into one category, hospital services. Differentiation between inpatient and outpatient and among service types are all combined under this broad category. In addition new procedures for hospital data collection identify a payor, diagnosis, and the payor's reimbursement arrangement from selected hospital bills.

A new geographic sample and item structure were introduced in January 1998 and expenditure weights were updated to 1993–95. Pricing of a new housing sample using computer-assisted data collection started in June 1998. In January 1999 the index was rebased from the 1982–84 time period to 1993–95.

For more information, see: Bureau of Labor Statistics, *Handbook of Methods*, BLS Bulletin 2490, U.S. Department of Labor, Washington, DC. April 1997; Revising the Consumer Price Index, *Monthly Labor Review*, Dec 1996. U.S. Department of Labor, Bureau of Labor Statistics, Washington, DC; IK Ford and D Ginsburg, Medical Care and the Consumer Price Index, National Bureau of Economic Research, Research Studies in Income and Wealth vol. 62; or visit the BLS/CPI Web site at www.bls.gov/cpi/home.htm.

Current Population Survey (CPS)

Bureau of the Census

Bureau of Labor Statistics

The Current Population Survey (CPS) is a household sample survey of the civilian noninstitutionalized population conducted monthly by the U.S. Bureau of the Census for the Department of Labor, Bureau of Labor Statistics (BLS). CPS provides estimates of employment, unemployment, and other characteristics of the general labor force, the population as a whole, and various other population subgroups. Estimates of health insurance coverage are derived from the Annual Demographic Supplement (ADS), which includes a series of questions asked each March in addition to regular CPS questions. The ADS is also known as the "March Supplement."

The CPS sample is located in 754 sample areas, with coverage in every State and the District of Columbia. Beginning with 2001 estimates are based on interviews of an expanded sample of 60,000 households per month. Prior to 2001 estimates were based on 50,000 households per month. Also starting in 2001 the State Children's Health Insurance Program (SCHIP) sample expansion was introduced, which increased the March sample to approximately 72,000 households in order to produce statistically reliable State data on the number of low income children who do not have health insurance coverage. The expanded sample for the March Supplement also improved reliability of other national estimates. In an average month the nonresponse rate is about 6–7 percent. In 1994 major changes were introduced, which included a complete redesign of the questionnaire

including new health insurance questions, and the introduction of computer-assisted interviewing for the entire survey. In addition, there were revisions to some of the labor force concepts and definitions. Prior to the redesign, CPS data were primarily collected using a paper-and-pencil form.

The estimation procedure used involves inflation by the reciprocal of the probability of selection, adjustment for nonresponse, and ratio adjustment. Beginning in 1994 new population controls that were based on the 1990 census adjusted for the estimated population undercount were used. Starting with *Health, United States, 2003*, poverty estimates for 2000 were recalculated based on the expanded SCHIP sample, and beginning with 2000 data census 2000-based population controls were implemented.

For more information, visit the CPS Web site at www.bls.census.gov/cps/cpsmain.htm.

Department of Veterans Affairs Databases

Department of Veterans Affairs

The Department of Veterans Affairs (VA) maintains the *National Patient Care Database* (NPCD) and the *National Enrollment Database* (NED). Data are collected locally at each VA medical center and are transmitted electronically to the VA Austin Automation Center for use in providing nationwide statistics, reports, and comparisons.

The NPCD is a nationwide system that contains a statistical record for each episode of care provided under VA auspices in VA and non-VA hospitals, nursing homes, and domiciliaries, and in VA outpatient clinics. Three major extracts from the NPCD are the patient treatment file (PTF), the patient census file, and the outpatient clinic file (OPC).

The *Patient Treatment File (PTF)* collects data at the time of the patient's discharge on each episode of inpatient care provided to patients at VA hospitals, VA nursing homes, VA domiciliaries, community nursing homes, and other non-VA facilities. The PTF record contains the scrambled social security number, dates of inpatient treatment, date of birth, State and county of residence, type of disposition, place of disposition after discharge, as well as the ICD-9-CM diagnostic and procedure or operative codes for each episode of care.

The *Patient Census File* collects data on each patient remaining in a VA medical facility at midnight at the end of each quarter of the fiscal year. The census record includes information similar to that reported in the patient treatment file record.

The *Outpatient Clinic File (OPC)* collects data on each instance of medical treatment provided to a veteran in an outpatient setting. The OPC record includes the age, scrambled social security number, State and county of residence, VA eligibility code, clinic(s) visited, purpose of visit, and the date of visit for each episode of care.

The VA also maintains the *National Enrollment Database* (NED) as the official repository of enrollment information for each veteran enrolled in the VA health care system. In addition, an extract containing selected information from the NPCD, the NED, and the cost distribution system is also produced by the Austin Automation Center.

For more information, write: Department of Veterans Affairs, Office of Policy, Planning, and Preparedness, Policy Analysis Service, 810 Vermont Ave., NW, Washington, DC 20420; or visit the National Patient Care Database at www.virec.research.med.va.gov/DATABASES/NPCD/NPCD.HTM.

Drug Abuse Warning Network (DAWN)

Substance Abuse and Mental Health Services Administration

The Drug Abuse Warning Network (DAWN) is a large-scale, ongoing drug abuse data collection system based on information from hospital emergency departments (EDs) and medical examiner jurisdictions. The major objectives of the DAWN data system include monitoring of drug-abuse patterns and trends, identification of substances associated with drug-abuse episodes, and assessment of drug-related consequences and other health hazards. Estimates reported in this publication are from the hospital ED component of DAWN.

Hospitals eligible for DAWN are non-Federal, short-stay general hospitals that have a 24-hour emergency department. Since 1988 the DAWN emergency department data have been collected from a representative sample of eligible hospitals located throughout the coterminous United States, including 21 oversampled metropolitan areas. Within each

facility, a designated DAWN reporter is responsible for identifying eligible drug-abuse episodes by reviewing emergency department records and abstracting and submitting data on each reportable case. To be included in DAWN, the patient presenting to the ED must meet all of the following four criteria: (a) patient was between ages 6 and 97 years and was treated in the hospital's ED; (b) patient's presenting problem(s) for the ED visit was induced by or related to drug use, regardless of when drug use occurred; (c) episode involved use of an illegal drug or use of a legal drug or other chemical substance contrary to directions; (d) patient's reason for using the substance(s) was dependence, suicide attempt or gesture, and/or psychic effect.

The data from the DAWN sample are used to generate estimates of the total number of emergency department drug-abuse episodes and drug mentions in all eligible hospitals in the coterminous United States and in the 21 metropolitan areas. Overall, a response rate of 81 percent of sample hospitals was obtained in the 2001 survey.

For further information, see Substance Abuse and Mental Health Services Administration, Office of Applied Studies. Emergency Department Trends from the Drug Abuse Warning Network, Preliminary Estimates January–June 2001 with Revised Estimates 1994 to 2001, DAWN Series D-21, DHHS Publication No. (SMA) 02-3635, Rockville, MD. 2002; or write: Office of Applied Studies, Substance Abuse and Mental Health Services Administration, Room 16-105, 5600 Fishers Lane, Rockville, MD 20857; or visit the SAMHSA Web site at www.drugabusestatistics.samhsa.gov.

Employee Benefits Survey—See *National Compensation Survey*.

Inventory of Mental Health Organizations (IMHO)

Substance Abuse and Mental Health Services Administration (SAMHSA)

The Survey and Analysis Branch of SAMHSA's Center for Mental Health Services conducted a biennial Inventory of Mental Health Organizations and General Hospital Mental Health Services (IMHO/GHMHS) from 1986 until 1994. The core questionnaire included versions designed for specialty mental health organizations and another for non-Federal general hospitals with separate psychiatric services.

IMHO/GHMHS has been the primary source for Center for Mental Health Services data included in *Health, United States*. The data system was based on questionnaires mailed every other year to mental health organizations in the United States, including psychiatric hospitals, non-Federal general hospitals with psychiatric services, Department of Veterans Affairs psychiatric services, residential treatment centers for emotionally disturbed children, freestanding outpatient psychiatric clinics, partial care organizations, freestanding day-night organizations, and multiservice mental health organizations, not elsewhere classified.

IMHO/GHMHS was a redesign of three previous inventory systems with more complicated data collection procedures. In 1998 the IMHO/GHMHS was replaced by the Survey of Mental Health Organizations, General Hospital Mental Health Services, and Managed Behavioral Health Care Organizations (SMHO). A brief 100 percent inventory of organizations was conducted by postcard and used to provide basic information on all organizations and as a sampling frame from which to draw a sample for a more in-depth sample survey. The sample survey questionnaire differed from the previous core questionnaires mainly by inclusion of questions relating to managed behavioral health care organizations.

For more information, write: Survey and Analysis Branch, Division of State and Community Systems Development, Center for Mental Health Services, Room 15C-04, 5600 Fishers Lane, Rockville, MD 20857. For further information on mental health and data from the 1997 Client/Patient Sample Survey, see: Center for Mental Health Services, *Mental Health, United States, 2000*. Manderscheid R, Henderson MJ, eds. DHHS Pub. No. (SMA) 01-3537. Washington, DC; or visit the Center for Mental Health Services Web site at www.samhsa.gov/centers/cmhs/cmhs.html.

Medicaid Data System

Centers for Medicare & Medicaid Services

The primary data sources for Medicaid statistical data are the Medicaid Statistical Information System (MSIS) and the CMS-64 reports.

MSIS is the basic source of State-reported eligibility and claims data on the Medicaid population, their characteristics, utilization, and payments. Beginning in FY1999, as a result of legislation enacted from the Balanced Budget Act of 1997, States are required to submit individual eligibility and claims data tapes to CMS quarterly through the Medicaid Statistical Information System (MSIS). Prior to FY1999, States were required to submit an annual HCFA-2082 report, designed to collect aggregated statistical data on eligibles, recipients, services, and expenditures during a Federal fiscal year (October 1 through September 30). The data reported for each year represented people on the Medicaid rolls, recipients of Medicaid services and payments for claims adjudicated during the year. The data reflected bills adjudicated or processed during the year, rather than services used during the year. States summarized and reported the data processed through their own Medicaid claims processing and payment operations, unless they opted to participate in MSIS, in which case the 2082 report was produced by HCFA (Health Care Financing Administration, the predecessor to CMS).

The CMS-64 is a product of the financial budget and grant system. The CMS-64 is a statement of expenditures for the Medicaid program that States submit to CMS 30 days after each quarter. The report is an accounting statement of actual expenditures made by the States for which they are entitled to receive Federal reimbursement under title XIX for that quarter. The amount claimed on the CMS-64 is a summary of expenditures derived from source documents such as invoices, cost reports and eligibility records.

The CMS-64 shows the disposition of Medicaid grant funds for the quarter being reported and previous years, the recoupments made or refunds received, and income earned on grant funds. The data on the CMS-64 are used to reconcile the monetary advance made on the basis of States' funding estimates filed prior to the beginning of the quarter on the CMS-37. As such, the CMS-64 is the primary source for making adjustments for any identified overpayments and underpayments to the States. Also incorporated into this process are disallowance actions forwarded from other Federal financial adjustments. Finally, the CMS-64 provides information that forms the basis for a series of Medicaid financial reports and budget analyses. Additionally included are third party liability (TPL) collections tables. Third party liability refers to the legal obligation of certain health care sources to pay the medical claims of Medicaid recipients before Medicaid pays these claims. Medicaid pays only after the TPL sources have met their legal obligation to pay.

Users of Medicaid data may note apparent inconsistencies that are primarily due to the difference in the information captured in MSIS versus CMS-64 reports. The most substantive difference is due to payments made to "disproportionate share hospitals." Payments to disproportionate share hospitals do not appear in MSIS since States directly reimburse these hospitals and there is no fee-for-service billing. Other less significant differences between MSIS and the CMS-64 occur because adjudicated claims data are used in MSIS versus the reporting of actual payments reflected in the CMS-64. Differences also may occur because of internal State practices for capturing and reporting these data through two separate systems. Finally, national totals for the CMS-64 are different because they include other jurisdictions, such as the Northern Mariana Islands and American Samoa.

For further information on Medicaid data, visit the CMS Web site at www.cms.gov/medicaid/datasources.asp or the Research Data Center (ResDAC) Web site at www.resdac.umn.edu/medicaid/data_available.asp. Also see Appendix II, *Medicaid*.

Medical Expenditure Panel Survey (MEPS)

Agency for Healthcare Research and Quality

The Medical Expenditure Panel Survey (MEPS) is a national probability survey conducted on an annual basis since 1996. The survey is designed to produce nationally representative estimates of healthcare use, expenditures, sources of payment, insurance coverage, and quality of care for the U.S. civilian noninstitutionalized population. The panel design of the survey features several rounds of interviewing covering 2 full calendar years. The MEPS consists of three components.

The Household Component (HC) is a nationally representative survey of the civilian noninstitutionalized population drawn from a subsample of households that participated in the prior year's National Health Interview Survey conducted by the National Center for Health Statistics. The sample sizes for the HC are approximately 10,000 families in 1996 and 1998–2000, 13,500 families in 1997 and 2001, and 15,000 families annually beginning in 2002. The full-year response rate has generally been about 66 percent. Missing expenditure data were imputed using data collected in the Medical Provider Component whenever possible.

Data are collected in the Medical Provider Component (MPC) to improve the accuracy of expenditure estimates derived solely from the Household Component (HC). The MPC is particularly useful in obtaining expenditure information for persons enrolled in managed care plans and Medicaid recipients. The MPC collects data from hospitals, physicians, and home health providers that were reported in the HC as providing care to MEPS sample persons. Sample sizes for the MPC vary from year to year depending on the HC sample size and the MPC sampling rates for providers.

The Insurance Component (IC) consists of two subcomponent samples, a household sample and list sample. The household sample collects detailed information from employers on the health insurance held by and offered to respondents to the MEPS HC. The list sample collects data on the types and costs of workplace health insurance from a total of about 40,000 business establishments and governments each year.

The Medical Expenditure Panel Surveys (MEPS) update the 1987 National Medical Expenditure Survey (NMES). The Household Survey (HS) and the Medical Provider Survey (MPS) components of the 1987 NMES were designed to provide nationally representative estimates of the health status, health insurance coverage, and health care use and expenditures for the U.S. civilian noninstitutionalized population for the calendar year 1987. The HS consisted of four rounds of household interviews. Income was collected in a special supplement administered early in 1988. Events under the scope of the MPS included medical services provided by or under the direction of a physician, all hospital events, and home health care. The sample of events included in the MPS was all events for persons covered by Medicaid and for a 25 percent sample of HS respondents. For the first core household interview, 17,500 households were selected. The 12-month joint core questionnaire/health questionnaire/access supplement response rate for the household component of the NMES was 80 percent. Missing expenditure data were imputed.

For further information about the National Medical Expenditure Survey, see: Hahn B and Lefkowitz D. Annual expenses and sources of payment for health care services (AHRQ Pub. No. 93-0007). National Medical Expenditure Survey Research Findings 14, Agency for Healthcare Research and Quality. Rockville, MD. Public Health Service. Nov. 1992. For further information on the MEPS, visit the MEPS Web site at www.meps.ahrq.gov.

Medicare Administrative Data

Centers for Medicare & Medicaid Services

CMS collects and synthesizes a broad range of quantitative information on its programs, from estimates of future Medicare spending to enrollment, spending, and claims data. The Claims and Utilization Data files contain extensive utilization information at various levels of summarization for a variety of providers and services. There are many types and levels of these files, including but not limited to the National Claims History (NCH) files, the Standard Analytic Files (SAF), Stay Records files, Part B Medicare files, and various other files.

The National Claims History 100 Percent Nearline File contains all institutional and noninstitutional claims, and provides records of every Medicare claim submitted, including adjustment claims. The Standard Analytical Files (SAFs) contain final action claims data in which all adjustments have been resolved. These files contain information collected by Medicare to pay for health care services provided to a Medicare beneficiary. SAFs are available for each institutional (inpatient, outpatient, skilled nursing facility, hospice, or home health agency) and noninstitutional (physician and durable medical equipment providers) claim type. The record unit of SAFs is the claim (some episodes of care may have more than one claim). SAF files include the Inpatient SAF, the Skilled Nursing Facility SAF, the Outpatient SAF, the Home Health Agency SAF, the Hospice SAF, the Clinical Laboratory SAF, the Durable Medical Equipment SAF, and a 5-Percent Beneficiary File SAF.

Medicare Provider and Analysis Review (MedPAR) files contain inpatient hospital and skilled nursing facility (SNF) final action stay records. Each MedPAR record represents a stay in an inpatient hospital or SNF. An inpatient "stay" record summarizes all services rendered to a beneficiary from the time of admission to a facility through discharge. Each MedPAR record may represent one claim or multiple claims, depending on the length of a beneficiary's stay and the amount of inpatient services used throughout the stay.

The Denominator File contains demographic and enrollment information about each beneficiary enrolled in Medicare during a calendar year. The information in the Denominator File is 'frozen' in March of the following calendar year. Some of the information contained in this file includes the beneficiary unique identifier, State and county codes, ZIP Code, date of birth, date of death, sex, race, age, monthly entitlement indicators (for Medicare Part A, Medicare Part B, or Part A and Part B), reasons for entitlement, State buy-in indicators, and monthly managed care indicators (yes/no). The Denominator File is used to determine beneficiary demographic characteristics, entitlement, and beneficiary participation in Medicare Managed Care Organizations.

The Vital Status File contains demographic information about each beneficiary ever entitled to Medicare. Some of the information contained in this file includes the beneficiary unique identifier, State and county codes, ZIP Code, date of birth, date of death, sex, race, and age. Often the Vital Status File is used to obtain recent death information for a cohort of Medicare beneficiaries.

The Group Health Plan (GHP) Master File contains data on beneficiaries who are currently enrolled or have ever been enrolled in a Managed Care Organization (MCO) under contract with CMS. Each record represents one beneficiary and each beneficiary has one record. Some of the information contained in this file includes the Beneficiary Unique Identifier number, date of birth, date of death, State and county, and managed care enrollment information such as dates of membership and MCO contract number. The GHP Master File is used to identify the exact MCO in which beneficiaries were enrolled.

Medicare claims are linked to survey-reported events to produce the Cost and Use file that provides complete expenditure and source of payment data on all health care services, including those not covered by Medicare. Data are also combined to produce estimates of expenditures, per-beneficiary utilization, and other statistics.

For more information about Medicare data files, see CMS' Research Data Center (ResDAC) Web site at www.resdac.umn.edu/medicare/data_available.asp or the CMS Web site at http://cms.hhs.gov/data/default.asp. Also see Appendix II, *Medicare*.

Medicare Current Beneficiary Survey (MCBS)

Centers for Medicare & Medicaid Services

The Medicare Current Beneficiary Survey (MCBS) is a continuous survey of a nationally representative sample of about 18,000 aged and disabled Medicare beneficiaries enrolled in Medicare Part A (hospital insurance), or Part B (medical insurance), or both, and residing in households or long-term care facilities. The survey provides comprehensive time-series data on utilization of health services, health and functional status, health care expenditures, and health insurance and beneficiary information (such as income, assets, living arrangement, family assistance, and quality of life). The longitudinal design of the survey allows each sample person to be interviewed three times a year for 4 years, whether he or she resides in the community or a facility or moves between the two settings, using the version of the questionnaire appropriate to the setting. Sample persons in the community are interviewed using computer-assisted personal interviewing (CAPI) survey instruments. Because long-term care facility residents often are in poor health, information about institutionalized patients is collected from proxy respondents such as nurses and other primary care givers affiliated with the facility. The sample is selected from the Medicare enrollment files with oversampling among disabled persons under age 65 and among persons 80 years of age and over.

Medicare claims are linked to survey-reported events to produce the Cost and Use file that provides complete expenditure and source of payment data on all health care services, including those not covered by Medicare. The Access to Care file contains information on beneficiaries' access to health care, satisfaction with care, and usual source of care. The sample for this file represents the "always enrolled" population, those who participated in the Medicare program for the entire year. In contrast, the Cost and Use file represents the "ever enrolled" population, including the experience of those who enter Medicare during the year and those who died.

For more information about the MCBS, see: A profile of the Medicare Current Beneficiary Survey, by GS Adler. Health Care Financing Review, vol 15 no 4. Health Care Financing Administration. Washington, DC. Public Health Service. 1994. For further information on the MCBS, visit the MCBS Web site at www.cms.hhs.gov/mcbs/default.asp.

Monitoring the Future Study (MTF)

National Institute on Drug Abuse

Monitoring the Future Study (MTF) is a large-scale epidemiological survey of drug use and related attitudes. It has been conducted annually since 1975 under a series of investigator-initiated research grants from the National Institute on Drug Abuse to the University of Michigan's Institute for Social Research. MTF is composed of three substudies: (a) annual survey of high school seniors initiated in 1975; (b) ongoing panel studies of representative samples from each graduating class that have been conducted by mail since 1976; and (c) annual surveys of 8th and 10th graders initiated in 1991.

The survey design is a multistage random sample with stage one being selection of particular geographic areas, stage two selection of one or more schools in each area, and stage three selection of students within each school. Data are collected using self-administered questionnaires conducted in the classroom by representatives of the Institute for Social Research. Dropouts and students who are absent on the day of the survey are excluded (about 18 percent of high school seniors, about 12 percent of 10th graders, and about 10 percent of 8th graders in 2001). Recognizing that the dropout population is at higher risk for drug use, this survey was expanded to include similar nationally representative samples of 8th and 10th graders in 1991. Statistics that are published in the *Dropout Rates in the United States: 2000* (published by the National Center for Educational Statistics, Pub. No. NCES 2002-114) stated that among persons 15–16 years of age, 2.9 percent have dropped out of school while the dropout rate increases to 3.5 percent for persons 17 years of age, 6.1 percent for persons 18 years of age, and 9.6 percent for persons 19 years of age. Therefore, surveying eighth graders (where dropout rates are much lower than for high school seniors) should be effective for picking up students at higher risk for drug use. Although the prevalence of drug use is slightly underestimated due to the exclusion of dropouts and absentees, the methodology is consistent over time and trend estimates are little affected.

Approximately 44,300 8th, 10th, and 12th graders in 394 schools were surveyed in 2002. In 2002 the annual senior samples comprised roughly 13,500 seniors in 120 public and private high schools nationwide, selected to be representative of all seniors in the continental United States. The 10th-grade samples involved about 14,700 students in 133 schools in 2002, and the 2002 8th-grade samples had approximately 15,500 students in 141 schools. Response rates of 83 percent, 85 percent, and 91 percent for 12th, 10th, and 8th graders in 2002 have been relatively constant across time. Absentees constitute virtually all of the nonrespondents.

Estimates of substance use for youth based on the National Household Survey on Drug Abuse (NHSDA) are generally lower than estimates based on the MTF and the Youth Risk Behavior Surveillance System (YRBSS). In addition to the fact that the MTF excludes dropouts and absentees, rates are not directly comparable across these surveys due to differences in populations covered, sample design, questionnaires, interview setting, and statistical approaches to make the survey estimates generalizable to the entire population. The NHSDA survey collects data in homes, whereas the MTF and YRBSS collect data in school classrooms. The NHSDA estimates are tabulated by age, while the MTF and YRBSS estimates are tabulated by grade, representing different ages as well as different populations. See Cowan CD. Coverage, Sample Design, and Weighting in Three Federal Surveys. Journal of Drug Issues 31(3), 595–614, 2001.

For further information on Monitoring the Future Study, see: National Institute on Drug Abuse, Monitoring the Future National Survey Results on Drug Use, 1975–2001. Volume I, Secondary School Students, NIH Pub. No. 02-5106. Bethesda, MD: Public Health Service, August 2002; or visit the NIDA Web site at www.nida.nih.gov or the Monitoring the Future Web site at www.monitoringthefuture.org/.

National Ambulatory Medical Care Survey (NAMCS)

Centers for Disease Control and Prevention

National Center for Health Statistics

The National Ambulatory Medical Care Survey (NAMCS), initiated in 1973, is a continuing national probability sample of ambulatory medical encounters. The scope of the survey covers patient encounters in the offices of non-Federally employed physicians classified by the

American Medical Association or American Osteopathic Association as "office-based, patient care" physicians. Patient encounters with physicians engaged in prepaid practices—health maintenance organizations (HMOs), independent practice organizations (IPAs), and other prepaid practices—are included in NAMCS. Excluded are visits to hospital-based physicians, visits to specialists in anesthesiology, pathology, and radiology, and visits to physicians who are principally engaged in teaching, research, or administration. Telephone contacts and nonoffice visits are also excluded.

A multistage probability design is employed. The first-stage sample consists of 84 primary sampling units (PSUs) in 1985 and 112 PSUs in 1992 selected from about 1,900 such units into which the United States has been divided. In each sample PSU, a sample of practicing non-Federal office-based physicians is selected from master files maintained by the American Medical Association and the American Osteopathic Association. The final stage involves systematic random samples of office visits during randomly assigned 7-day reporting periods. In 1985 the survey excluded Alaska and Hawaii. Starting in 1989 the survey included all 50 States.

In 1999 a sample of 2,499 physicians was selected, 1,728 were in scope, and 1,087 participated in the survey for a response rate of 63 percent. Data were provided on 20,760 records. In the 2000 survey a sample of 3,000 physicians was selected, 2,049 were in scope, and 1,388 participated for a response rate of 68 percent. Data were provided on 27,369 records. Data are collected on providers seen; reason for the visit; diagnoses; waiting time; drugs ordered, provided, or continued; and selected procedures and tests performed during the visit.

The estimation procedure used in NAMCS has three basic components: inflation by the reciprocal of the probability of selection, adjustment for nonresponse, and ratio adjustment to fixed totals.

For more detailed information on NAMCS, see: Cherry DK. National Ambulatory Medical Care Survey: 2000 summary. Advance data from vital and health statistics; no. 328. Hyattsville, MD: National Center for Health Statistics. 2002; or visit the NHCS section of the NCHS Web site at www.cdc.gov/nchs/nhcs.htm.

National Compensation Survey

Bureau of Labor Statistics

The National Compensation Survey (NCS) is conducted quarterly by The Bureau of Labor Statistics' Office of Compensation and Working Conditions and provides comprehensive measures of occupational earnings, compensation cost trends, benefit incidence, and detailed plan provisions. Detailed occupational earnings are available for metropolitan and nonmetropolitan areas, broad geographic regions, and on a national basis. The Employment Cost Index (ECI) and Employer Costs for Employee Compensation (ECEC) are compensation measures derived from the National Compensation Survey (NCS). ECI measures changes in labor costs. Average hourly employer cost for employee compensation is presented in the ECEC. Data from the March survey are presented in *Health, United States*.

In separate surveys the National Compensation Survey covers the incidence and detailed provisions of selected employee benefit plans in small private establishments (in even years), medium and large private establishments (in odd years), and State and local governments (in even years). National benefits data are presented for three broad occupational groupings: professional, technical, and related; clerical and sales; and blue-collar and service employees. Broad incidence data were also available by goods- and service-producing, union affiliation, and full- and part-time status.

The Employment Cost Index (ECI) is a quarterly measure of changes in labor costs. It is one of the principal economic indicators used by the Federal Reserve Bank. ECI data show changes in wages, salaries, benefit costs, and total compensation for all workers and separately for private industry and State and local government workers; report compensation changes by industry, occupational group, union and nonunion status, region, and metropolitan/nonmetropolitan status; provide seasonally adjusted and unadjusted data; and present historical data on changes in labor costs.

The Employer Costs for Employee Compensation (ECEC) product is produced quarterly and shows the employers' average hourly cost for total compensation and its components. The key features of ECEC include:

■ Compensation costs for wages and salaries and benefits

■ Cost data in dollar amounts and as percentages of compensation

■ Data on Civilian workers and State and local government workers

■ Compensation costs by major occupation, industry, region, union and nonunion status, establishment size, and full- or part-time status

■ Reflects today's labor force composition

The sample for the NCS is selected using a three-stage design. The first stage involves the selection of areas. The NCS sample consists of 154 metropolitan and nonmetropolitan areas that represent the Nation's 326 metropolitan statistical areas and the remaining portions of the 50 States. In the second stage, establishments are systematically selected with probability of selection proportionate to their relative employment size within the industry. Use of this technique means that the larger an establishment's employment, the greater its chance of selection.

The third stage of sampling is a probability sample of occupations within a sampled establishment. This step is performed by the BLS field economist during an interview with the respondent establishment in which selection of an occupation is based on probability of selection proportionate to employment in the establishment. Each occupation is classified under its corresponding major occupational group using the Occupational Classification System Manual (OCSM) and the Census Occupation Index, which are based on the 1990 U.S. Census.

Data collection is conducted by BLS field economists. Data are gathered from each establishment on the primary business activity of the establishment, types of occupations, number of employees, wages and salaries and benefits, hours of work, and duties and responsibilities. Wage data obtained by occupation and work level allows NCS to publish occupational wage statistics for localities, census divisions, and the Nation.

The methodology and procedures used to make estimates vary by product line. For the wage series, individual wage rates are weighted by number of workers; sample weight, adjusted for nonresponding establishments and other factors; and the occupation work schedule (hourly, weekly, or annual). The benefit series has three weight-adjustment factors applied to the data to account for establishment nonresponse, occupational nonresponse, and to adjust the estimated employment totals to actual counts of employment by industry for the survey reference date.

To measure compensation costs free from the influence of employment shifts among occupations and industries, the ECI is calculated with fixed employment weights unlike the method with which wage series and benefit series are calculated. Since December 1994, 1990 employment counts from the Bureau's Occupational Employment Survey have been used. The ECI is a standard Laspeyres fixed-weighted index.

The ECEC estimates are based on data collected for the ECI. Unlike the ECI, ECEC estimates are weighted by the most recently available industry and occupational employment mix derived from data produced by the BLS Current Employment Statistics (CES) program.

For more information, see: U.S. Department of Labor, Bureau of Labor Statistics, *Employment Cost Indexes 1975–99*, Bulletin 2532, Oct. 2000; and visit the BLS Web site at www.bls.gov/ncs/home.htm.

National Health Accounts

Centers for Medicare & Medicaid Services

Estimates of expenditures for health based on National Health Accounts are compiled annually by type of expenditure and source of funds by the Office of the Actuary. The American Hospital Association (AHA) data on hospital finances are the primary source for estimates relating to hospital care. The salaries of physicians and dentists on the staffs of hospitals, hospital outpatient clinics, hospital-based home health agencies, and nursing home care provided in the hospital setting are considered to be components of hospital care. Expenditures for home health care and for services of health professionals (for example, doctors, chiropractors, private duty nurses, therapists, and podiatrists) are estimated primarily using a combination of data from the U.S. Bureau of the Census Services Annual Survey and the quinquennial Census of Service Industries.

The estimates of retail spending for prescription drugs are based on household and industry data on prescription drug transactions. Expenditures for other medical nondurables and vision products and other medical durables purchased in retail outlets are based on estimates of personal consumption

expenditures prepared by the U.S. Department of Commerce's Bureau of Economic Analysis, U.S. Bureau of Labor Statistics/Consumer Expenditure Survey; the 1987 National Medical Expenditure Survey and the 1996 Medical Expenditure Panel Survey conducted by the Agency for Healthcare Research and Quality; and spending by Medicare and Medicaid. Those durable and nondurable products provided to inpatients in hospitals or nursing homes, and those provided by licensed professionals or through home health agencies are excluded here, but are included with the expenditure estimates of the provider service category.

Nursing home expenditures cover care rendered in establishments providing inpatient nursing and health-related personal care through active treatment programs for medical and health-related conditions. These establishments cover skilled nursing and intermediate care facilities, including those for the mentally retarded. Spending estimates are primarily based upon data from the U.S. Bureau of the Census Services Annual Survey and the quinquennial Census of Service Industries.

Expenditures for construction include those spent on the erection or renovation of hospitals, nursing homes, medical clinics, and medical research facilities, but not for private office buildings providing office space for private practitioners. Expenditures for noncommercial research (the cost of commercial research by drug companies is assumed to be imbedded in the price charged for the product; to include this item again would result in double counting) are developed from information gathered by the National Institutes of Health and the National Science Foundation.

Source of funding estimates likewise come from a multiplicity of sources. Data on the Federal health programs are taken from administrative records maintained by the servicing agencies. Among the sources used to estimate State and local government spending for health are the U.S. Bureau of the Census' Government Finances, and the National Academy of Social Insurance reports on State-operated Workers' Compensation programs. Federal and State-local expenditures for education and training of medical personnel are excluded from these measures where they are separable. For the private financing of health care, data on the financial experience of health insurance organizations come from special Centers for Medicare & Medicaid Services analyses of private health insurers, and from the Bureau of Labor Statistics' survey on the cost of employer-sponsored health insurance and on consumer expenditures. Information on out-of-pocket spending from the U.S. Bureau of the Census Services Annual Survey; U.S. Bureau of Labor Statistics Consumer Expenditure Survey; the 1987 National Medical Expenditure Survey and the Medical Expenditure Panel Surveys conducted by the Agency for Healthcare Research and Quality; and from private surveys conducted by the American Hospital Association, American Medical Association, American Dental Association, and IMS Health, an organization that collects data from the pharmaceutical industry, is used to develop estimates of direct spending by customers.

For more specific information on definitions, sources, and methods used in the National Health Accounts contact: Office of the Actuary, Centers for Medicare & Medicaid Services, 7500 Security Blvd., Baltimore, MD 21244-1850; or visit the Centers for Medicare & Medicaid Services National Health Accounts Web site at http://cms.hhs.gov/statistics/nhe.

State Health Expenditures

Estimates of personal health care spending by State are created using the same definitions of health care sectors used in producing the National Health Expenditures (NHE). The same data sources used in creating NHE are also used to create State estimates whenever possible. Additional sources are employed when surveys used to create valid national estimates lack sufficient sample size to create valid State-level estimates. State-level data are used to estimate the State-by-State distribution of health spending, and the NHE national totals for the specific type of service or source of funds are used to control the level of State-by-State distributions. This procedure implicitly assumes that national spending estimates can be created more accurately than State-specific expenditures.

The NHE data that were used as national totals for these State estimates were published in Health, United States, 2001, and differ from the sum of State estimates because national totals included expenditures for persons living in U.S. territories and for military and Federal civilian employees and their families stationed overseas. The sum of the State-level expenditures exclude health spending for those groups. Starting with Health, United States, 2002, NHE reflect new data and benchmark revisions incorporated after completion of the State estimates, and incorporate a conceptual revision to exclude spending for persons living in U.S. territories and military and Federal civilian employees and their families living overseas.

Starting in Health, United States, 2002, State estimates are based on the location of the beneficiary's residence. This differs from previous estimates published in Health, United States, which presented spending based on the health care provider's location. State estimates were first constructed based on the provider's location because data available to estimate spending by State primarily comes from providers and represents the State-of-provider location. However, the most useful unit for analyzing spending trends and differences are per capita units, which are based on spending estimates for the State in which people reside. Therefore, State-of-provider-based expenditures are adjusted to a State-of-residence basis using interstate border-crossing flow patterns that represent travel patterns across State borders for health care.

Data for the interstate border-crossing flow patterns are based on Medicare claims. Medicare is the only comprehensive source upon which to base interstate flows of spending between State-of-provider and State-of-beneficiary residence. Data for non-Medicare payers (excluding Medicaid) are also based on Medicare flow patterns, but are further adjusted for age-specific service mix variation in hospital and physician services. Medicaid services are not adjusted because it is assumed that care provided to eligible State residents is most often provided by in-State providers and further assumed that spending by Medicaid is identical on a residence and provider basis.

In addition to differences noted earlier, national totals for residence-based State health expenditures may differ slightly from national totals for provider-based expenditures due to inflows and outflows of health care spending to the U.S. territories. Because flow patterns are based on Medicare data, we are able to adjust for services that Medicare beneficiaries receive outside of the United States, and for services received by Medicare beneficiaries in the United States who either live in the U.S. territories or in other countries. Similar adjustments for the non-Medicare, non-Medicaid population are not possible.

For more information contact: Office of the Actuary, Centers for Medicare & Medicaid Services, 7500 Security Blvd., Baltimore, MD 21244-1850; or visit the Centers for Medicare & Medicaid Services National Health Expenditures Web site at http://cms.hhs.gov/statistics/nhe/#state.

National Health Care Survey (NHCS)

Centers for Disease Control and Prevention

National Center for Health Statistics

The National Health Care Survey is a family of surveys that collect data from health care providers and establishments about the utilization of health services and characteristics of providers and their patients. The components of the NHCS represent the major sectors of the U.S. health care system providing data on ambulatory, inpatient, and long-term care settings. Each survey in the family is based on a multistage sampling design that includes the health care facilities or providers and their records. Data are collected through abstraction of medical records, completion of encounter forms, compilation of data from State and professional associations, purchase of data from commercial abstraction services, and surveys of providers. Data from all survey components are collected from the establishment, and in no case is information received directly from the person receiving care. This family of surveys includes the following components:

- National Ambulatory Medical Care Survey (NAMCS)
- National Hospital Ambulatory Medical Care Survey (NHAMCS)
- National Hospital Discharge Survey (NHDS)
- National Survey of Ambulatory Surgery (NSAS)
- National Home and Hospice Care Survey (NHHCS)
- National Nursing Home Survey (NHHS)

National Health and Nutrition Examination Survey (NHANES)

Centers for Disease Control and Prevention

National Center for Health Statistics

The NHANES program of the National Center for Health Statistics includes a series of cross-sectional nationally representative health examination surveys beginning in 1960. Each cross-sectional survey provides a national estimate for the U.S. population at the time of the survey, enabling examination of trends over time in the U.S. population. In each survey a nationally representative sample of the U.S. population was selected using a complex, stratified, multistage probability cluster sampling design.

For the first program or cycle of the National Health Examination Survey (NHES I), 1960–62, data were collected on the total prevalence of certain chronic diseases as well as the distributions of various physical and physiological measures, including blood pressure and serum cholesterol levels. For that program, a highly stratified, multistage probability sample of 7,710 adults, of whom 86.5 percent were examined, was selected to represent the 111 million civilian noninstitutionalized adults 18–79 years of age in the United States at that time. The sample areas consisted of 42 primary sampling units (PSUs) from the 1,900 geographic units.

NHES II (1963–65) and NHES III (1966–70) examined probability samples of the Nation's noninstitutionalized children ages 6–11 years (NHES II) and 12–17 years (NHES III) focusing on factors related to growth and development. Both cycles were multistage, stratified probability samples of clusters of households in land-based segments and used the same 40 PSUs. NHES II sampled 7,417 children with a response rate of 96 percent. NHES III sampled 7,514 youth with a response rate of 90 percent.

For more information on NHES I, see: Gordon T, Miller HW. Cycle I of the Health Examination Survey: Sample and response, United States, 1960–62. National Center for Health Statistics. Vital Health Stat 11(1). 1974. For more information on NHES II, see: Plan, operation, and response results of a program of children's examinations. National Center for Health Statistics. Vital Health Stat 1(5). 1967. For more information on NHES III, see: Schaible WL. Quality control in a National Health Examination Survey. National Center for Health Statistics. Vital Health Stat 2(44). 1972.

In 1971 a nutrition surveillance component was added and the survey name was changed to the National Health and Nutrition Examination Survey (NHANES). In NHANES I, conducted from 1971 to 1974, a major purpose was to measure and monitor indicators of the nutrition and health status of the American people through dietary intake data, biochemical tests, physical measurements, and clinical assessments for evidence of nutritional deficiency. Detailed examinations were given by dentists, ophthalmologists, and dermatologists with an assessment of need for treatment. In addition, data were obtained for a subsample of adults on overall health care needs and behavior, and more detailed examination data were collected on cardiovascular, respiratory, arthritic, and hearing conditions.

The NHANES I target population was the civilian noninstitutionalized population 1–74 years of age residing in the coterminous United States, except for people residing on any of the reservation lands set aside for the use of American Indians. The sample design was a multistage, stratified probability sample of clusters of persons in land-based segments. The sample areas consisted of 65 PSUs selected from the 1,900 PSUs in the coterminous United States. A subsample of persons 25–74 years of age was selected to receive the more detailed health examination. Groups at high risk of malnutrition were oversampled at known rates throughout the process. Household interviews were completed for more than 96 percent of the 28,043 persons selected for the NHANES I sample, and about 75 percent (20,749) were examined.

For NHANES II, conducted from 1976 to 1980, the nutrition component was expanded. In the medical area primary emphasis was placed on diabetes, kidney and liver functions, allergy, and speech pathology. The NHANES II target population was the civilian noninstitutionalized population 6 months–74 years of age residing in the United States, including Alaska and Hawaii.

NHANES II used a multistage probability design that involved selection of PSUs, segments (clusters of households) within PSUs, households, eligible persons, and finally, sample persons. The sample design provided for oversampling among persons 6 months–5 years of age, 60–74 years of age, and those living in poverty areas. A sample of 27,801 persons was selected for NHANES II. Of this sample 20,322 (73.1 percent) were examined. Race information for NHANES I and NHANES II was determined primarily by interviewer observation.

The estimation procedure used to produce national statistics for NHANES I and NHANES II involved inflation by the reciprocal of the probability of selection, adjustment for nonresponse, and poststratified ratio adjustment to population totals. Sampling errors also were estimated to measure the reliability of the statistics.

For more information on NHANES I, see: Miller HW. Plan and operation of the Health and Nutrition Examination Survey, United States, 1971–73. National Center for Health Statistics. Vital Health Stat 1(10a) and 1(10b). 1977 and 1978; and Engel A, Murphy RS, Maurer K, Collins E. Plan and operation of the NHANES I Augmentation Survey of Adults 25–74

years, United States, 1974–75. National Center for Health Statistics. Vital Health Stat 1(14). 1978.

For more information on NHANES II, see: McDowell A, Engel A, Massey JT, Maurer K. Plan and operation of the second National Health and Nutrition Examination Survey, 1976–80. National Center for Health Statistics. Vital Health Stat 1(15). 1981. For information on nutritional applications of these surveys, see: Yetley E, Johnson C. Nutritional applications of the Health and Nutrition Examination Surveys (HANES). Ann Rev Nutr 7:441–63. 1987.

The Hispanic Health and Nutrition Examination Survey (HHANES), conducted during 1982–84, was similar in content and design to the previous National Health and Nutrition Examination Surveys. The major difference between HHANES and the previous national surveys is that HHANES used a probability sample of three special subgroups of the population living in selected areas of the United States rather than a national probability sample. The three HHANES universes included approximately 84, 57, and 59 percent of the respective 1980 Mexican-, Cuban-, and Puerto Rican-origin populations in the continental United States. Hispanic ethnicity of these populations was determined by self-report.

In the HHANES three geographically and ethnically distinct populations were studied: Mexican Americans living in Texas, New Mexico, Arizona, Colorado, and California; Cuban Americans living in Dade County, Florida; and Puerto Ricans living in parts of New York, New Jersey, and Connecticut. In the Southwest 9,894 persons were selected (75 percent or 7,462 were examined), in Dade County 2,244 persons were selected (60 percent or 1,357 were examined), and in the Northeast 3,786 persons were selected (75 percent or 2,834 were examined).

For more information on HHANES, see: Maurer KR. Plan and operation of the Hispanic Health and Nutrition Examination Survey, 1982–84. National Center for Health Statistics. Vital Health Stat 1(19). 1985.

The third National Health and Nutrition Examination Survey (NHANES III) was a 6-year survey covering the years 1988–94. Over the 6-year period, 39,695 persons were selected for the survey of which 30,818 (77.6 percent) were examined in the mobile examination center. The NHANES III target population was the civilian noninstitutionalized population 2 months of age and over. The sample design provided for oversampling among children 2–35 months of age, persons 70 years of age and over, black Americans, and Mexican Americans. Race was reported for the household by the respondent.

For more information on NHANES III, see: Ezzati TM, Massey JT, Waksberg J, et al. Sample design: Third National Health and Nutrition Examination Survey. National Center for Health Statistics. Vital Health Stat 2(113). 1992; Plan and operation of the Third National Health and Nutrition Examination Survey, 1988–94. National Center for Health Statistics. Vital Health Stat 1(32). 1994; or visit the NCHS Web site at www.cdc.gov/nchs/nhanes.htm.

Beginning in 1999, NHANES became a continuous, annual survey that can be linked to related Federal Government surveys of the general U.S. population, specifically, the National Health Interview Survey (NHIS) and, in the future, the U.S. Department of Agriculture's (USDA) Continuing Survey of Food Intakes by Individuals (CSFII). The new design also allows increased flexibility in survey content. Since April 1999, NHANES collects data every year from a representative sample of the U.S. population, newborns and older, by in-home personal interviews and physical examinations in the mobile examination center.

The major objectives of continuous NHANES are to:

■ estimate the national prevalence of selected diseases and risk factors

■ monitor trends in the prevalence, awareness, treatment, and control of selected diseases

■ monitor trends in risk behaviors and environmental exposures

■ analyze risk factors for selected diseases

■ study the relationship between diet, nutrition, and health

■ explore emerging public health issues and new technologies

■ establish a national probability sample of genetic material for future genetic testing

The sample frame for continuous NHANES is the list of PSUs selected for the current design of the National Health Interview Survey (NHIS). For the current NHIS design, there are 358 PSUs in the annual sample, divided into four panels with each of the four panels comprising a nationally representative sample. Two of the four panels are available for use by the NHANES. Of the approximately 200 PSUs available in the two national panels for the first stage-

sampling frame for the NHANES, 120 NHIS PSUs were selected to comprise six annual national samples, and 20 PSUs were randomly assigned to each year in 1999–2004. For each year, a subset of 15 PSUs was selected with the remaining five PSUs held in reserve. With 15 PSUs per year, approximately 5,000 sample persons can be examined.

For 1999, due to a delay in the start of data collection, there were only 12 distinct PSUs. For the purpose of variance estimation, the 1999–2000 survey is considered to have 26 PSUs. In the sample selection for NHANES 1999–2000, there were 22,839 households screened. Of these, 6,005 households had at least one eligible sample person identified for interviewing. There were a total of 12,160 eligible sample persons identified. Of these 9,965 were interviewed and 9,282 were examined. The overall response rate for those interviewed was 81.9 percent (9,965 out of 12,160) and the response rate for those examined was 76.3 percent (9,282 out of 12,160).

With only 2 years of data in NHANES 1999–2000, instead of the 6 years for NHANES III, sample size is smaller and number of geographic units in the sample is more limited. Due to smaller sample sizes, standard errors for a variable in NHANES 1999–2000 will be approximately 70 percent greater than for the corresponding variable in NHANES III.

NHANES 1999–2000 includes oversampling of low-income persons, adolescents 12–19 years, persons 60 years of age and over, African Americans, and Mexican Americans. The sample is not specifically designed to give a nationally representative sample for the total population of Hispanics residing in the United States.

For more information on NHANES 1999–2000, visit the NHANES Web site at www.cdc.gov/nchs/about/major/nhanes/nhanes99-02.htm.

National Health Interview Survey (NHIS)

Centers for Disease Control and Prevention

National Center for Health Statistics

The National Health Interview Survey (NHIS), initiated in 1957, is a continuing nationwide sample survey of the civilian noninstitutionalized population. Data are collected through household interviews. Information is obtained on personal and demographic characteristics including race and ethnicity by self-report or as reported by an informant. Information is also obtained on illnesses, injuries, impairments, chronic conditions, utilization of health resources, and other health topics.

The sample design plan of NHIS follows a multistage probability design that permits a continuous sampling of the civilian noninstitutionalized population residing in the United States. The survey is designed in such a way that the sample scheduled for each week is representative of the target population, and the weekly samples are additive over time.

In 1985 NHIS adopted several new sample design features although, conceptually, the sampling plan remained the same as the previous design. Two major changes included reducing the number of primary sampling locations from 376 to 198 for sampling efficiency and oversampling the black population to improve the precision of the statistics. The sample was designed so that a typical NHIS sample for the data collection years 1985–94 consisted of approximately 7,500 segments containing about 59,000 assigned households. Of these households, an expected 10,000 were vacant, demolished, or occupied by persons not in the target population of the survey. The expected sample of 49,000 occupied households yielded a probability sample of about 127,000 persons. In 1994 the sample numbered 116,179 persons.

In 1995 the NHIS sample was redesigned again. Major design changes included increasing the number of primary sampling units from 198 to 358 and oversampling the black and Hispanic populations to improve the precision of the statistics. The sample was designed so that a typical NHIS sample for the data collection years 1995–2004 would consist of approximately 7,000 segments. The expected sample of 44,000 occupied respondent households will yield a probability sample of about 106,000 persons. In 1997 the sample numbered 103,477 persons; 98,785 persons in 1998, 97,059 persons in 1999, 100,618 persons in 2000, and 100,760 persons in 2001.

The NHIS questionnaire fielded from 1982 to 1996 consisted of two parts: a set of basic health and demographic items known as the Core questionnaire and one or more sets of questions on current health topics (supplements). Information was collected from responsible family members residing in the household. Proxy responses were acceptable for Core and Supplement questionnaires when family members were not present at the time of interview. Data for children were collected from proxy respondents.

In 1997 the NHIS questionnaire was redesigned and from 1997 through the present consists of three parts: a basic module, a periodic module, and a topical module. The basic module functions as the new Core questionnaire and comprises three components (Family Core, Sample Adult Core, Sample Child Core). For the Family Core, information is obtained about all members of the family by interviewing any adult members of the household who are present and who may respond for themselves and as proxies for other members of the family. Information is obtained by asking respondents or proxy respondents a series of questions in an unfolding family style. For example, questions on activity limitation are asked as follows: "Are you/any family members limited in activities?" If so, "Who is this?" For the Sample Adult Core, one adult in the household is randomly selected to participate; proxy respondents are not used in this component. For families with children under 18 years of age, one child in the household is randomly selected for participation in the Sample Child Core. Data for this component are collected from a knowledgeable adult in the household. Starting with 1998 periodic and topical modules are incorporated into selected years of the NHIS.

In the 1997 NHIS questionnaire redesign the measurement of some basic concepts was changed and some concepts were measured in different ways. While some questions remain the same over time, they may be preceded by different questions or topics. For some questions, there was a change in the reference period for reporting an event or condition.

Also in 1997 the collection methodology changed from paper and pencil questionnaires to computer-assisted personal interviewing (CAPI). Because of the extensive redesign of the questionnaire in 1997 and introduction of the CAPI method of data collection, data from 1997 and later years may not be comparable with data from earlier years.

The household response rate for the ongoing portion of the survey (core) has been between 94 and 98 percent over the years. In recent years the total household response rate was 92 percent in 1997, 90 percent in 1998, 88 percent in 1999, and 89 percent in 2000 and 2001. Response rates for special health topics (supplements) have generally been lower. For example, the response rate was 80 percent for the 1994 Year 2000 Supplement, which included questions about cigarette smoking and use of such preventive services as mammography. In 1997 the final response rate for the sample adult supplement was 80 percent, 74 percent in 1998, 70 percent in 1999, 72 percent in 2000, and 74 percent in

2001. In 1997 the final response rate for the sample child supplement was 84 percent, 82 percent in 1998, 78 percent in 1999, 79 percent in 2000, and 81 percent in 2001.

For more information about the survey design, methods used in estimation, and general qualifications of the data obtained from the survey, see: Botman SL, Moore TF, Moriarity CL, and Parsons VL. Design and estimation for the National Health Interview Survey, 1995–2004. National Center for Health Statistics. Vital Health Stat 2(130). 2000; Massey JT, Moore TF, Parsons VL, Tadros W. Design and estimation for the National Health Interview Survey, 1985–94. National Center for Health Statistics. Vital Health Stat 2(110). 1989; Kovar MG, Poe GS. The National Health Interview Survey design, 1973–84, and procedures, 1975–83. National Center for Health Statistics. Vital Health Stat 1(18). 1985; Blackwell DL, Tonthat L. Summary Health Statistics for U.S. Children: National Health Interview Survey, 1998. National Center for Health Statistics. Vital Health Stat 10(208). 2002; Blackwell DL, Tonthat L. Summary Health Statistics for the U.S. Population: National Health Interview Survey, 1998. National Center for Health Statistics. Vital Health Stat 10(207). 2002; Pleis JR, Coles R. Summary Health Statistics for U.S. Adults: National Health Interview Survey, 1998. National Center for Health Statistics. Vital Health Stat 10(209). 2002; or visit the NHIS section of the NCHS Web site at www.cdc.gov/nchs/nhis.htm.

National Health Provider Inventory (NHPI)

Centers for Disease Control and Prevention

National Center for Health Statistics

The National Master Facility Inventories (NMFIs), forerunners of the National Health Provider Inventory (NHPI), were a series of inventories of inpatient health facilities in the United States conducted by NCHS. The inventories included hospitals, nursing and related-care homes, and other custodial care facilities. The last NMFI was conducted in 1982. In 1986 the inventory was changed to the Inventory of Long-Term Care Places (ILTCP) and included nursing and related-care homes and facilities for the mentally retarded. In 1991 the inventory was again changed to NHPI and included nursing homes, board and care homes, home health agencies, and hospices. The NHPI has not been repeated since 1991. The

NMFI, ILTCP, and NHPI served as sampling frames for the NCHS National Nursing Home Survey and National Home and Hospice Care Survey.

National Home and Hospice Care Survey (NHHCS)

Centers for Disease Control and Prevention

National Center for Health Statistics

The National Home and Hospice Care Survey (NHHCS) is a sample survey of health agencies and hospices. Initiated in 1992, it was also conducted in 1993, 1994, 1996, 1998, and 2000. The original sampling frame consisted of all home health care agencies and hospices identified in the 1991 National Health Provider Inventory (NHPI). The 1992 sample contained 1,500 agencies. These agencies were revisited during the 1993 survey (excluding agencies that had been found to be out of scope for the survey). In 1994 in-scope agencies identified in the 1993 survey were revisited, along with 100 newly identified agencies added to the sample. In 1996 the universe was again updated and a new sample of 1,200 agencies was drawn. In 1998 a sample of 1,350 agencies was selected. In 2000, 1,800 agencies were sampled and the response rate was 96.4 percent.

The sample design for the 1992–94 NHHCS was a stratified three-stage probability design. Primary sampling units were selected at the first stage, agencies were selected at the second stage, and current patients and discharges were selected at the third stage. The sample design for the 1996, 1998, and 2000 NHHCS was a two-stage probability design, in which agencies were selected at the first stage and current patients and discharges were selected at the second stage. Current patients were those on the rolls of the agency as of midnight the day before the survey. Discharges were selected to estimate the number of discharges from the agency during the year before the survey. After the samples were selected, a patient questionnaire was completed for each current patient and discharge by interviewing the staff member most familiar with the care provided to the patient. The respondent was requested to refer to the medical records for each patient.

For additional information see: Haupt BJ. Development of the National Home and Hospice Care Survey. National Center for

Health Statistics. Vital Health Stat 1(33). 1994; and visit the National Health Care Survey (NHCS) Web site at www.cdc.gov/nchs/nhcs.htm.

National Hospital Ambulatory Medical Care Survey (NHAMCS)

Centers for Disease Control and Prevention

National Center for Health Statistics

The National Hospital Ambulatory Medical Care Survey (NHAMCS), initiated in 1992, is a continuing annual national probability sample of visits by patients to emergency departments (EDs) and outpatient departments (OPDs) of non-Federal, short-stay, or general hospitals. Telephone contacts are excluded.

A four-stage probability sample design is used in NHAMCS, involving samples of primary sampling units (PSUs), hospitals with EDs and/or OPDs within PSUs, EDs within hospitals and/or clinics within OPDs, and patient visits within EDs and/or clinics. In 1999 the hospital response rate for NHAMCS was 93 percent for EDs and 86 percent for OPDs. In 2000 the hospital response rate was 94 percent for EDs and 88 percent for OPDs. Hospital staff were asked to complete Patient Record Forms (PRF) for a systematic random sample of patient visits occurring during a randomly assigned 4-week reporting period. On the PRF, up to three physicians' diagnoses were collected and coded by NCHS to the *International Classification of Diseases, Clinical Modification* (ICD-9-CM). Additionally, if the cause-of-injury check box was marked on the PRF, up to three external causes of injury were coded by NCHS to the ICD-9-CM Supplementary Classification of External Causes of Injury and Poisoning. In 1999 the number of PRFs completed for EDs was 21,103 and for OPDs 29,487. In 2000 the number of PRFs completed for EDs was 25,622 and for OPDs 27,510.

For more detailed information on NHAMCS, see: McCaig LF, McLemore T. Plan and operation of the National Hospital Ambulatory Medical Care Survey. National Center for Health Statistics. Vital Health Stat 1(34). 1994; and visit the National Health Care Survey (NHCS) section of the NCHS Web site at www.cdc.gov/nchs/nhcs.htm.

National Hospital Discharge Survey (NHDS)

Centers for Disease Control and Prevention

National Center for Health Statistics

The National Hospital Discharge Survey (NHDS), which has been conducted annually since 1965, is a national probability survey designed to meet the need for information on characteristics of inpatients discharged from non-Federal short-stay hospitals in the United States. The survey is conducted in all 50 States and the District of Columbia. Only hospitals with an average length of stay of fewer than 30 days for all patients, general hospitals, or children's general hospitals are included in the survey. Federal, military, and Department of Veterans Affairs hospitals, as well as hospital units of institutions (such as prison hospitals), and hospitals with fewer than six beds staffed for patient use, are excluded. All discharged patients from in-scope hospitals are included in the survey; however, discharged newborn infants are not included in *Health, United States*.

The original sample was selected in 1964 from a frame of short-stay hospitals listed in the National Master Facility Inventory. A two-stage stratified sample design was used, with hospitals stratified according to bed size and geographic region. Sample hospitals were selected with probabilities ranging from certainty for the largest hospitals to 1 in 40 for the smallest hospitals. Within each sample hospital, a systematic random sample of discharges was selected from the daily listing sheet. Initially, the within-hospital sampling rates for selecting discharges varied inversely with the probability of hospital selection, so that the overall probability of selecting a discharge was approximately the same across the sample. Those rates were adjusted for individual hospitals in subsequent years to control the reporting burden of those hospitals.

In 1985, for the first time, two data-collection procedures were used for the survey. The first was the traditional manual system of sample selection and data abstraction. In the manual system, sample selection and transcription of information from the hospital records to abstract forms were performed by either the hospital staff or representatives of NCHS or both. The second was an automated method, used in approximately 17 percent of the sample hospitals in 1985, involving the purchase of data tapes from commercial abstracting services. These tapes were then subjected to the NCHS sampling, editing, and weighting procedures.

In 1988 NHDS was redesigned. The hospitals with the most beds and/or discharges annually were selected with certainty, but the remaining sample was selected using a three-stage stratified design. The first stage is a sample of PSUs used by the National Health Interview Survey. Within PSUs, hospitals were stratified or arrayed by abstracting status (whether subscribing to a commercial abstracting service) and within abstracting status arrayed by type of service and bed size. Within these strata and arrays, a systematic sampling scheme with probability proportional to the annual number of discharges was used to select hospitals. The rates for systematic sampling of discharges within hospitals varied inversely with probability of hospital selection within the PSU. Discharge records from hospitals submitting data via commercial abstracting services and selected State data systems (approximately 40 percent of sample hospitals) were arrayed by primary diagnoses, patient sex and age group, and date of discharge before sampling. Otherwise, the procedures for sampling discharges within hospitals were the same as those used in the prior design.

In 2000 the hospital sample was updated by continuing the sampling process among hospitals that were NHDS-eligible for the sampling frame in 2000 but not in 1997. The additional hospitals were added at the end of the list for the strata where they belonged, and the systematic sampling was continued as if the additional hospitals had been present during the initial sample selection. Hospitals that were no longer NHDS-eligible were deleted. A similar updating process occurred in 1991, 1994, and 1997.

The basic unit of estimation for NHDS is the sample patient abstract. The estimation procedure involves inflation by the reciprocal of the probability of selection, adjustment for nonresponding hospitals and missing abstracts, and ratio adjustments to fixed totals. In 2000, 509 hospitals were selected, 481 were within scope, 434 participated (90 percent), and 313,259 medical records were abstracted. In 2001, the sample consisted of 504 hospitals, of which 477 were within scope and 448 of those participated, providing data for approximately 330,000 discharges.

Hospital utilization rates per 1,000 population were computed using estimates of the civilian population of the United States as of July 1 of each year. Rates for 1990 through 1999 use postcensal estimates of the civilian population based on the

1990 census adjusted for net underenumeration using the 1990 National Population Adjustment Matrix from the U.S. Bureau of the Census. These estimates will differ from estimates that calculate discharge rates for 1990–1999 based on estimates of the civilian population that incorporate information from the census 2000 (intercensal estimates—not currently available) thereby adjusting for the "error of closure." The estimates for 2000 that appeared in *Health, United States, 2002* were computed using postcensal civilian population estimates based on the 1990 Census adjusted for net underenumeration. The estimates for 2000 and 2001 that appear in *Health, United States, 2003* were calculated using estimates of the civilian population based on census 2000, and therefore are not directly comparable with rates calculated for the 1990s. See related *Population Census and Population Estimates*.

For more detailed information on the design of NHDS and the magnitude of sampling errors associated with NHDS estimates, see: Hall MJ, DeFrances CJ. 2001 National Hospital Discharge Summary Advance data from vital and health statistics; no 332. Hyattsville, MD: National Center for Health Statistics. 2003; Dennison C, Pokras R. Design and operation of the National Hospital Discharge Survey: 1988 redesign. National Center for Health Statistics. Vital Health Stat 1(39). 2000; and visit the National Health Care Survey Web site at www.cdc.gov/nchs/nhcs.htm.

National Household Survey on Drug Abuse (NHSDA)

Substance Abuse and Mental Health Services Administration

The National Household Survey on Drug Abuse (NHSDA), sponsored by the Substance Abuse and Mental Health Services Administration (SAMHSA), collects data on use of tobacco, alcohol, and illicit drugs among persons 12 years of age and over in the civilian noninstitutionalized population in the United States. This includes civilians living on military bases and persons living in noninstitutionalized group quarters, such as college dormitories, rooming houses, and shelters. Persons excluded from the survey include homeless people who do not use shelters, active military personnel, and residents of institutional group quarters, such as jails and hospitals.

The NHSDA survey has been conducted since 1971. In 1999 the NHSDA underwent a major redesign affecting the method of data collection, sample design, sample size, and oversampling. Because of the differences in methodology and impact of the new design on data collection, comparisons should not be made between data from the redesigned surveys (1999 onward) and data obtained from surveys prior to 1999. Beginning in 1999 the survey used a combination of computer-assisted personal interview (CAPI) conducted by the interviewer and a computer-assisted self-interview (ACASI). Use of ACASI is designed to provide the respondent with a highly private and confidential means of responding to questions and to increase the level of honest reporting of illicit drug use and other sensitive behaviors.

A 5-year sample design provides State estimates for years 1999 through 2003. The sample employs a 50-State design with an independent, multistage area probability sample for each of the 50 States and the District of Columbia. The eight States with the largest population (which together account for 48 percent of the total U.S. population age 12 years and over) were designated as large sample States (California, Florida, Illinois, Michigan, New York, Ohio, Pennsylvania, and Texas). For these States the design provided a sample large enough to support direct State estimates. For the remaining 42 States and the District of Columbia, smaller, but adequate, samples were selected to support State estimates using small-area estimation techniques. The design also oversamples youths and young adults so that each State's sample is approximately equally distributed among three major age groups: 12–17 years, 18–25 years, and 26 years and over.

Each State was stratified into regions (48 regions in each of 8 large States, 12 regions in each of 42 small States and the District of Columbia). At the first stage of sampling, 8 area segments were selected in each region, for a total of 7,200 sample units nationally. In these segments, 171,519 addresses were screened and 89,745 persons were interviewed within the screened addresses in 2001. Weighted response rates for household screening and for interviewing were 91.9 percent and 73.3 percent, respectively, for an overall weighted response rate of 67.3 percent. A description of the methodology can be found in Summary of Findings from the 2001 National Household Survey on Drug Abuse, available from SAMHSA's Web site.

Direct survey estimates considered to be unreliable due to unacceptably large sampling errors are not shown in table 62 in this report, and are noted by asterisks (*). The criterion used for suppressing all direct survey estimates was based on the relative standard error (RSE), which is defined as the ratio of the standard error (se) over the estimate. Proportion estimates (p) within the range [0<p<1], rates, and corresponding estimated number of users were suppressed if:

$$[se(p) / p] / [-ln(p)] > 0.175 \text{ when } p < 0.5$$

or

$$[se(p) / (1-p)] / [-ln(1-p)] > 0.175 \text{ when } p \geq 0.5$$

The separate formulae for $p<0.5$ and $p\leq0.5$ produces a symmetric suppression rule; that is, if p is suppressed, then so will 1−p. This is an ad hoc rule that requires an effective sample size in excess of 50. When $0.05<p<0.95$, the symmetric properties of the rule produce a local maximum effective sample size of 68 at $p=0.5$. Thus, estimates with these values of p along with effective sample sizes falling below 68 are suppressed. A local minimum effective sample size of 50 occurs at $p=0.2$ and again at $p=0.8$ within this same interval; so, estimates are suppressed for values of p with effective sample sizes below 50. A minimum effective sample size of 68 was added to the suppression criteria in the 2000 NHSDA. As p approaches 0.00 or 1.00 outside the interval (0.05, 0.95), the suppression criteria will still require increasingly larger effective sample sizes. Also new to the 2000 survey is a minimum nominal sample size suppression criteria ($n=100$) that protects against unreliable estimates caused by small design effects and small nominal sample sizes. Prevalence estimates are also suppressed if they are close to zero or 100 percent (i.e., if $p<.00005$ or if $p>.99995$).

Estimates of substance use for youth based on the NHSDA are generally lower than estimates based on Monitoring the Future (MTF) and Youth Risk Behavior Surveillance System (YRBSS). In addition to the fact that the MTF excludes dropouts and absentees, rates are not directly comparable across these surveys, due to differences in populations covered, sample design, questionnaires, interview setting, and statistical approaches to make the survey estimates generalizable to the entire population. The NHSDA survey collects data in homes, whereas the MTF and YRBSS collect data in school classrooms. The NHSDA estimates are tabulated by age, while the MTF and YRBSS estimates are tabulated by grade, representing different ages as well as different populations. See Cowan CD. Coverage, Sample

Design, and Weighting in Three Federal Surveys. Journal of Drug Issues 31(3), 595–614, 2001.

For more information on the National Household Survey on Drug Abuse (NHSDA), see: NHSDA Series: H-13 Summary of Findings from the 2000 National Household Survey on Drug Abuse, DHHS Pub No (SMA) 01-3549; or write: Office of Applied Studies, Substance Abuse and Mental Health Services Administration, Room 16C-06, 5600 Fishers Lane, Rockville, MD 20857; for the 2001 NHSDA Summary of National Findings, visit the SAMHSA Web site at www.drugabusestatistics.samhsa.gov.

National Immunization Survey (NIS)

Centers for Disease Control and Prevention

National Center for Health Statistics and National Immunization Program

The National Immunization Survey (NIS) is a continuing nationwide telephone sample survey to gather data on children 15–35 months of age. Estimates of vaccine-specific coverage are available for national, State, and 28 urban areas considered to be high risk for undervaccination.

NIS uses a two-phase sample design. First, a random-digit-dialing (RDD) sample of telephone numbers is drawn. When households with age-eligible children are contacted, the interviewer collects information on the vaccinations received by all age-eligible children. In 2001 the overall response rate was 70 percent, yielding data for 33,437 children aged 15–35 months. The interviewer also collects information on the vaccination providers. In the second phase, all vaccination providers are contacted by mail. The vaccination information from providers was obtained for 72 percent of all children who were eligible for provider followup in 2001. Providers' responses are combined with information obtained from the households to provide a more accurate estimate of vaccination coverage levels. Final estimates are adjusted for households without telephones.

For more information about the survey design and methods used in estimation, see: Zell ER, Ezzati-Rice TM, Battaglia PM, Wright RA. National Immunization Survey: The Methodology of a Vaccination Surveillance System. Public Health Reports 115:65–77. 2000; or visit the NCHS Web site at www.cdc.gov/nis.

National Medical Expenditure Survey (NMES)—See Medical Expenditure Panel Survey.

National Notifiable Diseases Surveillance System (NNDSS)

Centers for Disease Control and Prevention

Epidemiology Program Office

The Epidemiology Program Office (EPO) of CDC, in partnership with the Council of State and Territorial Epidemiologists (CSTE), operates the National Notifiable Diseases Surveillance System. The primary purpose of this system is to provide weekly provisional information on the occurrence of diseases defined as notifiable by CSTE. The system also provides annual summaries of the data. State epidemiologists report cases of notifiable diseases to EPO who tabulates and publishes these data in the Morbidity and Mortality Weekly Report (MMWR) and the Summary of Notifiable Diseases, United States (entitled Annual Summary before 1985). Notifiable disease surveillance is conducted by public health practitioners at local, State, and national levels to support disease prevention and control activities.

Notifiable disease reports are received from health departments in the 50 States, 5 territories, New York City, and the District of Columbia. Policies for reporting notifiable disease cases can vary by disease or reporting jurisdiction, depending on case status classification (i.e., confirmed, probable, or suspect). CSTE and CDC annually review the status of national infectious disease surveillance and recommend additions or deletions to the list of nationally notifiable diseases based on the need to respond to emerging priorities. For example, Q fever and tularemia became nationally notifiable in 2000. However, reporting nationally notifiable diseases to CDC is voluntary. Reporting is currently mandated by law or regulation only at the local and State level. Therefore, the list of diseases that are considered notifiable varies slightly by State. For example, reporting of cyclosporiasis to CDC is not done by some States in which this disease is not notifiable to local or State authorities. More information regarding notifiable diseases, including case definitions for these conditions, is available on the Web at www.cdc.gov/epo/dphsi/phs.htm.

Notifiable disease data are useful for analyzing disease trends and determining relative disease burdens. However, these data must be interpreted in light of reporting practices. Some diseases that cause severe clinical illness (for example, plague and rabies) are most likely reported accurately if diagnosed by a clinician. However, persons who have diseases that are clinically mild and infrequently associated with serious consequences (for example, salmonellosis) might not seek medical care from a health care provider. Even if these less severe diseases are diagnosed, they are less likely to be reported.

The degree of completeness of data reporting also is influenced by the diagnostic facilities available; the control measures in effect; public awareness of a specific disease; and the interests, resources, and priorities of State and local officials responsible for disease control and public health surveillance. Finally, factors such as changes in case definitions for public health surveillance, introduction of new diagnostic tests, or discovery of new disease entities can cause changes in disease reporting that are independent of the true incidence of disease.

For more information, see: Centers for Disease Control and Prevention, Summary of Notifiable Diseases, United States, 2001 *Morbidity and Mortality Weekly Report* 50(53) Public Health Service, DHHS, Atlanta, GA, 2003; or write: Chief, Surveillance Systems Branch, Division of Public Health Surveillance and Informatics. Epidemiology Program Office, Centers for Disease Control and Prevention, 4770 Buford Highway, MS K74, Atlanta, GA 30341-3717; or visit the EPO Web site at www.cdc.gov/epo/.

National Nursing Home Survey (NNHS)

Centers for Disease Control and Prevention

National Center for Health Statistics

NCHS conducted six National Nursing Home Surveys (NNHS), the first survey from August 1973–April 1974; the second from May–December 1977; the third from August 1985–January 1986; the fourth from July–December 1995; the fifth from July–December 1997; and the sixth from July–December 1999. The next NNHS, which has undergone a major redesign, is scheduled to be conducted during calendar year 2004.

For the initial NNHS conducted in 1973–74, the universe included nursing homes that provided some level of nursing care and excluded homes providing only personal or

domiciliary care. The sample of 2,118 homes was selected from the 17,685 homes listed in the 1971 National Master Facility Inventory (NMFI) or those that opened for business in 1972. Data were obtained from about 20,600 staff and 19,000 residents. Response rates were 97 percent for facilities, 88 percent for expenses, 82 percent for staff, and 98 percent for residents.

The 1977 NNHS encompassed all types of nursing homes, including personal care and domiciliary care homes. The sample of about 1,700 facilities was selected from 23,105 nursing homes in the sampling frame, which consisted of all homes listed in the 1973 NMFI and those opening for business between 1973 and December 1976. Data were obtained from about 13,600 staff, 7,000 residents, and 5,100 discharged residents. Response rates were 95 percent for facilities, 85 percent for expenses, 81 percent for staff, 99 percent for residents, and 97 percent for discharges.

The 1985 NNHS was similar to the 1973–74 survey in that it excluded personal or domiciliary care homes. The sample of 1,220 homes was selected from a sampling frame of 20,479 nursing and related-care homes. The frame consisted of all homes in the 1982 NMFI; homes identified in the 1982 Complement Survey of NMFI "missing" from the 1982 NMFI; facilities that opened for business between 1982 and June 1984; and hospital-based nursing homes obtained from the Centers for Medicare & Medicaid Services. Information on the facility was collected through a personal interview with the administrator. Accountants were asked to complete a questionnaire on expenses or provide a financial statement. Resident data were provided by a nurse familiar with the care provided to the resident. The nurse relied on the medical record and personal knowledge of the resident. In addition to employee data that were collected during the interview with the administrator, a sample of registered nurses completed a self-administered questionnaire. Discharge data were based on information recorded in the medical record. Additional data about current and discharged residents were obtained in telephone interviews with next of kin. Data were obtained from 1,079 facilities, 2,763 registered nurses, 5,243 current residents, and 6,023 discharges. Response rates were 93 percent for facilities, 68 percent for expenses, 80 percent for registered nurses, 97 percent for residents, 95 percent for discharges, and 90 percent for next of kin.

The 1995, 1997, and 1999 NNHS also included only nursing homes that provided some level of nursing care, and excluded homes providing only personal or domiciliary care, similar to the 1985 and 1973–74 surveys. The 1995 sample of 1,500 homes was selected from a sampling frame of 17,500 nursing homes. The frame consisted of an updated version of the 1991 National Health Provider Inventory (NHPI). Data were obtained from about 1,400 nursing homes and 8,000 current residents. Data on current residents were provided by a staff member familiar with the care received by residents and from information contained in residents' medical records.

The 1997 sample of 1,488 nursing homes was the same basic sample used in 1995. Excluded were out-of-scope and out-of-business places identified in the 1995 survey. Included were a small number of additions to the sample from a supplemental frame of places not in the 1995 frame. The 1997 NNHS included the discharge component not available in the 1995 survey.

The 1999 sample of 1,423 nursing homes was selected from a sampling frame of 18,419 possible facilities from the most current National Health Provider Inventory. A supplemental frame was used to add facilities not in the 1997 frame. Like the 1995 and 1997 surveys, the 1999 survey excluded out-of-scope and out-of-business nursing homes identified in 1997. The 1999 NNHS also included a discharge resident component.

Statistics for the National Nursing Home Surveys are derived by a multistage estimation procedure that provides essentially unbiased national estimates and has three major components: (a) inflation by the reciprocals of the probabilities of sample selection, (b) adjustment for nonresponse, and (c) ratio adjustment to fixed totals. The surveys are adjusted for three types of nonresponse: (1) when an eligible nursing facility did not respond; (2) when the facility failed to complete the sampling lists; and (3) when the facility did not complete the facility questionnaire but did complete the questionnaire for residents in the facility.

For more information on the 1973–74 NNHS, see: Meiners MR. Selected operating and financial characteristics of nursing homes, United States, 1973–74 National Nursing Home Survey. National Center for Health Statistics. Vital Health Stat 13(22). 1975. For more information on the 1977 NNHS, see: Van Nostrand JF, Zappolo A, Hing E, et al. The National Nursing Home Survey, 1977 summary for the United States. National Center for Health Statistics. Vital Health Stat 13(43). 1979. For more information on the 1985 NNHS, see: Hing E, Sekscenski E, Strahan G. The National Nursing

Home Survey: 1985 summary for the United States. National Center for Health Statistics. Vital Health Stat 13(97). 1989. For more information on the 1995 NNHS, see: Strahan G. An overview of nursing homes and their current residents: Data from the 1995 National Nursing Home Survey. Advance data from vital and health statistics; no 280. Hyattsville, MD: National Center for Health Statistics. 1997. For more information on the 1997 NNHS, see: The National Nursing Home Survey: 1997 summary. National Center for Health Statistics. Vital Health Stat 13(147). 2000. For more information on the 1999 NNHS, see: Jones A. The National Nursing Home Survey: 1999 summary. National Center for Health Statistics. Vital Health Stat 13(152). 2002. Information about the 1995, 1997, 1999, and 2001 NNHS is also available at the National Health Care Survey Web site at www.cdc.gov/nchs/nhcs.htm.

National Survey of Ambulatory Surgery (NSAS)

Centers for Disease Control and Prevention

National Center for Health Statistics

The National Survey of Ambulatory Surgery (NSAS) is a nationwide sample survey of ambulatory surgery patient discharges from short-stay non-Federal hospitals and freestanding surgery centers. NSAS was conducted in 1994, 1995, and 1996. The sample consisted of eligible hospitals listed in the 1993 SMG Hospital Market Database and the 1993 SMG Freestanding Outpatient Surgery Center Database or Medicare Provider-of-Service files. Facilities specializing in dentistry, podiatry, abortion, family planning, or birthing were excluded.

A three-stage stratified cluster design was used, and facilities were stratified according to primary sampling unit (PSU). The second stage consisted of the selection of facilities from sample PSUs, and the third stage consisted of a systematic random sample of cases from all locations within a facility where ambulatory surgery was performed. Locations within hospitals dedicated exclusively to dentistry, podiatry, pain block, abortion, or small procedures (sometimes referred to as "lump and bump" rooms) were not included. In 1996, of the 751 hospitals and freestanding ambulatory surgery centers selected for the survey, 601 were in-scope and 488 responded for an overall response rate of 81 percent. These facilities provided information for approximately 125,000 ambulatory surgery discharges. Up to six procedures were coded to the *International Classification of Diseases, 9th Revision, Clinical Modification*. Estimates were derived using a multistage estimation procedure: inflation by reciprocals of the probabilities of selection; adjustment for nonresponse; and population weighting ratio adjustments.

For more detailed information on the design of NSAS, see: McLemore T, Lawrence L. Plan and operation of the National Survey of Ambulatory Surgery. National Center for Health Statistics. Vital Health Stat 1(37). 1997; and visit the National Health Care Survey Web site at www.cdc.gov/nchs/nhcs.htm.

National Survey of Family Growth (NSFG)

Centers for Disease Control and Prevention

National Center for Health Statistics

Data from the National Survey of Family Growth (NSFG) are based on samples of women ages 15–44 years in the civilian noninstitutionalized population of the United States. The first and second cycles, conducted in 1973 and 1976, excluded most women who had never been married. The third, fourth, and fifth cycles, conducted in 1982, 1988, and 1995, included all women ages 15–44 years.

The purpose of the survey is to provide national data on factors affecting birth and pregnancy rates, adoption, and maternal and infant health. These factors include sexual activity, marriage, divorce and remarriage, unmarried cohabitation, contraception and sterilization, infertility, breastfeeding, pregnancy loss, low birthweight, and use of medical care for family planning and infertility.

Interviews are conducted in person by professional female interviewers using a standardized questionnaire. In 1973–88 the average interview length was about 1 hour. In 1995 the average interview lasted about 1 hour and 45 minutes. In all cycles black women were sampled at higher rates than white women, so that detailed statistics for black women could be produced.

Interviewing for Cycle 1 of NSFG was conducted from June 1973 to February 1974. Counties and independent cities of the United States were sampled to form a frame of primary sampling units (PSUs), and 101 PSUs were selected. From these 101 PSUs, 10,879 women 15–44 years of age were selected, 9,797 of these were interviewed. Most never-married women were excluded from the 1973 NSFG.

Interviewing for Cycle 2 of NSFG was conducted from January to September 1976. From 79 PSUs, 10,202 eligible women were identified; of these, 8,611 were interviewed. Again, most never-married women were excluded from the sample for the 1976 NSFG.

Interviewing for Cycle 3 of NSFG was conducted from August 1982 to February 1983. The sample design was similar to that in Cycle 2: 31,027 households were selected in 79 PSUs. Household screener interviews were completed in 29,511 households (95.1 percent). Of the 9,964 eligible women identified, 7,969 were interviewed. For the first time in NSFG, Cycle 3 included women of all marital statuses.

Interviewing for Cycle 4 was conducted between January and August 1988. The sample was obtained from households that had been interviewed in the National Health Interview Survey in the 18 months between October 1, 1985 and March 31, 1987. For the first time, women living in Alaska and Hawaii were included so that the survey covered women from the noninstitutionalized population of the entire United States. The sample was drawn from 156 PSUs; 10,566 eligible women ages 15–44 years were sampled. Interviews were completed with 8,450 women.

Between July and November 1990, 5,686 women were interviewed by telephone in the first NSFG telephone reinterview. The average length of interview in 1990 was 20 minutes. The response rate for the 1990 telephone reinterview was 68 percent of those responding to the 1988 survey and still eligible for the 1990 survey.

Interviewing for Cycle 5 of NSFG was conducted between January and October 1995. The sample was obtained from households that had been interviewed in 198 PSUs in the National Health Interview Survey in 1993. Of the 13,795 eligible women in the sample, 10,847 were interviewed. For the first time, Hispanic as well as black women were sampled at a higher rate than other women.

In order to make national estimates from the sample for the millions of women ages 15–44 years in the United States, data for the interviewed sample women were (a) inflated by the reciprocal of the probability of selection at each stage of sampling (for example, if there was a 1 in 5,000 chance that a woman would be selected for the sample, her sampling weight was 5,000), (b) adjusted for nonresponse, and (c) forced to agree with benchmark population values based on data from the Current Population Survey of the U.S. Bureau of the Census (this last step is called "poststratification").

Quality control procedures for selecting and training interviewers, and coding, editing, and processing data were built into NSFG to minimize nonsampling error.

More information on the methodology of NSFG is available in the following reports: French DK. National Survey of Family Growth, Cycle I: Sample design, estimation procedures, and variance estimation. National Center for Health Statistics. Vital Health Stat 2(76). 1978; Grady WR. National Survey of Family Growth, Cycle II: Sample design, estimation procedures, and variance estimation. National Center for Health Statistics. Vital Health Stat 2(87). 198l; Bachrach CA, Horn MC, Mosher WD, Shimizu I. National Survey of Family Growth, Cycle III: Sample design, weighting, and variance estimation. National Center for Health Statistics. Vital Health Stat 2(98). 1985; Judkins DR, Mosher WD, Botman SL. National Survey of Family Growth: Design, estimation, and inference. National Center for Health Statistics. Vital Health Stat 2(109). 1991; Goksel H, Judkins DR, Mosher WD. Nonresponse adjustments for a telephone followup to a National In-Person Survey. Journal of Official Statistics 8(4):417–32. 1992; Kelly JE, Mosher WD, Duffer AP, Kinsey SH. Plan and operation of the 1995 National Survey of Family Growth. Vital Health Stat 1(36). 1997; Potter FJ, Iannacchione VG, Mosher WD, Mason RE, Kavee JD. Sampling weights, imputation, and variance estimation in the 1995 National Survey of Family Growth. Vital Health Stat 2(124). 1998; or visit the NCHS Web site at www.cdc.gov/nchs/nsfg.htm.

National Survey of Substance Abuse Treatment Services (N-SSATS)

Substance Abuse and Mental Health Services Administration

The National Survey of Substance Abuse Treatment Services (N-SSATS) is part of the Drug and Alcohol Services Information System (DASIS) maintained by the Substance Abuse and Mental Health Services Administration (SAMHSA). N-SSATS is a census of all known substance abuse treatment facilities. It seeks information from all specialized facilities that treat substance abuse. These include facilities that treat only substance abuse, as well as specialty substance abuse units operating within larger mental health facilities (for example, community mental health centers), general health (for example, hospitals), social service (for

example, family assistance centers), and criminal justice (for example, probation departments) agencies. N-SSATS solicits data concerning facility and client characteristics for a specific reference day (October 1 in 1998 and 2000 and March 29 in 2002) including number of individuals in treatment, substance of abuse (alcohol, drugs, or both), and types of services. Public and private facilities are included.

Treatment facilities contacted through N-SSATS are identified from the Inventory of Substance Abuse Treatment Services (I-SATS) that lists all known substance abuse treatment facilities. Response rates to the surveys were 91, 94, and 95 percent in 1998, 2000, and 2002, respectively. The full survey was not conducted in 1999 or 2001.

For further information on N-SSATS, contact: Office of Applied Studies, Substance Abuse and Mental Health Services Administration, Room 16-105, 5600 Fishers Lane, Rockville, MD 20857; or visit the OAS statistical information section of the SAMHSA Web site at www.drugabusestatistics.samhsa.gov.

National Vital Statistics System

Centers for Disease Control and Prevention

National Center for Health Statistics

Through the National Vital Statistics System, the National Center for Health Statistics (NCHS) collects and publishes data on births, deaths, marriages, and divorces in the United States. Fetal deaths are classified and tabulated separately from other deaths. The Division of Vital Statistics obtains information on births and deaths from the registration offices of all States, New York City, the District of Columbia, Puerto Rico, the U.S. Virgin Islands, and Guam. Geographic coverage for births and deaths has been complete since 1933. Trend tables in this book show data for the aggregate of 50 States, New York City, and the District of Columbia, as well as for each individual State and the District of Columbia.

Until 1972 microfilm copies of all death certificates and a 50-percent sample of birth certificates were received from all registration areas and processed by NCHS. In 1972 some States began sending their data to NCHS through the Cooperative Health Statistics System (CHSS). States that participated in the CHSS program processed 100 percent of their death and birth records and sent the entire data file to NCHS on computer tapes. Currently, data are sent to NCHS through the Vital Statistics Cooperative Program (VSCP), following the same procedures as CHSS. The number of participating States grew from 6 in 1972 to 46 in 1984. Starting in 1985 all 50 States and the District of Columbia participated in VSCP.

U.S. Standard Certificates—U.S. Standard Live Birth and Death Certificates and Fetal Death Reports are revised periodically, allowing careful evaluation of each item and addition, modification, and deletion of items. Beginning with 1989 revised standard certificates replaced the 1978 versions. The 1989 revision of the birth certificate includes items to identify the Hispanic parentage of newborns and to expand information about maternal and infant health characteristics. The 1989 revision of the death certificate includes items on educational attainment and Hispanic origin of decedents, as well as changes to improve the medical certification of cause of death. Standard certificates recommended by NCHS are modified in each registration area to serve the area's needs. However, most certificates conform closely in content and arrangement to the standard certificate, and all certificates contain a minimum data set specified by NCHS.

Birth File

The birth file is comprised of demographic and medical information from birth certificates. Demographic information, such as race and ethnicity, is provided by the mother at the time of birth. Medical and health information is based on hospital records. The number of States reporting information on maternal education, Hispanic origin, marital status, and tobacco use during pregnancy has increased over the years spanned by this report. Interpretation of trend data should take into consideration expansion of reporting areas and immigration. See Appendix II for methodologic and reporting area changes for the following birth certificate items: *Age* (maternal age); *Education* (maternal education); *Hispanic origin; Marital status; Prenatal care; Race; Tobacco use.*

For more information, see: National Center for Health Statistics, *Vital Statistics of the United States*, Vol. I Natality, Technical Appendix, available at the NCHS Web site at www.cdc.gov/nchs/births.htm.

Mortality File

The mortality data file is comprised of demographic and medical information from death certificates. Demographic information is provided by the funeral director based on information supplied by an informant. Medical certification of cause of death is provided by a physician, medical examiner, or coroner. The mortality data file is a fundamental source of cause-of-death information by demographic characteristics and for geographic areas, such as States. The mortality file is one of the few sources of comparable health-related data for smaller geographic areas in the United States and over a long time period. Mortality data can be used not only to present the characteristics of those dying in the United States, but also to determine life expectancy and to compare mortality trends with other countries. Data for the entire United States refer to events occurring within the United States; data for geographic areas are by place of residence. See Appendix II for methodologic and reporting area changes for the following death certificate items: *Education; Hispanic origin; Race.*

For more information, see: Grove RD, Hetzel AM. *Vital statistics rates in the United States, 1940–60.* Washington: U.S. Government Printing Office, 1968; and National Center for Health Statistics, *Vital Statistics of the United States*, Vol. II Mortality Part A, Technical Appendix, available at the NCHS Web site at www.cdc.gov/nchs/datawh/statab/pubd/ta.htm.

Multiple Cause of Death File

The National Center for Health Statistics (NCHS) is responsible for compiling and publishing annual national statistics on causes of death. In carrying out this responsibility, NCHS adheres to the World Health Organization Nomenclature Regulations. These Regulations require that (1) cause of death be coded in accordance with the applicable revision of the *International Classification of Diseases* (ICD) (see Appendix II, table IV and ICD); and (2) underlying cause of death be selected in accordance with international rules. Traditionally, national mortality statistics have been based on a count of deaths with one underlying cause assigned for each death. National single-cause mortality statistics go back to the year 1900.

Starting with data year 1968, electronic files exist with multiple cause of death information. These files contain codes for all diagnostic terms and related codable information recorded on the death certificate. These codes comprise the entity axis, and are the input for a software program called TRANSAX. The TRANSAX program eliminates redundant entity axis codes and combines other entity axis codes to create the best set of ICD codes for a record. The output of the TRANSAX program is the record axis. Record axis data are generally used for research and analysis of multiple or nonunderlying cause of death. Because the function of the TRANSAX program is not to select a single underlying cause of death, record axis data may or may not include the underlying cause. Tabulations of underlying and nonunderlying cause of death in table 48 (selected occupational diseases) are compiled by searching both underlying cause of death and record axis data.

For more information, see www.cdc.gov/nchs/products/ elec_prods/subject/mortmcd.htm.

Linked Birth/Infant Death Data Set

National linked files of live births and infant deaths are data sets for research on infant mortality. To create these data sets, death certificates are linked with corresponding birth certificates for infants who die in the United States before their first birthday. Linked data files include all variables on the national natality file, including the more accurate racial and ethnic information, as well as variables on the national mortality file, including cause of death and age at death. The linkage makes available for the analysis of infant mortality extensive information from the birth certificate about the pregnancy, maternal risk factors, and infant characteristics and health items at birth. Each year 97–98 percent of infant death records are linked to their corresponding birth records.

National linked files of live births and infant deaths were first produced for the 1983 birth cohort. Birth cohort linked file data are available for 1983–91 and period linked file data for 1995–2000. Period linked file data starting with 1995 are not strictly comparable with birth cohort data for 1983–91. While birth cohort linked files have methodological advantages, their production incurs substantial delays in data availability, since it is necessary to wait until the close of a second data year to include all infant deaths to the birth cohort.

Starting with data year 1995, more timely linked file data are produced in a period data format preceding the release of the corresponding birth cohort format. Other changes to the data set starting with 1995 data include addition of record weights to correct for the 2.2–2.5 percent of records that could not be linked and addition of an imputation for not stated birthweight. The 1995–2000 weighted mortality rates are less than 1 percent to 4.1 percent higher than unweighted rates for the same period. The 1995–2000 weighted mortality rates with imputed birthweight are less than 1 percent to 6.3 percent

higher than unweighted rates with imputed birthweight for the same period.

For more information, see: Mathews TJ, Menacker F, MacDorman MF. Infant mortality statistics from the 2000 period linked birth/infant death data set. National vital statistics reports; vol 50 no 12. Hyattsville, MD: National Center for Health Statistics. 2002; or visit the NCHS Web site at www.cdc.gov/nchs/linked.htm.

Compressed Mortality File

The Compressed Mortality File (CMF) used to compute death rates by urbanization level is a county-level national mortality and population database. The mortality database of CMF is derived from the detailed mortality files of the National Vital Statistics System starting with 1968. The population database of CMF is derived from intercensal and postcensal population estimates and census counts of the resident population of each U.S. county by age, race, and sex. Counties are categorized according to level of urbanization based on an NCHS-modified version of the 1993 rural-urban continuum codes for metropolitan and nonmetropolitan counties developed by the Economic Research Service, U.S. Department of Agriculture. See Appendix II, *Urbanization*.

For more information about the CMF, contact: D. Ingram, Office of Analysis, Epidemiology, and Health Promotion, National Center for Health Statistics, 3311 Toledo Road, Mailstop 6226, Hyattsville, MD 20782.

Nurse Supply Estimates

Health Resources and Services Administration (HRSA)

Nurse supply estimates in this report are based on a model developed by HRSA's Bureau of Health Professions to meet the requirements of Section 951, P.L. 94-63. The model estimates for each State (a) population of nurses currently licensed to practice; (b) supply of full- and part-time practicing nurses (or available to practice); and (c) full-time equivalent supply of nurses practicing full time plus one-half of those practicing part time (or available on that basis). The three estimates are divided into three levels of highest educational preparation—associate degree or diploma, baccalaureate, and master's and doctorate. Among the factors considered are new graduates, changes in educational status, nursing employment rates, age, migration patterns, death rates, and licensure phenomena. The base data for the model are derived from the National Sample Surveys of Registered Nurses, conducted by the Division of Nursing, Bureau of Health Professions, HRSA. Other data sources include National League for Nursing for data on nursing education and National Council of State Boards of Nursing for data on licensure. For further information, visit HRSA's Division of Nursing Web site at www.bhpr.hrsa.gov/nursing/.

Online Survey Certification and Reporting Database (OSCAR)

Centers for Medicare & Medicaid Services

The Online Survey Certification and Reporting (OSCAR) database has been maintained by the Centers for Medicare & Medicaid Services (CMS), formerly the Health Care Financing Administration (HCFA), since 1992. OSCAR is an updated version of the Medicare and Medicaid Automated Certification System that has been in existence since 1972. OSCAR is an administrative database containing detailed information on all Medicare and Medicaid health care providers in addition to all currently certified Medicare and Medicaid nursing home facilities in the United States and Territories. (Data for the Territories are not shown in this report.) The purpose of the nursing home facility survey certification process is to ensure that nursing facilities meet the current CMS long-term care requirements and thus can participate in serving Medicare and Medicaid beneficiaries. Included in the OSCAR database are all certified nursing facilities, certified hospital-based nursing homes, and certified units for other types of nursing home facilities (for example, life-care communities or board and care homes). Facilities not included in OSCAR are all noncertified facilities (that is, facilities that are only licensed by the State and are limited to private payment sources) and nursing homes that are part of the Department of Veterans Affairs. Also excluded are nursing homes that are intermediate care facilities for the mentally retarded.

Information on the number of beds, residents, and resident characteristics is collected during an inspection of all certified facilities. The information in OSCAR is based on each facility's own administrative record system in addition to interviews with key administrative staff members.

All certified nursing homes are inspected by representatives of the State survey agency (generally the department of health) at least once every 15 months. Therefore a complete census must be based on a 15-month reporting cycle rather than a 12-month cycle. Some nursing homes are inspected twice or more often during any given reporting cycle. In order to avoid overcounting, the data must be edited and duplicates removed. Data editing and compilation were performed by Cowles Research Group and published in the group's *Nursing Home Statistical Yearbook* series

For more information, see: Cowles CM, 1995; 1996; 1997 Nursing Home Statistical Yearbook. Anacortes, WA: Cowles Research Group (CRG), 1995; 1997; 1998; Cowles CM, 1998; 1999; 2000; 2001 Nursing Home Statistical Yearbook. Washington, DC: American Association of Homes and Services for the Aging (AAHSA), 1999; 2000; 2001; 2002; HCFA: OSCAR Data Users Reference Guide, 1995, available from CMS, Health Standards and Quality Bureau, HCFA/HSQB S2 11-07, 7500 Security Boulevard, Baltimore, MD 21244; and visit the CMS Web site at www.cms.gov or the CRG Web site at www.longtermcareinfo.com/crg or the AAHSA Web site at www.aahsa.org.

Population Census and Population Estimates

Bureau of the Census

Decennial Census

The census of population (decennial census) has been held in the United States every 10 years since 1790. The decennial census has enumerated the resident population as of April 1 of the census year ever since 1930. Data on sex, race, age, and marital status are collected from 100 percent of the enumerated population. More detailed information such as income, education, housing, occupation, and industry are collected from a representative sample of the population.

Race Data on the 1990 Census

The question on race on the 1990 census was based on the Office of Management and Budget's (OMB) "1977 Statistical Policy Directive 15, Race and Ethnicity Standards for Federal Statistics and Administrative Reporting." This document specified rules for the collection, tabulation, and reporting of race and ethnicity data within the Federal statistical system. The 1977 standards required Federal agencies to report race-specific tabulations using four single-race categories: American Indian or Alaska Native, Asian or Pacific Islander, black, and white. Under the 1977 standards, race and ethnicity were considered to be two separate and distinct concepts. Thus, persons of Hispanic origin may be of any race.

Race Data on the 2000 Census

The question on race on the 2000 census was based on OMB's 1997 "Revisions of the Standards for the Classification of Federal Data on Race and Ethnicity" (see Appendix II, *Race*). The 1997 standards incorporated two major changes in the collection, tabulation, and presentation of race data. First, the 1997 standards increased from four to five the minimum set of categories to be used by Federal agencies for identification of race: American Indian or Alaska Native, Asian, Black or African American, Native Hawaiian or Other Pacific Islander, and White. Second, the 1997 standards included the requirement that Federal data collection programs allow respondents to select one or more race categories when responding to a query on their racial identity. This provision means that there are potentially 31 race groups, depending on whether an individual selects one, two, three, four, or all five of the race categories. The 1997 standards continue to call for use, when possible, of a separate question on Hispanic or Latino ethnicity and specify that the ethnicity question should appear before the question on race. Thus under the 1997 standards, as under the 1977 standards, Hispanics may be of any race.

Modified Decennial Census Files

For several decades the Census Bureau has produced modified decennial census files. These modified files incorporate adjustments to the 100 percent April 1 count data for (1) errors in the census data discovered subsequent to publication, (2) misreported age data, and (3) nonspecified race.

For the 1990 census, the Census Bureau modified the age, race, and sex data on the census and produced the Modified Age Race Sex (MARS) file. The differences between the population counts on the original census file and the MARS file are primarily due to modification of the race data. Of the 248.7 million persons enumerated in 1990, 9.8 million persons did not specify their race (over 95 percent were of Hispanic origin). For the 1990 MARS file, these persons were assigned the race reported by a nearby person with an identical response to the Hispanic origin question.

For the 2000 census, the Census Bureau modified the race data on the census and produced the Modified Race Data Summary File. For this file, persons who reported "Some

other race" as part of their race response were assigned to one of the 31 race groups, which are the single- and multiple-race combinations of the five race categories specified in the 1997 race and ethnicity standards. Persons who did not specify their race were assigned to one of the 31 race groups using imputation. Of the 18.5 million persons who reported "Some other race" as part of their race response or who did not specify their race, 16.8 million (90.4 percent) were of Hispanic origin.

Bridged-Race Population Estimates for Census 2000

Race data on the 2000 census are not comparable with race data on other data systems that are continuing to collect data using the 1977 standards on race and ethnicity during the transition to full implementation of the 1997 standards. For example, most of the States in the Vital Statistics Cooperative Program will revise their birth and death certificates to conform to the 1997 standards after 2000. Thus, population estimates for 2000 and beyond with race categories comparable to the 1977 categories are needed so that race-specific birth and death rates can be calculated. To meet this need, NCHS, in collaboration with the U.S. Census Bureau, developed methodology to bridge the 31 race groups in census 2000 to the four single-race categories specified under the 1977 standards.

The bridging methodology was developed using information from the 1997–2000 National Health Interview Survey (NHIS) (Ingram DD, Weed JA, Parker JD, et al. U.S. census 2000 population with bridged race categories. Vital Health Stat 2. Forthcoming, 2003.) The NHIS is an annual survey sponsored by NCHS and conducted by the Census Bureau (see *National Health Interview Survey*). The NHIS provides a unique opportunity to investigate multiple-race groups because since 1982, the NHIS has allowed respondents to choose more than one race but has also asked respondents reporting multiple races to choose a "primary" race. The bridging methodology developed by NCHS involved the application of regression models relating person-level and county-level covariates to the selection of a particular primary race by the multiple-race respondents. Bridging proportions derived from these models were applied by the U.S. Census Bureau to the Census 2000 Modified Race Data Summary File. This application resulted in bridged counts of the April 1, 2000 resident single-race populations for four racial groups, American Indian or Alaska Native, Asian or Pacific Islander, black, and white.

For more information about bridged-race population estimates, see www.cdc.gov/nchs/about/major/dvs/popbridge/popbridge.htm.

Postcensal Population Estimates

Postcensal population estimates are estimates made for the years following a census, before the next census has been taken. National postcensal population estimates are derived by updating the resident population enumerated in the decennial census using a components of population change approach. The following formula is used to update the decennial census counts:

(1) decennial census enumerated resident population

(2) + births to U.S. resident women,

(3) − deaths to U.S. residents,

(4) + net international migration,

(5) + net movement of U.S. Armed Forces and civilian citizens of the U.S.

State postcensal estimates are based on similar data and a variety of other data series, including school statistics from State departments of education and parochial school systems. The postcensal estimates are consistent with official decennial census figures and do not reflect estimated decennial census underenumeration.

The Census Bureau has produced a postcensal series of estimates of the July 1 resident population of the United States based on census 2000 by applying the components of change methodology to the Modified Race Data Summary File. These postcensal estimates have race data for 31 race groups, in accordance with the 1997 race and ethnicity standards. So that the race data for the 2000-based postcensal estimates would be comparable with race data on vital records, the Census Bureau applied the NHIS bridging methodology to the 31-race group postcensal population estimates to obtain postcensal estimates for the four single-race categories (American Indian or Alaska Native, Asian or Pacific Islander, black, and white). Bridged-race postcensal population estimates are available at www.cdc.gov/nchs/about/major/dvs/popbridge/popbridge.htm.

Note that before the bridged-race April 1, 2000 population counts and the bridged-race 2000-based postcensal estimates were available, the Census Bureau extended their postcensal

series of estimates based on the 1990 census (with the four single-race categories needed to compute vital rates) to July 1, 2001. NCHS initially calculated vital rates for 2000 using 1990-based July 1, 2000 postcensal population estimates and vital rates for 2001 using 1990-based July 1, 2001 postcensal estimates. Vital rates for 2000 have been revised using the bridged-race April 1, 2000 population counts and vital rates for 2001 have been revised using the 2000-based bridged-race July 1, 2001 postcensal population estimates.

Intercensal Population Estimates

The further from the census year on which the postcensal estimates are based, the less accurate are the postcensal estimates. With the completion of the decennial census at the end of the decade, intercensal estimates for the preceding decade were prepared to replace the less accurate postcensal estimates. Intercensal population estimates take into account the census of population at the beginning and end of the decade. Thus intercensal estimates are more accurate than postcensal estimates as they correct for the "error of closure" or difference between the estimated population at the end of the decade and the census count for that date. The "error of closure" at the national level was quite small for the 1960s (379,000). However, for the 1970s it amounted to almost 5 million, for the 1980s, 1.5 million, and for the 1990s, about 6 million. The error of closure differentially affects age, race, sex, and Hispanic origin subgroup populations as well as the rates based on these populations. Vital rates that were calculated using postcensal population estimates are routinely revised when intercensal estimates become available because the intercensal estimates correct for the error of closure.

Intercensal estimates for the 1990s with race data comparable to the 1977 standards have been derived so that vital rates for the 1990s could be revised to reflect census 2000. Calculation of the intercensal population estimates for the 1990s was complicated by the incomparability of the race data on the 1990 and 2000 censuses. The Census Bureau, in collaboration with National Cancer Institute and NCHS, derived race-specific intercensal population estimates for the 1990s using the 1990 MARS file as the beginning population base and the bridged-race population estimates for April 1, 2000 as the ending population base. Bridged-race intercensal population estimates are available at www.cdc.gov/nchs/about/major/dvs/popbridge/popbridge.htm.

Revised bridged-race population estimates for women aged 15–17 and 18–19 years based on the 2000 census for computing teenage birth rates in table 3 were not available from the U.S. Census Bureau when this report was prepared. The 1991–99 population estimates for these teenage subgroups were prepared by the Division of Vital Statistics, National Center for Health Statistics (NCHS). The NCHS population estimates were prepared by applying proportions derived from the 1990-based population estimates (according to data year, race, and Hispanic origin for the teenage population) to the 2000-based population of women aged 15–19 years within each race/Hispanic origin group, and adjusting the sum of the population estimates to be consistent with the total population of women aged 15–19 years for each race/Hispanic origin group (2000 based). Rates based on these population estimates are intended as interim measures and caution should be used in interpreting the rates and trends. When the necessary intercensal population estimates based on the 2000 census become available from the U.S. Bureau of the Census, the rates for women aged 15–17 and 18–19 years in table 3 will be revised on the Web site at www.cdc.gov/nchs/hus.htm.

Special Population Estimates

Special population estimates are prepared for the education reporting area for mortality statistics because educational attainment of decedent is not reported by all 50 States. The Housing and Household Economics Statistics Division of the U.S. Bureau of the Census currently produces unpublished estimates of populations by age, race, sex, and educational attainment for NCHS. These population estimates are based on the Current Population Survey, adjusted to resident population controls. The control totals used for July 1, 1994–96 are 1990-based population estimates for 45 reporting States and the District of Columbia (DC); for July 1, 1997–2000, 1990-based population estimates for 46 reporting States and DC; and for July 1, 2001, 2000-based population estimates for 47 reporting States and DC. See Appendix II, *Education.*

For more information about the population census and population estimates, visit the U.S. Bureau of the Census Web site at www.census.gov/.

Sexually Transmitted Disease (STD) Surveillance

Centers for Disease Control and Prevention

National Center of HIV, STD, and TB Prevention

The Division of STD Prevention (DSTD) of the National Center of HIV, STD, and TB Prevention (NCHSTP), Centers for Disease Control and Prevention (CDC) compiles sexually transmitted disease (STD) surveillance information from the following sources of data: (1) case reports from STD project areas; (2) prevalence data from the Regional Infertility Prevention Program, the National Job Training Program (formerly the Job Corps), the Jail STD Prevalence Monitoring Projects, the adolescent Women Reproductive Health Monitoring Project, the Men Who Have Sex With Men (MSM) Prevalence Monitoring Project, and the Indian Health Service; (3) sentinel surveillance of gonococcal antimicrobial resistance from the Gonococcal Isolate Surveillance Project (GISP); and (4) national sample surveys implemented by federal and private organizations.

Case reports of STDs are reported to CDC by STD surveillance systems operated by State and local STD control programs and health departments in 50 States, the District of Columbia, selected cities, 3,139 U.S. counties, and outlying areas comprised of U.S. dependencies and possessions, and independent nations in free association with the United States. Case report data is the source of statistical data in table 52. Because of incomplete diagnosis and reporting, the number of STD cases reported to CDC is less than the actual number of cases occurring among the United States population. Data from outlying areas are not included in table 52.

STD data are submitted to CDC on a variety of hardcopy summary reporting forms (monthly, quarterly, and annually) and electronic summary or individual case-specific (line-listed) formats via the National Electronic Telecommunications System for Surveillance (NETSS). Reports and corrections sent to CDC on hardcopy forms and for NETSS electronic data through May 3, 2002, are included in table 52.

Crude incidence rates (new cases/population) were calculated on an annual basis per 100,000 civilian population. The 2001 rates for the United States were calculated by dividing the number of cases reported in 2001 by the post-1990 estimated 2000 population.

For more information, see: Centers for Disease Control and Prevention. *Sexually Transmitted Disease Surveillance, 2001.* Atlanta, GA: U.S. Department of Health and Human Services, September 2002; or visit the STD Prevention Web site at: www.cdc.gov/std/stats/.

Surveillance, Epidemiology, and End Results Program (SEER)

National Cancer Institute

In the Surveillance, Epidemiology, and End Results (SEER) Program, the National Cancer Institute (NCI) contracts with population-based registries throughout the United States to provide data on all residents diagnosed with cancer during the year and to provide current followup information on all previously diagnosed patients.

Analysis of cancer survival rates in this report covers residents at the time of the initial diagnosis of cancer in the following SEER 9 registries: Atlanta, Georgia; Connecticut; Detroit, Michigan; Hawaii; Iowa; New Mexico; San Francisco-Oakland; Seattle-Puget Sound; and Utah. Analysis of cancer incidence covers residents in the following SEER 12 registries: the SEER 9 registries plus Los Angeles and San Jose-Monterey, California and the Alaska Native Tumor Registry.

Population estimates (1990-based postcensal estimates) used to calculate incidence rates are obtained from the U.S. Bureau of the Census. NCI uses estimation procedures as needed to obtain estimates for years and races not included in data provided by the U.S. Bureau of the Census. Rates presented in this report may differ somewhat from previous reports due to revised population estimates and the addition and deletion of small numbers of incidence cases.

Life tables used to determine normal life expectancy when calculating relative survival rates were obtained from NCHS and in-house calculations. Separate life tables are used for each race-sex-specific group included in the SEER Program.

For further information, see: Ries LAG, Eisner MP, Kosary CL, et al. (eds). *SEER Cancer Statistics Review 1973–99.* National Cancer Institute. Bethesda, MD. 2002; or visit the SEER Web site at www.seer.cancer.gov.

Survey of Occupational Injuries and Illnesses (SOII)

Bureau of Labor Statistics

Since 1971 the Bureau of Labor Statistics (BLS) has conducted an annual survey of establishments in the private sector to collect statistics on occupational injuries and illnesses. The Survey of Occupational Injuries and Illnesses is a Federal/State program in which employer reports are collected from about 169,000 private industry establishments and processed by State agencies cooperating with BLS. Data for the mining industry and for railroad activities are provided by Department of Labor's Mine Safety and Health Administration and Department of Transportation's Federal Railroad Administration. Excluded from the survey are self-employed individuals; farmers with fewer than 11 employees; private households; Federal Government agencies; and employees in State and local government agencies. Establishments are classified in industry categories based on the 1987 Standard Industrial Classification (SIC) Manual, as defined by the Office of Management and Budget.

Survey estimates of occupational injuries and illnesses are based on a scientifically selected probability sample, rather than a census of the entire population. An independent sample is selected for each State and the District of Columbia that represents industries in that jurisdiction. BLS includes all the State samples in the national sample.

Establishments included in the survey are instructed in a mailed questionnaire to provide summary totals of all entries for the previous calendar year to its Log and Summary of Occupational Injuries and Illnesses (OSHA No. 200 form). Additionally, from the selected establishments, approximately 550,000 injuries and illnesses with days away from work are sampled to obtain demographic and detailed case characteristic information. An occupational injury is any injury such as a cut, fracture, sprain, or amputation that results from a work-related event or from a single instantaneous exposure in the work environment. An occupational illness is any abnormal condition or disorder other than one resulting from an occupational injury, caused by exposure to factors associated with employment. It includes acute and chronic illnesses or diseases that may be caused by inhalation, absorption, ingestion, or direct contact. Lost workday cases involve days away from work, days of restricted work activity, or both. The response rate is about 92 percent.

The number of injuries and illnesses reported in any given year can be influenced by the level of economic activity, working conditions and work practices, worker experience and training, and the number of hours worked. Long-term latent illnesses caused by exposure to carcinogens are believed to be understated in the survey's illness measures. In contrast, new illnesses such as contact dermatitis and carpal tunnel syndrome are easier to relate directly to workplace activity.

For more information, see: Bureau of Labor Statistics, Workplace Injuries and Illnesses in 2001, Washington, DC. U.S. Department of Labor, December 2002; or visit the BLS occupational safety and health Web site at www.bls.gov/iif/home.htm.

Youth Risk Behavior Survey (YRBS)

Centers for Disease Control and Prevention

National Center for Chronic Disease Prevention and Health Promotion

The national Youth Risk Behavior Survey (YRBS) is conducted by the Centers for Disease Control and Prevention's National Center for Chronic Disease Prevention and Health Promotion to monitor the prevalence of priority health risk behaviors among high school students in grades 5–12 that contribute to morbidity and mortality in both adolescence and adulthood.

The national YRBS of high school students was conducted in 1990, 1991, 1993, 1995, 1997, 1999, and 2001. The national YRBS school-based surveys employ a three-stage cluster sample design to produce a nationally representative sample of students in grades 5–12 attending public and private high schools. The first-stage sampling frame contains primary sampling units (PSUs) consisting of large counties or groups of smaller, adjacent counties. The PSUs are then stratified based on degree of urbanization and relative percent of black and Hispanic students in the PSU. The PSUs are selected from these strata with probability proportional to school enrollment size. At the second sampling stage, schools are selected with probability proportional to school enrollment size. To enable separate analysis of data for black and Hispanic students, schools with substantial numbers of black and Hispanic students are sampled at higher rates than all other schools. The third stage of sampling consists of randomly selecting one or two intact classes of a required subject from grades 5–12 at each chosen school. All students in the selected classes are eligible to participate in the survey. A weighting factor is applied to each student record to adjust for nonresponse and for the varying probabilities of selection, including those resulting from the oversampling of black and Hispanic students. The sample size for the 2001 YRBS was 13,601. The school response rate was 75 percent, and the student response rate was 83 percent, for an overall response rate of 63 percent.

National YRBS data are subject to at least two limitations. First, these data apply only to adolescents who attend regular high school. These students may not be representative of all persons in this age group because those who have dropped out of high school or attend an alternative high school are not surveyed. Second, the extent of underreporting or overreporting cannot be determined, although the survey questions demonstrate good test-retest reliability.

Estimates of substance use for youth based on the YRBS differ from the National Household Survey on Drug Abuse (NHSDA) and Monitoring the Future (MTF). Rates are not directly comparable across these surveys due to differences in populations covered, sample design, questionnaires, interview setting, and statistical approaches to make the survey estimates generalizable to the entire population. The NHSDA survey collects data in homes, whereas the MTF and YRBS collect data in school classrooms. The NHSDA estimates are tabulated by age, while the MTF and YRBS estimates are tabulated by grade, representing different ages as well as different populations. See Cowan CD. Coverage, Sample Design, and Weighting in Three Federal Surveys. Journal of Drug Issues 31(3), 595–614, 2001.

For further information on the YRBS, see: CDC. Youth risk behavior surveillance—United States, 1999. CDC surveillance summaries, June 9, 2000. MMWR 2000:49(SS-05); CDC. Youth risk behavior surveillance—United States, 2001. CDC surveillance summaries, June 21, 2002. MMWR 2002:51(SS-04); or write: Director, Division of Adolescent and School Health, National Center for Chronic Disease Prevention and Health Promotion, Centers for Disease Control and Prevention, 4770 Buford Highway NE, Mail Stop K-32, Atlanta, GA 30341-3717; or visit the Division of Adolescent and School Health Web site at www.cdc.gov/nccdphp/dash/.

Private and Global Sources

Alan Guttmacher Institute Abortion Survey

The Alan Guttmacher Institute (AGI) conducts periodic surveys of abortion providers. Data are collected from clinics, physicians, and hospitals identified as potential providers of abortion services. For 1999 and 2000, 2,442 facilities were surveyed. In addition, State health statistics agencies were contacted, requesting all available data reported by providers to each State health agency on the number of abortions performed in 1999 and 2000. For States that provide data to AGI, the health agency figures were used for providers who did not respond to the survey. Of the 2,442 potential providers, 1,931 performed abortions between January 1999 and June 2001. Of the abortions reported for 2000, 77 percent were reported by the providers, 10 percent came from health department data, 11 percent were estimated by knowledgeable sources, and 2 percent were projections or other estimates.

The number of abortions estimated by AGI through the mid- to late-1980s was about 20 percent higher than the number reported to the Centers for Disease Control and Prevention (CDC). Between 1989 and 1997 the AGI estimates were about 12 percent higher than those reported by CDC. Beginning in 1998, health departments of four States did not report abortion data to CDC. The four reporting areas (the largest of which was California) that did not report abortions to CDC in 1998 accounted for 18 percent of all abortions tallied by AGI's 1995–96 survey.

For more information, write: The Alan Guttmacher Institute, 120 Wall Street, New York, NY 10005; or visit AGI's Web site at www.agi-usa.org.

American Association of Colleges of Osteopathic Medicine

The American Association of Colleges of Osteopathic Medicine (AACOM) compiles data on various aspects of osteopathic medical education for distribution to the profession, the government, and the public. Questionnaires are sent annually to schools of osteopathic medicine requesting information on characteristics of applicants and students, curricula, faculty, grants, contracts, revenues, and expenditures. The response rate is 100 percent.

For more information, see: *2001 Annual Report on Osteopathic Medical Education*, American Association of Colleges of Osteopathic Medicine: 5550 Friendship Blvd, Suite 310, Chevy Chase, Maryland 20815; or visit the AACOM Web site at www.aacom.org.

American Association of Colleges of Pharmacy

The American Association of Colleges of Pharmacy (AACP) compiles data on the Colleges of Pharmacy, including information on student enrollment and types of degrees conferred. Data are collected through an annual survey; the response rate is 100 percent.

For further information, see: *Profile of Pharmacy Students*. The American Association of Colleges of Pharmacy, 1426 Prince Street, Alexandria, VA; or visit the AACP Web site at www.aacp.org.

American Association of Colleges of Podiatric Medicine

The American Association of Colleges of Podiatric Medicine (AACPM) compiles data on the Colleges of Podiatric Medicine, including information on the schools and enrollment. Data are collected annually through written questionnaires. The response rate is 100 percent.

For further information, write: The American Association of Colleges of Podiatric Medicine, 1350 Piccard Drive, Suite 322, Rockville, MD 20850-4307; or visit the AACPM Web site at www.aacpm.org.

American Dental Association

The Division of Educational Measurement of the American Dental Association (ADA) conducts annual surveys of predoctoral dental educational institutions. The questionnaire, mailed to all dental schools, collects information on student characteristics, financial management, and curricula.

For more information, see: American Dental Association, *1999–2000 Survey of Predoctoral Dental Educational Institutions*. Chicago, IL. 2001; or visit the ADA Web site at www.ada.org.

American Hospital Association Annual Survey of Hospitals

Data from the American Hospital Association (AHA) annual survey are based on questionnaires sent to all AHA-registered and nonregistered hospitals in the United States and its associated areas. U.S. Government hospitals located outside the United States are excluded. Overall, the average response rate over the past 5 years has been approximately 83 percent. For nonreporting hospitals and for the survey questionnaires of reporting hospitals on which some information was missing, estimates are made for all data except those on beds, bassinets, and facilities. Data for beds and bassinets of nonreporting hospitals are based on the most recent information available from those hospitals. Data for facilities and services are based only on reporting hospitals.

Estimates of other types of missing data are based on data reported the previous year, if available. When unavailable, estimates are based on data furnished by reporting hospitals similar in size, control, major service provided, length of stay, and geographic and demographic characteristics.

For more information on the AHA Annual Survey of Hospitals, see: Health Forum, LLC, an American Hospital Association Company. Hospital Statistics, 2002. Chicago, IL. 2002; or visit the AHA Web site at www.aha.org.

American Medical Association Physician Masterfile

A masterfile of physicians has been maintained by the American Medical Association (AMA) since 1906. The Physician Masterfile contains data on almost every physician in the United States, members and nonmembers of the AMA, and on those graduates of American medical schools temporarily practicing overseas. The file also includes graduates of international medical schools who are in the United States and meet education standards for primary recognition as physicians.

A file is initiated on each individual upon entry into medical school or, in the case of international graduates, upon entry into the United States. Between 1965–85 a mail questionnaire survey was conducted every 4 years to update the file information on professional activities, self-designated area of specialization, and present employment status. Since 1985

approximately one-third of all physicians are surveyed each year.

For more information on the AMA Physician Masterfile, see: Division of Survey and Data Resources, American Medical Association, *Physician Characteristics and Distribution in the U.S., 2002–2003* ed. Chicago, IL. 2002; or visit the AMA Web site at www.ama-assn.org.

Association of American Medical Colleges

The Association of American Medical Colleges (AAMC) collects information on student enrollment in medical schools through the annual Liaison Committee on Medical Education questionnaire, the fall enrollment questionnaire, and the American Medical College Application Service (AMCAS) data system. Other data sources are the institutional profile system, the premedical students questionnaire, the minority student opportunities in medicine questionnaire, the faculty roster system, data from the Medical College Admission Test, and one-time surveys developed for special projects.

For more information, see: Association of American Medical Colleges, *Statistical Information Related to Medical Education*, Washington, DC. 2001; or visit the AAMC Web site at www.aamc.org.

Association of Schools and Colleges of Optometry

The Association of Schools and Colleges of Optometry (ASCO) compiles data on various aspects of optometric education including data on schools and enrollment. Questionnaires are sent annually to all schools and colleges of optometry. The response rate is 100 percent.

For further information, write: Annual Survey of Optometric Educational Institutions, Association of Schools and Colleges of Optometry, 6110 Executive Blvd., Suite 510, Rockville, MD 20852; or visit the ASCO Web site at www.opted.org.

Association of Schools of Public Health

The Association of Schools of Public Health (ASPH) compiles data on schools of public health in the United States and Puerto Rico. Questionnaires are sent annually to all member schools. The response rate is 100 percent.

Unlike health professional schools that emphasize specific clinical occupations, schools of public health offer study in specialty areas such as biostatistics, epidemiology, environmental health, occupational health, health administration, health planning, nutrition, maternal and child health, social and behavioral sciences, and other population-based sciences.

For further information, write: Association of Schools of Public Health, 1101 15th Street, NW, Suite 910, Washington, DC 20005; or visit the ASPH Web site at www.asph.org.

European Health for All Database

World Health Organization Regional Office for Europe

The WHO Regional Office for Europe (WHO/Europe) provides country-specific and topic-specific health information via the Internet for people who influence health policy in the WHO European Region and the media.

WHO/Europe collects statistics on health and makes them widely available through:

■ The European health for all database (HFA-DB) that contains data on about 600 health indicators collected from national counterparts in 51 European countries, and data from other WHO technical programs and some international organizations.

■ Highlights on health in countries in the WHO European Region that give an overview of the health situation in each country in comparison with other countries. Highlights complement the public health reports produced by a number of member States in the region.

■ Health status overview for countries of central and eastern Europe that are candidates for accession to the European Union (Bulgaria, the Czech Republic, Estonia, Hungary, Latvia, Lithuania, Poland, Romania, Slovakia and Slovenia).

WHO/Europe helps countries strengthen their national health information systems, particularly by supporting:

■ the development of national health indicator databases

■ the exchange of experience on national public health reports between countries; a database of public health reports is maintained and available for consultation and networking

■ implementation of international classifications and definitions in countries

■ regional networks of health information professionals

For more information, visit the European health for all database at http://hfadb.who.dk/hfa/.

InterStudy National Health Maintenance Organization Census

From 1976 to 1980 the Office of Health Maintenance Organizations conducted a census of health maintenance organizations (HMOs). Since 1981 InterStudy has conducted the census. A questionnaire is sent to all HMOs in the United States asking for updated enrollment, profit status, and Federal qualification status. New HMOs are also asked to provide information on model type. When necessary, information is obtained, supplemented, or clarified by telephone. For nonresponding HMOs State-supplied information or the most current available data are used.

In 1985 a large increase in the number of HMOs and enrollment was partly attributable to a change in the categories of HMOs included in the census: Medicaid-only and Medicare-only HMOs have been added. Also component HMOs, which have their own discrete management, can be listed separately, whereas, previously the oldest HMO reported for all of its component or expansion sites, even when the components had different operational dates or were different model types.

For further information, see: *The InterStudy Competitive Edge.* InterStudy Publications, St. Paul, MN. 2002; or visit the InterStudy Web site at www.hmodata.com.

National League for Nursing

The division of research of the National League for Nursing (NLN) conducts The Annual Survey of Schools of Nursing in October of each year. Questionnaires are sent to all graduate nursing programs (master's and doctoral), baccalaureate programs designed exclusively for registered nurses, basic registered nursing programs (baccalaureate, associate degree, and diploma), and licensed practical nursing programs. Data on enrollments, first-time admissions, and graduates are completed for all nursing education programs. Response rates of approximately 80 percent are achieved for other areas of inquiry.

For more information, see: National League for Nursing, *Nursing Data Review* 1997, New York, NY. 1997; or visit the NLN Web site at www.nln.org.

Organization for Economic Cooperation and Development Health Data

The Organization for Economic Cooperation and Development (OECD) provides annual data on statistical indicators on health and economic policies collected from 30 member countries since the 1960s. The international comparability of health expenditure estimates depends on the quality of national health accounts in OECD member countries. In recent years the OECD health accounts have become an informal standard for reporting on health care systems. Additional limitations in international comparisons include differing boundaries between health care and other social care particularly for the disabled and elderly, and underestimation of private expenditures on health.

The OECD was established in 1961 with a mandate to promote policies to achieve the highest sustainable economic growth and a rising standard of living among member countries. The Organization now comprises 30 member countries: Australia, Austria, Belgium, Canada, Czech Republic, Denmark, Finland, France, Germany, Greece, Hungary, Iceland, Ireland, Italy, Japan, Korea, Luxembourg, Mexico, Netherlands, New Zealand, Norway, Poland, Portugal, Slovak Republic, Spain, Sweden, Switzerland, Turkey, the United Kingdom, and the United States.

As part of its mission, the OECD has developed a number of activities in relation to health and health care systems. The main aim of OECD work on health policy is to conduct cross-national studies of the performance of OECD health systems and to facilitate exchanges between member countries of their experiences of financing, delivering, and managing health services. To support this work, each year the OECD compiles cross-country data in OECD Health Data, one of the most comprehensive sources of comparable health-related statistics. OECD Health Data is an essential tool to carry out comparative analyses and draw lessons from international comparisons of diverse health care systems. This international database now incorporates the first results arising from the implementation of the OECD manual, A System of Health Accounts (2000), which provide a standard framework for producing a set of comprehensive, consistent, and internationally comparable data on health spending. The

OECD collaborates with other international organizations such as the WHO.

For further information, see www.oecd.org/health.

United Nations Demographic Yearbook

The Statistical Office of the United Nations prepares the *Demographic Yearbook*, a comprehensive collection of international demographic statistics.

Questionnaires are sent annually and monthly to more than 220 national statistical services and other appropriate government offices. Data forwarded on these questionnaires are supplemented, to the extent possible, by data taken from official national publications and by correspondence with the national statistical services. To ensure comparability, rates, ratios, and percents have been calculated in the statistical office of the United Nations.

Lack of international comparability among estimates arises from differences in concepts, definitions, and time of data collection. The comparability of population data is affected by several factors, including (a) definitions of the total population, (b) definitions used to classify the population into its urban and rural components, (c) difficulties relating to age reporting, (d) extent of over- or underenumeration, and (e) quality of population estimates. The completeness and accuracy of vital statistics data also vary from one country to another. Differences in statistical definitions of vital events may also influence comparability.

International demographic trend data are available on a CD-ROM entitled United Nations, 2000. Demographic Yearbook—Historical Supplement 1948–97. CD-ROM Special Issue. United Nations publication sales number E/F.99.XIII.12.

For more information, see: United Nations, *Demographic Yearbook 2000*, United Nations, New York, 2002; or visit the United Nations Web site at www.un.org or their Web site locator at www.unsystem.org.

World Health Statistics Annual

World Health Organization

The World Health Organization (WHO) prepares the *World Health Statistics Annual*, an annual volume of information on vital statistics and causes of death designed for use by the medical and public health professions. Each volume is the result of a joint effort by the national health and statistical administrations of many countries, the United Nations, and WHO. United Nations estimates of vital rates and population size and composition, where available, are reprinted directly in the *Statistics Annual*. For those countries for which the United Nations does not prepare demographic estimates, primarily smaller populations, the latest available data reported to the United Nations and based on reasonably complete coverage of events are used.

Information published on infant mortality is based entirely on official national data either reported directly or made available to WHO.

Selected life table functions are calculated from the application of a uniform methodology to national mortality data provided to WHO, in order to enhance their value for international comparisons. The life table procedure used by WHO may often lead to discrepancies with national figures published by countries, due to differences in methodology or degree of age detail maintained in calculations.

The international comparability of estimates published in the *World Health Statistics Annual* is affected by the same problems as is the United Nations *Demographic Yearbook*. Cross-national differences in statistical definitions of vital events, in the completeness and accuracy of vital statistics data, and in the comparability of population data are the primary factors affecting comparability.

For more information, see: World Health Organization, *World Health Statistics Annual 2000*, World Health Organization, Geneva, 2002; World Health Statistics 1997–99 at www.who.int/whosis; or visit the WHO Web site at www.who.int.

Appendix II

Definitions and Methods

Appendix II is an alphabetical listing of terms used in *Health, United States*. It includes cross-references to related terms and synonyms. It also describes the methods used for calculating age-adjusted rates, average annual rate of change, relative standard error, birth rates, death rates, and years of potential life lost. Appendix II includes standard populations used for age adjustment (tables I, II, and III); *International Classification of Diseases* (ICD) codes for cause of death from the Sixth through Tenth Revisions and the years when the Revisions were in effect (tables IV and V); comparability ratios between ICD–9 and ICD–10 for selected causes (table VI); ICD-9-CM codes for external cause-of-injury, diagnostic, and procedure categories (tables VII, IX, and X); and industry codes from the Standard Industrial Classification Manual (table VIII). New standards for presenting Federal data on race and ethnicity are described under *Race* and sample tabulations of National Health Interview Survey (NHIS) data comparing the 1977 and 1997 Standards for Federal data on race and Hispanic origin are presented in tables XI and XII.

Abortion—The Centers for Disease Control and Prevention's (CDC) surveillance system counts legal induced abortions only. For surveillance purposes, legal abortion is defined as a procedure performed by a licensed physician or someone acting under the supervision of a licensed physician to voluntarily terminate a pregnancy.

Acquired immunodeficiency syndrome (AIDS)—All 50 States and the District of Columbia report AIDS cases to CDC using a uniform surveillance case definition and case report form. The case reporting definitions were expanded in 1985 *(MMWR 1985; 34:373–5)*; 1987 *(MMWR 1987; 36 (supp. no. 1S): 1S–15S)*; 1993 for adults and adolescents *(MMWR 1992; 41 (no. RR-17): 1–19)*; and 1994 for pediatric cases *(MMWR 1994; 43 (no. RR-12): 1–19)*. The revisions incorporated a broader range of AIDS-indicator diseases and conditions and used HIV diagnostic tests to improve the sensitivity and specificity of the definition. The 1993 expansion of the case definition caused a temporary distortion of AIDS incidence trends. In 1995 new treatments for HIV and AIDS (protease inhibitors) were approved. These therapies have prevented or delayed the onset of AIDS and premature death among many HIV-infected persons, which should be considered when interpreting trend data. AIDS surveillance data are published annually by CDC in the HIV/AIDS Surveillance Report at www.cdc.gov/hiv/stats/hasrlink.htm. See related *Human immunodeficiency virus (HIV) infection*.

Active physician—See *Physician*.

Activities of daily living (ADL)—Activities of daily living are activities related to personal care and include bathing or showering, dressing, getting in or out of bed or a chair, using the toilet, and eating. In the National Health Interview Survey respondents were asked about needing the help of another person with personal care because of a physical, mental, or emotional problem. Respondents are considered to have an ADL limitation if any condition causing the respondent to need help with the specific activities was chronic.

In the Medicare Current Beneficiary Survey (table 136), if a sample person had any difficulty performing an activity by him or herself and without special equipment, or did not perform the activity at all because of health problems, the person was categorized as having a limitation in that activity. The limitation may have been temporary or chronic at the time of the interview. In the *Chartbook on Trends in Health of Americans, 2003*, a sample person was categorized as having a limitation in their activities of daily living if, in addition to having any difficulty performing an activity or not performing the activity because of health problems, the sample person also received help or supervision with at least one of the following six activities: bathing or showering, dressing, eating, getting in or out of bed or chairs, walking, and using the toilet. Sample persons who were administered a community interview answered health status and functioning questions themselves, if able to do so. A proxy such as a nurse answered questions about the sample person's health status and functioning for those in a long-term care facility. Beginning in 1997, interview questions for persons in long-term care facilities were changed slightly from those administered to persons in the community in order to differentiate residents who were independent from those who received supervision or assistance with transferring, locomotion on unit, dressing, eating, toilet use, and bathing. See related *Condition; Instrumental activities of daily living (IADL); Limitation of activity*.

Addition—An addition to a mental health organization is defined by the Substance Abuse and Mental Health Services Administration's Center for Mental Health Services as a new admission, a readmission, a return from long-term leave, or a transfer from another service of the same organization or another organization. See related *Mental health organization; Mental health service type.*

Admission—The American Hospital Association defines admissions as persons, excluding newborns, accepted for inpatient services during the survey reporting period. See related *Days of care; Discharge; Inpatient.*

Age—Age is reported as age at last birthday, that is, age in completed years, often calculated by subtracting date of birth from the reference date, with the reference date being the date of the examination, interview, or other contact with an individual.

Mother's (maternal) age is reported on the birth certificate by all States. Birth statistics are presented for mother's age 10–49 years through 1996 and 10–54 years starting in 1997, based on mother's date of birth or age as reported on the birth certificate. The age of mother is edited for upper and lower limits. When the age of the mother is computed to be under 10 years or 55 years or over (50 years or over in 1964–96), it is considered not stated and imputed according to the age of the mother from the previous birth record of the same race and total birth order (total of fetal deaths and live births). Before 1963 not stated ages were distributed in proportion to the known ages for each racial group. Beginning in 1997 the birth rate for the maternal age group 45–49 years includes data for mother's age 50–54 years in the numerator and is based on the population of women 45–49 years in the denominator.

Age adjustment—Age adjustment is used to compare risks of two or more populations at one point in time or one population at two or more points in time. Age-adjusted rates should be viewed as relative indexes rather than actual measures of risk. Age-adjusted rates are computed by the direct method by applying age-specific rates in a population of interest to a standardized age distribution, in order to eliminate differences in observed rates that result from age differences in population composition.

Age-adjusted rates are calculated by the direct method as follows:

Table I. United States standard population and proportion distribution by age for age adjusting death rates

Age	Population	Proportion distribution (weights)	Standard million
Total	274,634,000	1.000000	1,000,000
Under 1 year	3,795,000	0.013818	13,818
1–4 years	15,192,000	0.055317	55,317
5–14 years	39,977,000	0.145565	145,565
15–24 years	38,077,000	0.138646	138,646
25–34 years	37,233,000	0.135573	135,573
35–44 years	44,659,000	0.162613	162,613
45–54 years	37,030,000	0.134834	134,834
55–64 years	23,961,000	0.087247	87,247
65–74 years	18,136,000	0.066037	66,037
75–84 years	12,315,000	*0.044842	44,842
85 years and over	4,259,000	0.015508	15,508

*Figure is rounded up instead of down to force total to 1.0.

SOURCE: Anderson RN, Rosenberg HM. Age Standardization of Death Rates: Implementation of the Year 2000 Standard. National vital statistics reports; vol 47 no 3. Hyattsville, Maryland: National Center for Health Statistics. 1998.

Table II. Numbers of live births and mother's age groups used to adjust maternal mortality rates to live births in the United States in 1970

Mother's age	Number
All ages	3,731,386
Under 20 years	656,460
20–24 years	1,418,874
25–29 years	994,904
30–34 years	427,806
35 years and over	233,342

SOURCE: U.S. Bureau of the Census: Population estimates and projections. *Current Population Reports.* Series P-25, No. 499. Washington, D.C.: U.S. Government Printing Office, May 1973.

$$\sum_{i=1}^{n} r_i \times (p_i / P)$$

where r_i = rate in age group i in the population of interest

p_i = standard population in age group i

$$P = \sum_{i=1}^{n} p_i$$

n = total number of age groups over the age range of the age-adjusted rate

Age adjustment by the direct method requires use of a standard age distribution. The standard for age adjusting death rates and estimates from surveys in *Health, United States* is the projected year 2000 U.S. resident population. Starting with *Health, United States, 2001*, the year 2000 U.S. standard population replaces the 1940 U.S. population for age adjusting mortality statistics. The U.S. standard population also replaces the 1970 civilian noninstitutionalized population and 1980 U.S. resident population, which previously had been used as standard age distributions for age adjusting estimates from NCHS surveys.

Changing the standard population has implications for racial and ethnic differentials in mortality. For example, the mortality ratio for the black to white populations is reduced from 1.6 using the 1940 standard to 1.4 using the 2000 standard, reflecting the greater weight that the 2000 standard gives to the older population where race differentials in mortality are smaller.

For more information on implementing the new population standard for age adjusting death rates, see Anderson RN, Rosenberg HM. Age Standardization of Death Rates: Implementation of the Year 2000 Standard. National vital statistics reports; vol 47 no 3. Hyattsville, Maryland: National Center for Health Statistics. 1998. For more information on the derivation of age adjustment weights for use with NCHS survey data, see Klein RJ, Schoenborn CA. Age Adjustment Using the 2000 Projected U.S. Population. Healthy People Statistical Notes no 20. Hyattsville, Maryland: National Center for Health Statistics. 2001. Both reports are available through the NCHS home page at www.cdc.gov/nchs. The United States standard population is available through the Bureau of the Census home page at www.census.gov/prod/1/pop/p25-1130/, table 2.

Mortality data—Death rates are age adjusted to the year 2000 U.S. standard population (table I). Age-adjusted rates are calculated using age-specific death rates per 100,000 population rounded to 1 decimal place. Adjustment is based on 11 age groups with two exceptions. First, age-adjusted death rates for black males and black females in 1950 are based on nine age groups, with under 1 year and 1–4 years of age combined as one group and 75–84 years and 85 years of age combined as one group. Second, age-adjusted death rates by educational attainment for the age group 25–64 years are based on four 10-year age groups (25–34 years, 35–44 years, 45–54 years, and 55–64 years).

Age-adjusted rates for years of potential life lost (YPLL) before age 75 years also use the year 2000 standard population and are based on eight age groups (under 1 year, 1–14 years, 15–24 years, and 10-year age groups through 65–74 years).

Maternal mortality rates for pregnancy, childbirth, and the puerperium are calculated as the number of deaths per 100,000 live births. These rates are age adjusted to the 1970 distribution of live births by mother's age in the United States as shown in table II. See related *Rate: Death and related rates; Years of potential life lost.*

National Health and Nutrition Examination Survey— Estimates based on the National Health Examination Survey (NHES) and the National Health and Nutrition Examination Survey (NHANES) are age adjusted to the year 2000 U.S. standard population using five age groups: 20–34 years, 35–44 years, 45–54 years, 55–64 years, and 65–74 years. Beginning in 1999–2000 estimates are age adjusted using three age groups (20–39 years, 40–59 years, and 60–74 years or 60 years and over) due to a smaller sample size; however, use of three rather than five groups had virtually no effect on age-adjusted estimates (see table III). Prior to the 2000 edition of *Health, United States*, these estimates were age adjusted to the 1980 U.S. resident population.

National Health Care Surveys—Estimates based on the National Hospital Discharge Survey (NHDS), the National Survey of Ambulatory Surgery (NSAS), the National Ambulatory Medical Care Survey (NAMCS), the National Hospital Ambulatory Medical Care Survey (NHAMCS), the National Nursing Home Survey (NNHS) (resident rates table), and the National Home and Hospice Care Survey (NHHCS) are age adjusted to the year 2000 U.S. standard population (table III). Information on the age groups used in the age adjustment procedure is contained in the footnotes to the relevant tables.

National Health Interview Survey—Estimates based on the National Health Interview Survey (NHIS) are age adjusted to the year 2000 U.S. standard population (table III). Information on the age groups used in the age adjustment procedure is contained in the footnotes on the relevant tables. Prior to the 2000 edition of *Health, United States* these estimates were age adjusted to the 1970 civilian noninstitutionalized population.

AIDS—See *Acquired immunodeficiency syndrome.*

Alcohol abuse treatment clients—See *Substance abuse treatment clients.*

Alcohol consumption—Alcohol consumption is measured differently in various data systems.

Monitoring the Future Study—This school-based survey of secondary school students collects information on alcohol use using self-completed questionnaires. Information on consumption of alcoholic beverages, defined as beer, wine, wine coolers, and liquor, is based on the following question: "On how many occasions (if any) have you had alcohol to drink- more than just a few sips- in the last 30 days?" Students responding affirmatively are then asked "How many times have you had five or more drinks in a row in the last two weeks?" For this question, a "drink" means a 12-ounce can (or bottle) of beer, a 4-ounce glass of wine, a 12-ounce bottle (or can) of wine cooler, or a mixed drink or shot of liquor.

National Health Interview Survey (NHIS)—Starting with the 1997 NHIS, information on alcohol consumption is collected in the sample adult questionnaire. Adult respondents are asked two screening questions about lifetime alcohol consumption: "In any one year, have you had at least 12 drinks of any type of alcoholic beverage? In your entire life, have you had at least 12 drinks of any type of alcoholic beverage?" Persons who report at least 12 drinks in a lifetime are then asked a series of questions about alcohol consumption in the past year: "In the past year, how often did you drink any type of alcoholic beverage? In the past year, on those days that you drank alcoholic beverages, on the average, how many drinks did you have? In the past year, on how many days did you have 5 or more drinks of any alcoholic beverage?"

National Household Survey on Drug Abuse (NHSDA)— Starting in 1999 NHSDA information about the frequency of the consumption of alcoholic beverages in the past 30 days has been obtained for all persons surveyed who are 12 years of age and over. An extensive list of examples of the kinds of beverages covered was given to respondents prior to the question administration. A "drink" is defined as a can or bottle of beer, a glass of

Table III. United States standard population and age groups used to age adjust survey data

Survey and age	Number in thousands
NHIS, NAMCS, NHAMCS, NHHCS, NNHS, NHDS, and NSAS	
All ages	274,634
18 years and over	203,851
25 years and over	117,593
40 years and over	118,180
65 years and over	34,710
Under 18 years	70,783
2–17 years	63,229
18–44 years	108,150
18–24 years	26,258
25–34 years	37,233
35–44 years	44,659
45–64 years	60,991
45–54 years	37,030
55–64 years	23,961
65–74 years	18,136
75 years and over	16,574
18–49 years	127,956
40–64 years:	
40–49 years	42,285
50–64 years	41,185
NHES and NHANES I–III	
20–74 years	179,276
20–34 years	55,490
35–44 years	44,659
45–54 years	37,030
55–64 years	23,961
65–74 years	18,136
NHANES (1999–2000)	
20–74 years or 20 years and over:	
20–39 years	77,670
40–59 years	72,816
60–74 years	28,790
or	
60 years and over	45,364
SAMHSA's DAWN	
6 years and over	251,751
6–11 years	24,282
12–17 years	23,618
18–25 years	29,679
26–34 years	33,812
35 years and over	140,360

SOURCE: U.S. Bureau of Census: Current Population Reports. P25–1130. Population Projections of the United States by Age, Sex, Race, and Hispanic Origin, table 2. U.S. Government Printing Office, Washington, DC, 1996.

wine or a wine cooler, a shot of liquor, or a mixed drink with liquor in it. Those times when the respondent had only a sip or two from a drink are not considered consumption. Alcohol use is based on the following questions: "During the past 30 days, on how many days did you drink one or more drinks of an alcoholic beverage?", "On the days that you drank during the past 30 days, how many drinks did you usually have?", and "During the past 30 days, on how many days did you have 5 or more drinks on the same occasion?"

Ambulatory care—In the National Ambulatory Medical Care Survey and National Hospital Ambulatory Medical Care Survey, ambulatory care is health care provided to persons in physician offices, hospital outpatient departments, and hospital emergency departments without their admission to a health facility. See related *Emergency department; Office visit; Outpatient department*.

Ambulatory surgery—According to the National Survey of Ambulatory Surgery (NSAS), ambulatory surgery refers to previously scheduled surgical and nonsurgical procedures performed on an outpatient basis in a hospital or freestanding ambulatory surgery center's general or main operating rooms, satellite operating rooms, cystoscopy rooms, endoscopy rooms, cardiac catheterization labs, and laser procedure rooms. Procedures performed in locations dedicated exclusively to dentistry, podiatry, abortion, pain block, or minor procedures are not included. In NSAS, data on up to six surgical and nonsurgical procedures are collected and coded. See related *Outpatient surgery; Procedure*.

Average annual rate of change (percent change)—In *Health, United States* average annual rates of change or growth rates are calculated as follows:

$$[(P_n / P_o)^{1/N} - 1] \times 100$$

where P_n = later time period

P_o = earlier time period

N = number of years in interval.

This geometric rate of change assumes that a variable increases or decreases at the same rate during each year between the two time periods.

Average length of stay—In the National Health Interview Survey, average length of stay per discharged inpatient is computed by dividing the total number of hospital days for a specified group by the total number of discharges for that group. Similarly, in the National Hospital Discharge Survey, average length of stay is computed by dividing the total number of days of care, counting the date of admission but

not the date of discharge, by the number of patients discharged. The American Hospital Association computes average length of stay by dividing the number of inpatient days by the number of admissions. See related *Days of care; Discharge; Inpatient*.

Bed—For the American Hospital Association the bed count is the number of beds, cribs, and pediatric bassinets that are set up and staffed for use by inpatients on the last day of the reporting period. In the Center for Medicare & Medicaid Service's Online Survey Certification and Reporting (OSCAR) database, all beds in certified facilities are counted on the day of certification inspection. The World Health Organization defines a hospital bed as one regularly maintained and staffed for the accommodation and full-time care of a succession of inpatients and situated in a part of the hospital where continuous medical care for inpatients is provided. The Center for Mental Health Services counts the number of beds set up and staffed for use in inpatient and residential treatment services on the last day of the survey reporting period. See related *Hospital; Mental health organization; Mental health service type; Occupancy rate*.

Birth cohort—A birth cohort consists of all persons born within a given period of time, such as a calendar year.

Birth rate—See *Rate: Birth and related rates*.

Birthweight—The first weight of the newborn obtained after birth. Low birthweight is defined as less than 2,500 grams or 5 pounds 8 ounces. Very low birthweight is defined as less than 1,500 grams or 3 pounds 4 ounces. Before 1979 low birthweight was defined as 2,500 grams or less and very low birthweight as 1,500 grams or less.

Body mass index (BMI)—BMI is a measure that adjusts bodyweight for height. It is calculated as weight in kilograms divided by height in meters squared. Overweight for children and adolescents is defined as BMI at or above the sex- and age-specific 95th percentile BMI cut points from the 2000 CDC Growth Charts (www.cdc.gov/growthcharts/). Healthy weight for adults is defined as a BMI of 18.5 to less than 25; overweight, as greater than or equal to a BMI of 25; and obesity, as greater than or equal to a BMI of 30. BMI cut points are defined in the Report of the Dietary Guidelines Advisory Committee on the Dietary Guidelines for Americans, 2000. U.S. Department of Agriculture, Agricultural Research Service, Dietary Guidelines Advisory Committee, p.23, or access on the Internet at www.health.gov/dietaryguidelines/dgac/; NHLBI Obesity Education Initiative Expert Panel on the Identification, Evaluation, and Treatment of Overweight and Obesity in Adults. Clinical Guidelines on the Identification, Evaluation, and Treatment of Overweight and Obesity in Adults—The Evidence Report. Obes Res 1998;6:51S-209S or access on the Internet at www.nhlbi.nih.gov/guidelines/obesity/ob_gdlns.htm; and in U.S. Department of Health and Human Services. *Tracking Healthy People 2010*. Washington, DC: U.S. Government Printing Office, November 2000. Objectives 19.1, 19.2, and 19.3, or access on the Internet at www.health.gov/healthypeople/document/html/volume2/19nutrition.htm.

Cause of death—For the purpose of national mortality statistics, every death is attributed to one underlying condition, based on information reported on the death certificate and using the international rules for selecting the underlying cause of death from the conditions stated on the death certificate. The underlying cause is defined by the World Health Organization (WHO) as the disease or injury that initiated the train of events leading directly to death, or the circumstances of the accident or violence, which produced the fatal injury. Generally more medical information is reported on death certificates than is directly reflected in the underlying cause of death. The conditions that are not selected as underlying cause of death constitute the nonunderlying cause of death, also known as multiple cause of death.

Cause of death is coded according to the appropriate revision of the *International Classification of Diseases* (ICD) (see table IV). Effective with deaths occurring in 1999, the United States began using the Tenth Revision of the ICD (ICD-10); during the period 1979–98, causes of death were coded and classified according to the Ninth Revision (ICD-9). Table V lists ICD codes for the Sixth through Tenth Revisions for causes of death shown in *Health, United States*.

Each of these revisions has produced discontinuities in cause-of-death trends. These discontinuities are measured using comparability ratios. These measures of discontinuity are essential to the interpretation of mortality trends. For further discussion, see the Mortality Technical Appendix available on the NCHS web site at www.cdc.gov/nchs/about/major/dvs/mortdata.htm. See related *Comparability ratio; International Classification of Diseases; Appendix I, National Vital Statistics System, Multiple Cause of Death File.*

Table IV. Revision of the *International Classification of Diseases (ICD)* according to year of conference by which adopted and years in use in the United States

Revision of the International Classification of Diseases	Year of conference by which adopted	Years in use in United States
First	1900	1900–1909
Second	1909	1910–1920
Third	1920	1921–1929
Fourth	1929	1930–1938
Fifth	1938	1939–1948
Sixth	1948	1949–1957
Seventh	1955	1958–1967
Eighth	1965	1968–1978
Ninth	1975	1979–1998
Tenth	1992	1999–

Cause-of-death ranking—Selected causes of death of public health and medical importance comprise tabulation lists and are ranked according to the number of deaths assigned to these causes. The top-ranking causes determine the leading causes of death. Certain causes on the tabulation lists are not ranked if, for example, the category title represents a group title (such as Major cardiovascular diseases and Symptoms, signs, and abnormal clinical and laboratory findings, not elsewhere classified); or the category title begins with the words "Other" and "All other." In addition when one of the titles that represents a subtotal (such as Malignant neoplasms) is ranked, its component parts are not ranked. The tabulation lists used for ranking in the *Tenth Revision of the International Classification of Diseases* (ICD) include the List of 113 Selected Causes of Death, which replaces the ICD-9 List of 72 Selected Causes, HIV infection and Alzheimer's disease; and the ICD-10 List of 130 Selected Causes of Infant Death, which replaces the ICD-9 List of 60 Selected Causes of Infant Death and HIV infection. Causes that are tied receive the same rank; the next cause is assigned the rank it would have received had the lower-ranked causes not been tied, i.e., skip a rank. See related *International Classification of Diseases*.

Chronic condition—See *Condition.*

Cigarette smoking—Cigarette smoking and related tobacco use are measured in several different data systems.

Birth File—Information on cigarette smoking of the mother during pregnancy is based on Yes No responses to the birth certificate item "Other risk factors for this

Table V. Cause-of-death codes, according to applicable revision of *International Classification of Diseases (ICD)*

Cause of death (Tenth Revision titles)	Sixth and Seventh Revisions	Eighth Revision	Ninth Revision	Tenth Revision
Communicable diseases	. . .	. . .	001–139, 460–466, 480–487, 771.3	A00–B99, J00–J22
Chronic and noncommunicable diseases	. . .	. . .	140–459, 470–478, 490–799	C00–I99, J30–R99
Injuries	. . .	. . .	E800–E869, E880–E929, E950–E999	V01–Y34, Y85–Y87, Y89
Meningococcal Infection	. . .	. . .	036	A39
Septicemia	. . .	. . .	038	A40–A41
Human immunodeficiency virus (HIV) disease[1]	. . .	. . .	*042–*044	B20–B24
Malignant neoplasms	140–205	140–209	140–208	C00–C97
Colon, rectum, and anus	153–154	153–154	153, 154	C18–C21
Trachea, bronchus, and lung	162–163	162	162	C33–C34
Breast	170	174	174–175	C50
Prostate	177	185	185	C61
In situ neoplasms and benign neoplasms	. . .	. . .	210–239	D00–D48
Diabetes mellitus	260	250	250	E10–E14
Anemias	. . .	. . .	280–285	D50–D64
Meningitis	. . .	. . .	320–322	G00, G03
Alzheimer's disease	. . .	. . .	331.0	G30
Diseases of heart	6th: 410–443 7th: 400–402, 410–443	390–398, 402, 404, 410–429	390–398, 402, 404, 410–429	I00–I09, I11, I13, I20–I51
Ischemic heart disease	. . .	. . .	410–414, 429.2	I20–I25
Cerebrovascular diseases	330–334	430–438	430–434, 436–438	I60–I69
Atherosclerosis	. . .	. . .	440	I70
Influenza and pneumonia	480–483, 490–493	470–474, 480–486	480–487	J10–J18
Chronic lower respiratory diseases	241, 501, 502, 527.1	490–493, 519.3	490–494, 496	J40–J47
Chronic liver disease and cirrhosis	581	571	571	K70, K73–K74
Nephritis, nephrotic syndrome, and nephrosis	. . .	. . .	580–589	N00–N07, N17–N19, N25–N27
Pregnancy, childbirth, and the puerperium	640–689	630–678	630–676	A34, O00–O95, O98–O99
Congenital malformations, deformations, and chromosomal abnormalities	. . .	. . .	740–759	Q00–Q99
Certain conditions originating in the perinatal period	. . .	. . .	760–779	P00–P96
Newborn affected by maternal complications of pregnancy	. . .	. . .	761	P01
Newborn affected by complications of placenta, cord, and membranes	. . .	. . .	762	P02
Disorders related to short gestation and low birthweight, not elsewhere classified	. . .	. . .	765	P07
Birth trauma	. . .	. . .	767	P10–P15
Intrauterine hypoxia and birth asphyxia . . .	. . .	. . .	768	P20–P21
Respiratory distress of newborn	. . .	. . .	769	P22
Sudden infant death syndrome	. . .	. . .	798.0	R95
Unintentional injuries[2]	E800–E936, E960–E965	E800–E929, E940–E946	E800–E869, E880–E929	V01–X59, Y85–Y86
Motor vehicle-related injuries[2]	E810–E835	E810–E823	E810–E825	V02–V04, V09.0, V09.2, V12–V14, V19.0–V19.2, V19.4–V19.6, V20–V79, V80.3–V80.5, V81.0–V81.1, V82.0–V82.1, V83–V86, V87.0–V87.8, V88.0–V88.8, V89.0, V89.2
Suicide	E963, E970–E979	E950–E959	E950–E959	X60–X84, Y87.0
Homicide	E964, E980–E983	E960–E969	E960–E969	X85–Y09, Y87.1
Injury by firearms	. . .	E922, E955, E965, E970, E985	E922, E955.0–E955.4, E965.0–E965.4, E970, E985.0–E985.4	W32–W34, X72–X74, X93–X95, Y22–Y24, Y35.0

. . . Cause-of-death code numbers are not provided for causes not shown in *Health, United States*.

[1]Categories for coding human immunodeficiency virus infection were introduced in 1987. The * indicates codes are not part of the Ninth Revision.

[2]In the public health community, the term "unintentional injuries" is preferred to "accidents" and "motor vehicle-related injuries" to "motor vehicle accidents."

pregnancy: Tobacco use during pregnancy." See related *Tobacco use*.

Monitoring the Future Survey—Information on current cigarette smoking is obtained for high school seniors (starting in 1975) and eighth and tenth graders (starting in 1991) based on the following question: "How frequently have you smoked cigarettes during the past 30 days?"

National Health Interview Survey (NHIS)—Information about cigarette smoking is obtained for adults 18 years of age and over. Starting in 1993 current smokers are identified based on the following two questions: "Have you smoked at least 100 cigarettes in your entire life?" and "Do you now smoke cigarettes every day, some days, or not at all?" Persons who smoked 100 cigarettes and who now smoke every day or some days are defined as current smokers. Before 1992 current smokers were identified based on positive responses to the following two questions: "Have you smoked 100 cigarettes in your entire life?" and "Do you smoke now?" (traditional definition). In 1992 the definition of current smoker in the NHIS was modified to specifically include persons who smoked on "some days." (revised definition). In 1992 cigarette smoking data were collected for a half-sample with half the respondents (one-quarter sample) using the traditional smoking questions and the other half of respondents (one-quarter sample) using the revised smoking question ("Do you smoke every day, some days, or not at all?"). An unpublished analysis of the 1992 traditional smoking measure revealed that the crude percent of current smokers 18 years of age and over remained the same as 1991. The statistics for 1992 combine data collected using the traditional and the revised questions.

In 1993–95 estimates of cigarette smoking prevalence were based on a half-sample. Smoking data were not collected in 1996. Starting in 1997 smoking data were collected in the sample adult questionnaire. For further information on survey methodology and sample sizes pertaining to the NHIS cigarette smoking data for data years 1965–92 and other sources of cigarette smoking data available from the National Center for Health Statistics, see: National Center for Health Statistics, *Bibliographies and Data Sources, Smoking Data Guide*, no. 1, DHHS pub. no. (PHS) 91-1308-1, Public Health

Service. Washington, DC: U.S. Government Printing Office. 1991.

National Household Survey on Drug Abuse—Information on current cigarette smoking is obtained for all persons surveyed who are 12 years of age and over based on the following question: "During the past 30 days, have you smoked part or all of a cigarette?"

Youth Risk Behavior Survey—Information on current cigarette smoking is obtained from high school students (starting in 1991) based on the following question: "During the past 30 days, on how many days did you smoke cigarettes?"

Civilian noninstitutionalized population; Civilian population—See *Population*.

Cocaine-related emergency department episodes—The Drug Abuse Warning Network monitors selected adverse medical consequences of cocaine and other drug abuse episodes by measuring contacts with hospital emergency departments. Contacts may be for drug overdose, unexpected drug reactions, chronic abuse, detoxification, or other reasons in which drug use is known to have occurred.

Cohort fertility—Cohort fertility refers to the fertility of the same women at successive ages. Women born during a 12-month period constitute a birth cohort. Cohort fertility for birth cohorts of women is measured by central birth rates, which represent the number of births occurring to women of an exact age divided by the number of women of that exact age. Cumulative birth rates by a given exact age represent the total childbearing experience of women in a cohort up to that age. Cumulative birth rates are sums of central birth rates for specified cohorts and show the number of children ever born up to the indicated age. For example, the cumulative birth rate for women exactly 30 years of age as of January 1, 1960, is the sum of the central birth rates for the 1930 birth cohort for the years 1944 (when its members were age 14) through 1959 (when they were age 29). Cumulative birth rates are also calculated for specific birth orders at each exact age of woman. The percent of women who have not had at least one live birth by a certain age is found by subtracting the cumulative first birth rate for women of that age from 1,000 and dividing by 10. For method of calculation, see Heuser RL. *Fertility tables for birth cohorts by color:*

United States, 1917–73. Rockville, Maryland: NCHS. 1976. See related *Rate: Birth and related rates.*

Community hospitals—See *Hospital.*

Comparability ratio—About every 10–20 years the *International Classification of Diseases* (ICD) is revised to stay abreast of advances in medical science and changes in medical terminology. Each of these revisions produces breaks in the continuity of cause-of-death statistics. Discontinuities across revisions are due to changes in classification and rules for selecting underlying cause of death. Classification and rule changes impact cause-of-death trend data by shifting deaths away from some cause-of-death categories and into others. Comparability ratios measure the effect of changes in classification and coding rules. For causes shown in table VI, comparability ratios range between 0.9754 and 1.0588, except for influenza and pneumonia, with a comparability ratio of 0.6982, indicating that influenza and pneumonia is about 30 percent less likely to be selected as the underlying cause of death in ICD-10 than in ICD-9; and HIV disease with a comparability ratio of 1.1448, indicating that HIV disease is more than 14 percent more likely to be selected as the underlying cause using ICD-10 coding.

Another factor also contributes to discontinuities in death rates across revisions. For selected causes of death, the ICD-9 codes used to calculate death rates for 1980 through 1998 differ from the ICD-9 codes most nearly comparable with the corresponding ICD-10 cause-of-death category. Examples of these causes are ischemic heart disease, cerebrovascular diseases, trachea, bronchus and lung cancer, unintentional injuries, and homicide. To address this source of discontinuity, mortality trends for 1980–98 were recalculated using ICD-9 codes that are more comparable with codes for corresponding ICD-10 categories. Table V shows the ICD-9 codes used for these causes. While this modification may lessen the discontinuity between the Ninth and Tenth Revisions, the effect on the discontinuity between the Eighth and Ninth Revisions is not measured.

Preliminary comparability ratios shown in table VI are based on a comparability study in which the same deaths were coded by both the Ninth and Tenth Revisions. The comparability ratio was calculated by dividing the number of deaths classified by ICD-10 by the number of deaths classified by ICD-9. The resulting ratios represent the net effect of the Tenth Revision on cause-of-death statistics and can be used to adjust mortality statistics for causes of death

classified by the Ninth Revision to be comparable with cause-specific mortality statistics classified by the Tenth Revision.

The application of comparability ratios to mortality statistics helps to make the analysis of change between 1998 and 1999 more accurate and complete. The 1998 comparability-modified death rate is calculated by multiplying the comparability ratio by the 1998 death rate. Comparability-modified rates should be used to estimate mortality change between 1998 and 1999.

Caution should be taken when applying the comparability ratios presented in table VI to age-, race-, and sex-specific mortality data. Demographic subgroups may sometimes differ with regard to their cause-of-death distribution, and this would result in demographic variation in cause-specific comparability ratios.

For more information, see Anderson RN, Minino AM, Hoyert DL, Rosenberg HM. Comparability of cause of death between ICD-9 and ICD-10: Preliminary estimates; and Kochanek KD, Smith BL, Anderson RN. Deaths: Preliminary data for 1999. National vital statistics reports. vol 49 no 2 and vol 49 no 3. Hyattsville, MD: National Center for Health Statistics. 2001. See related *Cause of death; International Classification of Diseases; tables* IV and V.

Compensation—See *Employer costs for employee compensation.*

Condition—A health condition is a departure from a state of physical or mental well-being. In the National Health Interview Survey, each condition reported as a cause of an individual's activity limitation has been classified as "chronic," "not chronic," or "unknown if chronic," based on the nature of the condition and/or the duration of the condition. Conditions that are not cured once acquired (such as heart disease, diabetes, and birth defects in the original response categories, and amputee and "old age" in the ad hoc categories) are considered chronic, while conditions related to pregnancy are always considered not chronic. Additionally, other conditions must have been present 3 months or longer to be considered chronic. An exception is made for children less than 1 year of age who have had a condition "since birth," as these conditions are always considered chronic. The National Nursing Home Survey uses a specific list of chronic conditions, disregarding time of onset.

Table VI. Comparability of selected causes of death between the Ninth and Tenth Revisions of the *International Classification of Diseases (ICD)*

Cause of death[1]	Preliminary comparability ratio[2]
Human immunodeficiency virus (HIV) disease	1.1448
Malignant neoplasms	1.0068
Colon, rectum, and anus	0.9993
Trachea, bronchus, and lung	0.9837
Breast	1.0056
Prostate	1.0134
Diabetes mellitus	1.0082
Diseases of heart	0.9858
Ischemic heart diseases	0.9990
Cerebrovascular diseases	1.0588
Influenza and pneumonia	0.6982
Chronic lower respiratory diseases	1.0478
Chronic liver disease and cirrhosis	1.0367
Pregnancy, childbirth, and the puerperium	*
Unintentional injuries	1.0305
Motor vehicle-related injuries	0.9754
Suicide	0.9962
Homicide	0.9983
Injury by firearms	0.9973
Chronic and noncommunicable diseases	1.0100
Injuries	1.0117
Communicable diseases	0.8536
HIV disease	1.1448
Other communicable diseases	0.8023

*Figure does not meet standards of reliability or precision.
[1]See table V for ICD-9 and ICD-10 cause-of-death codes.
[2]Ratio of number of deaths classified by ICD-10 to number of deaths classified by ICD-9.
SOURCE: Anderson RN, Miniño AM, Hoyert DL, Rosenberg HM. Comparability of cause-of-death classification between ICD-9 and ICD-10: Preliminary estimates. National Vital Statistics Reports. Vol 49 No 2. Hyattsville, Maryland: National Center for Health Statistics. 2001.

Consumer Price Index (CPI)—The CPI is prepared by the U.S. Bureau of Labor Statistics. It is a monthly measure of the average change in the prices paid by urban consumers for a fixed market basket of goods and services. The medical care component of CPI shows trends in medical care prices based on specific indicators of hospital, medical, dental, and drug prices. A revision of the definition of CPI has been in use since January 1988. See related *Gross domestic product; Health expenditures, national; Appendix I, Consumer Price Index.*

Crude birth rate; Crude death rate—See *Rate: Birth and related rates; Rate: Death and related rates.*

Days of care—Days of care is defined similarly in different data systems. See related *Admission; Average length of stay; Discharge; Hospital; Hospital Utilization; Inpatient.*

American Hospital Association—Days, hospital days, or inpatient days are the number of adult and pediatric days of care rendered during the entire reporting period. Days of care for newborns are excluded.

National Health Interview Survey (NHIS)—Hospital days during the year refer to the total number of hospital days occurring in the 12-month period before the interview week. A hospital day is a night spent in the hospital for persons admitted as inpatients. Starting in 1997 hospitalization data from NHIS are for all inpatient stays, whereas estimates for prior years published in *Health, United States* excluded hospitalizations for deliveries and newborns.

National Hospital Discharge Survey—Days of care refers to the total number of patient days accumulated by inpatients at the time of discharge from non-Federal short-stay hospitals during a reporting period. All days from and including the date of admission but not including the date of discharge are counted.

Death rate—See *Rate: Death and related rates.*

Dental visit—Starting in 1997 National Health Interview Survey respondents were asked "About how long has it been since you last saw or talked to a dentist? Include all types of dentists, such as orthodontists, oral surgeons, and all other dental specialists as well as hygienists." Starting in 2001 the question was modified slightly to ask respondents how long has it been since they last saw a dentist. Questions about dental visits were not asked for children under 2 years of age for years 1997–99 and under 1 year of age for 2000 and beyond. Estimates are presented for persons with a dental visit in the past year. Prior to 1997 dental visit estimates were based on a 2-week recall period.

Diagnosis—See *First-listed diagnosis.*

Diagnostic and other nonsurgical procedures—See *Procedure.*

Discharge—The National Health Interview Survey defines a hospital discharge as the completion of any continuous period of stay of 1 night or more in a hospital as an inpatient. According to the National Hospital Discharge Survey, a discharge is a completed inpatient hospitalization. A hospitalization may be completed by death or by releasing the patient to the customary place of residence, a nursing home, another hospital, or other locations. See related *Admission; Average length of stay; Days of care; Inpatient.*

Domiciliary care homes—See *Nursing home.*

Drug abuse—See *Illicit drug use.*

Drug abuse treatment clients—See *Substance abuse treatment clients.*

Education—Several approaches to defining educational categories are used in this report. In survey data educational categories are based on information about educational credentials, such as diplomas and degrees. In vital statistics educational attainment is based on years of school completed.

Birth File—Information on educational attainment of mother is based on number of years of school completed, as reported by the mother on the birth certificate. Between 1970 and 1992 the reporting area for maternal education expanded.

Mother's education was reported on the birth certificate by 38 States in 1970. Data were not available from Alabama, Arkansas, California, Connecticut, Delaware, District of Columbia, Georgia, Idaho, Maryland, New Mexico, Pennsylvania, Texas, and Washington. In 1975 these data became available from four additional States, Connecticut, Delaware, Georgia, Maryland, and the District of Columbia, increasing the number of States reporting mother's education to 42 and the District of Columbia. Between 1980 and 1988 only three States, California, Texas, and Washington, did not report mother's education. In 1988 mother's education was also missing from New York State outside New York City. In 1989–91 mother's education was missing only from Washington and New York State outside New York City. Starting in 1992 mother's education was reported by all 50 States and the District of Columbia.

Mortality File—Information on educational attainment of decedent became available for the first time in 1989 due to revision of the U.S. Standard Certificate of Death. Decedent's educational attainment is reported on the death certificate by the funeral director based on information provided by an informant such as next of kin. Mortality data by educational attainment for 1989 were based on data from 20 States and by 1994–96 increased

to 45 States and the District of Columbia. In 1994–96 the following States either did not report educational attainment on the death certificate or the information was more than 20 percent incomplete: Georgia, Kentucky, Oklahoma, Rhode Island, and South Dakota. In 1997–2000 information on decedent's education was available from Oklahoma, increasing the reporting area to 46 States and the District of Columbia (DC). With the addition of Kentucky in 2001, the reporting area increased to 47 States and DC.

Calculation of unbiased death rates by educational attainment based on the National Vital Statistics System requires that the reporting of education on the death certificate be complete and consistent with the reporting of education on the Current Population Survey, the source of population estimates for denominators for death rates. Death records that are missing information about decedent's education are not included in the calculation of rates. Therefore the levels of death rates by educational attainment shown in this report are underestimated by approximately the percent with not stated education, which ranges from 3 to 9 percent.

The validity of information about the decedent's education was evaluated by comparing self-reported education obtained in the Current Population Survey with education on the death certificate for decedents in the National Longitudinal Mortality Survey (NLMS). (Sorlie PD, Johnson NJ: Validity of education information on the death certificate, Epidemiology 7(4):437–9, 1996.) Another analysis compared self-reported education collected in the first National Health and Nutrition Examination Survey (NHANES I) with education on the death certificate for decedents in the NHANES I Epidemiologic Followup Study. (Makuc DM, Feldman JJ, Mussolino ME: Validity of education and age as reported on death certificates, American Statistical Association. 1996 Proceedings of the Social Statistics Section, 102–6, 1997.) Results of both studies indicated that there is a tendency for some people who did not graduate from high school to be reported as high school graduates on the death certificate. This tendency results in overstating the death rate for high school graduates and understating the death rate for the group with less than 12 years of education. The bias was greater among older than younger decedents and somewhat greater among black than white decedents.

In addition, educational gradients in death rates based on the National Vital Statistics System were compared with those based on the NLMS, a prospective study of persons in the Current Population Survey. Results of these comparisons indicate that educational gradients in death rates based on the National Vital Statistics System were reasonably similar to those based on NLMS for white persons 25–64 years of age and black persons 25–44 years of age. The number of deaths for persons of Hispanic origin in NLMS was too small to permit comparison for this ethnic group. For further information on measurement of education, see: Kominski R and Siegel PM. Measuring education in the Current Population Survey. *Monthly Labor Review*, September 1993: 34–38.

National Health Interview Survey (NHIS)—Beginning in 1997 the NHIS questionnaire was changed to ask "What is the highest level of school ___ has completed or the highest degree received?" Responses were used to categorize individuals according to educational credentials (for example, no high school diploma or general educational development (GED) high school equivalency diploma; high school diploma or GED; some college, no bachelor's degree; bachelor's degree or higher).

Prior to 1997 the education variable in NHIS was measured by asking, "What is the highest grade or year of regular school ___ has ever attended?" and "Did ___ finish the grade/year?" Responses were used to categorize individuals according to years of education completed (for example, less than 12 years, 12 years, 13–15 years, and 16 or more years).

Data from the 1996 and 1997 NHIS were used to compare distributions of educational attainment for adults 25 years of age and over using categories based on educational credentials (1997) with categories based on years of education completed (1996). A larger percent of persons reported "some college" than "13–15 years" of education and a correspondingly smaller percent reported "high school diploma or GED" than "12 years of education." In 1997, 19 percent of adults reported no high school diploma, 31 percent a high school diploma or GED, 26 percent some college, and 24 percent a bachelor's degree or higher. In 1996, 18 percent of adults reported less than 12 years of education,

37 percent 12 years of education, 20 percent 13–15 years, and 25 percent 16 or more years of education.

Emergency department—According to the National Hospital Ambulatory Medical Care Survey (NHAMCS), an emergency department is a hospital facility that provides unscheduled outpatient services to patients whose conditions require immediate care and is staffed 24 hours a day. Off-site emergency departments open less than 24 hours are included if staffed by the hospital's emergency department. See related *Emergency department visit; Outpatient department.*

Emergency department visit—Starting with the 1997 National Health Interview Survey, respondents to the sample adult and sample child questionnaires are asked about the number of visits to hospital emergency rooms during the past 12 months, including visits that resulted in hospitalization. In the National Hospital Ambulatory Medical Care Survey an emergency department visit is a direct personal exchange between a patient and a physician or other health care providers working under the physician's supervision, for the purpose of seeking care and receiving personal health services. See related *Emergency department; Injury-related visit.*

Employer costs for employee compensation—This is a measure of the average cost per employee hour worked to employers for wages and salaries and benefits. Wages and salaries are defined as the hourly straight-time wage rate, or for workers not paid on an hourly basis, straight-time earnings divided by the corresponding hours. Straight-time wage and salary rates are total earnings before payroll deductions, excluding premium pay for overtime and for work on weekends and holidays, shift differentials, nonproduction bonuses, and lump-sum payments provided in lieu of wage increases. Production bonuses, incentive earnings, commission payments, and cost-of-living adjustments are included in straight-time wage and salary rates. Benefits covered are paid leave—paid vacations, holidays, sick leave, and other leave; supplemental pay—premium pay for overtime and work on weekends and holidays, shift differentials, nonproduction bonuses, and lump-sum payments provided in lieu of wage increases; insurance benefits—life, health, and sickness and accident insurance; retirement and savings benefits—pension and other retirement plans and savings and thrift plans; legally required benefits—social security, railroad retirement and supplemental retirement, railroad unemployment insurance, Federal and State unemployment insurance, workers' compensation, and other benefits required by law, such as State temporary disability insurance; and other benefits—severance pay and supplemental unemployment plans. See related *Appendix I, National Compensation Survey*.

Environmental Protection Agency Standards—The Federal Clean Air Act of 1970, amended in 1977 and 1990, requires the Environmental Protection Agency (EPA) to establish National Ambient Air Quality Standards. EPA has set specific standards for each of six major pollutants: carbon monoxide, lead, nitrogen dioxide, ozone, sulfur dioxide, and particulate matter whose aerodynamic size is equal to or less than 10 microns (PM-10). Each pollutant standard represents a maximum concentration level (micrograms per cubic meter) that cannot be exceeded during a specified time interval. For more information, see www.epa.gov/oar/oaqps.

Ethnicity—See *Hispanic origin*.

Expenditures—See *Health expenditures, national; Appendix I, National Health Accounts*.

Family income—For purposes of the National Health Interview Survey (NHIS) and National Health and Nutrition Examination Survey (NHANES), all people within a household related to each other by blood, marriage, or adoption constitute a family. Each member of a family is classified according to the total income of the family. Unrelated individuals are classified according to their own income. In the NHIS (in years prior to 1997) and NHANES, family income was the total income received by members of a family (or by an unrelated individual) in the 12 months before the interview. Starting in 1997 the NHIS collected family income data for the calendar year prior to the interview (for example, 1997 family income data were based on 1996 calendar year information). Family income includes wages, salaries, rents from property, interest, dividends, profits and fees from their own businesses, pensions, and help from relatives. Family income data are used in the computation of poverty level. For data years 1990–96, about 16–18 percent of persons had missing data on poverty level. Missing values were imputed for family income using a sequential hot deck within matrix cells imputation approach. A detailed description of the imputation procedure as well as data files with imputed annual family income for 1990–96 are available from NCHS on CD-ROM NHIS Imputed Annual Family Income 1990–96, series 10, no 9A. See related *Poverty level*.

Federal hospitals—See *Hospital*.

Federal physicians—See *Physician*.

Fee-for-service health insurance—This is private (commercial) health insurance that reimburses health care providers on the basis of a fee for each health service provided to the insured person. It is also known as indemnity health insurance. Medicare Parts A and B are sometimes referred to as "Medicare fee-for-service." See related *Health insurance coverage; Medicare*.

Fertility rate—See *Rate: Birth and related rates*.

Fetal death—A fetal death is death before the complete expulsion or extraction from its mother, irrespective of the duration of pregnancy; the death is indicated by the fact that after such separation, the fetus does not breathe or show any other evidence of life, such as beating of the heart, pulsation of the umbilical cord, or definite movement of voluntary muscles. For statistical purposes, fetal deaths are classified according to gestational age. In this report tabulations are shown for fetal deaths with stated or presumed gestation of 20 weeks or more and of 28 weeks or more, the latter gestational age group also known as late fetal deaths. See related *Gestation; Live birth; Rate: Death and related rates*.

First-listed diagnosis—In the National Hospital Discharge Survey, this is the first recorded diagnosis on the medical record face sheet (summary sheet).

First-listed external cause of injury—In the National Hospital Ambulatory Medical Care Survey, this is the first-listed external cause of injury coded from the Patient Record Form (PRF). Up to three causes of injury can be reported on the PRF. Injuries are coded by NCHS to the *International Classification of Diseases, Ninth Revision, Clinical Modification* Supplementary Classification of External Causes of Injury and Poisoning. See table VII for a listing of injury categories and codes. See related *Injury-related visit*.

General hospitals—See *Hospital*.

General hospital psychiatric services—See *Mental health organization*.

Figure I. Census Bureau: Four Geographic Regions and 9 Divisions of the United States

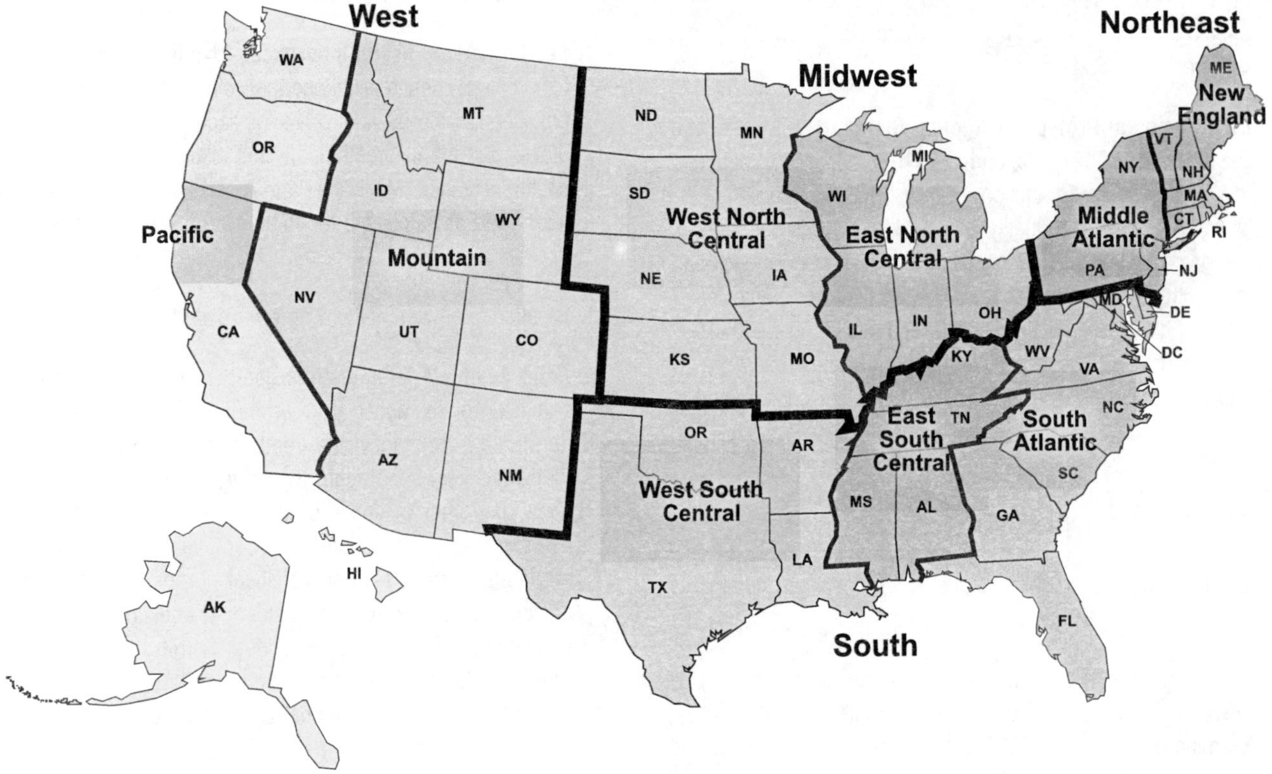

Geographic region and division—The U.S. Bureau of the Census groups the 50 States and the District of Columbia for statistical purposes into four geographic regions—Northeast, Midwest, South, and West—and nine divisions, based on geographic proximity. See figure I.

The Department of Commerce's Bureau of Economic Analysis (BEA) groups States into eight regions based on their homogeneity with respect to income characteristics, industrial

composition of the employed labor force, and such noneconomic factors as demographic, social, and cultural characteristics. See figure II.

Three Census Bureau divisions—West North Central, East North Central, and New England—and three BEA regions—Plains, Great Lakes, and New England—are composed of the same States. The States composing the remaining Census Bureau divisions differ from those composing the corresponding BEA regions.

Gestation—For the National Vital Statistics System and the Centers for Disease Control and Prevention's Abortion Surveillance, the period of gestation is defined as beginning with the first day of the last normal menstrual period and ending with the day of birth or day of termination of pregnancy. See related *Abortion; Fetal death; Live birth.*

Gross domestic product (GDP)—GDP is the market value of the goods and services produced by labor and property located in the United States. As long as the labor and property are located in the United States, the suppliers (that

Table VII. Codes for first-listed external causes of injury from the *International Classification of Diseases, Ninth Revision, Clinical Modification*

External cause of injury category	E-Code numbers
Unintentional	E800–E869, E880–E929
Motor vehicle traffic	E810–E819
Falls	E880–E886, E888
Struck by or against objects or persons	E916–E917
Caused by cutting and piercing instruments or objects	E920
Intentional (suicide and homicide)	E950–E969

Figure II. **Bureau of Economic Analysis:** Eight Geographic Regions of the United States

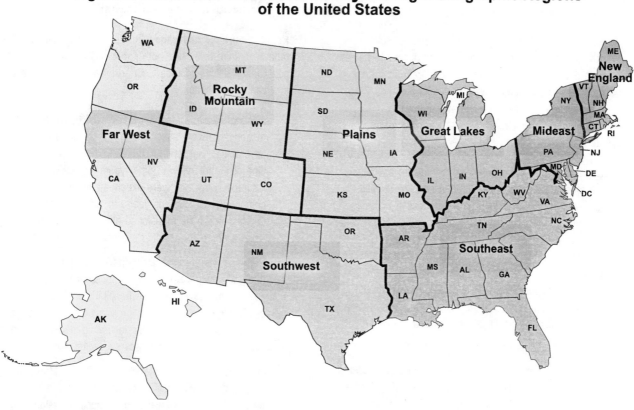

is, the workers and, for property, the owners) may be U.S. residents or residents of other countries. See related *Consumer Price Index; Health expenditures, national.*

Health care contact—Starting in 1997 the National Health Interview Survey has been collecting information on health care contacts with doctors and other health care professionals using the following questions: "During the past 12 months, how many times have you gone to a hospital emergency room about your own health?"; "During the past 12 months, did you receive care at home from a nurse or other health care professional? What was the total number of home visits received?" "During the past 12 months, how many times have you seen a doctor or other health care professional about your own health at a doctor's office, a clinic, or some other place? Do not include times you were hospitalized overnight, visits to hospital emergency rooms, home visits, or telephone calls." Beginning in 2000 this question was amended to also exclude dental visits. For each question respondents were shown a flashcard with response categories of 0, 1, 2–3, 4–9, 10–12, or 13 or more visits in 1997–99. Starting in 2000

response categories were expanded to: 0, 1, 2–3, 4–5, 6–7, 8–9, 10–12, 13–15, 16 or more. Analyses of the percent of persons with health care visits were tabulated as follows: For tabulation of the 1997–99 data, responses of 2–3 were recoded to 2 and responses of 4–9 were recoded to 6. Starting in 2000 tabulation of responses of 2–3 were recoded to 2 and other responses were recoded to the midpoint of the range. A summary measure of health care visits was constructed by adding recoded responses for these questions and categorizing the sum as: none, 1–3, 4–9, or 10 or more health care visits in the past 12 months.

Analyses of the percent of children without a health care visit are based upon the following question: "During the past 12 months, how many times has ___ seen a doctor or other health care professional about (his/her) health at a doctor's office, a clinic, or some other place? Do not include times ____was hospitalized overnight, visits to hospital emergency rooms, home visits, or telephone calls." See related *Emergency department visit; Home visit.*

Health expenditures, national—See related *Consumer price index; Gross domestic product.*

Health services and supplies expenditures—These are outlays for goods and services relating directly to patient care plus expenses for administering health insurance programs and government public health activities. This category is equivalent to total national health expenditures minus expenditures for research and construction.

National health expenditures—This measure estimates the amount spent for all health services and supplies and health-related research and construction activities consumed in the United States during the calendar year. Detailed estimates are available by source of expenditures (for example, out-of-pocket payments, private health insurance, and government programs), and by type of expenditures (for example, hospital care, physician services, and drugs), and are in current dollars for the year of report. Data are compiled from a variety of sources.

Nursing home expenditures—These cover care rendered in establishments primarily engaged in providing inpatient nursing and rehabilitative services and continuous personal care services to persons requiring nursing care (skilled nursing and intermediate care facilities, including those for the mentally retarded) and continuing care retirement communities with on-site nursing care facilities. The costs of long-term care provided by hospitals are excluded.

Personal health care expenditures—These are outlays for goods and services relating directly to patient care. The expenditures in this category are total national health expenditures minus expenditures for research and construction, expenses for administering health insurance programs, and government public health activities.

Private expenditures—These are outlays for services provided or paid for by nongovernmental sources—consumers, insurance companies, private industry, philanthropic, and other nonpatient care sources.

Public expenditures—These are outlays for services provided or paid for by Federal, State, and local government agencies or expenditures required by governmental mandate (such as workmen's compensation insurance payments).

Health insurance coverage—The term "health insurance" is broadly defined to include both public and private payors who cover medical expenditures incurred by a defined population in a variety of settings.

National Health Interview Survey (NHIS)—NHIS respondents were asked about their health insurance coverage in the previous month in 1993–96 and at the time of the interview in other years. Questions on health insurance coverage were expanded starting in 1993 compared with previous years. In 1997 the entire questionnaire was redesigned and data were collected using a computer-assisted personal interview (CAPI).

Respondents are covered by private health insurance if they indicate private health insurance or if they are covered by a single-service hospital plan, except in 1997 and 1998 when no information on single-service plans was obtained. Private health insurance includes managed care such as health maintenance organizations (HMOs).

Until 1996 persons were defined as having Medicaid or other public assistance coverage if they indicated that they had either Medicaid or other public assistance, or if they reported receiving Aid to Families with Dependent Children (AFDC) or Supplemental Security Income (SSI). After welfare reform in late 1996, Medicaid was delinked from AFDC and SSI. Starting in 1997 persons have been considered covered by Medicaid if they report Medicaid or a State-sponsored health program. Starting in 1998 persons are considered covered by Medicaid if they report being covered by the State Children's Health Insurance Program (SCHIP). Medicare or military health plan coverage is also determined in the interview and, starting in 1997, other government-sponsored program coverage is determined as well.

If respondents do not report coverage under one of the above types of plans and they have unknown coverage under either private health insurance or Medicaid, they are considered to have unknown coverage.

The remaining respondents are considered uninsured. The uninsured are persons who do not have coverage under private health insurance, Medicare, Medicaid, public assistance, a State-sponsored health plan, other government-sponsored programs, or a military health plan. Persons with only Indian Health Service coverage are considered uninsured. Estimates of the percent of persons who are uninsured based on the NHIS (table 129) may differ slightly from those based on the March Current Population Survey (CPS) (table 151) due to differences in survey questions, recall period, and other aspects of survey methodology.

In 2001 in the NHIS 1.3 percent of persons age 65 years and over had no health insurance but the small sample size precludes the presentation of separate estimates for this population. Therefore the term "uninsured" refers only to the population under age 65.

See related *Fee-for-service health insurance; Health maintenance organization; Managed care; Medicaid; Medicare; State Children's Health Insurance Program (SCHIP); Uninsured.*

Health maintenance organization (HMO)—An HMO is a health care system that assumes or shares both the financial risks and the delivery risks associated with providing comprehensive medical services to a voluntarily enrolled population in a particular geographic area, usually in return for a fixed, prepaid fee. Pure HMO enrollees use only the prepaid capitated health services of the HMO panel of medical care providers. Open-ended HMO enrollees use the prepaid HMO health services but, in addition may receive medical care from providers who are not part of the HMO panel. There is usually a substantial deductible, copayment, or coinsurance associated with use of nonpanel providers.

HMO model types are:

Group model HMO—An HMO that contracts with a single multi-specialty medical group to provide care to the HMO's membership. The group practice may work exclusively with the HMO, or it may provide services to non-HMO patients as well. The HMO pays the medical group a negotiated per capita rate, which the group distributes among its physicians, usually on a salaried basis.

Staff model HMO—A type of closed-panel HMO (where patients can receive services only through a limited number of providers) in which physicians are employees of the HMO. The providers see members in the HMO's own facilities.

Network model HMO—An HMO model that contracts with multiple physician groups to provide services to HMO members; may involve large single and multi-specialty groups.

Individual practice association (IPA)—A type of healthcare provider organization composed of a group of independent practicing physicians who maintain their own offices and band together for the purpose of contracting their services to HMOs, PPOs (preferred provider organizations), and insurance companies. An IPA may contract with and provide services to both HMO and non-HMO plan participants.

Mixed model HMO—An HMO that combines features of more than one HMO model.

See related *Managed care; Point-of-service plan; Preferred provider organization.*

Health services and supplies expenditures—See *Health expenditures, national.*

Health status, respondent-assessed—Health status was measured in the National Health Interview Survey by asking the respondent "Would you say ____'s health is excellent, very good, good, fair, or poor?"

Healthy People 2010—Healthy People 2010 is the prevention agenda for the Nation. It is a statement of national health objectives designed to identify the most significant preventable threats to health and to establish national goals to reduce these threats. Healthy People 2010 is a set of health objectives for the Nation to achieve over the first decade of the new century. More information on Healthy People 2010 is available at www.health.gov/healthypeople. See related *Leading Health Indicators.*

Hispanic origin—Hispanic or Latino origin includes persons of Mexican, Puerto Rican, Cuban, Central and South American, and other or unknown Latin American or Spanish origins. Persons of Hispanic origin may be of any race. In the National Health Interview Survey questionnaire, questions on Hispanic origin are self-reported and precede questions on race.

Birth File—The reporting area for an Hispanic-origin item on the birth certificate expanded between 1980 and 1993. Trend data on births of Hispanic and non-Hispanic parentage in this report are affected by expansion of the reporting area and by immigration. These two factors affect numbers of events, composition of the Hispanic population, and maternal and infant health characteristics.

In 1980 and 1981 information on births of Hispanic parentage was reported on the birth certificate by the following 22 States: Arizona, Arkansas, California, Colorado, Florida, Georgia, Hawaii, Illinois, Indiana, Kansas, Maine, Mississippi, Nebraska, Nevada, New Jersey, New Mexico, New York, North Dakota, Ohio, Texas, Utah, and Wyoming. In 1982 Tennessee, and in 1983 the District of Columbia began reporting this information. Between 1983 and 1987 information on births of Hispanic parentage was available for 23 States and the District of Columbia. In 1988 this information became available for Alabama, Connecticut, Kentucky, Massachusetts, Montana, North Carolina, and Washington, increasing the number of States reporting information on births of Hispanic parentage to 30 States and the District of Columbia. In 1989 this information became available from an additional 17 States, increasing the number of Hispanic-reporting States to 47 and the District of Columbia. In 1989 only Louisiana, New Hampshire, and Oklahoma did not report Hispanic parentage on the birth certificate. With the inclusion of Oklahoma in 1989 and Louisiana in 1990 as Hispanic-reporting States, 99 percent of birth records included information on mother's origin. Hispanic origin of the mother was reported on the birth certificates of 49 States and the District of Columbia in 1991 and 1992; only New Hampshire did not provide this information. Starting in 1993 Hispanic origin of mother was reported by all 50 States and the District of Columbia.

Mortality File—The reporting area for an Hispanic-origin item on the death certificate expanded between 1985 and 1997. In 1985 mortality data by Hispanic origin of decedent were based on deaths to residents of the following 17 States and the District of Columbia whose data on the death certificate were at least 90 percent complete on a place-of-occurrence basis and of comparable format: Arizona, Arkansas, California, Colorado, Georgia, Hawaii, Illinois, Indiana, Kansas, Mississippi, Nebraska, New York, North Dakota, Ohio, Texas, Utah, and Wyoming. In 1986 New Jersey began reporting Hispanic origin of decedent, increasing the

number of reporting States to 18 and the District of Columbia in 1986 and 1987. In 1988 Alabama, Kentucky, Maine, Montana, North Carolina, Oregon, Rhode Island, and Washington were added to the reporting area, increasing the number of States to 26 and the District of Columbia. In 1989 an additional 18 States were added, increasing the Hispanic reporting area to 44 States and the District of Columbia. In 1989 only Connecticut, Louisiana, Maryland, New Hampshire, Oklahoma, and Virginia were not included in the reporting area. Starting with 1990 data in this book, the criterion was changed to include States whose data were at least 80 percent complete. In 1990 Maryland, Virginia, and Connecticut, in 1991 Louisiana, and in 1993 New Hampshire were added, increasing the reporting area for Hispanic origin of decedent to 47 States and the District of Columbia in 1990, 48 States and the District of Columbia in 1991 and 1992, and 49 States and the District of Columbia in 1993–96. Only Oklahoma did not provide this information in 1993–96. Starting in 1997 Hispanic origin of decedent was reported by all 50 States and the District of Columbia. Based on data from the U.S. Bureau of the Census, the 1990 reporting area encompassed 99.6 percent of the U.S. Hispanic population. In 1990 more than 96 percent of death records included information on Hispanic origin of decedent.

See related *Race*.

HIV—See *Human immunodeficiency virus (HIV) disease*.

Home health care—Home health care as defined by the National Home and Hospice Care Survey is care provided by a home health care agency to individuals and families in their place of residence for promoting, maintaining, or restoring health; or for minimizing the effects of disability and illness including terminal illness.

Home visit—Starting in 1997 the National Health Interview Survey has been collecting information on home visits received during the past 12 months. Respondents are asked "During the past 12 months, did you receive care at home from a nurse or other health care professional? What was the total number of home visits received?" These data are combined with data on visits to doctors' offices, clinics, and emergency departments to provide a summary measure of health care visits. See related *Emergency department visit; Health care contact*.

Hospice care—Hospice care as defined by the National Home and Hospice Care Survey is a program of palliative and supportive care services providing physical, psychological, social, and spiritual care for dying persons, their families, and other loved ones by a hospice program or agency. Hospice services are available in home and inpatient settings.

Hospital—According to the American Hospital Association, hospitals are licensed institutions with at least six beds whose primary function is to provide diagnostic and therapeutic patient services for medical conditions by an organized physician staff, and have continuous nursing services under the supervision of registered nurses. The World Health Organization considers an establishment to be a hospital if it is permanently staffed by at least one physician, can offer inpatient accommodation, and can provide active medical and nursing care. Hospitals may be classified by type of service, ownership, size in terms of number of beds, and length of stay. In the National Hospital Ambulatory Medical Care Survey, hospitals include all those with an average length of stay for all patients of less than 30 days (short-stay) or hospitals whose specialty is general (medical or surgical) or children's general. Federal hospitals and hospital units of institutions and hospitals with fewer than six beds staffed for patient use are excluded. See related *Average length of stay; Bed; Days of care; Emergency department; Inpatient; Outpatient department.*

Community hospital, based on the American Hospital Association definition, includes all non-Federal short-term general and special hospitals whose facilities and services are available to the public. Special hospitals include obstetrics and gynecology; eye, ear, nose, and throat; rehabilitation; orthopedic; and other specialty services. Short-term general and special childrens hospitals are also considered to be community hospitals. A hospital may include a nursing-home-type unit and still be classified as short-term, provided that the majority of its patients are admitted to units where the average length of stay is less than 30 days. Hospital units of institutions such as prisons and college infirmaries that are not open to the public and are contained within a nonhospital facility are not included in the category of community hospitals. Traditionally the definition included all non-Federal short-stay hospitals except facilities for the mentally retarded. In a revised definition the following additional sites were excluded: hospital units of

institutions, and alcoholism and chemical dependency facilities.

Federal hospitals are operated by the Federal Government.

For profit hospitals are operated for profit by individuals, partnerships, or corporations.

General hospitals provide diagnostic, treatment, and surgical services for patients with a variety of medical conditions. According to the World Health Organization, these hospitals provide medical and nursing care for more than one category of medical discipline (for example, general medicine, specialized medicine, general surgery, specialized surgery, and obstetrics). Excluded are hospitals, usually in rural areas, that provide a more limited range of care.

Nonprofit hospitals are controlled by nonprofit organizations, including religious organizations, fraternal societies, and others.

Psychiatric hospitals are ones whose major type of service is psychiatric care. See related *Mental health organization.*

Registered hospitals are hospitals registered with the American Hospital Association. About 98 percent of hospitals are registered.

Short-stay hospitals in the National Hospital Discharge Survey are those in which the average length of stay is less than 30 days. The National Health Interview Survey defines short-stay hospitals as any hospital or hospital department in which the type of service provided is general; maternity; eye, ear, nose, and throat; childrens; or osteopathic.

Specialty hospitals, such as psychiatric, tuberculosis, chronic disease, rehabilitation, maternity, and alcoholic or narcotic, provide a particular type of service to the majority of their patients.

Hospital-based physician—See *Physician.*

Hospital days—See *Days of care.*

Hospital utilization—Estimates of hospital utilization (such as hospital discharge rate, days of care rate, and average length of stay) presented in *Health, United States* are based on data from two different sources—the National Health Interview Survey (NHIS) and the National Hospital Discharge Survey (NHDS). Estimates of hospital utilization from these two surveys may differ because NHIS data are based on household interviews of the civilian noninstitutionalized population whereas NHDS data are based on hospital discharge records of all persons. Starting in 1997 hospital utilization data from the NHIS are for all hospital discharges whereas estimates for prior years excluded hospitalizations for delivery and newborns. NHDS includes hospital discharge records for all persons discharged alive or deceased and institutionalized persons, and excludes data for newborn infants. Differences in hospital utilization estimated by the two surveys are particularly evident for children and the elderly. For children NHIS estimates are higher than NHDS estimates due to inclusion of data for newborns. For the elderly NHDS estimates are higher than NHIS estimates because of inclusion of data for institutionalized persons and persons who died while hospitalized. See related *Average length of stay; Days of care; Discharge; Appendix I, National Health Interview Survey, National Hospital Discharge Survey.*

Human immunodeficiency virus (HIV) disease—Mortality and morbidity coding for HIV disease are similar and have evolved over time.

Mortality coding—Starting with data year 1999 and the introduction of the Tenth Revision of the *International Classification of Diseases* (ICD-10), the title for this cause of death was changed to "HIV disease" from "HIV infection" and the ICD codes changed to B20-B24. Beginning with data for 1987, NCHS introduced category numbers *042-*044 for classifying and coding HIV infection as a cause of death in ICD-9. The asterisk before the category numbers indicates that these codes were not part of the original ICD-9. HIV infection was formerly referred to as human T-cell lymphotropic virus-III/lymphadenopathy-associated virus (HTLV-III/LAV) infection. Before 1987 deaths involving HIV infection were classified to Deficiency of cell-mediated immunity (ICD-9 279.1) contained in the title All other diseases; to Pneumocystosis (ICD-9 136.3) contained in the title All other infectious and parasitic diseases; to Malignant neoplasms, including neoplasms of lymphatic and hematopoietic tissues; and to a number of other causes. Therefore, before 1987, death statistics for HIV infection

are not strictly comparable with data for 1987 and later years, and are not shown in this report.

Morbidity coding—The National Hospital Discharge Survey codes diagnosis data using the *International Classification of Diseases, Ninth Revision, Clinical Modification* (ICD-9-CM). Discharges with diagnosis of HIV as shown in *Health, United States* have at least one HIV diagnosis listed on the face sheet of the medical record and are not limited to the first-listed diagnosis. During 1984 and 1985 only data for AIDS (ICD-9-CM 279.19) were included. In 1986–94 discharges with the following diagnoses were included: acquired immunodeficiency syndrome (AIDS), human immunodeficiency virus (HIV) infection and associated conditions, and positive serological or viral culture findings for HIV (ICD-9-CM 042–044, 279.19, and 795.8). Beginning in 1995 discharges with the following diagnoses were included: human immunodeficiency virus (HIV) disease and asymptomatic human immunodeficiency virus (HIV) infection status (ICD-9-CM 042 and V08).

See related *Acquired immunodeficiency syndrome; Cause of death; International Classification of Diseases; International Classification of Diseases, Ninth Revision, Clinical Modification.*

ICD; ICD codes—See *Cause of death; International Classification of Diseases.*

Illicit drug use—Illicit drug use refers to use and misuse of illegal and controlled drugs.

Monitoring the Future Study—In this school-based survey of secondary school students, information on marijuana use is collected using self-completed questionnaires. The information is based on the following questions: "On how many occasions (if any) have you used marijuana in the last 30 days?" and "On how many occasions (if any) have you used hashish in the last 30 days?" Questions on cocaine use include the following: "On how many occasions (if any) have you taken "crack" (cocaine in chunk or rock form) during the last 30 days?" and "On how many occasions (if any) have you taken cocaine in any other form during the last 30 days.

National Household Survey on Drug Abuse—Information on illicit drug use is collected for all persons 12 years of age and over. Information on any illicit drug use, including marijuana or hashish, cocaine, heroin, hallucinogens, and nonmedical use of prescription drugs is based on the following question: "During the past 30 days, on how many days did you use (specific illicit drug)?" See related *Substance use.*

Incidence—Incidence is the number of cases of disease having their onset during a prescribed period of time. It is often expressed as a rate (for example, the incidence of measles per 1,000 children 5–15 years of age during a specified year). Incidence is a measure of morbidity or other events that occur within a specified period of time. See related *Prevalence.*

Income—See *Family Income.*

Individual practice association (IPA)—See *Health maintenance organization (HMO).*

Industry of employment—Industries are classified according to the *Standard Industrial Classification (SIC) Manual* of the Office of Management and Budget. Two editions of the SIC are used for coding industry data in *Health, United States*: the 1977 supplement to the 1972 edition and the 1987 edition. The changes between versions include a few detailed titles created to correct or clarify industries or to recognize changes within the industry. Codes for major industry divisions (table VIII) were not changed between versions.

Health data by industry shown in *Health, United States* are from two different surveys conducted by the Bureau of Labor Statistics, the Census of Fatal Occupational Injuries (CFOI) and the Survey of Occupational Injuries and Illnesses (SOII).

Table VIII. Codes for industries, according to the *Standard Industrial Classification (SIC) Manual*

Industry	Code numbers
Agriculture, forestry, and fishing	01–09
Mining	10–14
Construction	15–17
Manufacturing	20–39
Transportation and public utilities	40–49
Wholesale trade	50–51
Retail trade	52–59
Finance, insurance, and real estate	60–67
Services	70–89
Public administration	91–97

Establishments engaged in the same kind of economic activity are classified by the same industry code, regardless of whether ownership is by corporations or sole proprietorships in the private sector, or government agencies. The category "private sector" includes all industry divisions except public administration and military, which are in the public sector. The category "not classified" is used when there is insufficient information to determine a specific industry classification. Data from CFOI are presented separately for private sector and government. Data from SOII are presented for the private sector only and exclude the self-employed.

Infant death—An infant death is the death of a live-born child before his or her first birthday. Age at death may be further classified according to neonatal and postneonatal. Neonatal deaths are those that occur before the 28th day of life; postneonatal deaths are those that occur between 28 and 365 days of age. See related *Live birth; Rate: Death and related rates.*

Injury—See *First-listed external cause of injury.*

Injury-related visit—In the National Hospital Ambulatory Medical Care Survey an emergency department visit was considered injury related if, on the Patient Record Form (PRF), the checkbox for injury was indicated. In addition, injury visits were identified if the physician's diagnosis was injury related (ICD-9-CM code of 800–999), an external cause-of-injury code was present (ICD-9-CM E800–E999), or the patient's reason for visit code was injury related. See related *Emergency department visit; First-listed external cause of injury.*

Inpatient—An inpatient is a person who is formally admitted to the inpatient service of a hospital for observation, care, diagnosis, or treatment. See related *Admission; Average length of stay; Days of care; Discharge; Hospital.*

Inpatient care—See *Mental health service type.*

Inpatient days—See *Days of care.*

Instrumental activities of daily living (IADL)—Instrumental activities of daily living are activities related to independent living and include preparing meals, managing money, shopping for groceries or personal items, performing light or heavy housework, and using a telephone. In the Medicare Current Beneficiary Survey if a sample person had any difficulty performing an activity by him or herself and without special equipment, or did not perform the activity at all because of health problems, the person was categorized as having a limitation in that activity. The limitation may have been temporary or chronic at the time of the interview. Sample persons in the community answered health status and functioning questions themselves, if able to do so. For sample persons in a long-term care facility, a proxy such as a nurse answered questions about the sample person's health status and functioning.

In the National Health Interview Survey (NHIS) respondents are asked about needing the help of another person for handling routine IADL needs due to a physical, mental, or emotional problem. Persons are considered to have an IADL limitation in the NHIS if any causal condition is chronic.

See related *Activities of daily living (ADL); Limitation of activity.*

Insured—See *Health insurance coverage.*

Intermediate care facilities—See *Nursing home.*

International Classification of Diseases—The ICD provides the ground rules for coding and classifying cause-of-death data. The ICD is developed collaboratively between the World Health Organization (WHO) and 10 international centers, one of which is housed at NCHS. The purpose of the ICD is to promote international comparability in the collection, classification, processing, and presentation of health statistics. Since the beginning of the century, the ICD has been modified about once every 10 years, except for the 20-year interval between ICD-9 and ICD-10 (see table IV). The purpose of the revisions is to stay abreast with advances in medical science. New revisions usually introduce major disruptions in time series of mortality statistics (see tables V and VI). For more information, see www.cdc.gov/nchs/about/major/dvs/icd10des.htm. See related *Cause of death; Comparability ratio; International Classification of Diseases, Ninth Revision, Clinical Modification.*

International Classification of Diseases, Ninth Revision, Clinical Modification (ICD-9-CM)—The ICD-9-CM is based on and is compatible with the World Health Organization's *International Classification of Diseases, Ninth Revision* (ICD-9). The United States currently uses ICD-9-CM to code morbidity diagnoses and inpatient procedures. ICD-9-CM consists of three volumes. Volumes 1 and 2 contain the diagnosis tabular list and index. Volume 3 contains the procedure classification (tabular and index combined).

ICD-9-CM is divided into 17 chapters and 2 supplemental classifications. The chapters are arranged primarily by body system. In addition there are chapters for infectious and parasitic diseases; neoplasms; endocrine, nutritional, and metabolic diseases; mental disorders; complications of pregnancy, childbirth and puerperium; certain conditions originating in the perinatal period; congenital anomalies; and symptoms, signs and ill-defined conditions. The two supplemental classifications are for factors influencing health status and contact with health service and external causes of injury and poisoning. For additional information about ICD-9-CM, see www.cdc.gov/nchs/icd9.htm. See related *International Classification of Diseases.*

In *Health, United States* morbidity data are classified using ICD-9-CM. Diagnostic categories and codes for ICD-9-CM are shown in table IX; ICD-9-CM procedure categories and codes are shown in table X. Starting with data year 1999 the United States began using ICD-10 to code mortality data.

Late fetal death rate—See *Rate: Death and related rates.*

Leading causes of death—See *Cause-of-death ranking.*

Leading Health Indicators—Leading Health Indicators (LHIs) are used to measure important determinants of the Nation's health during the first decade of the twenty-first century. Five of the indicators relate primarily to individual behaviors including physical activity, overweight and obesity, tobacco use, substance abuse, and responsible sexual behavior. The other five address mental health, injury and violence, environmental quality, immunization, and access to health care. More information on the LHIs is available at www.health.gov/healthypeople/LHI/. See related *Healthy People 2010.*

Length of stay—See *Average length of stay.*

Life expectancy—Life expectancy is the average number of years of life remaining to a person at a particular age and is based on a given set of age-specific death rates, generally the mortality conditions existing in the period mentioned. Life expectancy may be determined by race, sex, or other characteristics using age-specific death rates for the population with that characteristic. See related *Rate: Death and related rates.*

Table IX. Codes for diagnostic categories from the *International Classification of Diseases, Ninth Revision, Clinical Modification*

Diagnostic category	Code numbers
Females with delivery	V27
Human immunodeficiency virus (HIV) (1984–85)	279.19
(1986–94)	042–044, 279.19, 795.8
(Beginning in 1995)	042, V08
Malignant neoplasms	140–208
Large intestine and rectum	153–154, 197.5
Trachea, bronchus, and lung	162, 197.0, 197.3
Breast	174–175, 198.81
Prostate	185
Diabetes	250
Alcohol and drug	291–292, 303–305
Serious mental illness	295–298
Diseases of the nervous system and sense organs	320–389
Diseases of the circulatory system	390–459
Diseases of heart	391–392.0, 393–398, 402, 404, 410–416, 420–429
Ischemic heart disease	410–414
Acute myocardial infarction	410
Congestive heart failure	428.0
Cerebrovascular diseases	430–438
Diseases of the respiratory system	460–519
Pneumonia	466.1, 480–487.0
Asthma	493
Hyperplasia of prostate	600
Decubitus ulcers	707.0
Diseases of the musculoskeletal system and connective tissue	710–739
Osteoarthritis	715
Intervertebral disc disorders	722
Injuries and poisoning	800–999
Fracture, all sites	800–829
Fracture of neck of femur (hip)	820

Table X. Codes for procedure categories from the *International Classification of Diseases, Ninth Revision, Clinical Modification*

Procedure category	Code numbers
Extraction of lens	13.1–13.6
Insertion of prosthetic lens (pseudophakos)	13.7
Myringotomy with insertion of tube	20.01
Tonsillectomy, with or without adenoidectomy	28.2–28.3
Coronary angioplasty (Prior to 1997)	36.0
(Beginning in 1997)	36.01–36.05, 36.09
Coronary artery bypass graft	36.1
Cardiac catheterization	37.21–37.23
Pacemaker insertion or replacement	37.7–37.8
Carotid endarterectomy	38.12
Endoscopy of large or small intestine with or without biopsy	45.11–45.14, 45.16, 45.21–45.25
Cholecystectomy	51.2
Prostatectomy	60.2–60.6
Bilateral destruction or occlusion of fallopian tubes	66.2–66.3
Hysterectomy	68.3–68.7, 68.9
Cesarean section	74.0–74.2, 74.4, 74.99
Repair of current obstetrical laceration	75.5–75.6
Reduction of fracture	76.7, 79.0–79.3
Arthroscopy of knee	80.26
Excision or destruction of intervertebral disc	80.5
Total hip replacement	81.51
Lumpectomy	85.21
Mastectomy	85.4
Angiocardiography with contrast material	88.5

Limitation of activity—In the National Health Interview Survey limitation of activity refers to a long-term reduction in a person's capacity to perform the usual kind or amount of activities associated with his or her age group due to a chronic condition. Limitation of activity is assessed by asking respondents a series of questions about limitations in their ability to perform activities usual for their age group because of a physical, mental, or emotional problem. Respondents are asked about limitations in activities of daily living, instrumental activities of daily living, play, school, work, difficulty walking or remembering, and any other activity limitations. For reported limitations, the causal health conditions are determined and respondents are considered limited if one or more of these conditions is chronic. See related *Activities of daily living; Condition; Instrumental activities of daily living.*

Live birth—A live birth is the complete expulsion or extraction of the neonate from its mother, irrespective of the duration of the pregnancy, which, after such separation, breathes or shows any other evidence of life such as heartbeat, umbilical cord pulsation, or definite movement of voluntary muscles, whether the umbilical cord has been cut or the placenta is attached. Each product of such a birth is considered live born. See related *Gestation; Rate: Birth and related rates.*

Live-birth order—In the National Vital Statistics System this item from the birth certificate refers to the total number of live births the mother has had, including the present birth as recorded on the birth certificate. Fetal deaths are excluded. See related *Live birth.*

Long term care facility—See *Nursing home.*

Low birthweight—See *Birthweight.*

Mammography—Mammography is an x-ray image of the breast used to detect irregularities in breast tissue. In the National Health Interview Survey questions concerning use of mammography differed slightly across the years for which data are shown. In 1987 and 1990 women were asked to report when they had their last mammogram. In 1991 women were asked whether they had a mammogram in the past 2 years. In 1993 and 1994 women were asked whether they had a mammogram within the past year, between 1 and 2 years ago, or over 2 years ago. In 1998 women were asked whether they had a mammogram a year ago or less, more than 1 year but not more than 2 years, or more than 2 years

ago. In 1999 women were asked when they had their most recent mammogram in days, weeks, months, or years. In 1999, 10 percent of women in the sample responded "2 years ago" and in this analysis these women were coded as "within the past 2 years" although a response of "2 years ago" may include women whose last mammogram was more than 2 but less than 3 years ago. Thus estimates for 1999 are overestimated to some degree in comparison with estimates in previous years. In 2000 women were asked when they had their most recent mammogram (give month and year). Women who did not respond were given a followup question that used the 1999 wording and women who did not answer the followup question were asked a second followup question that used the 1998 wording. In 2000, 2 percent of women in the sample answered "2 years ago" using the 1999 wording and they were coded as "within the past 2 years." Thus estimates for 2000 may be slightly overestimated in comparison with estimates for years prior to 1999.

Managed care—A term originally used to refer to the prepaid health care sector (e.g., health maintenance organizations or HMOs) where care is provided under a fixed budget and costs are therein capable of being "managed." Increasingly, the term is being used to include preferred provider organizations (PPOs) and even forms of indemnity insurance coverage (or fee-for-service insurance) that incorporate preadmission certification and other utilization controls. See related *Health maintenance organization; Preferred provider organization.*

Marital status—Marital status is classified through self-reporting into the categories married and unmarried. The term married encompasses all married people including those separated from their spouses. Unmarried includes those who are single (never married), divorced, or widowed. The abortion surveillance program classified separated people as unmarried before 1978.

> *Birth File*—In 1970, 39 States and the District of Columbia (DC) and in 1975, 38 States and DC included a direct question about mother's marital status on the birth certificate. Since 1980 national estimates of births to unmarried women have been based on two methods for determining marital status, a direct question in the birth registration process and inferential procedures. In 1980–96 marital status was reported on the birth certificates of 41–45 States and DC; with the addition of California in 1997, 46 States and DC; and in 1998–2001,

48 States and DC. In 1997, all but four States (Connecticut, Michigan, Nevada, and New York) and, in 1998, all but two States (Michigan and New York) included a direct question about mother's marital status on their birth certificates. In 1998–2001 marital status was imputed as "married" on those 0.03–0.05 percent of birth records with missing information in the 48 States and DC where this information was obtained by a direct question.

For States lacking a direct question, marital status was inferred. Before 1980 the incidence of births to unmarried women in States with no direct question on marital status was assumed to be the same as the incidence in reporting States in the same geographic division. Starting in 1980 for States without a direct question, marital status was inferred by comparing the parents' and child's surnames. Inferential procedures in current use depend on the presence of a paternity acknowledgment or missing information on the father. Changes in reporting procedures by some States in 1995 and 1997 had little effect on national totals, but did affect trends for age groups and some State trends. Details of the changes in reporting procedures are described in Ventura SJ, Bachrach CA. Nonmarital Childbearing in the United States, 1940–99. National vital statistics reports; vol 48 no 16. Hyattsville, Maryland: National Center for Health Statistics. 2000, available at www.cdc.gov/nchs/births.htm.

Maternal age—See *Age*.

Maternal death—Maternal death is defined by the World Health Organization as the death of a woman while pregnant or within 42 days of termination of pregnancy, irrespective of the duration and site of the pregnancy from any cause related to or aggravated by the pregnancy or its management, but not from accidental or incidental causes. A maternal death is one for which the certifying physician has designated a maternal condition as the underlying cause of death. Maternal conditions are those assigned to pregnancy, childbirth, and the puerperium, ICD-10 codes A34, O00-O95, O98-O99 (see table V). Changes have been made in the classification and coding of maternal deaths between ICD-9 and ICD-10, effective with mortality data for 1999. ICD-10 changes pertain to indirect maternal causes and timing of death relative to pregnancy. If only indirect maternal causes of death (i.e., a previously existing disease or a disease that developed during pregnancy which was not due to direct obstetric causes but

was aggravated by physiologic effects of pregnancy) are reported in Part I of the death certificate and pregnancy is reported in either Part I or Part II, ICD-10 classifies this as a maternal death. ICD-9 only classified the death as maternal if pregnancy was reported in Part I. Some State death certificates include a separate question regarding pregnancy status. A positive response to the question is interpreted as "pregnant" being reported in Part II of the cause-of-death section of the death certificate. If the medical certifier did not specify when death occurred relative to the pregnancy, it is assumed that the pregnancy terminated 42 days or less prior to death. Under ICD-10 a new category has been added for deaths from maternal causes that occurred more than 42 days after delivery or termination of pregnancy (O96-O97). In 1999 there were 15 such deaths and in 2000, there were 8. See related *Rate: Death and related rates*.

Maternal education—See *Education*.

Maternal mortality rate—See *Rate: Death and related rates*.

Medicaid—Medicaid was authorized by Title XIX of the Social Security Act in 1965 as a jointly funded cooperative venture between the Federal and State governments to assist States in the provision of adequate medical care to eligible needy persons. Within broad Federal guidelines, each of the States establishes its own eligibility standards; determines the type, amount, duration, and scope of services; sets the rate of payment for services; and administers its own program.

Medicaid is the largest program providing medical and health-related services to America's poorest people. However, Medicaid does not provide medical assistance for all poor persons. Under the broadest provisions of the Federal statute, Medicaid does not provide health care services even for very poor persons unless they are in a designated group, which include:

■ Individuals who meet the requirements for the Aid to Families with Dependent Children (AFDC) program that were in effect in their State on July 16, 1996, or, at State option, more liberal criteria (with some exceptions).

■ Children under age 6 whose family income is at or below 133 percent of the Federal poverty level.

■ Pregnant women whose family income is below 133 percent of the Federal poverty level (services to these women are limited to those related to pregnancy, complications of pregnancy, delivery, and postpartum care).

■ Supplemental Security Income (SSI) recipients in most States (some States use more restrictive Medicaid eligibility requirements that predate SSI).

■ Recipients of adoption or foster care assistance under Title IV of the Social Security Act.

■ Special protected groups (typically individuals who lose their cash assistance due to earnings from work or from increased Social Security benefits, but who may keep Medicaid for a period of time).

■ All children born after September 30, 1983, who are under age 19 and in families with incomes at or below the Federal poverty level (this process phases in coverage).

■ Certain Medicare beneficiaries (low income is only one test for Medicaid eligibility for those within these groups; their resources also are tested against threshold levels, as determined by each State within Federal guidelines).

States also have the option of providing Medicaid coverage for other "categorically related" groups.

Medicaid operates as a vendor payment program. States may pay health care providers directly on a fee-for-service basis, or States may pay for Medicaid services through various prepayment arrangements, such as health maintenance organizations (HMOs) or other forms of managed care. Within Federally imposed upper limits and specific restrictions, each State for the most part has broad discretion in determining the payment methodology and payment rate for services. Thus, the Medicaid program varies considerably from State to State, as well as within each State over time. See related *Health expenditures, national; Health insurance coverage; Health maintenance organization; Managed care; Appendix I, Medicaid Data System*.

Medical specialties—See *Physician specialty*.

Medical vendor payments—Under the Medicaid program, medical vendor payments are payments (expenditures) to medical vendors from the State through a fiscal agent or to a health insurance plan. Adjustments are made for Indian Health Service payments to Medicaid, cost settlements, third party recoupments, refunds, voided checks, and other financial settlements that cannot be related to specific provided claims. Excluded are payments made for medical care under the emergency assistance provisions, payments made from State medical assistance funds that are not federally matchable, disproportionate share hospital payments,

cost sharing or enrollment fees collected from recipients or a third party, and administration and training costs.

Medicare—This is a nationwide health insurance program providing health insurance protection to people 65 years of age and over, people entitled to social security disability payments for 2 years or more, and people with end-stage renal disease, regardless of income. The program was enacted July 30, 1965, as Title XVIII, *Health Insurance for the Aged of the Social Security Act*, and became effective on July 1, 1966. From its inception, it has included two separate but coordinated programs, hospital insurance (Part A) and supplementary medical insurance (Part B). In 1999, additional choices were allowed for delivering Medicare Part A and Part B benefits. Medicare+Choice (Part C) is an expanded set of options for the delivery of health care under Medicare, created in the Balanced Budget Act passed by Congress in 1997. The term Medicare+Choice refers to options other than original Medicare. While all Medicare beneficiaries can receive their benefits through the original fee-for-service (FFS) program, most beneficiaries enrolled in both Part A and Part B can choose to participate in a Medicare+Choice plan instead. Organizations that seek to contract as Medicare+Choice plans must meet specific organizational, financial, and other requirements. Most Medicare+Choice plans are coordinated care plans, which include health maintenance organizations (HMOs), provider-sponsored organizations (PSOs), preferred provider organizations (PPOs), and other certified coordinated care plans and entities that meet the standards set forth in the law. The Medicare+Choice program also includes Medical savings account (MSA) plans, which provide benefits after a single high deductible is met, and private, unrestricted FFS plans, which allow beneficiaries to select certain private providers. These programs are available in only a limited number of States. For those providers who agree to accept the plan's payment terms and conditions, this option does not place the providers at risk, nor does it vary payment rates based on utilization. Only the coordinated care plans are considered "managed care" plans. Except for MSA plans, all Medicare+Choice plans are required to provide at least the current Medicare benefit package, excluding hospice services. Plans may offer additional covered services and are required to do so (or return excess payments) if plan costs are lower than the Medicare payments received by the plan.

In the National Health Interview Survey (NHIS), the category "Medicare HMO" is defined as persons who are age 65 years or over and who responded "yes" when asked if they were under a Medicare managed care arrangement such as an HMO. This is a subset of Medicare Part C. Respondents who stated they had Medicare coverage but did not answer yes to the "managed care arrangement such as an HMO" are included in the Medicare fee-for-service category. "Medicare fee-for-service" is defined as Medicare Part A and/or Part B.

See related *Fee-for-service health insurance; Health insurance coverage; Health maintenance organization; Managed care; Appendix I, Medicare Administrative Data.*

Mental health organization—The Center for Mental Health Services of the Substance Abuse and Mental Health Services Administration defines a mental health organization as an administratively distinct public or private agency or institution whose primary concern is provision of direct mental health services to the mentally ill or emotionally disturbed. Excluded are private office-based practices of psychiatrists, psychologists, and other mental health providers; psychiatric services of all types of hospitals or outpatient clinics operated by Federal agencies other than the Department of Veterans Affairs (for example, Public Health Service, Indian Health Service, Department of Defense, and Bureau of Prisons); general hospitals that have no separate psychiatric services but admit psychiatric patients to nonpsychiatric units; and psychiatric services of schools, colleges, halfway houses, community residential organizations, local and county jails, State prisons, and other human service providers. The major types of mental health organizations are described below.

Freestanding psychiatric outpatient clinics provide only outpatient mental health services on either a regular or emergency basis. A psychiatrist generally assumes the medical responsibility for services.

Psychiatric hospitals (public or private) primarily provide 24-hour inpatient care and treatment in a hospital setting to persons with mental illnesses. Psychiatric hospitals may be under State, county, private for profit, or private nonprofit auspices.

General hospital psychiatric services provide psychiatric services with assigned staff for 24-hour inpatient or residential care and/or less than 24-hour outpatient care in a separate ward, unit, floor, or wing of the hospital.

Department of Veterans Affairs medical centers are hospitals operated by the Department of Veterans Affairs (formerly Veterans Administration) and include Department of Veterans Affairs general hospital psychiatric services (including large neuropsychiatric units) and Department of Veterans Affairs psychiatric outpatient clinics.

Residential treatment centers for emotionally disturbed children must meet all of the following criteria: (a) Provide 24-hour residential services; (b) Are not licensed as a psychiatric hospital and have the primary purpose of providing individually planned mental health treatment services in conjunction with residential care; (c) Include a clinical program directed by a psychiatrist, psychologist, social worker, or psychiatric nurse with a graduate degree; (d) Serve children and youth primarily under the age of 18; and (e) Have the primary diagnosis as mental illness, classified as other than mental retardation, developmental disability, or substance-related disorders, according to DSM-II/ICDA-8 or DSM-IIIR/ICD-9-CM codes, for the majority of admissions.

Multiservice mental health organizations provide services in both 24-hour and less than 24-hour settings and are not classifiable as a psychiatric hospital, general hospital, or residential treatment center for emotionally disturbed children. (The classification of a psychiatric or general hospital or residential treatment center for emotionally disturbed children takes precedence over a multiservice classification, even if two or more services are offered.)

Partial care organizations provide a program of ambulatory mental health services, or rehabilitation, habitation, or education programs.

See related *Addition; Mental health service type.*

Mental health service type—This term refers to the following types of mental health services:

24-hour mental health care, formerly called inpatient care, provides care in a mental health hospital setting.

Less than 24-hour care, formerly called outpatient or partial care treatment, provides mental health services on an ambulatory basis.

Residential treatment care provides overnight mental health care in conjunction with an intensive treatment program in a setting other than a hospital. Facilities may offer care to emotionally disturbed children or mentally ill adults.

See related *Addition; Mental health organization*.

Metropolitan statistical area (MSA)—The Office of Management and Budget (OMB) defines metropolitan areas according to published standards that are applied to Census Bureau data. The collective term "metropolitan area" includes metropolitan statistical areas (MSAs), consolidated metropolitan statistical areas (CMSAs), and primary metropolitan statistical areas (PMSAs). An MSA is a county or group of contiguous counties that contains at least one city with a population of 50,000 or more or a Census Bureau-defined urbanized area of at least 50,000 with a metropolitan population of at least 100,000. In addition to the county or counties that contain all or part of the main city or urbanized area, an MSA may contain other counties that are metropolitan in character and are economically and socially integrated with the main city. If an MSA has a population of 1 million or more and meets requirements specified in the standards, it is termed a CMSA, consisting of two or more major components, each of which is recognized as a PMSA. In New England, cities and towns, rather than counties, are used to define MSAs. Counties that are not within an MSA are considered to be nonmetropolitan.

For National Health Interview Survey (NHIS) data before 1995, metropolitan population is based on MSAs as defined by OMB in 1983 using the 1980 Census. Starting with the 1995 NHIS, metropolitan population is based on MSAs as defined by OMB in 1993 using the 1990 Census. For further information on metropolitan areas, see U.S. Department of Commerce, Bureau of the Census, *State and Metropolitan Area Data Book*. See related *Urbanization*.

Multiservice mental health organizations—See *Mental health organization*.

National ambient air quality standards—See *Environmental Protection Agency Standards*.

Neonatal mortality rate—See *Rate: Death and related rates*.

Non-Federal physicians—See *Physician*.

Nonpatient revenues—Nonpatient revenues are those revenues received for which no direct patient care services are rendered. The most widely recognized source of nonpatient revenues is philanthropy. Philanthropic support may be direct from individuals or may be obtained through philanthropic fund-raising organizations such as the United Way. Support may also be obtained from foundations or corporations. Philanthropic revenues may be designated for direct patient care use or may be contained in an endowment fund where only the current income may be tapped.

Nonprofit hospitals—See *Hospital*.

Notifiable disease—A notifiable disease is one that, when diagnosed, health providers are required, usually by law, to report to State or local public health officials. Notifiable diseases are those of public interest by reason of their contagiousness, severity, or frequency.

Nursing care—The following definition of nursing care applies to data collected in National Nursing Home Surveys through 1977. Nursing care is provision of any of the following services: application of dressings or bandages; bowel and bladder retraining; catheterization; enema; full bed bath; hypodermic, intramuscular, or intravenous injection; irrigation; nasal feeding; oxygen therapy; and temperature-pulse-respiration or blood pressure measurement. See related *Nursing home*.

Nursing care homes—See *Nursing home*.

Nursing home—In the Online Survey Certification and Reporting database, a nursing home is a facility that is certified and meets the Center for Medicare & Medicaid Services' long-term care requirements for Medicare and Medicaid eligibility.

In the National Master Facility Inventory (NMFI), which provided the sampling frame for 1973–74, 1977, and 1985 National Nursing Home Surveys, a nursing home was an establishment with three or more beds that provided nursing or personal care services to the aged, infirm, or chronically ill. The following definitions of nursing home types applied to facilities listed in the NFMI. The 1977 National Nursing Home Survey included personal care homes and domiciliary care homes while the National Nursing Home Surveys of 1973–74, 1985, 1995, 1997, and 1999 excluded them.

Nursing care homes employ one or more full-time registered or licensed practical nurses and provide nursing care to at least one-half the residents.

Personal care homes with nursing have fewer than one-half the residents receiving nursing care. In addition, such homes employ one or more registered or licensed practical nurses or provided administration of medications and treatments in accordance with physicians' orders, supervision of self-administered medications, or three or more personal services.

Personal care homes without nursing have no residents who receive nursing care. These homes provide administration of medications and treatments in accordance with physicians' orders, supervise self-administered medications, or provide three or more personal services.

Domiciliary care homes primarily provide supervisory care but also provided one or two personal services.

The following definitions of certification levels apply to data collected in National Nursing Home Surveys of 1973–74, 1977, and 1985:

Skilled nursing facilities provide the most intensive nursing care available outside a hospital. Facilities certified by Medicare provide posthospital care to eligible Medicare enrollees. Facilities certified by Medicaid as skilled nursing facilities provide skilled nursing services on a daily basis to individuals eligible for Medicaid benefits.

Intermediate care facilities are certified by the Medicaid program to provide health-related services on a regular basis to Medicaid eligibles who do not require hospital or skilled nursing facility care but do require institutional care above the level of room and board.

Not certified facilities are not certified as providers of care by Medicare or Medicaid.

Beginning with the 1995 through 1999 National Nursing Home Surveys, nursing homes have been defined as facilities that routinely provide nursing care services and have three or

more beds set up for residents. Facilities may be certified by Medicare or Medicaid or not certified but licensed by the State as a nursing home. The facilities may be freestanding or a distinct unit of a larger facility.

After October 1, 1990, long-term care facilities which met the Omnibus Budget Reconciliation Act of 1987 (OBRA 87) nursing home reform requirements that were formerly certified under the Medicaid program as skilled nursing, nursing home, or intermediate care facilities were reclassified as "nursing facilities." The Medicare program continues to certify skilled nursing facilities, but not intermediate care facilities. State Medicaid programs can certify intermediate care facilities for the mentally retarded or developmentally disabled. Nursing facilities must also be certified to participate in the Medicare program in order to be certified for participation in Medicaid, with the exception of those facilities that have obtained waivers. Thus most nursing home care is now provided in skilled care facilities.

See related *Nursing care; Resident.*

Nursing home expenditures—See *Health expenditures, national.*

Obesity—See *Body mass index (BMI).*

Occupancy rate—In American Hospital Association statistics, hospital occupancy rate is calculated as the average daily census divided by the number of hospital beds, cribs, and pediatric bassinets set up and staffed on the last day of the reporting period, expressed as a percent. Average daily census is calculated by dividing the total annual number of inpatients, excluding newborns, by 365 days to derive the number of inpatients receiving care on an average day during the annual reporting period. The occupancy rate for facilities other than hospitals is calculated as the number of residents at the facility reported on the day of the interview divided by the number of reported beds. In the Online Survey Certification and Reporting database, occupancy is determined as of the day of certification inspection as the total number of residents on that day divided by the total number of beds on that day.

Office—In the National Ambulatory Medical Care Survey, a physician's ambulatory practice (office) can be in any location other than in a hospital, nursing home, other extended care facility, patients' home, industrial clinic, college clinic, or family planning clinic. Offices in health maintenance organizations and private offices in hospitals are included. See related *Office visit; Outpatient visit; Physician.*

Office-based physician—See *Physician.*

Office visit—In the National Ambulatory Medical Care Survey, an office visit is any direct personal exchange between an ambulatory patient and a physician or members of his or her staff for the purposes of seeking care and rendering health services. See related *Outpatient visit.*

Operations—See *Procedure.*

Outpatient department—According to the National Hospital Ambulatory Medical Care Survey (NHAMCS), an outpatient department (OPD) is a hospital facility where nonurgent ambulatory medical care is provided. The following types of OPDs are excluded from the NHAMCS: ambulatory surgical centers, chemotherapy, employee health services, renal dialysis, methadone maintenance, and radiology. See related *Emergency department; Outpatient visit.*

Outpatient surgery—According to the American Hospital Association, outpatient surgery is a surgical operation, whether major or minor, performed on patients who do not remain in the hospital overnight. Outpatient surgery may be performed in inpatient operating suites, outpatient surgery suites, or procedure rooms within an outpatient care facility. A surgical operation involving more than one surgical procedure is considered one surgical operation. See related *Ambulatory surgery; Procedure.*

Outpatient visit—The American Hospital Association defines outpatient visits as visits for receipt of medical, dental, or other services at a hospital by patients who are not lodged in the hospital. Each appearance by an outpatient to each unit of the hospital is counted individually as an outpatient visit, including all clinic visits, referred visits, observation services, outpatient surgeries, and emergency department visits. In the National Hospital Ambulatory Medical Care Survey an outpatient department visit is a direct personal exchange between a patient and a physician or other health care provider working under the physician's supervision for the purpose of seeking care and receiving personal health services. See related *Emergency department visit; Outpatient department.*

Overweight—See *Body mass index (BMI).*

Ozone—See *Environmental Protection Agency Standards.*

Pap smear—A Pap smear (also known as a Papanicolaou smear or Pap test) is a microscopic examination of cells scraped from the cervix that is used to detect cancerous or precancerous conditions of the cervix or other medical conditions. In the National Health Interview Survey questions concerning use of Pap smear differed slightly across the years for which data are shown. In 1987 women were asked to report when they had their most recent Pap smear in days, weeks, months, or years. Women who did not respond were asked a followup question, "Was it 3 years ago or less, between 3 and 5 years, or 5 years or more ago?" In 1993 and 1994 women were asked whether they had a Pap smear within the past year, between 1 and 3 years ago, or more than 3 years ago. In 1998 women were asked whether they had a Pap smear 1 year ago or less, more than 1 year but not more than 2 years, more than 2 years but not more than 3 years, more than 3 years but not more than 5 years, or more than 5 years ago. In 1999 women were asked when they had their most recent Pap smear in days, weeks, months, or years. In 1999, 4 percent of women in the sample responded "3 years ago." In this analysis these women were coded as "within the past 3 years," although a response of "3 years ago" may include women whose last Pap smear was more than 3 but less than 4 years ago. Thus estimates for 1999 are overestimated to some degree in comparison with estimates for previous years. In 2000 women were asked when they had their most recent Pap smear (give month and year). Women who did not respond were given a followup question that used the 1999 wording and women who did not answer the followup question were asked a second followup question that used the 1998 wording. In 2000 less than 1 percent of women in the sample answered "3 years ago" using the 1999 wording and they were coded as "within the past 3 years." Thus estimates for 2000 may be slightly overestimated in comparison with estimates for years prior to 1999.

Partial care organization—See *Mental health organization.*

Partial care treatment—See *Mental health service type.*

Patient—See *Ambulatory care; Home health care; Hospice care; Inpatient; Office visit; Outpatient visit.*

Percent change—See *Average annual rate of change.*

Perinatal mortality rate; ratio—See *Rate: Death and related rates.*

Personal care homes with or without nursing—See *Nursing home.*

Personal health care expenditures—See *Health expenditures, national.*

Physician—Data on physician characteristics are obtained through physician self-report for the American Medical Association's Physician Masterfile. The AMA tabulates data only for doctors of medicine (MDs), but some tables in *Health, United States* include data for both MDs and doctors of osteopathy (DOs).

> *Active (or professionally active) physicians* are currently engaged in patient care or other professional activity for a minimum of 20 hours per week. Other professional activity includes administration, medical teaching, research, and other activities, such as employment with insurance carriers, pharmaceutical companies, corporations, voluntary organizations, medical societies, and the like. Physicians who are retired, semi-retired, working part-time, or not practicing are classified as inactive and are excluded. Also excluded are physicians with address unknown and physicians who did not provide information on type of practice or present employment (not classified).

> *Federal physicians* are those employed full time by the Federal Government, including the Army, Navy, Air Force, Veterans' Administration, Public Health Service, and other federally-funded agencies. The majority of U.S. physicians are employed outside the Federal Government (97.4 percent).

> *Hospital-based physicians* are employed under contract with hospitals to provide direct patient care and include physicians in residency training (including clinical fellows) and full-time members of the hospital staff.

> *Office-based physicians* are engaged in seeing patients in solo practice, group practice, two-physician practice, other patient care employment, or inpatient services such as those provided by pathologists and radiologists.

Data for physicians are presented by type of education (doctors of medicine and doctors of osteopathy); place of education (U.S. medical graduates and international medical graduates); activity status (professionally active and inactive); employment setting (Federal and non-Federal); area of specialty; and geographic area. See related *Office; Physician specialty.*

Physician specialty—A physician specialty is any specific branch of medicine in which a physician may concentrate. Data are based on physician self-reports of their primary area of specialty. Physician data are broadly categorized into two areas of practice: generalists and specialists.

> *Primary care generalists* practice in the general fields of family and general practice, general internal medicine, and general pediatrics. They specifically exclude primary care specialists.

> *Primary care specialists* practice in the subspecialties of general and family practice, internal medicine, and pediatrics. Family practice subspecialties include geriatric medicine and sports medicine. Internal medicine subspecialties include diabetes, endocrinology and metabolism, hematology, hepatology, cardiac electrophysiology, infectious diseases, diagnostic laboratory immunology, geriatric medicine, sports medicine, nephrology, nutrition, medical oncology, and rheumatology. Pediatric subspecialties include adolescent medicine, critical care pediatrics, neonatal-perinatal medicine, pediatric allergy, pediatric cardiology, pediatric endocrinology, pediatric pulmonology, pediatric emergency medicine, pediatric gastroenterology, pediatric hematology/oncology, diagnostic laboratory immunology, pediatric nephrology, pediatric rheumatology, and sports medicine.

> *Specialist physicians* practice in the primary care specialties, in addition to all other specialist fields not included in the generalist definition. Specialist fields include allergy and immunology, aerospace medicine, anesthesiology, cardiovascular diseases, child and adolescent psychiatry, colon and rectal surgery, dermatology, diagnostic radiology, forensic pathology, gastroenterology, general surgery, medical genetics, neurology, nuclear medicine, neurological surgery, obstetrics and gynecology, occupational medicine, ophthalmology, orthopedic surgery, otolaryngology, psychiatry, public health and general preventive medicine, physical medicine and rehabilitation, plastic

surgery, anatomic and clinical pathology, pulmonary diseases, radiation oncology, thoracic surgery, urology, addiction medicine, critical care medicine, legal medicine, and clinical pharmacology.

See related *Physician.*

Point-of-service (POS) plan—A health plan that allows members to choose to receive services from a participating or non-participating network provider, usually with a financial disincentive for going outside the network. More of a product than an organization, POS plans can be offered by HMOs, PPOs, or self-insured employers. See related *Health maintenance organization; Managed care; Preferred provider organization.*

Population—The U.S. Bureau of the Census collects and publishes data on populations in the United States according to several different definitions. Various statistical systems then use the appropriate population for calculating rates. See also *Appendix I, Population Census and Population Estimates.*

Total population is the population of the United States, including all members of the Armed Forces living in foreign countries, Puerto Rico, Guam, and the U.S. Virgin Islands. Other Americans abroad (for example, civilian Federal employees and dependents of members of the Armed Forces or other Federal employees) are not included.

Resident population includes persons whose usual place of residence (that is, the place where one usually lives and sleeps) is in one of the 50 States or the District of Columbia. It includes members of the Armed Forces stationed in the United States and their families. It excludes international military, naval, and diplomatic personnel and their families located in this country and residing in embassies or similar quarters. Also excluded are international workers and international students in this country and Americans living abroad. The resident population is the denominator for calculating birth and death rates and incidence of disease.

Civilian population is the resident population excluding members of the Armed Forces. However, families of members of the Armed Forces are included. This population is the denominator in rates calculated for the National Hospital Discharge Survey, the National Home and Hospice Care Survey, the National Nursing Home Survey, and the National Survey of Ambulatory Surgery.

Civilian noninstitutionalized population is the civilian population not residing in institutions such as correctional institutions, detention homes, and training schools for juvenile delinquents; homes for aged and dependent persons (for example, nursing homes and convalescent homes); homes for dependent and neglected children; homes and schools for mentally or physically handicapped persons; homes for unwed mothers; psychiatric, tuberculosis, and chronic disease hospitals; and residential treatment centers. Census Bureau estimates of the civilian noninstitutionalized population are used to calculate sample weights for the National Health Interview Survey, National Health and Nutrition Examination Survey, and National Survey of Family Growth, and as denominators in rates calculated for the National Ambulatory Medical Care Survey and the National Hospital Ambulatory Medical Care Survey.

Introduction of census 2000 population estimates—Health United States, 2003 marks the transition to the use of year 2000 resident population estimates based on the 2000 census for calculation of rates. Previously 1991–2000 rates were based on post-1990 population estimates. Birth rates and death rates for 1991–99 were revised using intercensal population estimates based on the 2000 census. Rates for 2000 were revised using census 2000 counts. Data systems and surveys that use civilian and civilian noninstitutionalized population estimates as denominators for computation of rates for the period 1991–99 may be updated in future Health, U.S. reports, but have not been updated in the 2003 report. See *Appendix I, Population Census and Population Estimates.*

Postneonatal mortality rate—See *Rate: Death and related rates.*

Poverty level—Poverty statistics are based on definitions originally developed by the Social Security Administration. These include a set of money income thresholds that vary by family size and composition. Families or individuals with income below their appropriate thresholds are classified as below the poverty level. These thresholds are updated annually by the U.S. Bureau of the Census to reflect changes in the Consumer Price Index for all urban consumers (CPI-U). For example, the average poverty threshold for a family of four was $17,603 in 2000 and $13,359 in 1990. For more information, see U.S. Bureau of the Census: *Consumer Income and Poverty 2001*. Series P-60. Washington, DC: U.S. Government Printing Office. Also see www.census.gov/hhes/www/poverty.html.

National Health Interview Survey—Poverty level, for years prior to 1997, was based on family income and family size using Bureau of the Census poverty thresholds. Beginning in 1997 poverty status is based on family income, family size, number of children in the family, and for families with two or fewer adults, the age of the adults in the family. See related *Consumer Price Index; Family income; Appendix I, Current Population Survey; National Health Interview Survey.*

Preferred provider organization (PPO)—A PPO is a type of medical plan where coverage is provided to participants through a network of selected health care providers (such as hospitals and physicians). The enrollees may go outside the network, but they would pay a greater percentage of the cost of coverage than within the network. See related *Health maintenance organization; Managed care; Point-of-service plan.*

Prenatal Care—Information on when pregnancy care began is recorded on the birth certificate. Between 1970 and 1980 the reporting area for prenatal care expanded. In 1970, 39 States and the District of Columbia reported prenatal care on the birth certificate. Data were not available from Alabama, Alaska, Arkansas, Connecticut, Delaware, Georgia, Idaho, Massachusetts, New Mexico, Pennsylvania, and Virginia. In 1975 these data were available from three additional States, Connecticut, Delaware, and Georgia, increasing the number of States reporting prenatal care to 42 and the District of Columbia. Starting in 1980 prenatal care information was available for the entire United States.

Prevalence—Prevalence is the number of cases of a disease, infected persons, or persons with some other attribute present during a particular interval of time. It is often expressed as a rate (for example, the prevalence of diabetes per 1,000 persons during a year). See related *Incidence.*

Primary admission diagnosis—In the National Home and Hospice Care Survey the primary admission diagnosis is the first-listed diagnosis at admission on the patient's medical

record as provided by the agency staff member most familiar with the care provided to the patient.

Primary care specialties—See *Physician specialty.*

Private expenditures—See *Health expenditures, national.*

Procedure—The National Hospital Discharge Survey (NHDS) and the National Survey of Ambulatory Surgery (NSAS) define a procedure as a surgical or nonsurgical operation, diagnostic procedure, or therapeutic procedure (such as respiratory therapy) recorded on the medical record of discharged patients. A maximum of four procedures per discharge is recorded in NHDS and up to six procedures per discharge in NSAS. Procedures are coded according to the *International Classification of Diseases, Ninth Revision, Clinical Modification* (see table X). In *Health, United States, 1998* and earlier editions, procedures were categorized as surgical operations and diagnostic and other nonsurgical procedures. The distinction between surgical and diagnostic procedures has become less meaningful due to development of noninvasive and minimally invasive surgery. Thus the practice of classifying procedures as surgical or diagnostic has been discontinued. See related *Ambulatory surgery; Outpatient surgery.*

Proprietary hospitals—See *Hospital.*

Psychiatric hospitals—See *Hospital; Mental health organization.*

Public expenditures—See *Health expenditures, national.*

Public health activities—Public health activities may include any of the following essential services of public health—surveillance, investigations, education, community mobilization, workforce training, research, and personal care services delivered or funded by governmental agencies.

Race—In 1977 the Office of Management and Budget (OMB) issued Race and Ethnicity Standards for Federal Statistics and Administrative Reporting in order to promote comparability of data among Federal data systems. The 1977 Standards called for the Federal Government's data systems to classify individuals into the following four racial groups: American Indian or Alaska Native, Asian or Pacific Islander, black, and white. Depending on the data source, the classification by race was based on self-classification or on observation by an interviewer or other person filling out the questionnaire.

In 1997 new standards were announced for classification of individuals by race within the Federal Government's data systems (*Federal Register*, 62FR58781–58790). The 1997 Standards have five racial groups: American Indian or Alaska Native, Asian, Black or African American, Native Hawaiian or Other Pacific Islander, and White. These five categories are the minimum set for data on race in Federal statistics. The 1997 Standards also offer an opportunity for respondents to select more than one of the five groups, leading to many possible multiple race categories. As with the single race groups, data for the multiple race groups are to be reported when estimates meet agency requirements for reliability and confidentiality. The 1997 Standards allow for observer or proxy identification of race but clearly state a preference for self-classification. The Federal Government considers race and Hispanic origin to be two separate and distinct concepts. Thus Hispanics may be of any race. Federal data systems are required to comply with the 1997 Standards by 2003.

National Health Interview Survey (NHIS)—Starting with *Health, United States, 2002* and data year 1999, race-specific estimates based on the NHIS are tabulated using the 1997 Standards and are not strictly comparable with estimates for earlier years. The 1997 Standards specify five single race categories plus multiple race categories. Estimates for specific race groups are shown when they meet requirements for statistical reliability and confidentiality. The race categories "White only," "Black or African American only," "American Indian and Alaska Native only," "Asian only," and "Native Hawaiian and Other Pacific Islander only" include persons who reported only one racial group; the category "2 or more races" includes persons who reported more than one of the five racial groups in the 1997 Standards or one of the five racial groups and "Some other race." Prior to data year 1999, data were tabulated according to the 1977 Standards with four racial groups and the category "Asian only" included Native Hawaiian and Other Pacific Islander. Estimates for single race categories prior to 1999 included persons who reported one race or, if they reported more than one race, identified one race as best representing their race. Differences between estimates tabulated using the two Standards for data year 1999 are discussed in the footnotes for each NHIS table.

Tables XI and XII illustrate NHIS data tabulated by race and Hispanic origin according to the 1997 and 1977 Standards for two health statistics (cigarette smoking and private health insurance coverage). In these illustrations, three separate tabulations using the 1997 Standards are shown: (1) Race: mutually exclusive race groups, including several multiple race combinations; (2) Race, any mention: race groups that are not mutually exclusive because each race category includes all persons who mention that race; and (3) Hispanic origin and race: detailed race and Hispanic origin with a multiple race total category. Where applicable, comparison tabulations by race and Hispanic origin are shown based on the 1977 Standards. Because there are more race groups with the 1997 Standards, the sample size of each race group under the 1997 Standards is slightly smaller than the sample size under the 1977 Standards. Only those few multiple race groups with sufficient numbers of observations to meet standards of statistical reliability are shown. Tables XI and XII also illustrate changes in labels and group categories in the 1997 Standards. The race designation of Black was changed to Black or African American and the ethnicity designation of Hispanic was changed to Hispanic or Latino.

Data systems included in *Health, United States*, other than the National Health Interview Survey (NHIS), the National Health and Examination Survey (NHANES), and the National Household Survey of Drug Abuse (NHSDA), generally do not permit tabulation of estimates for the detailed race and ethnicity categories shown in tables XI and XII, either because race data based on the 1997 standard categories are not yet available, or because there are insufficient numbers of observations to meet statistical reliability or confidentiality requirements.

National Health and Nutrition Examination Survey (NHANES)—Starting with *Health, United States, 2003* race-specific estimates based on NHANES are tabulated using the 1997 Standards for data years 1999 and beyond. Prior to data year 1999, the 1977 Standards were used. Because of the differences between the two Standards, the race-specific estimates shown in trend tables based on the NHANES for 1999–2000 are not strictly comparable with estimates for earlier years. Each trend table based on the NHANES includes a footnote that discusses differences between estimates tabulated using the two Standards for survey years 1999–2000.

Table XI. Current cigarette smoking by persons 18 years of age and over, according to race and Hispanic origin under the 1977 and 1997 Standards for Federal data on race and ethnicity: United States, average annual 1993–95

1997 Standards	Sample size	Percent	Standard error	1977 Standards	Sample size	Percent	Standard error
				Race			
White only	46,228	25.2	0.26	White	46,664	25.3	0.26
Black or African American only	7,208	26.6	0.64	Black	7,334	26.5	0.63
American Indian and Alaska Native only	416	32.9	2.53	American Indian and Alaska Native	480	33.9	2.38
Asian only	1,370	15.0	1.19	Asian and Pacific Islander	1,411	15.5	1.22
2 or more races total	786	34.5	2.00				
Black or African American; White	83	*21.7	6.05				
American Indian and Alaska Native; White	461	40.0	2.58				
				Race, any mention			
White, any mention	46,882	25.3	0.26				
Black or African American, any mention	7,382	26.6	0.63				
American Indian and Alaska Native, any mention	965	36.3	1.71				
Asian, any mention	1,458	15.7	1.20				
Native Hawaiian and Other Pacific Islander, any mention	53	*17.5	5.10				
				Hispanic origin and race			
Not Hispanic or Latino:				Non-Hispanic:			
White only	42,421	25.8	0.27	White	42,976	25.9	0.27
Black or African American only	7,053	26.7	0.65	Black	7,203	26.7	0.64
American Indian and Alaska Native only	358	33.5	2.69	American Indian and Alaska Native	407	35.4	2.53
Asian only	1,320	14.8	1.21	Asian and Pacific Islander	1,397	15.3	1.24
2 or more races total	687	35.6	2.15				
Hispanic or Latino	5,175	17.8	0.65	Hispanic	5,175	17.8	0.65

*Relative standard error 20–30 percent.

NOTES: The 1997 Standards for Federal data on race and ethnicity set five single race groups (White, Black, American Indian or Alaska Native, Asian, and Native Hawaiian or Other Pacific Islander) and allow respondents to report one or more race groups. Estimates for single race and multiple race groups not shown above do not meet standards for statistical reliability or confidentiality (relative standard error greater than 30 percent). Race groups under the 1997 Standards were based on the question, "What is the group or groups which represents _____ race?" For persons who selected multiple groups, race groups under the 1977 Standards were based on the additional question, "Which of those groups would you say best represents _____ race?" Race-specific estimates in this table were calculated after excluding respondents of other and unknown race. Other published race-specific estimates are based on files in which such responses have been edited. Percents are age adjusted to the year 2000 standard using three age groups: Under 18 years, 18–44 years, and 45–64 years of age. See Appendix II, Age adjustment.

SOURCE: Centers for Disease Control and Prevention, National Center for Health Statistics. National Health Interview Survey.

The NHANES sample was designed to provide estimates specifically for persons of Mexican origin and not for all Hispanic-origin persons in the United States. Persons of Hispanic-origin other than Mexicans were entered into the sample with different selection probabilities that are not nationally representative of the total U.S. Hispanic population. Estimates are shown for non-Hispanic white, non-Hispanic black, and Mexican. Although data were collected according to the 1997 Standards, there are insufficient numbers of observations to meet statistical reliability or confidentiality requirements for reporting estimates for additional race categories.

National Household Survey of Drug Abuse (NHSDA)— Race-specific estimates based on NHSDA are tabulated using the 1997 Standards. Estimates in the NHSDA trend table begin with the data year 1999. Estimates for specific race groups are shown when they meet requirements for statistical reliability and confidentiality. The race categories "White only," "Black or African American only," "American Indian and Alaska Native only," "Asian only," and "Native Hawaiian and Other Pacific Islander only" include persons who reported only one racial group; and the category "2 or more races" includes persons who reported more than one of the five racial groups in the 1997 Standards or one of the five racial groups and "Some other race."

*National Vital Statistics System—*Most of the States in the Vital Statistics Cooperative Program are still revising

Table XII. Private health care coverage for persons under 65 years of age, according to race and Hispanic origin under the 1977 and 1997 Standards for Federal data on race and ethnicity: United States, average annual 1993–95

1997 Standards	Sample size	Percent	Standard error	1977 Standards	Sample size	Percent	Standard error
			Race				
White only	168,256	76.1	0.28	White	170,472	75.9	0.28
Black or African American only	30,048	53.5	0.63	Black	30,690	53.6	0.63
American Indian and Alaska Native only	2,003	44.2	1.97	American Indian and Alaska Native	2,316	43.5	1.85
Asian only	6,896	68.0	1.39	Asian and Pacific Islander	7,146	68.2	1.34
Native Hawaiian and Other Pacific Islander only	173	75.0	7.43				
2 or more races total	4,203	60.9	1.17				
Black or African American; White	686	59.5	3.21				
American Indian and Alaska Native; White	2,022	60.0	1.71				
Asian; White	590	71.9	3.39				
Native Hawaiian and Other Pacific Islander; White	56	59.2	10.65				
			Race, any mention				
White, any mention	171,817	75.8	0.28				
Black or African American, any mention	31,147	53.6	0.62				
American Indian and Alaska Native, any mention	4,365	52.4	1.40				
Asian, any mention	7,639	68.4	1.27				
Native Hawaiian and Other Pacific Islander, any mention	283	68.7	6.23				
			Hispanic origin and race				
Not Hispanic or Latino:				Non-Hispanic:			
White only	146,109	78.9	0.27	White	149,057	78.6	0.27
Black or African American only	29,250	53.9	0.64	Black	29,877	54.0	0.63
American Indian and Alaska Native only	1,620	45.2	2.15	American Indian and Alaska Native	1,859	44.6	2.05
Asian only	6,623	68.2	1.43	Asian and Pacific Islander	6,999	68.4	1.40
Native Hawaiian and Other Pacific Islander only	145	76.4	7.79				
2 or more races total	3,365	62.6	1.18				
Hispanic or Latino	31,040	48.8	0.74	Hispanic	31,040	48.8	0.74

NOTES: The 1997 Standards for Federal data on race and ethnicity set five single race groups (White, Black, American Indian or Alaska Native, Asian, and Native Hawaiian or Other Pacific Islander) and allow respondents to report one or more race groups. Estimates for single race and multiple race groups not shown above do not meet standards for statistical reliability or confidentiality (relative standard error greater than 30 percent). Race groups under the 1997 Standards were based on the question, "What is the group or groups which represents _____ race?" For persons who selected multiple groups, race groups under the 1977 Standards were based on the additional question, "Which of those groups would you say best represents _____ race?" Race-specific estimates in this table were calculated after excluding respondents of other and unknown race. Other published race-specific estimates are based on files in which such responses have been edited. Percents are age adjusted to the year 2000 standard using three age groups: Under 18 years, 18–44 years, and 45–64 years of age. See Appendix II, Age adjustment.

SOURCE: Centers for Disease Control and Prevention, National Center for Health Statistics. National Health Interview Survey.

their birth and death records to conform to the 1997 standards on race and ethnicity. During the transition to full implementation of the 1997 standards, vital statistics data will continue to be presented for the four major race groups, white, black or African American, American Indian or Alaska Native, and Asian or Pacific Islander, in accordance with 1977 standards.

Birth File—Information about the race and Hispanic ethnicity of the mother and father are provided by the mother at the time of birth and recorded on the birth certificate and fetal death record. Since 1980, birth rates, birth characteristics, and fetal death rates for live born infants and fetal deaths are presented in this report according to race of mother. Before 1980 data were tabulated by race of newborn and fetus, taking into account the race of both parents. If the parents were of different races and one parent was white, the child was classified according to the race of the other parent. When neither parent was white, the child was classified according to father's race, with one exception: if either parent was Hawaiian, the child was classified Hawaiian. Before 1964, if race was unknown, the birth was classified as white. Beginning in 1964 unknown race was classified according to information on the previous record.

Mortality File—Information about the race and Hispanic ethnicity of the decedent is reported by the funeral director as provided by an informant, often the surviving next of kin, or, in the absence of an informant, on the basis of observation. Death rates by race and Hispanic origin are based on information from death certificates (numerators of the rates) and on population estimates from the Census Bureau (denominators). Race and ethnicity information from the census is by self-report. To the extent that race and Hispanic origin are inconsistent between these two data sources, death rates will be biased. Studies have shown that persons self-reported as American Indian, Asian, or Hispanic on census and survey records may sometimes be reported as white or non-Hispanic on the death certificate, resulting in an underestimation of deaths and death rates for the American Indian, Asian, and Hispanic groups. Bias also results from undercounts of some population groups in the census, particularly young black and young white males and elderly persons, resulting in an overestimation of death rates. The net effects of misclassification and undercoverage result in overstated death rates for the white population and black population estimated to be 1 percent and 5 percent, respectively; and understated death rates for other population groups estimated as follows: American Indians, 21 percent; Asian or Pacific Islanders, 11 percent; and Hispanics, 2 percent. For more information, see Rosenberg HM, Maurer JD, Sorlie PD, Johnson NJ, et al. Quality of death rates by race and Hispanic origin: A summary of current research, 1999. National Center for Health Statistics. Vital Health Stat 2(128). 1999.

Denominators for infant and maternal mortality rates are based on number of live births rather than population estimates. Race information for the denominator is supplied from the birth certificate. Before 1980, child's race took into account the races of both parents. Starting in 1980, race was based solely on race of mother. Race information for the numerator is the race of the deceased child or mother, as recorded on the death certificate.

Vital event rates for the American Indian or Alaska Native population shown in this book are based on the total U.S. resident population of American Indians and Alaska Natives, as enumerated by the U.S. Bureau of Census. In contrast the Indian Health Service calculates vital event rates for this population based on U.S. Bureau of Census county data for American Indians and Alaska Natives who reside on or near reservations. Interpretation of trends for the American Indian and Alaska Native population should take into account that population estimates for these groups increased by 45 percent between 1980 and 1990, partly due to better enumeration techniques in the 1990 decennial census and to the increased tendency for people to identify themselves as American Indian in 1990.

Interpretation of trends for the Asian population in the United States should take into account that this population more than doubled between 1980 and 1990, primarily due to immigration.

For more information on coding race using vital statistics, see: National Center for Health Statistics, Technical Appendix, *Vital Statistics of the United States,* Vol. I, Natality, and Vol. II Mortality, Part A available on the NCHS home page at www.cdc.gov/nchs/nvss.htm. See related *Hispanic origin; Appendix I, Population Census and Population Estimates.*

Rate—A rate is a measure of some event, disease, or condition in relation to a unit of population, along with some specification of time. See related *Age adjustment; Population.*

■ *Birth and related rates*

Birth rate is calculated by dividing the number of live births in a population in a year by the midyear resident population. For census years, rates are based on unrounded census counts of the resident population, as of April 1. For the noncensus years 1981–89, rates were based on national estimates of the resident population, as of July 1, rounded to 1,000s. Rounded population estimates for 5-year age groups were calculated by summing unrounded population estimates before rounding to 1,000s. Starting in 1991 rates were based on unrounded national population estimates. Beginning in 1997 the birth rate for the maternal age group 45–49 years includes data for mother's age 50–54 years in the numerator and is based on the population of women 45–49 years in the denominator. Birth rates are expressed as the number of live births per 1,000 population. The rate may be restricted to births to women of specific age, race, marital status, or geographic location (specific rate), or it may be related to the entire population (crude rate). See related *Cohort fertility; Live birth.*

Fertility rate is the total number of live births, regardless of age of mother, per 1,000 women of reproductive age, 15–44 years.

■ *Death and related rates*

Death rate is calculated by dividing the number of deaths in a population in a year by the midyear resident population. For census years, rates are based on unrounded census counts of the resident population, as of April 1. For the noncensus years 1981–89, rates were based on national estimates of the resident population, as of July 1, rounded to 1,000s. Rounded population estimates for 10-year age groups were calculated by summing unrounded population estimates before rounding to 1,000s. Starting in 1991 rates were based on unrounded national population estimates. Rates for the Hispanic and non-Hispanic white populations in each year are based on unrounded State population estimates for States in the Hispanic reporting area. Death rates are expressed as the number of deaths per 100,000 population. The rate may be restricted to deaths in specific age, race, sex, or geographic groups or from specific causes of death (specific rate) or it may be related to the entire population (crude rate).

Fetal death rate is the number of fetal deaths with stated or presumed gestation of 20 weeks or more divided by the sum of live births plus fetal deaths, per 1,000 live births plus fetal deaths. *Late fetal death rate* is the number of fetal deaths with stated or presumed gestation of 28 weeks or more divided by the sum of live births plus late fetal deaths, per 1,000 live births plus late fetal deaths. See related *Fetal death; Gestation.*

Infant mortality rate based on period files is calculated by dividing the number of infant deaths during a calendar year by the number of live births reported in the same year. It is expressed as the number of infant deaths per 1,000 live births. *Neonatal mortality rate* is the number of deaths of children under 28 days of age, per 1,000 live births. *Postneonatal mortality rate* is the number of deaths of children that occur between 28 days and 365

days after birth, per 1,000 live births. See related *Infant death.*

Birth cohort infant mortality rates are based on linked birth and infant death files. In contrast to period rates in which the births and infant deaths occur in the same period or calendar year, infant deaths constituting the numerator of a birth cohort rate may have occurred in the same year as, or in the year following, the year of birth. The birth cohort infant mortality rate is expressed as the number of infant deaths per 1,000 live births. See related *Birth cohort.*

Perinatal relates to the period surrounding the birth event. Rates and ratios are based on events reported in a calendar year. *Perinatal mortality rate* is the sum of late fetal deaths plus infant deaths within 7 days of birth divided by the sum of live births plus late fetal deaths, per 1,000 live births plus late fetal deaths. *Perinatal mortality ratio* is the sum of late fetal deaths plus infant deaths within 7 days of birth divided by the number of live births, per 1,000 live births.

Maternal mortality rate is defined as the number of maternal deaths per 100,000 live births. The maternal mortality rate is a measure of the likelihood that a pregnant woman will die from maternal causes. The number of live births used in the denominator is a proxy for the population of pregnant women who are at risk of a maternal death. See related *Maternal death.*

Region—See *Geographic region and division.*

Registered hospitals—See *Hospital.*

Registered nursing education—Registered nursing data are shown by level of educational preparation. Baccalaureate education requires at least 4 years of college or university; associate degree programs are based in community colleges and are usually 2 years in length; and diploma programs are based in hospitals and are usually 3 years in length.

Registration area—The United States has separate registration areas for birth, death, marriage, and divorce statistics. In general, registration areas correspond to States and include two separate registration areas for the District of Columbia and New York City. All States have adopted laws that require registration of births and deaths and reporting of fetal deaths. It is believed that more than 99 percent of births and deaths occurring in this country are registered.

The *death registration area* was established in 1900 with 10 States and the District of Columbia, and the *birth registration area* was established in 1915, also with 10 States and the District of Columbia. Beginning with 1933, all States were included in the birth and death registration areas. The specific States added year by year are shown in "History and Organization of the Vital Statistics System," reprinted from *Vital Statistics of the United States Vol I, 1950*, chapter 1, National Center for Health Statistics, 1978. Currently, Puerto Rico, U.S. Virgin Islands, and Guam each constitutes a separate registration area, although their data are not included in statistical tabulations of U.S. resident data. See related *Reporting area*.

Relative standard error—The relative standard error (RSE) is a measure of an estimate's reliability. The RSE of an estimate is obtained by dividing the standard error of the estimate ($SE(r)$) by the estimate itself (r). This quantity is expressed as a percent of the estimate and is calculated as follows: $RSE=100 \times (SE(r)/r)$. Estimates with large RSEs are considered unreliable. In *Health, United States* most statistics with large RSEs are preceded by an asterisk or not presented.

Relative survival rate—The relative survival rate is the ratio of the observed survival rate for the patient group to the expected survival rate for persons in the general population similar to the patient group with respect to age, sex, race, and calendar year of observation. The 5-year relative survival rate is used to estimate the proportion of cancer patients potentially curable. Because over one-half of all cancers occur in persons 65 years of age and over, many of these individuals die of other causes with no evidence of recurrence of their cancer. Thus, because it is obtained by adjusting observed survival for the normal life expectancy of the general population of the same age, the relative survival rate is an estimate of the chance of surviving the effects of cancer.

Reporting area—In the National Vital Statistics System, the reporting area for such basic items on the birth and death certificates as age, race, and sex, is based on data from residents of all 50 States in the United States and the District of Columbia (DC). The reporting area for selected items such as Hispanic origin, educational attainment, and marital status,

is based on data from those States that require the item to be reported, whose data meet a minimum level of completeness (such as 80 or 90 percent), and are considered to be sufficiently comparable to be used for analysis. In 1993–96 the reporting area for Hispanic origin of decedent on the death certificate included 49 States and DC. Starting in 1997 the Hispanic reporting area includes all 50 States and DC. See related *Registration area; Appendix I, National Vital Statistics System.*

Resident—In the Online Survey Certification and Reporting database, all residents in certified facilities are counted on the day of certification inspection. In the National Nursing Home Survey, a resident is a person on the roster of the nursing home as of the night before the survey. Included are all residents for whom beds are maintained even though they may be on overnight leave or in a hospital. See related *Nursing home.*

Resident population—See *Population.*

Residential treatment care—See *Mental health service type.*

Residential treatment centers for emotionally disturbed children—See *Mental health organization.*

Rural—See *Urbanization.*

Self-assessment of health—See *Health status, respondent-assessed.*

Short-stay hospital—See *Hospital.*

Skilled nursing facility—See *Nursing home.*

Smoker—See *Cigarette smoking; Tobacco use.*

Specialty hospital—See *Hospital.*

State health agency—The agency or department within State government headed by the State or territorial health official. Generally, the State health agency is responsible for setting statewide public health priorities, carrying out national and State mandates, responding to public health hazards, and assuring access to health care for underserved State residents.

State Children's Health Insurance Program (SCHIP)—Title XXI of the Social Security Act, known as the State Children's Health Insurance Program (SCHIP), is a program initiated by the Balanced Budget Act of 1997 (BBA). In addition to allowing States to craft or expand an existing State insurance program, SCHIP provides more Federal funds for States to expand Medicaid eligibility to include a greater number of children who are currently uninsured. With certain exceptions, these are low-income children who would not qualify for Medicaid based on the plan that was in effect on April 15, 1997. Funds from SCHIP also may be used to provide medical assistance to children during a presumptive eligibility period for Medicaid. This is one of several options from which States may select to provide health care coverage for more children, as prescribed within the BBA's Title XXI program. See related *Health insurance coverage; Medicaid*.

Substance use—refers to the use of selected substances including alcohol, tobacco products, drugs, inhalants, and other substances that can be consumed, inhaled, injected, or otherwise absorbed into the body with possible detrimental effects.

The Monitoring the Future Study (MTF)—The MTF collects information on use of selected substances using self-completed questionnaires to a school-based survey of secondary school students. MTF has tracked 12th graders' illicit drug use and attitudes towards drugs since 1975. In 1991, 8th and 10th graders were added to the study. The survey includes questions on abuse of substances including (but not limited to) marijuana, inhalants, illegal drugs, alcohol, cigarettes, and other tobacco products. A standard set of three questions is used to assess use of the substances in the past month. "Past month" refers to an individual's use of a substance at least once during the month preceding their response to the survey. See related *Appendix I, Monitoring the Future Study*.

National Household Survey of Drug Abuse (NHSDA)— The NHSDA conducts in-person interviews of a sample of individuals 12 years of age and older at their place of residence. For illicit drug use, alcohol use, and tobacco use, information is collected about use in past month. For information on illicit drug use, respondents in the NHSDA are asked about use of marijuana/hashish, cocaine (including crack), inhalants, hallucinogens, heroin, and prescription-type drugs used nonmedically (pain relievers, tranquilizers, stimulants, and sedatives). A series of questions is asked about each substance: "Have you ever, even once, used [e.g., Ecstasy, also

known as MDMA/substance]?" "Think specifically about the past 30 days, from [date] up to and including today. During the past 30 days, on how many days did you use [substance]?" Numerous probes and checks are included in the computer-assisted interview system. Nonprescription medications and legitimate uses under a doctor's supervision are not included in the survey. Summary measures such as "any illicit drug use" are produced. See related *Appendix I, National Household Survey of Drug Abuse*.

See related *Alcohol consumption; Cigarette smoking; Illicit drug use*.

Substance abuse treatment clients—In the Substance Abuse and Mental Health Services Administration's National Survey of Substance Abuse Treatment Services, substance abuse treatment clients have been admitted to treatment and have been seen on a scheduled appointment basis at least once in the month before the survey reference date or were inpatients on the survey reference date. Types of treatment include 24-hour detoxification, 24-hour rehabilitation or residential care, and outpatient care.

Suicidal ideation—Suicidal ideation is having thoughts of suicide or of taking action to end one's own life. Suicidal ideation includes all thoughts of suicide, both when the thoughts include a plan to commit suicide and when they do not include a plan. Suicidal ideation is measured in the Youth Risk Behavior Survey by the question "During the past 12 months, did you ever seriously consider attempting suicide?"

Surgical operation—See *Procedure*.

Surgical specialty—See *Physician specialty*.

Tobacco use—Information on tobacco use during pregnancy became available on birth certificates for the first time in 1989 with revision of the U.S. Standard Birth Certificate. In 1989, 43 States and the District of Columbia collected data on tobacco use. The following States did not require the reporting of tobacco use in the standard format on the birth certificate: California, Indiana, Louisiana, Nebraska, New York, Oklahoma, and South Dakota. In 1990 information on tobacco use became available from Louisiana and Nebraska, increasing the number of reporting States to 45 and the District of Columbia. In 1991–93, with the addition of Oklahoma to the reporting area, information on tobacco use was available for 46 States and the District of Columbia; in 1994–98, 46 States, the District of Columbia, and New York City reported tobacco use; in 1999 information on tobacco use became available from Indiana and New York, increasing the number of reporting States to 48 and the District of Columbia; and in 2000–01, with the addition of South Dakota, the reporting area included 49 States and the District of Columbia. During 1989–2001 California did not require the reporting of tobacco use in the standard format on the birth certificate. The areas reporting tobacco use comprised 87 percent of the U.S. births in 1999–2001. See related *Cigarette smoking*.

Uninsured—In the Current Population Survey (CPS) persons are considered uninsured if they do not have coverage through private health insurance, Medicare, Medicaid, State Children's Health Insurance Program, military or Veterans coverage, another government program, a plan of someone outside the household, or other insurance. In addition, if the respondent has missing Medicaid information but has income from certain low income public programs, then Medicaid coverage is imputed. The questions on health insurance are administered in March and refer to the previous calendar year.

In the National Health Interview Survey (NHIS), the uninsured are persons who do not have coverage under private health insurance, Medicare, Medicaid, public assistance, a State-sponsored health plan, other government-sponsored programs, or a military health plan. Persons with only Indian Health Service coverage are considered uninsured. Estimates of the percent of persons who are uninsured based on the NHIS (table 129) may differ slightly from those based on the March CPS (table 151) due to differences in survey questions, recall period, and other aspects of survey methodology. In 2001 in the NHIS, 1.3 percent of persons age 65 years and over had no health insurance but the small sample size precludes the presentation of separate estimates for this population. Therefore the term "uninsured" refers only to the population under age 65.

See related *Health insurance coverage; Appendix I, Current Population Survey*.

Urbanization—In this report death rates are presented according to the urbanization level of the decedent's county of residence. Counties and county equivalents were assigned to one of five urbanization levels based on their classification

in the Urban Influence code system (December 1996 Revision) developed by the Economic Research Service, U.S. Department of Agriculture. There are three levels for metropolitan counties and two levels for nonmetropolitan counties. The categorization of counties as metropolitan or nonmetropolitan in the Urban Influence code system is based on the June 1993 OMB definition of metropolitan areas (the application of the 1990 metropolitan area standards to the 1990 decennial census data). Metropolitan areas include metropolitan statistical areas (MSAs), consolidated metropolitan statistical areas (CMSAs), and primary metropolitan statistical areas (PMSAs). See *Metropolitan statistical area* for definitions of metropolitan and nonmetropolitan counties.

The Urban Influence code system classifies metropolitan counties as either large metro (counties in MSA/PMSAs of 1 million or more population) or small metro (counties in MSA/PMSAs of less than 1 million population). For this report, the large metro category of the Urban Influence code system was divided into two urbanization levels: large central metro and large fringe metro. Thus, metropolitan counties were assigned to one of three metropolitan urbanization levels: (a) *large central*—counties in large (1 million or more population) MSA/PMSAs that contain all or part of the largest central city of the MSA/PMSA; (b) *large fringe*—counties in large (1 million or more population) MSA/PMSAs that do not contain any part of the largest central city of the MSA/PMSA (counties in a few PMSAs with less than 1 million population were assigned to the large fringe urbanization level because the PMSA in which they are located is adjacent to a large central county of the CMSA); and (c) *small*—counties in small (less than 1 million population) MSA/PMSAs.

The Urban Influence code system divides nonmetropolitan counties into seven categories based on adjacency to a metropolitan area and size of the largest city. A county is considered to have a city with a specified size if it includes all or part of the city. The seven categories were collapsed into two categories: (d) *nonmetro counties with a city of 10,000 or more population* and (e) *nonmetro counties without a city of 10,000 or more population*.

Usual source of care—Usual source of care was measured in the National Health Interview Survey (NHIS) in 1993 and 1994 by asking the respondent "Is there a particular person or place that ____ usually goes to when ____ is sick or needs advice about ___ health?" In the 1995 and 1996 NHIS, the respondent was asked "Is there one doctor, person, or place that ____ usually goes to when ____ is sick or needs advice about ____ health?" Starting in 1997 the respondent was asked "Is there a place that ____ usually goes when he/she is sick or you need advice about (his/her) health?" Persons who report the emergency department as their usual source of care are defined as having no usual source of care in this report.

Wages and salaries—See *Employer costs for employee compensation*.

Years of potential life lost—Years of potential life lost (YPLL) is a measure of premature mortality. Starting with *Health, United States, 1996–97*, YPLL is presented for persons under 75 years of age because the average life expectancy in the United States is over 75 years. YPLL-75 is calculated using the following eight age groups: under 1 year, 1–14 years, 15–24 years, 25–34 years, 35–44 years, 45–54 years, 55–64 years, 65–74 years. The number of deaths for each age group is multiplied by years of life lost, calculated as the difference between age 75 years and the midpoint of the age group. For the eight age groups, the midpoints are 0.5, 7.5, 19.5, 29.5, 39.5, 49.5, 59.5, and 69.5. For example, the death of a person 15–24 years of age counts as 55.5 years of life lost. Years of potential life lost is derived by summing years of life lost over all age groups. In *Health, United States, 1995* and earlier editions, YPLL was presented for persons under 65 years of age. For more information, see Centers for Disease Control. *MMWR*. Vol 35 no 25S, suppl. 1986.

Appendix III

Additional Data Years Available

For trend tables spanning long periods, only selected data years are shown to highlight major trends. Additional years of data are available for some of the tables in electronic spreadsheets available through the Internet and on CD-ROM.

To access the files on the Internet, go to the *Health, United States* Web site at www.cdc.gov/nchs/hus.htm and scroll down to "Spreadsheet files."

Downloadable spreadsheet files for trend tables, many of which include more data years than are shown in the printed report, are available in Excel. Spreadsheet files for selected trend tables with National Health Interview Survey data also include standard errors.

Spreadsheet files in Excel are also available on a CD-ROM. A limited supply of CD-ROMs are available from the National Center for Health Statistics upon request, while supplies last, or CD-ROMs may be purchased from the Government Printing Office.

Table number	Table topic	Additional data years available
1	Resident population	1981–89, 1991–99
2	Poverty	1986–89, 1991–93, 1996
3	Fertility rates and birth rates	1981–84, 1986–89, 1991–94
5	Live births	1971–74, 1976–79, 1981–84, 1986–89, 1991–94, 1996–98
6	Prenatal care	1981–84, 1986–89, 1991–94
8	Teenage childbearing	1981–84, 1986–89, 1991–94
9	Nonmarital childbearing	1981–84, 1986–89, 1991–94
10	Maternal education	1981–84, 1986–89, 1991–94
11	Maternal smoking	1991–94
12	Low birthweight	1981–84, 1986–89, 1991–94
13	Low birthweight	1991–94
16	Abortions	1981–84, 1986–89, 1991–93
19	Infant mortality rates	1984, 1986–89, 1991
20	Infant mortality rates	1984, 1985–89, 1991, 1996–97
21	Infant mortality rates	1984, 1986–88
22	Infant mortality rates	1981–84, 1986–89, 1991–94
27	Life expectancy	1975, 1981–84, 1986–89
29	Age-adjusted death rates for selected causes	1981–89, 1991–94, 1996
30	Years of potential life lost	1991–94, 1996–97; Crude 1999
35	Death rates for all causes	1981–89, 1991–94, 1996
36	Diseases of heart	1981–89, 1991–94, 1996–98
37	Cerebrovascular diseases	1981–89, 1991–94, 1996–98
38	Malignant neoplasms	1981–89, 1991–94, 1996–98
39	Malignant neoplasms of trachea, bronchus, and lung	1981–89, 1991–94, 1996–98
40	Malignant neoplasm of breast	1981–89, 1991–94, 1996–98
41	Chronic lower respiratory diseases	1981–89, 1991–94, 1996
42	Human immunodeficiency virus (HIV) disease	1988–89, 1991–94, 1996
43	Maternal mortality	1981–89, 1991–94, 1996
44	Motor vehicle–related injuries	1981–89, 1991–94, 1996–98
45	Homicide	1981–89, 1991–94, 1996–98
46	Suicide	1981–89, 1991–94, 1996–98
47	Firearm-related injuries	1981–89, 1991–94, 1996–98

48	Occupational diseases	1981–84, 1986–89, 1991–94, 1996
49	Occupational injury deaths	1983
50	Occupational injuries	1981–84, 1986–89, 1991–94, 1996
51	Leading Health Indicators	1991–94, 1996–97
52	Notifiable diseases	1985, 1988–89, 1991–94, 1996–97
59	Cigarette smoking	1987–88, 1991–94
60	Cigarette smoking	1987–88, 1991–94
61	Cigarette smoking	1993–95, 1994–97
63	Use of selected substances	1981–89, 1992–94, 1996–97
64	Cocaine-related emergency department episodes	1992–94
65	Alcohol consumption	1998–99
70	Health care visits	1998, 2000
73	No health care visits	1999–2000
74	No usual source of health care	1995–96 and 1999–2000
75	Emergency department visits	1998, 2000
76	No usual source of health care	1997–98
77	Emergency department visits	1998
78	Dental visits	1998, 2000
82	Ambulatory care visits	1997
83	Injury-related visits	1998–99
84	Ambulatory care visits	1997–99
89	Discharges	1998, 2000
90	Discharges	1991–96, 2000
91	Discharges	1988–89, 1991–94, 1996, 1998, 2000
92	Rates of discharges	1995–2000
93	Discharges	1995–99
94	Ambulatory and inpatient procedures	Total 1994–96; Inpatient 1997, 1999–2000
95	Hospital admissions	1985, 1991–94, 1996–98
96	Nursing home residents	1997
97	Nursing home residents	1997
98	Persons employed	1975, 1983–89, 1991–94, 1996
100	Physicians	1970, 1980, 1987, 1989, 1990, 1992–94, 1996
101	Primary care doctors of medicine	1994, 1996
103	Health professions schools	1998
106	Hospitals	1985, 1991–94, 1996–97
108	Community hospital beds	1985, 1988–89, 1995–99
109	Occupancy rates	1985, 1988–89, 1995–99
110	Nursing homes	1996–99
113	Consumer Price Index	1965, 1975, 1985, 1996, 1998
117	Expenditures for health care	1996
118	Sources of payment for health care	1996
121	Employers' costs and health insurance	1992–93, 1995–97, 1998–99
122	Hospital expenses	1975, 1985, 1991–94, 1996–97
123	Nursing home average monthly charges	1964, 1973–74
124	Nursing home average monthly charges	1977, 1997
127	Private health insurance	1994
128	Medicaid coverage	1994
129	No health insurance coverage	1994
130	Health care coverage	1984, 1994, 1996–97
132	Health maintenance organizations	1984–87, 1989, 1991–94
134	Medicare	1985, 1996
136	Medicare	1993–98
137	Medicaid	1975, 1985–89, 1991–94
138	Medicaid	1975, 1985–89, 1991–94

Index to Trend Tables

(Numbers refer to table numbers)

C

C—Con.

D

F

G

H

H—Con.

H—Con.

I

J

L

M

Table

M—Con.

Table

N

S—Con.

T

U

V

W

W